MERENESS'
ESSENTIALS OF PSYCHIATRIC NURSING

MERENESS'

ESSENTIALS OF PSYCHIATRIC NURSING

Cecelia Monat Taylor, Ph.D., R.N.

Director of Nursing,
Mohawk Valley Psychiatric Center, Utica, New York;
Formerly Professor of Nursing,
Syracuse University, Syracuse, New York

THIRTEENTH EDITION

THE C. V. MOSBY COMPANY

St. Louis • Baltimore • Philadelphia • Toronto 1990

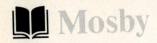

Editor: Linda L. Duncan
Developmental editor: Joanna May
Project manager: Teri Merchant
Designer: Susan E. Lane
Editing and production: CRACOM Corporation

THIRTEENTH EDITION

Printed in the United States of America

The C.V. Mosby Company
11830 Westline Industrial Drive, St. Louis, Missouri 63146

Library of Congress Cataloging in Publication Data

Taylor, Cecelia Monat.
    Mereness' essentials of psychiatric nursing.
    Includes bibliographical references.
    1. Psychiatric nursing.   I. Mereness, Dorothy A.
Essentials of psychiatric nursing.   II. Title.
III. Title: Essentials of psychiatric nursing.
[DNLM: 1. Psychiatric Nursing.   WY 160 T239m]
RC440.T38   1990   610.73'68   89-14276
ISBN 0-8016-5290-1

C/D/D   9   8   7   6   5   4   3

To those persons
hospitalized for mental illness over the past 50 years
and their nurses
upon whose shoulders stand the clients and nurses of today

Foreword
1940-1990
The evolution of a textbook

The publication of the thirteenth edition of this textbook is a milestone since this book will have been in continuous publication for half a century. In a sense, the development of this text, which has proved to be the most durable in the field, is the story of the development of psychiatric nursing itself. Since it has played an important role in my life throughout my entire professional career, I am pleased and privileged to tell its story within the context of the development of psychiatric nursing.

This text was first published by The C.V. Mosby Company in the spring of 1940 and carried the title *Psychiatry for Nurses*. The major author was Dr. Louis J. Karnosh, Professor of Nervous Diseases at the Medical School of Western Reserve University (now Case Western Reserve University) and Clinical Director of the Psychiatric Division of Cleveland City Hospital (now Cleveland Metropolitan General Hospital). Miss Edith Gage, Director of Nursing at the Psychiatric Division of City Hospital, was the nurse co-author.

Dr. Karnosh was a pioneer in psychiatry, having helped to establish in 1934 Engleside Hospital, a private psychiatric institution. His book was one of the earliest psychiatric texts for nurses. It became available just as I began a student experience in psychiatric nursing at City Hospital. As a student nurse at the Frances Payne Bolton School of Nursing at the former Western Reserve University, I was surprised that the curriculum included psychiatric nursing. Dr. Karnosh, who was interested in improving the nursing care of mentally ill persons, always gave a series of lectures to each group of student nurses. His lectures were a revelation, explaining much about human behavior which I had observed but did not understand. In addition, he was a fascinating speaker and a favorite of the students. I was intrigued by the lectures, the new textbook, and the psychiatric nursing experience.

Unfortunately, Dr. Karnosh was shot at his home and severely wounded by a distraught individual 2 weeks after the course began. He was able to give only two lectures to my student group. After 6 months he was able to return to work, but this was long after my experience at City Hospital had been concluded.

I was distressed because I had missed so many of Dr. Karnosh's lectures. After my psychiatric nursing experience was over, it was arranged at the School of Nursing and the University Hospital in Cleveland that I could be free on the day of his lectures to travel across the city by public transportation to hear the entire series. My classmates commented that I all but stood up and cheered during those lectures.

Edith Gage died about a year after the first edition of *Psychiatry for Nurses* had become available. Her position was filled by the instructor of psychiatric nursing. This created a vacancy about 6 months after I had completed the nursing curriculum at Western Reserve University. Dr. Karnosh suggested that I fill this vacancy. Although I had been a teacher before becoming a student nurse, and held a baccalaureate degree from a teachers' college, I knew nothing about teaching psychiatric nursing. The opportunity of working with Dr. Karnosh and learning more about psychiatric nursing overpowered my better judgment, and I accepted the position in November 1941. Within a month the United States declared war on Japan. I was declared an essential worker and frozen in my position. Thus began a 4-year stint of teaching an ever-growing student body without an assistant or vacations.

Because of the epidemic of mental illness that the experience with the Armed Forces precipitated among American youth, and because so few nurses at that time had had any experience in psychiatric nursing, our students were a precious commodity. Many of them were made head nurses and supervisors of psychiatric units as soon as they were inducted into the U.S. Nurse Corps.

In 1946 the U.S. Congress passed the Mental Health Act. That act was a direct result of the impact of the mental illness developed by many soldiers after serving in the Armed Forces during World War II. There was a paucity of professional workers to provide therapeutic approaches to the needs of those ill soldiers. When World War II ended, the Congress set about to rectify this serious weakness. Thus the Mental Health Act provided financial resources for the education of the members of the psychiatric team—psychiatrists, psychologists, psychiatric social workers, and psychiatric nurses. In the fall of 1947, six universities provided programs in psychiatric nursing for nurses interested in this field. The National Institute of Mental Health (NIMH) provided funding for these universities and the students recruited by them. This funding was increased as time progressed, and many more universities were added to the list of those which originally provided graduate programs in psychiatric nursing. NIMH continued to supply educational funding until today, although the amount of assistance has been drastically curtailed in recent years. In the future, funding for the education of psychiatric nurses from governmental sources will probably be nonexistent.

As a result of the Mental Health Act, many psychiatric nurses have developed clinical knowledge and expertise in teaching psychiatric nursing and in providing therapy for mentally distressed clients. Some of these nurses were able to complete a doctoral degree. Eventually, many of the educational leaders in the schools of nursing in this country were originally trained in psychiatric nursing.

It was not until the third edition of *Psychiatry for Nurses,* which appeared in 1949, that I was involved in a revision of the text. My name was included in the flyleaf as the collaborator. In that edition I was allowed to add only a few comments concerning nursing care at the end of each chapter. Dr. Karnosh wrote in the preface of the third edition that psychiatric nursing had come into its own following World War II. This revision emphasized the shock therapies. A long chapter on syphilis of the central nervous system was included, and a new chapter on psychosomatic disorders was added. The illustrations were pictures of actual patients, many of whom were unpleasant looking. Some purchasers of the text objected to these pictures. Since that time, a continuing effort has been made to identify meaningful illustrations for this text.

The fourth edition was published in 1953. During the 1950s NIMH also funded programs in schools of nursing that emphasized the integration of mental health concepts in all aspects of nursing. Thus the focus of nursing education on the psychosocial needs of patients was increased by this movement. These concepts were viewed as essential to the nursing care of all patients, regardless of their primary health problem. Unfortunately, in some current nursing education programs with integrated curriculums, study of psychopathology and the nursing care of psychiatric patients has disappeared entirely.

As a result of this lack of emphasis on psychiatric nursing at the undergraduate level, the number of applicants to graduate programs in psychiatric nursing is declining. If leadership in the field is to be continued, undergraduates must have an educational experience in psychiatric nursing to awaken their interest and encourage them to pursue graduate study in this area.

Dr. Karnosh retired in 1957. However, he maintained his private practice and for many years continued to present several of the lectures from the series which he had developed earlier as part of the educational program for students having a psychiatric nursing experience at City Hospital. He was much admired by students of the health care schools of the University for these unusually well-constructed and beautifully delivered lectures. Dr. Karnosh also wrote and privately published *A Psychiatrist's Anthology.* This book was popular for a long time among students of nursing and medicine in Cleveland. It was illustrated with his wood carvings, which depicted the physical expression of illness by individuals suffering from some of the major categories of mental illness. In addition, the book included a description of the thinking processes which are often experienced by these ill individuals.

The fifth edition of this text was published in 1958. The name of Dorothy Mereness appeared for the first time on the outside cover of the book. A chapter on psychopharmacology and a glossary were added.

About 30 years ago, while many nurses were being prepared as clinical specialists in psychiatric nursing, a new understanding developed about the impact of long-term care in large public institutions. Professional workers came to realize that long-term institutionalization was increasing the illness of many clients rather than improving their mental health. When this idea became widely understood among those responsible for long-term care, many clients who had been institutionalized for years were discharged.

Deinstitutionalization occurred without adequate planning, monitoring, or funding. The result was a lack of follow-up care and a high potential for the abuse of the mentally ill persons who were discharged into the community.

Many discharged individuals were not able to cope at all and returned again and again to the institution that discharged them, thus creating what was known as "the revolving door." Some individuals managed to live away from the institution more or less satisfactorily. A third group did not return to the institution, would not live with relatives or in group homes, and refused to accept any type of help. This group of homeless, destitute, emotionally ill people began living on the streets of many large cities and became known as the "street people." Their presence has been distressing to the public, but no real solution to this sociological problem has developed. As was forecast, the public is now demanding that facilities be provided for the physical and psychological care of these individuals.

Eventually, this attempt to change the pattern of hospitalization from large, impersonal, long-term care in public institutions resulted in the development of many smaller units in general hospitals and in small private agencies. All of these units provide intensive therapy and short-term hospitalization. In addition, smaller specialized units have begun to develop for the treatment of clients with special problems; examples include units for the treatment of emotionally disturbed children or for clients with alcohol or drug-related problems. Since people are living longer than in the past, a new specialty, geropsychiatry, has developed, which focuses on the treatment of the psychiatrically ill older client.

In 1965 I became Dean of the School of Nursing at the University of Pennsylvania. My days as Dean included the transition period when the University argued with itself about whether to continue to allow the Department of Nursing in the University to continue or to close it in favor of the diploma program which was controlled by the Hospital of the University of Pennsylvania. The hospital program had existed for many years and was strongly supported by the public. Eventually the University decided to support the college program in nursing, but we spent several years in fearful anticipation about our future.

My tenure as Dean included what is now referred to as "the Sixties." Students frequently visited the Dean's office to withdraw from school to "find themselves." Some came to weep loudly without being able to explain why. Entire classes sometimes descended on the Dean when they were concerned about the impact of an unfounded rumor. I often thought that my background in psychiatric nursing was one of the most valuable tools I had brought to the role of the Dean.

The seventh edition of this text appeared in 1966. My name was given the position as major author with Dr. Karnosh becoming the collaborator. The name of the text was changed to *Essentials of Psychiatric Nursing,* and the book was enlarged. This edition emphasized self-understanding on the part of the nurse and the development of psychiatric nursing skills. In 1968 this edition was published in the Philippines.

In 1970 the eighth edition was published. It carried my name as the only author. Chapters on children and adolescents, individuals with faulty intellectual development, and community psychiatry were added. Additional case histories were included in each chapter and discussed from the standpoint of the implications for nursing. Each chapter was concluded with a list of important concepts that the content of the chapter had covered. Finding appropriate illustrations continued to be a challenge. In the eighth edition pictures of nurses actively involved in patient activities were included.

The ninth edition, which appeared in 1974, introduced Cecelia Monat Taylor as the second author. Dr. Taylor completed the master's curriculum in Psychiatric Mental Health Nursing, which I developed and directed at New York University from 1955 to 1965. She and I had similar beliefs about psychiatric nursing and we worked together harmoniously. Dr. Taylor was actively involved in psychiatric nursing at Syracuse University at the time I had left the field to become the Dean of the School of Nursing at the University of Pennsylvania. In this edition the philosophy was revised, the entire content was reorganized, much of the book was rewritten, and all of it was updated. We attempted to emphasize the fact that a great deal of the treatment in psychiatry was being given outside an institution.

Dr. Karnosh died at age 85 in Cleveland in August 1977. He was survived by his wife and three daughters. At his death, he was Professor Emeritus of Neuropsychiatry at the Medical School of Case-Western Reserve University and an emeritus consultant at Cleveland Clinic. He had served as Chief of Neuropsychiatry at the old Cleveland City Hospital for over 20 years. Dr. Karnosh has been the single most influential person in my life.

Coincidentally, in 1977 I also concluded my tenure as Dean of the School of Nursing at the University of Pennsylvania. As my days of being a Dean were ending, the largess which nursing education had enjoyed from the federal government began to diminish, and fund-raising became a part of the Dean's role. The employment of a replacement for me in the spring of 1977 provided the opportunity of a sabbatical, part of which was spent as a consultant at the School of Nursing at King Abdul Aziz University in Jedda, Saudi Arabia.

The tenth edition of this text was published in 1978. The word *patient* was discarded in favor of *client* or *individual.* Again the book was enlarged. Emphasis was placed on understanding the psychodynamics of observed behavior, and the use of the nursing process was introduced.

In 1981 I became a full-time consultant for the State Board of Nursing in Harrisburg, Pennsylvania. This gave me the opportunity to visit almost all of the baccalaureate nursing programs in Pennsylvania.

In 1982 the eleventh edition of this text was released with Dr. Taylor as the sole author. Although this edition did not carry my name as one of the authors, Dr. Taylor and the publishers graciously changed the title to *Mereness' Essentials of Psychiatric Nursing*. For the first time the text was accompanied by a workbook, the author of which was and continues to be Carol Lofstedt, Professor of Nursing at Bronx Community College. Professor Lofstedt is a former student of mine and was Dr. Taylor's classmate at New York University. Her many years of experience teaching psychiatric nursing to associate degree students combined with her creativity has made the workbook a valuable addition. A workbook was considered vital to the productive use of the text because there was an increasing amount of information seen as "essential" to the effective practice of psychiatric nursing and a decreasing amount of time allocated to its study in most schools of nursing.

The broadened role of the psychiatric nurse was reflected in the 1982 American Nurses' Association (ANA) *Standards of Practice for Psychiatric/Mental Health Nursing*, which defined two levels of psychiatric nursing: the generalist and the specialist. Certification for both levels of practice, available through the ANA, is becoming increasingly popular as nurses attempt to demonstrate their competency and legitimize their practice. Peer review, another method of validating competency in practice, currently is being used by clinical specialists and nurses in private practice.

In 1984 I returned to Philadelphia from Harrisburg to work part-time as the Executive Director of the Philadelphia County District of the Pennsylvania Nurses' Association. Soon I must face the proposition that retirement cannot be denied indefinitely and that some specific plans for the future without employment must be made.

The twelfth edition of *Mereness' Essentials of Psychiatric Nursing* was published in 1986, and a separate chapter about the history of psychiatric nursing was deleted, although relevant historical information was included as an introduction to each chapter. Each chapter that discussed clinical issues was revised to include a detailed case study that was analyzed in terms of the nursing process. Selected nursing diagnostic categories and etiologic factors as approved by the Fifth National Conference on Nursing Diagnoses were cited for the first time. The perennial problem of illustrations was addressed by the sensitive ink drawings of Meri Bourgard, an artist who knew little about mental illness or the care of these persons.

Despite many positive changes over the years, the mental health system today is burdened with large numbers of both young and elderly clients with chronic psychiatric problems. The needs of this population place increasing demands on society to provide institutional, community mental health, and psychiatric nursing home facilities. There continue to be few programs for chronically mentally ill persons, limited funds for community services, and severe fragmentation of the system of delivering psychiatric care. Psychiatric nurses must become more involved in health policy planning to develop well-coordinated inpatient and outpatient supportive services for these clients.

Although the health care system continues to change rapidly and dramatically, it is reasonable to believe that in the foreseeable future there will continue to be many calls for the special skills of the psychiatric nurse. It is for this reason that a learning experience in psychiatric nursing is essential for all students of nursing. Thus this textbook is likely to continue to make a major contribution to the effective care of mentally ill persons.

Dorothy A. Mereness, Ed.D., R.N., F.A.A.N.
Philadelphia, Pennsylvania

Preface

It is a truism that the older one gets, the more quickly time seems to pass. As I contemplated the preparation of the thirteenth edition of *Mereness' Essentials of Psychiatric Nursing,* it seemed there would be little that required change from the last edition, published 4 short years ago. No prediction could have been more wrong!

Psychiatric nursing continues to be scrutinized as never before for its clinical effectiveness and cost efficiency. The number of nurses who are choosing to work in mental health settings, particularly public mental health settings, is decreasing commensurate with the decline in the number of individuals who are choosing to become nurses. At the same time, the treatment needs of those who are mentally ill are more numerous and complex than ever before. It is a rare day when the newpapers do not include at least one story about the plight of the mentally ill homeless or the tragedy of child abuse or present recently released statistics about the increase in the number of persons in need of mental health services. On the brighter side, the newspapers also report major advances in understanding the causes of major mental illnesses, particularly in regard to biological influences. All this is taking place in an educational context in which nursing programs are devoting less and less time to learning experiences with mentally ill persons.

Therefore, the challenge this revision presented was to provide accurate and necessary information to enable the student or entry level nurse to provide effective nursing care to mentally ill persons while simultaneously presenting this information in an understandable, challenging, and realistic manner. This challenge was made greater by my knowledge that this edition represents the fiftieth year of continuous publication of this textbook and my desire to have it continue to contribute to the successful preparation of nurses who will care for mentally ill persons.

I continue in the belief that all nurses should have sound theoretical and experiential preparation in the care of mentally ill persons. At the same time it is important to emphasize that students of nursing who are preparing for beginning professional practice should not be expected to become psychiatric nursing specialists. Instead they should be encouraged to use knowledge learned during earlier learning experiences and in turn to apply skills gained during the psychiatric nursing experience to the care of all persons. As a result, this edition retains material on concepts basic to psychiatric nursing, which includes topics such as personality development and the process of communication, the understanding of which is integral to the effective practice of nursing in any setting and with any client.

Two totally new chapters are included in this edition—Chapter 13 Biological Factors Influencing Mental Health and Mental Illness and Chapter 14 Cultural Factors Influencing Mental Health and Mental Illness. Their inclusion reflects an increasing professional awareness of the role of both biology and culture in the development, manifestation, and treatment of mental illness.

Although the entire book was reorganized and other chapters revised, the most major changes were made in Section Four The Consumers of Psychiatric Nursing. These nine chapters were completely rewritten so they would reflect a description of client behaviors which are aligned with the diagnostic criteria of the DSM-III-R. The ANA Classification of Human Responses of Concern for Psychiatric Mental Health Nursing Practice is introduced, along with the latest NANDA Diagnostic Categories, as a means of systematically organizing assessment and diagnostic data. Additional content in this section includes an expansion of the types of substance abuse and dependence in Chapter 19, a discussion of the needs of persons with borderline personality disorder in Chapter 20, additional information about the care of individuals with Alzheimer's disease in Chapter 21, the inclusion of mental retardation and developmental disorders of children in Chapter 22, and a section on the emotional needs of the person with AIDS in Chapter 23. Every chapter in this section has at least one case study which is analyzed according to the nursing process. Previous users of this text will notice that the "rationale" section in the nursing care plan has been deleted. I decided to omit this column to make the nursing care plan more similar to that which is used by practicing nurses, hoping to increase its applicability and relevance to the reality of nursing practice. Nevertheless, the rationale for each intervention can be found in the discussion entitled "Planning and Implementing Nursing Care."

Other less lengthy but equally significant additions include methods commonly used to increase self-awareness in Chapter 4 and Maslow's hierarchy of needs and Piaget's stages of cognitive development in Chapter 11. In general, I believe that this edition of *Mereness' Essentials of Psychiatric Nursing* includes the most current, accurate information available in a framework that reflects an orientation congruent with accepted standards of nursing practice.

Pedagogical changes in this edition include the addition of "Of Special Interest" boxes in some chapters, new figures and tables, and most important, marginal notes which summarize key points. As a result of the addition of marginal notes, the concluding statements which appeared in previous editions have been replaced with an "End Note" which succinctly summarizes the content of each chapter.

The plan of suggesting sources of additional information from easily obtained books and periodicals has been maintained. Thus relatively unknown sources of information have not been cited. In addition, references of several years ago have been retained when they are classics or still contain much currently valid information.

An attempt has been made to delete evidence of sexism in the language of this text; however, this has not always been possible. Therefore, for expediency and clarity, the client is often referred to in the third person, masculine gender, and the nurse is often referred to in the third person, feminine gender. Pronouns in quoted materials have not been changed.

The *Learning and Activity Guide* that accompanied the twelfth edition has been totally revised by its author, Carol Ruth Lofstedt, and continues to be a welcome and useful adjunct to this text. An instructor's guide and a test bank of questions correlated to each chapter is also available. I believe that the use of these additional materials, particularly the *Learning and Activity Guide,* will greatly enhance students' learning in a manner not possible within the constraints of a textbook.

In summary, I believe teachers and students of psychiatric nursing will find this edition of *Mereness' Essentials of Psychiatric Nursing* to be particularly useful in the teaching/learning processes. I trust it conveys my commitment to the care of mentally ill persons.

ACKNOWLEDGMENTS

In the preface to the last edition of this text I wrote "No revision of a textbook is ever accomplished without the indirect and direct support and assistance of many others." That statement was never as applicable as during this revision! At the beginning of my work on this revision, I fell and broke my left ankle in three places, which resulted in my having a full leg cast for 2 months and a short leg cast for the next 5 months. Therefore, for most of the time I worked on this edition I was confined to a wheelchair or needed a walker to navigate. Those who have not experienced such a situation may wonder why this should have been such a problem. I would encourage you to monitor the planning, time, and effort involved in retrieving a paper clip from the floor when encased in a twenty pound leg cast. You may also be interested to know that Carol Lofstedt, the author of the accompanying *Learning and Activity Guide,* also fell and broke her left shoulder in the midst of her revision of the workbook. I wonder what Freud would have to say about these incidents!

In addition to incurring an injury, I chose this time to change career paths and leave Syracuse University College of Nursing to become Director of Nursing at Mohawk Valley Psychiatric Center. Even the casual observer must conclude that I required much support and assistance during this period. I am blessed to have received them.

Specifically, I wish to acknowledge the administration of Syracuse University for granting me a sabbatical to work on this edition. Special thanks are due Marianne Miles, M.S., R.N., who contributed much to the new chapters on biological and cultural influences on mental health and mental illness. Finally, Linda Mueller, M.S., R.N., although not a psychiatric nurse, diligently and effectively searched the literature for recent publications which she identified and copied for my use. I thank her!

For a variety of reasons, I have never before acknowledged the assistance of the staff at The C. V. Mosby Company. This time, however, I would like to publicly recognize my Editor, Linda Duncan, and Developmental Editor, Joanna May, for their help and cheerful support throughout the entire process. Their substantive suggestions were exceeded only by their emotional support.

Readers may not know that many reviewers are involved in the production of a textbook. Such was the case with this text. A number of faculty from various regions in the country reviewed the content and organization of the last edition and made very helpful suggestions regarding reorganization and revision of content. I trust they will find many of their suggestions reflected in this edition. Other reviewers were asked by the publisher to critique the revisions as I prepared them. Because of ethical and professional reasons, I was not told their identity. Although all comments were welcomed and helpful, there were two reviewers who put an exceptional amount of time and effort into their critiques. Their experience, wisdom, and commitment to psychiatric nursing consistently illuminated their comments. Since the revisions are now complete, I have been told their names. They are Linda Nance Marks, Ed.D., R.N., Associate Professor, University of Texas at Arlington and Donna Fillingim Darty, M.S.N., R.N., Instructor, Psychiatric Nursing, Jefferson State Community College, Birmingham, Alabama. I thank you both from the bottom of my heart. Your comments were relevant, specific, helpful, and supportive.

Finally, I would like to acknowledge the continued interest and involvement of Dr. Dorothy A. Mereness in both the progress of this text and in the advancement of psychiatric nursing. Dr. Mereness generously agreed to rewrite the Forewords to the eleventh and twelfth editions as a Foreword to this historic thirteenth edition. Without Dr. Mereness this edition, in fact this book, would probably not have made the contribution it has. I *know* that my professional contributions would have been fewer if I had not been exposed to her guidance, friendship, and wisdom. Countless numbers of mentally ill persons owe her a great debt!

Faculty who have used this textbook since 1974 have indirectly followed the progress of my daughter, Corliss. You will be interested, and I hope pleased, to know that Corliss graduated from high school in June 1989 and began college in August 1989. If all goes well, the fourteenth edition of this text will coincide with her graduation from college.

My decision to change career paths to one which is more directly associated with the care of mentally ill persons has made me even more acutely aware of the need to prepare nurses to deliver expert psychiatric care. I trust that this edition will make a meaningful contribution to the education of nursing students, to the end that mentally ill individuals will benefit.

Cecelia Monat Taylor
Westdale, New York

Contents

The mental health delivery system and health care team

1

LEARNING OBJECTIVES

After studying this chapter the student will be able to:

- State the primary mode of mental health treatment during key periods from prehistoric times to the present.
- Identify the advantages and the disadvantages of the state mental hospital delivery system of the late nineteenth and early twentieth centuries.
- Discuss the federal legislation that led to the establishment of comprehensive community mental health centers as the system of mental health delivery.
- List the characteristics of a comprehensive community mental health center.
- State the origins of the health care specialties of psychiatric nursing, psychiatry, psychology, psychiatric social work, and activity therapies.
- Differentiate among the roles and functions of the psychiatrist, psychologist, psychiatric social worker, and activity therapist.

Human beings have always been concerned about behavior that is different from what is usually encountered in their society. At times the source of this concern has been compassion; at other times concern has stemmed from fear. At the same time, the labels applied to those who behave in a deviant manner have varied throughout the ages and include such terms as *sinner, lunatic, insane,* and *mentally ill.* The systems devised by the society to care for these persons have been strongly influenced by the prevailing beliefs about the cause and nature of

1

the deviant behavior. The responsibility for provision of care has shifted among the various subsystems of society, ranging from the family to the community as a whole to specialized agents of society such as the religious, political, and legal subsystems. The factors influencing this evolution are multiple and complex but include such variables as population density, availability of resources, religious beliefs and social practices, and the prevailing body of knowledge about human behavior.

Following is a history of the treatment of mentally ill persons, which is presented in the belief that the contemporary system of mental health delivery can be understood best if there is an appreciation of its historical roots.

HISTORICAL PERSPECTIVE
Prehistoric times

In prehistoric times, mentally ill persons were treated by tribal rites. If these failed, individuals were left to die of starvation or to be attacked by wild beasts.

The treatment of mentally ill persons during prehistoric times probably consisted of tribal rites designed to alter behavior. If these measures proved unsuccessful, the individual likely was abandoned to die of starvation or attack by wild animals. Critics of contemporary community-based mental health care point to the large number of mentally ill persons left to fend for themselves on the streets and in single-room occupancy dwellings of large cities as reflecting a slightly more sophisticated parallel to the measures used by primitive peoples of ancient times.

Early Greek and Roman era

Greek temples were often used to house mentally ill persons. Sometimes these people were treated with great kindness, while at other times treatment was harsh and barbaric.

The Golden Age of Greece was noted for its humane regard for the sick. The Greeks used as hospitals temples that had an abundance of fresh air, pure water, and sunshine. Theatricals, riding, walking, and listening to the sound of a waterfall were all recommended as methods to lift the mood. Despite this humane attitude, there were instances when the treatment was harsh; even in the best of the Greek temples, starving, chains, and flogging were advocated "because with these it was believed that when those who refused food began to eat, frequently the memory was also refreshed thereby."

There is little information about the Roman era in reference to mental illness. Galen, a Greek who practiced in Rome, based his treatment on the teachings of his Greek predecessors. Other physicians of the Roman era treated mentally ill persons by bleeding, purging, and sulfur baths.

Middle ages

In the Middle Ages, the treatment of mental illness was left to priests. Both harsh and humane treatments were used to drive out the "evil spirit."

With the collapse of Greek and Roman civilizations, the care of the sick, along with other cultural developments, suffered an almost complete eclipse. The treatment of mentally ill persons was left to priests, and superstitious belief flourished. The insane were flogged, fettered, scourged, and starved in the belief that the devils that possessed them could be driven out.

A few bright spots in this tragic picture were some monasteries or shrines where this technique of "exorcising" the evil spirit was performed by the gentle laying on of hands instead of the whip. Members of the nobility, self-appointed ascetics, and holy men of varying degrees of sincerity practiced this art, which at least was not physically cruel.

Sixteenth century

Although the treatment of mentally ill persons in the Middle Ages had little to recommend it, they fared even more poorly in the period that followed. When the church and the monastery gave up the care of the insane, it was gradually

In the sixteenth century, mentally ill persons were locked up in jails, dungeons, or lunatic asylums where the curious could pay to watch the "performance" of the sick inmates.

OF SPECIAL INTEREST

Out of the tradition and belief in the "holy" or "royal touch" arose several great shrines, of which the one at Gheel in Belgium is most famous. This legend tells of a king living in Ireland who was married to a beautiful woman and who became the father of an equally beautiful daughter. The good queen developed a fatal illness, and at her deathbed the daughter dedicated herself to a life of purity and service to the poor and the mentally bereft. The widowed king was overcome with grief and announced to his subjects that he must at once be cured of his sorrow by marrying the woman in his kingdom who most resembled the dead queen. No such person was found. But the devil came and whispered to the king that there was such a woman—his own daughter. The devil spurred the king to propose marriage to the girl, but she was appropriately outraged and fled across the English Channel to Belgium. There the king overtook her and, with Satan at his elbow, slew the girl and her faithful attendants. In the night an angel came, recapitated the body, and concealed it in the forest near the village of Gheel. Years later five mentally ill persons chained together spent the night with their keepers at a small wayside shrine near this Belgian village. According to the legend, all recovered overnight. Here indeed must be the place where the dead girl, reincarnated as St. Dymphna, was buried, and here was the sacred spot where her cures were effected.

In the fifteenth century, pilgrimages to Gheel from every part of the civilized world were organized for mentally sick persons. Many of the pilgrims remained in Gheel to live with the local people, and in the passing years it became the natural thing to accept them into the homes. Thus the first colony for mentally ill persons—and, for that matter, the only one that has been consistently successful—was formed. In 1851 the Belgian government took charge of this colony of mentally ill persons. It continues to the present. Hundreds of mentally ill individuals live in private homes, work with the townspeople, and suffer no particular restriction of freedom, except to refrain from visiting public places and from using alcohol and to report regularly to the supervising psychiatrist. Despite the success of the Gheel colony and its great humanizing value, most attempts at duplicating it elsewhere have been total or partial failures. The community mental health movement in the United States is, in a sense, an attempt to capture some of the values of community involvement demonstrated in Gheel.

taken over by the so-called almshouse, the contract house, and the secular asylum. The more violent persons were placed in jails and dungeons. In the sixteenth century Henry VIII officially dedicated Bethlehem Hospital in London as a lunatic asylum. It soon became the notorious "Bedlam" whose hideous practices were immortalized by Hogarth, the famous cartoonist. There keepers were allowed to exhibit the most boisterous of the patients for 2 pence a look, and the more harmless inmates were forced to seek charity on the streets of London as the "Bedlam beggars" of Shakespeare's *King Lear*.

Seventeenth century

The classic work, *Anatomy of Melancholy,* by Burton was published in 1621. Burton claimed that witches and magicians were both the cause and the cure of disease, while God and Satan battled continuously to possess the human soul.

Superstition about mental illness took a horrible turn in the seventeenth century. God and Satan were still thought to be engaged in a ceaseless battle for possession of one's soul. The year after the *Mayflower* sailed into Plymouth Harbor, Burton published his classic work *Anatomy of Melancholy,* wherein he stated that "witches and magicians can cure and cause most diseases." To seek out and execute witches became a sacred religious duty. At least 20,000 persons were said to have been burned in Scotland alone during the seventeenth century. Small wonder that Cotton Mather precipitated the witch mania in Salem, since he was merely subscribing to the beliefs of the day.

In those dark days, society was interested in its own self-security, not in the welfare of mentally ill persons. The almshouses were a combination of jail and asylum, and within their walls petty criminals and mentally ill persons were herded indiscriminately. In the seventeenth and eighteenth centuries the dungeons of Paris were the only places where violent mentally ill persons could be committed. Drastic purgings and bleedings were the favorite therapeutic procedures of the day, and "madshirts" and the whip were applied religiously by the cell keepers.

Eighteenth century

In 1792, Frenchman Philippe Pinel was instrumental in proving the error of treating mentally ill persons inhumanely. Pinel's pupil Esquirol continued his humane treatment and is regarded as the first teacher of psychiatry.

The political and social reformations in France toward the end of the eighteenth century influenced the hospitals and jails of Paris. In 1792 Philippe Pinel (1745–1826), a young physician who was medical director of the Bicêtre asylum outside Paris, was given permission by the Revolutionary Commune to liberate the inmates of two of the largest hospitals, some of whom had been in chains for 20 years. Had his experiment proved a failure he might well have lost his head by the guillotine. Fortunately he was right, and by his act he proved conclusively the fallacy of inhumane treatment of mentally ill persons. The reforms instituted by Pinel were continued by his pupil Esquirol, who founded no less than 10 asylums and was the first regular teacher of psychiatry. The Quakers, under the Brothers Tuke, had at this time established the York Retreat and effected the same epoch-making reforms in England.

In America the Pennsylvania Hospital was completed in 1756 under the guidance of Benjamin Franklin. One of the first two patients admitted was described as a "lunatic." Although mentally ill patients were relegated to the cellar, they were assured clean bedding and warm rooms. Benjamin Rush (1745–1813), a prime humanitarian and the "father of American psychiatry," began his duties at the Pennsylvania Hospital in 1783.

He believed that the phases of the moon influenced behavior (the lunar theory of insanity) and invented an inhumane restraining device called the "tranquilizer." At the same time, however, he insisted on more humane treatment of mentally ill patients and, as such, stands as a prominent transitional figure between the old era and the new.

Nineteenth century

The first public psychiatric hospital in America was built in Williamsburg, Virginia, in 1773 and is known today as the Eastern Psychiatric Hospital. Nevertheless, most of the states were still without special institutions for mentally ill persons in the first quarter of the nineteenth century.

The poorhouse or almshouse was still popular, but it invariably became a catchall for all types of offenders, and mentally ill people received the brunt of its manifold evils. Most shocking to people of today was placing the poor and the mildly demented on the auction block, where those with the strongest backs and the weakest minds were sold to the highest bidder, the returns from the sale being assigned to the township treasury.

About 1830 a vigorous movement for the erection of suitable state hospitals spread simultaneously through several states. The excellent results obtained by private institutions such as the Hartford Retreat, founded in 1818, probably served as an object lesson. Horace Mann took an enthusiastic interest in the plight of mentally ill persons, and the advantages of a state hospital system were publicized to promote construction of such institutions.

However, it remained for a sickly, 40-year-old schoolteacher to expose the sins of the poorhouse. From that day in 1841 when Dorothea Lynde Dix (1802–1887) described the hoarfrost on the walls of the cells of the East Somerville jail in Massachusetts to the day when she retreated into one of the very hospitals she was instrumental in creating, she effected reforms that shook the world. She so aroused the public conscience that millions of dollars were raised to build suitable hospitals, and 20 states responded directly to her appeals. She played an important part in the founding of St. Elizabeth's Hospital in Washington, D.C., directed the opening of two large institutions in Canada, completely reformed the asylum system in Scotland and in several other foreign countries, and rounded out a most amazing career by organizing the nursing forces of the northern armies during the Civil War. A resolution presented by the U.S. Congress in 1901 characterized her as "among the noblest examples of humanity in all history."

The state hospital system that rapidly developed throughout many states was limited almost solely to large institutions built in remote rural areas of the

---

In 1756 Benjamin Franklin founded the Pennsylvania Hospital where Benjamin Rush, the "father of American psychiatry," began working in 1783.

Eastern Psychiatric Hospital, Williamsburg, Virginia, was built in 1773 and is regarded as the first American public psychiatric hospital.

Dorothea Dix, an American schoolteacher in the mid-1800s, stirred public awareness of the evils of the poorhouse and raised money to erect suitable hospitals for mentally ill persons in parts of the United States, Canada, and Europe.

state and designed according to architectural plans developed by Dr. Thomas Kirkbride. The location of these institutions was determined by many considerations. For example, it was believed that the tranquil environment of the country would be soothing to disturbed individuals; rural land was inexpensive to purchase; and the remoteness of the setting effectively protected society from the inmates, both physically and emotionally.

The design of the institution resulted from a genuine desire to provide a homelike environment that would also be safe. However, because of the remoteness of the setting, such staff as there were had to live in adjoining quarters, and the institution had to produce its own food, heat, and other necessities. What evolved was a self-contained community where patients who were able worked on the farm; in the kitchen, laundry, and machine shop; and on the grounds and wards. For some patients, this responsibility proved therapeutic because it provided meaningful activity, thereby increasing their sense of self-esteem and group cohesiveness. In some state hospitals, selected patients were invited to share the Sunday dinner with the hospital superintendent. Many, if not all, were more comfortable than they would have been had they remained in their local community. On the other hand, there were abuses. At the very least, even the most able patient was taken advantage of, since he was not paid for his labor.

In addition to exploitation and perhaps not unrelated to it, another negative outcome of the state hospital system was the syndrome of *institutionalization*. Because of the remoteness of its location the state hospital was not accessible to the community, and families soon gave up any attempt to remain in contact with their hospitalized member. Having no contact with the outside world these patients adapted to their surroundings and their roles within the hospital to the extent that they resisted the few attempts made on their behalf to return them to their homes. Consequently, it was not uncommon for an individual, once admitted to the hospital, to spend the remainder of his life there.

By the middle of the nineteenth century the asylum, "the big house on the hill" surrounded by its landscaped park and topped by high towers and domes, became a familiar landmark. Although such matters as management, housing, and feeding of the patients were slowly attaining decent humanitarian standards, as late as 1840 there was no clear classification of mental disorders. A German teacher, Dr. Heinroth, was still advancing the theory that insanity and sin were identical. It was not until 1845 that the first authentic textbook on mental disease was published, aligning the treatment of mental illness with the treatment of other illnesses.

This self-contained state hospital system of mental health delivery, with all its advantages and disadvantages, might well have continued had it not been for the waves of immigrants to the United States in the mid-nineteenth century. The effect of this "population explosion" was an enlargement of the cities so that the state hospitals were no longer so geographically remote. In addition, and perhaps more important, the system was confronted with huge numbers of

Institutionalization
A syndrome wherein a person hospitalized for a long time adapts to the hospital environment to the extent of resisting discharge.

The first authentic textbook on psychiatric disorders was published in 1845; for the first time, discussion of mental illness paralleled that of other illnesses.

individuals who were believed to need mental health care. Because the cultural backgrounds and language of the immigrants were sufficiently different from those of the mainstream, the behavior of many was poorly tolerated by the society and the census of the state hospitals swelled. This made it impossible to continue the humane treatment delivered at an earlier time, and by the twentieth century the state hospital system had turned into an inefficient, expensive, and inhumane system able to do little more than protect inmates from each other and from society.

Twentieth century

Overt change in the state hospital system of mental health care began in 1908 when Clifford Beers, a psychiatric patient who was hospitalized several times, wrote a book entitled *A Mind That Found Itself.* Being of vivid colorful temperament, Mr. Beers had unlimited enthusiasm, which he directed to founding the National Committee for Mental Hygiene. Under the momentum of his leadership the movement became worldwide, and, for the first time, emphasis was placed on prevention of mental illness and early intervention.

Simultaneously with the mental hygiene movement came the astounding contributions of Sigmund Freud (1856–1939), which revolutionized the orthodox concepts of the mind, proposed a new technique for exploring it, and brought the subject of human behavior to the attention of every intelligent man and woman. Psychiatry at last left the closed doors of the asylums and participated in everyday human activity.

One of the most progressive actions the nation has ever taken in relation to mental illness was the passage of the National Mental Health Act in 1946. Among other accomplishments was the establishment of the National Institute of Mental Health (NIMH). A similar act was passed about the same time in Canada, and it had a similar effect in moving Canada into the forefront in the field of mental health. Both these acts provided for financing research and training programs. Through their enactment the governments expressed their belief that it was necessary to acquire more knowledge concerning the cause, prevention, and treatment of mental illness and that more professionally trained workers were needed to improve the care and treatment of mentally ill persons. Financial support for the education of psychologists, psychiatric social workers, psychiatrists, and psychiatric nurses was provided in the United States for many years through the National Mental Health Act.

The National Mental Health Act grew out of the experiences the nation had during World War II when more men in the Armed Forces were disabled by mental illness than by all the other problems related to actual military action. The many soldiers who were incapacitated by acute and chronic mental illness alerted the nation to the need for many more trained professional workers in the field, for greater knowledge about the cause and prevention of mental illness, and for greatly improved treatment techniques.

Publication of *A Mind That Found Itself* by a former mental patient, Clifford Beers, in 1908 brought about an emphasis on prevention of and early intervention in mental illness.

Sigmund Freud's theories brought the subject of human behavior to the attention of laypersons for the first time.

Therapeutic community
A specific use of the environment, or milieu, as a therapeutic tool. See Chapter 8 for more information on this treatment method.

Psychotropic drugs
Drugs that alter the chemistry of the brain and therefore the emotions and behavior of the person who takes them.

Because of the nation's increased attention to the problem of mental illness, the late 1940s and early 1950s saw the development of new methods for treating persons in need of mental health care. These methods included family diagnosis, short- and long-term treatment programs, and crisis-oriented therapy. At about the same time several new treatment methods were introduced into public psychiatric hospitals. Two of the most noteworthy were the therapeutic community, where the milieu was used as a specific therapeutic tool through examination of group processes and community self-regulation, and the open-door hospital, where the doors of the units were unlocked, allowing patients who were able to move freely within the hospital and the community. It is interesting to note that both these treatment modalities were first developed in England and were most successful with those patients who were not severely or chronically ill.

Major changes in the care of severely and chronically mentally ill persons were not possible until the development of psychotropic drugs, particularly the antipsychotic agents, which alter the chemistry of the brain and therefore the emotions and the behavior of those who take them. These medications were first used experimentally in 1953. By 1956 the number of patients in the state mental hospitals was reported to have fallen slightly, instead of increasing as had been the case for decades. This phenomenon was largely a result of the fact that, with the help of these medications, more individuals could control their behavior and thus could spend time outside the hospital in the community. Had it not been for these drugs, many individuals would never have been able to control their unusual behavior sufficiently to remain at home and receive continuing treatment on an outpatient basis.

In 1955 the Congress of the United States passed the Mental Health Study Act. This act provided funds for a 5-year study of the problem of mental illness in the United States. As a result of the act the Joint Commission on Mental Illness was established. On December 31, 1960, this commission submitted its final report to the Congress, to the Surgeon General of the Public Health Service, and to the governors of the 50 states. The published report was entitled *Action for Mental Health* and was available to the public in 1961. It was widely read, provided the necessary stimulus for developing more effective services for people in need of psychiatric help, and was the basis for additional legislation.

A milestone in the nation's developing awareness of the need for an improved approach to the problems of mental health and illness was reached on February 5, 1963, when President John F. Kennedy delivered his special message to the Congress on mental illness and mental retardation. In this speech he mentioned a few goals: "Central to a new mental health program is comprehensive community care. . . . The mentally ill can achieve . . . a constructive social adjustment. . . . The centers will focus on community resources. . . . Prevention as well as treatment will be a major activity." In that same year, 1963, the Community Mental Health Centers Act was passed, followed in 1965 by the

Staffing Act for the Community Mental Health Centers. These acts sought to revolutionize the provision of mental health care by emphasizing prevention and decentralized, local community treatment as opposed to institutional care for even those persons who manifest severe psychiatric difficulties. Federal funds to build and staff community mental health centers were appropriated and served as the force behind the rapid development of many such centers in a relatively short period. The first federally funded centers began operation in 1966, and thus began the deinstitutionalization of mentally ill persons.

In 1975 the Congress of the United States enacted the Community Mental Health Centers Amendments of 1975. This law provided for the continuation of federal funds to community mental health centers but also designated specific guidelines for services that must be provided. Specified in these guidelines were a full range of inpatient, outpatient, and emergency services. Certain population groups such as children and the elderly were targeted as particularly requiring services. Individuals suffering from drug and alcohol abuse and addiction and those persons being discharged from mental institutions also were included in the population groups given priority for services.

In 1977 President Jimmy Carter called for the development of a President's Commission on Mental Health, which was charged with identifying "the mental health needs of the nation." Nursing was represented on such a commission for

Deinstitutionalization The practice of discharging certain long-term mentally ill patients from the hospital to community-based treatment programs.

TABLE 1-1   *Locus of mental health care throughout history*

	Family/ community	Religious orders	Penal institutions/ almshouses	State mental hospitals	Community mental health centers	Yet to be determined
Prehistoric times	X					
Early Greek and Roman eras		X				
Middle Ages		X				
Sixteenth, seventeenth, eighteenth centuries			X			
Nineteenth century				X		
Twentieth century				X	X	?
Twenty-first century	?	?	?	?	?	?

the first time by Martha Mitchell, a nurse educator and clinical specialist in psychiatric-mental health nursing. The report of the 1977 commission recommended the development of a new federal grant program designed to strengthen existing community efforts and to develop new initiatives to address the mental health needs of communities. Special emphasis was placed on meeting the needs of underserved and high-risk populations such as the elderly, children, chronically mentally ill persons, cultural minorities, rural communities, and inner-city neighborhoods. The very timely issue of the economics of mental health care was addressed by a recommendation that mental health coverage be included in all health insurance and that this coverage not be limited to hospitalization. The commission also recommended that evaluation of federally funded community mental health centers be centralized.

In October 1980 Congress passed the Mental Health Systems Act of 1980. This legislation grew out of the commission's recommendations and it addressed, among other issues, research and training priorities and client's rights.

Unfortunately, before this legislation could be implemented, the political climate of the nation changed and a conservative administration was elected to the White House. In 1981 the Congress passed the Reagan administration's Omnibus Budget Reconciliation Act. This legislation drastically curtailed federal funding for all health services, including mental health services. Funds that were allocated were distributed to the states in the form of "block grants" in the belief that it is both the right and the responsibility of the state government to determine priorities for finite resources and to distribute these funds. The one exception has been the maintenance of federal funding for research, particularly biomedical research, about the causes and treatment of mental illness. Consequently, the short-term future of community mental health centers is highly dependent upon unpredictable state, local, and private funding and income from services provided. In many instances, this has meant a serious curtailment of innovative programming of mental health services and a marked decline in the training of mental health professionals.

THE CONTEMPORARY MENTAL HEALTH DELIVERY SYSTEM: COMPREHENSIVE COMMUNITY MENTAL HEALTH CENTERS

Despite a shift and reduction in funding, the public mental health delivery system model continues to be the comprehensive community mental health center. Each center is organized around a demographic unit with a population small enough to permit the development of comprehensive mental health services. It seeks to serve the people who reside in a specific geographic area, referred to as a *catchment area*. Depending upon population density, a catchment area may be as geographically small as a few square miles or as large as several counties. The staff of the community mental health center attempts to assist the communities in its catchment area to improve the mental health of its residents. Much emphasis is placed on assisting individuals and families who have developed emo-

Catchment area
The specific geographic area for which a particular institution, especially a community mental health center, is responsible.

TABLE 1-2   *Federal legislation leading to the establishment of comprehensive community mental health centers*

Year	Legislation	Effect
1946	National Mental Health Act	Established the National Institute of Mental Health (NIMH) Financed research and training programs
1955	Mental Health Study Act	Financed a 5-year study of mental illness in the United States Resulted in revolutionary report, *Action for Mental Health*
1963	Community Mental Health Centers Act	Emphasized prevention and decentralized, local community treatment Financed construction of community mental health centers
1965	Staffing Act for Community Mental Health Centers	Provided funding for staff for community mental health centers
1975	Community Mental Health Centers Amendments of 1975	Required inpatient, outpatient, and emergency services Specified target populations for priority services, including children, the elderly, drug and alcohol abusers, discharged mentally ill persons
1980	Mental Health Systems Act	Designed to strengthen existing community efforts and to develop new initiatives Never implemented due to 1981 legislation
1981	Omnibus Budget Reconciliation Act	Drastically curtailed federal funding for health care services Available funds allocated as "block grants" to states

tional problems to maintain their ties with the community and, when hospitalization is necessary, to return to community living as soon as possible. To achieve these goals it becomes essential that all helping agencies share information freely and cooperate effectively.

Specific requirements for a fully developed comprehensive community mental health center were identified in the law that made government funding available. When fully developed a comprehensive community mental health center was intended to include inpatient and outpatient services, day and night hospital units, crisis intervention centers, halfway houses, family therapy centers, rehabilitation centers, transitional facilities where individuals may receive board and care, and suicide prevention centers. In addition, it was expected to offer services to the community that included consultation to community agencies and professional personnel, diagnostic services, and rehabilitative services including vocational and educational programs. Finally, the comprehensive community mental health center was expected to provide training for professional and paraprofessional workers; to conduct research into the prevention, cause, and treatment of mental illness; and to evaluate the effectiveness of the programs offered.

Although some community mental health centers are able to provide all the above programs, only five services are currently required: outpatient care, partial hospitalization, 24-hour hospitalization and emergency care, consultation and education, and screening services. Despite the differences in services among community mental health centers, their practice shares some significant similarities:

1. Comprehensive and continuous service to the consumer. A person seeking help has immediate access to services, regardless of the time of day or week. Furthermore, every effort is made to link the individual with a service that would appropriately meet his needs, whether hospitalization or a community-based social program. Since many persons need more than one service, the community mental health center plays a major role in coordinating the provision of the required services.

2. Emphasis on treatments that utilize groups rather than relying entirely on individual one-to-one interventions. Thus the treatment focus is likely to be on family therapy, group therapy, milieu therapy, or crisis intervention.

3. Prevention of mental illness as a major focus. Thus consultation and educational activities become as important in the centers as treatment. Many of the professional workers spend more time in the consultation and educational aspects of their work than in the treatment aspects.

4. Planned social change. Professional workers are concerned not only with the individuals who seek help but also with the community itself, which is the incubator, in a sense of the word, of the mental health problems from which the population suffers. Thus the professional staff of the community mental health center works to improve the social systems that serve the population within the community, that is, the family, the churches, the schools, the hospitals, recreational facilities, the court system, housing, local government, industry, and so on.

5. Utilization of the services of individuals who are already working with the larger population in the catchment area. These individuals may include social service workers, police, clergy, teachers, public health nurses, and other community leaders who may serve on advisory boards or as consultants about the mental health needs of the community. In addition, some community mental health centers have involved individuals identified as indigenous workers. These people may lack formal education but have lived in the community and understand the unofficial community organization. They are aware of the real hopes, interests, and concerns of the people. In addition, they speak and understand the language commonly used by the people being served. With professional guidance the indigenous workers have been very successful in some community mental health centers because of their ability to relate in a meaningful way with the people seeking help and to offer it to them on a level that is acceptable and useful.

6. A commitment to an interdisciplinary treatment team approach. This practice is based on the belief that each mental health discipline has a necessary and valid perspective to contribute about the improvement of mental health and the prevention and treatment of mental illness. It is also believed that decisions and recommendations arrived at jointly are likely to be more effective than those derived by each discipline independently. Consequently, all disciplines share treatment responsibilities in these centers. The leadership of the treatment team may be held by any one of its members, depending on the background, experience, interests, and abilities of the individual team members.

The preceding is a description of the public community mental health system that provides the structure within which mentally ill persons are currently treated. Following is a discussion of the origins, roles, and functions of the professional disciplines that the interdisciplinary mental health team comprises.

THE INTERDISCIPLINARY MENTAL HEALTH TEAM

Four health care professions constitute the core mental health disciplines: psychiatric nursing, psychiatry, clinical psychology, and psychiatric social work. They all emerged as specialties within their respective professions during the last half of the nineteenth century at the time when behaviorally disturbed persons were generally viewed as being ill rather than as being possessed by demons or morally corrupt.

Psychiatric nursing

The first school of nursing in a psychiatric setting was established at McLean Hospital in 1882, 9 years after the first schools of nursing in the United States had been founded. Up to this time poorly trained, nonprofessional workers had dominated the care of patients in psychiatric institutions and the purpose of this school was to improve the care of mentally ill patients by upgrading the skills of attendants. The first class of 15 women graduated in 1886. By 1917 41 mental institutions were operating training schools for nurses. Unfortunately, the standards for admission and graduation established by most of these schools were much lower than those of schools of nursing in general hospitals. Beginning in 1906 nurse educators began to work toward establishing affiliations in psychiatric hospitals for students enrolled in schools of nursing in general hospitals, but it was not until 1955 that all schools of nursing offered an experience in psychiatric nursing as a required part of the curriculum. Schools of nursing in psychiatric hospitals no longer exist.

Nurses are professionals whose initial educational preparation is through an associate degree, baccalaureate degree, or diploma program. After this preparation the nurse becomes licensed as a registered nurse through successful completion of state board examinations. Without additional educational or experiential preparation this nurse can function as a generalist in any setting. An in-

Nurse generalist
A nurse whose education and experience are at the entry level, qualifying her to provide comprehensive care to patients with common health problems in any setting.

creasing number of nurses with baccalaureate degrees have continued their education to attain master's degrees in a particular clinical specialty. Nurses prepared as clinical specialists in psychiatric–mental health nursing at the graduate level have advanced preparation in promoting the mental health of individuals, groups, families, and communities, as well as in assisting these persons in increasing the effectiveness of their adaptations. The American Nurses Association (ANA) administers an examination process whereby psychiatric nurse generalists and psychiatric clinical nurse specialists both can document their expertise and become certified at the appropriate level. Although there is no legal requirement to hold ANA certification at this time, many psychiatric nurses are choosing to earn this credential. In addition, third-party providers are increasingly using certification as one determinant of eligibility for reimbursement for services provided. The specific roles and functions of the psychiatric nurse generalist are discussed in detail in Chapter 7.

Psychiatry

Although the superintendents of the asylums were physicians, the specialty of psychiatry was not known until 1846 when the practice of hospitalizing mentally ill persons made possible the systematic observation and study of mental disorders. It was not until after World War I that the specialty was given any significant attention in the curriculums of medical schools.

Psychiatrists are physicians who have had several years of supervised residency training in the medical specialty of psychiatry. The law does not require licensing beyond that necessary for any physician, but the medical profession makes available a voluntary examination in this clinical specialty. Physicians who successfully complete this examination are "board certified" and identify themselves as such. This designation helps to ensure the lay public of the services of a physician with advanced knowledge and experience in psychiatry. Psychiatrists function in private practice as well as treating hospitalized clients. In the latter instance the psychiatrist may be the leader of the treatment team, although there is a trend toward the treatment team leader being the person who is most knowledgeable about the client, regardless of professional discipline. The psychiatrist's unique function is prescribing medications and administering other somatic treatments such as electroconvulsive therapy. In addition the psychiatrist is the only professional equipped to make a medical diagnosis and is particularly skilled in identifying and treating persons whose problems have highly interrelated emotional and physiological components.

Clinical psychology

Unlike psychiatry, which had its origin in the practice setting, psychology began within the university as an academic, research-oriented discipline, devoted to the scholarly study of human behavior. The first psychological clinic was established in 1896 at the University of Pennsylvania, followed shortly by the estab-

---

Third-party providers
Providers of services rendered to a person in which an entity other than the giver or receiver of the service is responsible for the payment, e.g., insurance companies.

Somatic
Of or pertaining to the body.

Electroconvulsive therapy
The induction of a brief convulsion by passing an electric current through the brain for the treatment of affective disorders (i.e., acute depression) in patients resistant to psychotropic drug therapy.

lishment of psychological laboratories in such hospitals for mentally disturbed persons as McLean Hospital in Massachusetts, St. Elizabeth's Hospital in Washington, D.C., and Boston Psychopathic Hospital.

Psychologists are professionals who have advanced education in the study of mental processes and the treatment of mental disorders. They are not physicians but hold doctoral degrees. As is true in the fields of nursing and medicine, psychology has become such a broad discipline that most psychologists specialize. Those who are most directly involved in the diagnosis of mental illness and in the treatment of the emotionally ill are called *clinical psychologists*. Those clinical psychologists concerned with the diagnosis of mental illness have developed expertise in the use of inferential tools that are designed to assist in the diagnostic process and assessment of treatment effects. Such tools are projective techniques best exemplified by the Rorschach test, personality inventories such as the Minnesota Multiphasic Personality Inventory, and intelligence tests. Only clinical psychologists are trained in the use and interpretation of these highly complex instruments. Other clinical psychologists have chosen to develop expertise in the treatment of persons with a mental illness. Since the entire education of these psychologists has been geared to the study of human behavior, they are particularly effective when the problems of the individual or the family are clearly psychogenic in origin and manifestation. Most clinical psychologists work in close collaboration with a psychiatrist who assists in the treatment program if somatic therapies are indicated. Some states make legal certification mandatory for practice as a clinical psychologist.

Psychiatric social work

Social work began as an organized profession in the 1870s, but the specialty of psychiatric social work did not emerge until 1906 as a result of the aftercare movement, which was designed to provide adequate financial, medical, and moral assistance to patients released from mental hospitals. Mary C. Jarrett, believed to be the first psychiatric social worker, directed the first formal training course for psychiatric social workers at Smith College in 1918.

Social workers are health professionals, many of whom have educational preparation at the master's degree level. Although social workers are prepared to work with individuals and families who have a wide variety of physical, emotional, and social problems, some specialize in psychiatric social work. *Psychiatric social workers* are particularly skilled in assessing familial, environmental, and social factors that contribute to the dysfunctional behavior of the individual and the family. They also are major contributors to the planning and implementation of follow-up care.

Activity therapies

Although activity therapies are not considered a core mental health discipline, no discussion of the mental health team would be complete without mention of

Rorschach test
A projective personality assessment test developed by the Swiss psychiatrist Hermann Rorschach. It consists of ten pictures of ink-blots—five in black and white, three in black and red, and two multicolored—to which the subject responds by telling what images and emotions each design evokes. The test is designed to assess the degree to which intellectual and emotional factors are integrated into the subject's perception of the environment.

Psychogenic
Referring to any physical symptom, disease process, or emotional state that is of psychologic rather than physical origin.

them. The disciplines that make up the activity therapies include occupational therapy, recreational therapy, music therapy, rehabilitation counseling, educational therapy, and patient library services (bibliotherapy). Within these specialties other services may be provided, such as dance therapy, drama therapy, art therapy, horticulture therapy, and manual arts therapy. The history of occupational therapy, the oldest of the activity therapies, is cited here because of its intimate connection with nursing.

Occupational therapy
The use of purposeful activity with individuals who are limited by psychosocial dysfunction to maximize independence, prevent disability, and maintain health. The practice includes evaluation, treatment, and consultation.

The first book on the subject of occupational therapy was written by a nurse, Susan E. Tracy. This book, *Studies in Invalid Occupation,* was published in 1910. Miss Tracy also gave the first course of instruction on the subject in 1906 at the Adams Nervine in Boston. As such, nurses were the first occupational therapists, although that term was not used until 1921.

Some physicians also saw the potential therapeutic benefit of a planned activities program. As early as 1892 Dr. E.N. Brush wrote that even the most simple and routine tasks keep the mind occupied, awaken new trains of thought and interest, and divert the client from the delusions or hallucinations that harrass and annoy him. Dr. Brush particularly advocated the use of outdoor activities in the belief that physical exertion had a beneficial effect on the emotional health of the client. Since the nursing staff was responsible for initiating and supervising all client activities, a book titled *Occupation Therapy, a Manual for Nurses* was published in 1915. The author was Dr. William Rush Dunton, one of the earliest leaders in the field of occupational therapy. Dr. Dunton advised that the nurse "provide herself with an armamentarium which should consist at least of the following: playing cards, dominoes or card dominoes, cribbage board, scrap book with puzzles and catches, and one or more picture puzzles. . . . She is also urged to cultivate a particular craft in order that she may herself have a hobby and also that she may have special ability in instructing her client."*

All *activity therapists* are required to hold a minimum of a bachelor's degree in their field, and many have advanced degrees. A master's degree is required for entry into art therapy. Although each form of activity therapy has a specific focus, they share the principle that it is helpful to the emotionally disturbed person to be engaged in an activity that focuses on objects outside himself. The concept of *object relations* is fundamental in activity therapies. This concept includes not only the materials used in the therapy but also the setting, the therapist, and the other participants. These objects all have symbolic value, and through their use the individual expresses feelings, needs, and impulses. In this sense, all activity therapies are creative and therefore can be used in varying ways and for varied purposes. They are developed into a program based on psychodynamics but are highly individualized to meet the needs of the person for whom they are designed.

Psychodynamics
The influence of early childhood experiences on the behavior of the adult.

---

*Dunton, William Rush: Occupation therapy, a manual for nurses, Philadelphia, 1915, W.B. Saunders Co., p. 8.

The following four goals are common to all activity therapies in a mental health setting:

1. To provide opportunities for structured normal activities of daily living. Activities are designed to help the clients deal with their basic problems. In addition, the activities permit the maintenance as well as reinforcement of the healthy aspects of the client's personality.

2. To assist in diagnostic and personality evaluation. As trained members of the health care team, activity therapists can assist with diagnostic and personality evaluations through their observations of clients as they participate in activities. In addition, the process of participation, such as the type of activity chosen and the interaction that takes place between the client and the therapist and between the client and other participants, gives the therapist much valuable information about the personality structure of the client.

3. To enhance psychotherapy and other psychotherapeutic measures. The activity prescribed for the client often provides a nonverbal means for the client to express and resolve the feelings being discussed verbally in other settings. In addition, the interpersonal relationship established between the client and the therapist provides another vehicle for the provision of corrective emotional experiences.

4. To assist the client in making the transition from the sick role to becoming a contributing member of society. Some activities provide opportunity for work experience, often with the use of community resources. Through these activities the client is able to learn a skill that may be marketable. Other activities in this category focus on the development of the client's talents and interests so that he may learn to use his time in satisfying ways.

Psychotherapy
Any of a large number of related methods of treating mental and emotional disorders by psychologic techniques rather than by physical means.

All activity therapies have in common the fact that they are designed to achieve a specified goal, and the role of the therapist is to observe, direct, and guide the client in the activity. The therapist continuously assesses the client's reactions to the activity both as a means of providing information to other members of the treatment team and as a basis on which to alter the activity as the needs of the client change.

It should be noted that anyone may legally call himself or herself a psychotherapist or psychoanalyst, and these designations do not guarantee a level of expertise. All reputable therapists and analysts, however, have years of advanced education and supervised clinical training in their particular discipline.

END NOTE

This chapter traces the treatment of mentally ill individuals from prehistoric times to the present in the belief that an appreciation of the history of the treatment of mentally ill persons can aid in understanding the contemporary system of mental health delivery. The evolution of comprehensive community mental health centers is discussed in detail, since these centers are where mentally ill persons are currently treated. The similarities among community mental health centers include: comprehensive and continuous service to the consumer; emphasis on treatment in groups; prevention of mental illness as a major focus; planned social change; utilization of the services of individuals who are already working with the larger population in the catchment area; and a commitment to an interdisciplinary treatment team approach. The origins, roles, and functions of the professional disciplines that the interdisciplinary mental health team comprises are described.

SUGGESTED SOURCES OF ADDITIONAL INFORMATION

Adelson G and Leader M: The social worker's role: a study of private and voluntary hospitals, Hosp Commun Psychiatr 31:776, November 1980.

Beers C: A mind that found itself, New York, 1948, Doubleday & Co.

Carter EW: Psychiatric nursing: 1986, J Psychosoc Nurs 24(6):26, June 1986.

Chamberlain JC: The role of the federal government in the development of psychiatric nursing, J Psychosoc Nurs Ment Health Serv 21:11, April 1983.

Church O: From custody to community in psychiatric nursing, Nurs Res 36(6):48, January 1987.

Joint Commission on Mental Illness and Health: Action for mental health, New York, 1961, Basic Books, Inc.

Mark B: From "lunatic" to "client": 300 years of psychiatric patienthood, J Psychosoc Nurs Ment Health Serv 18(3):32, March 1980.

Moffie HS, et al: Paraprofessionals and psychiatric teams: an updated review, Hosp Commun Psychiatr 35:61, January 1984.

Morrissey J and Goldman H: Cycles of reform in the care of the chronically mentally ill, Hosp Commun Psychiatr 35:785, August 1984.

Rankin EADeS: Psychiatric/mental health nursing, Nurs Clin North Am 21(6):381, September 1986.

The mental health disciplines: notes on the development of 13 disciplines that play important roles in the treatment of the mentally disabled, Hosp Commun Psychiatr 27(7):495, 1976.

Thompson J, Bass R, and Witkin M: Fifty years of psychiatric services: 1940-1990, Hosp Commun Psychiatr 33:711, September 1982.

Two hundred years of mental health care in America: Hosp Commun Psychiatr 27(7): July 1976.

Waters H: All for one and one for all, Nurs Times 83(6):61, May 1987.

Psychiatric nursing and the law

2

LEARNING OBJECTIVES

After studying this chapter the student will be able to:

○ Differentiate between voluntary and involuntary admission for the treatment of mental illness.

○ Describe the usual procedure for involuntary admission.

○ Discuss the following client rights:
  1. The right to habeas corpus.
  2. The right to treatment.
  3. The right to informed consent.
  4. The right to confidentiality-privacy.
  5. The right to an independent psychiatric examination.
  6. The right to refuse treatment.
  7. The right to be free of restraints.

○ Discuss the professional accountability of the nurse as defined by law.

○ Discuss the medical specialty of forensic psychiatry.

Psychiatric nursing and the law both are primarily concerned with the behavior of human beings. Psychiatric nursing is concerned with assisting individuals, families, and community groups to achieve satisfying and productive patterns of living. The law provides rules for behavioral conduct to facilitate orderly social functioning while simultaneously protecting the rights of the individual. Thus psychiatric nursing and the law affect each other greatly. The nurse can practice effectively only if she is knowledgeable about the rudimentary principles of the law that concern mental illness, since she is accountable for providing care that is not only clinically sound but also protects both the society and the client.

Many authorities believe that the nurse can best fulfill this responsibility by assuming the role of client advocate where she assists the client to learn about his rights and how to protect and assert those rights within the health care system.

This chapter addresses those legal issues most likely to be encountered in the practice of psychiatric nursing in the hope that the nurse can satisfactorily fulfill the client advocate role.

METHODS OF PSYCHIATRIC ADMISSION

The detention of persons considered to be mentally ill is permitted by law, although the specifics of the law differ from state to state. However, all states assume the responsibility of segregating from society those persons whom psychiatrists deem dangerous or incompetent because of mental illness.

In 1953 the United States Public Health Service published the Draft Act Governing Hospitalization of the Mentally Ill. The following distinctions were suggested:

1. Voluntary admission is to be characterized by the individual's admission and discharge via his own signature.
2. Involuntary admission is undertaken by someone other than the client.

The least restrictive manner of obtaining treatment for mental illness is voluntary admission. Since many mentally ill individuals lack insight concerning their behavior and will not seek hospitalization of their own will, voluntary hospitalization is not always possible. The nurse must realize that a combination of overt behaviors and legal status, not a diagnostic category, determines whether an individual can be treated voluntarily or involuntarily. Suicidal, violent, acute psychotic, and antisocial behaviors in persons unwilling to be treated are the usual reasons for a person to be involuntarily admitted to a psychiatric treatment center.

Three types of involuntary admission result in commitment. The first is an *emergency commitment,* where the individual presents a "clear and present" danger to himself or to others. The length of this hospitalization is limited; in most states it is only for 3 to 5 days. The second type of involuntary admission is *temporary commitment,* where the individual can be involuntarily hospitalized for a longer period. In some states this time period is 6 months. The third type of commitment is called *extended* or *indefinite commitment,* which is valid for an unspecified period, usually subject to periodic judicial review. *Criminal commitment* is a form of extended or indefinite commitment allowing involuntary hospitalization of persons charged with crimes who are awaiting trial or who have been acquitted of a crime by reason of insanity.

Until recently, only state hospitals and some private psychiatric hospitals would admit persons who were on an involuntary status. Psychiatric units in general hospitals, in particular, were willing to admit only those individuals who voluntarily chose to be treated and could control their behavior sufficiently to be treated safely on an unlocked unit. This situation resulted in obvious and

A combination of overt behaviors and legal status, not a diagnostic category, determines whether an individual can be treated voluntarily or involuntarily.

Three types of involuntary admission resulting in commitment are: (1) *emergency,* (2) *temporary,* and (3) *extended.*

dramatic differences between the client populations treated in psychiatric hospitals and those treated in psychiatric units of general hospitals. Most recently, however, there is a trend in several states for psychiatric units to accept clients for treatment regardless of their admission status.

There is no uniformity of commitment methods among the states, but no one can be deprived of his liberty without due process of law. In general commitment proceedings consist of (1) application, (2) examination, (3) determination, and (4) detention if indicated. The action is usually initiated by relatives or friends, although any legally appointed officer of the law, members of charitable organizations, a public health official, or a private citizen may make the application, which will bring the matter to the attention of the proper court. In most states the court that settles matters of psychiatric commitment is the common pleas court or the probate court. Here the application is submitted, statements by interested parties are heard under oath, and all available information about the individual and his behavior is recorded.

Involuntary admission usually consists of: (1) application, (2) examination, (3) determination, and (4) detention, if indicated.

Frequently the application must be accompanied by the certificates of one or more physicians, or the judge may appoint one or two physicians to conduct a psychiatric examination. Some states require that at least one physician be a psychiatrist. The testimony of lay witnesses and of the examining physicians must be sufficient to convince a judge or jury that the person in question is potentially dangerous to himself or others and needs to be segregated and treated.

The issue of commitment is more than simply a legal and psychiatric question. Ideally, it is an issue of freedom of choice. Each nurse must decide whether to take a stand for or against commitment. It is imperative that nurses know and understand the commitment procedures in the states in which they practice. Furthermore they must work for the necessary legislative amendments that would facilitate appropriate reforms so as to fulfill the dictum *primum nil nocere*—we must minimize harm.

Nurses must know and understand the commitment procedures in the states in which they practice.

CLIENTS' RIGHTS

A right is the enjoyment of a privilege secured by law to a person. Mentally ill persons who are hospitalized may experience a double limitation on their rights—one created by the organization of the hospital system and the other created by their illness. While the individual's illness may limit him to some extent, prejudging his competency by the staff may be a greater obstacle to his exercising his rights. For example, a simple request to make a telephone call to his home is subject to interpretation, evaluation, and possible denial if it is not deemed to be in the best interest of the client and the hospital organization. Thus a tension exists in all psychiatric institutions between the client's need to exercise his civil rights and the hospital's need to provide care in an effective and efficient manner. When the hospital's organizational needs take precedence

A tension exists in all psychiatric institutions between the client's need to exercise civil rights and the hospital's need to provide care effectively and efficiently.

over the client's treatment needs or his civil rights, dehumanization, frustration, resignation, and despair occur.

If it is proved that the individual is incapable of conducting his affairs, a guardian may be appointed by the court or by state authorities to protect the individual's rights and property. In some states this property guardian is called a conservator. If the amount of the client's property warrants the expense of guardianship or if business involving such property must be transacted, the guardian's responsibilities are not trivial. A guardian is one who has direct responsibility for the individual's personal welfare. He is generally a near relative. He cannot confine the individual in an institution without permission or approval of the court, but he can dictate, within certain limits, the nature of the treatment and can sign a permit for a major operation. He may also have custody of the minor children of the individual if the other parent is absent or incapable of accepting this responsibility.

The wife or husband of a client rather than the parents is regarded as the natural guardian. Every guardian must give bond for the proper performance of his duties. At regular intervals the guardian is required to make an accounting of expenses and income. His first consideration must be the comfort of the client. The guardian is required to protect the client's welfare judiciously.

The law has defined certain rules for the control of human conduct, including protection from injury-producing situations. These rules have been developed from rights that pertain to each individual and may not be violated without legal repercussion, unless the individual consents to their invasion. The first 10 amendments to the U.S. Constitution, adopted in 1791, deal with human rights. Some of the rights included in these amendments are the freedom of speech, the right of protection from unreasonable search and seizure, the right to a speedy trial, and the right to due process of law before being denied life, liberty, or property.

A serious loss of civil rights was often the consequence of involuntary commitment to a psychiatric hospital. As a result, in many states the committed person was not able to make valid contracts, vote, marry, or divorce. However, in almost all legal jurisdictions legally committed individuals presently retain their constitutional and human rights, particularly those pertaining to their person, property, and civil liberties. Various rights have been listed in recent legislation, such as the following:

1. The right to keep clothing and personal effects
2. The right to communicate by telephone, to correspond, and to visit with persons outside the institution
3. The right to vote
4. The right to religious freedom
5. The right to enter contractual relationships
6. The right to make purchases

7. The right to make wills
8. The right to education
9. The right to habeas corpus
10. The right to be employed
11. The right to independent psychiatric examinations
12. The right to civil service status
13. The right to marry
14. The right to sue and to be sued
15. The right to retain licenses or permits established by law
16. The right not to be subjected to unnecessary mechanical restraint

In 1973 the American Hospital Association published a Patient's Bill of Rights (see Appendix A). The rights of clients are only as secure as the dedication of nurses and physicians who have the authority to protect them. These professionals must realize that most judges believe that personal freedom takes priority over endeavors to promote mental health that limit this freedom.

In 1976 the American Nurses Association (ANA) developed a Code for Nurses (see Appendix B). The code deals with issues of ethical nursing conduct. In developing the code the ANA recognized that the recipients of health care have basic rights that must not be intruded on by those who provide service. It is the responsibility of the nurse to recognize and respect the client's dignity as a human being by protecting his rights.

In 1977 the President's Commission on Mental Health recommended that each state have a bill of rights for all individuals who are being treated for mental illness. Furthermore, it urged that a copy of these rights be displayed in all psychiatric settings, be given to each client using the facilities, and be explained in an easily understandable manner. A model mental health client's bill of rights was included in the Mental Health Systems Act passed by the United States Congress in 1980. Although the Omnibus Budget Reconciliation Act of 1981 included the repeal of parts of the Mental Health Systems Act, it did retain the bill of rights except for the provisions and funding for protection and advocacy. A summary of the Mental Health Systems Act Bill of Rights is found in the box on p. 24.

Statements regarding clients' rights have been developed because of judicial disillusionment with the basic assumptions underlying the way mental health professionals have traditionally dealt with mentally ill individuals. It is imperative that judges and legislators continually reexamine fundamental assumptions that have gone unchallenged throughout the years. However, it is important to recognize that the mere enactment of legislation designed to protect clients' rights does not ensure enforcement. Nurses seeking employment in psychiatric institutions must be certain that these facilities have the proper internal structure to protect the client's rights. Facilities with no internal structure to enforce clients' rights are in a vulnerable position because clients may be forced

The nurse must be knowledgeable about the Patient's Bill of Rights published by the American Hospital Association in 1973.

The Code for Nurses developed in 1976 by the American Nurses' Association (ANA) deals with issues of ethical nursing conduct.

Mental Health Systems Act Bill of Rights

1. The right to appropriate treatment in the least restrictive setting.
2. The right to treatment based on a current, accurate, individualized, written treatment plan which includes a description of mental health services that may be needed after discharge.
3. The right to ongoing participation in the planning of treatment along with appropriate explanations of its objectives, potential adverse effects, and alternatives.
4. The right to refuse treatment, except in an emergency or as provided by law.
5. The right not to participate in experimentation. When consent is given, the patient has the right to have a full explanation of the procedure, its anticipated benefits, potential discomforts and risks, and alternative treatments, along with the right to revoke such consent at any time.
6. The right to freedom from restraint or seclusion, except in an emergency or when these are prescribed as a part of treatment.
7. The right to a humane treatment environment.
8. The right to confidentiality of the patient's mental health care records.
9. The right to access of the patient's own mental health care records, except to that information provided by third parties and that information deemed by a mental health professional to be detrimental to the patient's health.
10. The right to converse with others privately, to have convenient and reasonable access to the telephone and mails, and to see visitors during regularly scheduled hours, except when denied access to a particular visitor as part of the written treatment plan.
11. The right to be informed promptly about these rights.
12. The right to assert grievances regarding infringement of these rights, including the right to have such grievances heard in a fair, timely, and impartial manner.
13. The right to obtain assistance from designated or otherwise qualified advocates.
14. The right to exercise these rights without reprisal, including the denial of any appropriate, available treatment.
15. The right to referral to other providers of mental health services upon discharge.

to go outside the institution, possibly to court, to see that their rights are protected.

The right to habeas corpus

Habeas corpus
A writ requiring a person to be brought before a judge or a court, especially for investigation of restraint of the person's liberty.

The object of the right to habeas corpus is to ensure the speedy release of any individual who claims that he is being deprived of his liberty and being detained illegally. This fundamental right has not always been respected. Kenneth Donaldson, a client in a civil commitment case decided by the Supreme Court, was refused writs of habeas corpus 18 times during his 15 years of hospitalization before he finally won his chance to have a court hear his case.

The right to treatment

In 1960 Morton Birnbaum advocated the enforcement and recognition of the legal right of a mentally ill individual hospitalized in a public psychiatric institution to adequate medical treatment for psychiatric illness. Adequate treatment for institutionalized mentally ill and mentally retarded persons is a constitutional right. The U.S. Second Federal Appeals Court and the Alabama Federal District Court have elaborated the following legal doctrines: (1) persons in custody for mental illness have a right to treatment, (2) they may not be held without treatment, and (3) treatment can be legally defined.

In 1971 the guardians of committed patients and some employees of Bryce State Mental Hospital filed a class action suit against the Commissioner of Mental Health, members of the Alabama Mental Health Board, and others (*Wyatt vs Stickney*). The defendants were charged with providing inadequate treatment to approximately 5000 mentally ill persons. The court based its decision on the constitutional guarantee of a right to treatment. In 1972 the court issued an order that detailed criteria for adequate treatment: (1) a humane psychological and physical environment, (2) qualified staff in sufficient numbers to administer adequate treatment, and (3) individualized treatment plans.

> Adequate treatment consists of: (1) a humane psychological and physical environment, (2) qualified staff in sufficient numbers to administer adequate treatment, and (3) individualized treatment plans.

The right to informed consent

If clients consent to treatment, their consent must be informed by staff explanation. It is important to understand what consent means. For a consent to be valid it must be based on adequate knowledge and information and must be given by a person who has the legal capacity to consent. Furthermore it must be voluntarily given. A rapidly growing mental health doctrine requires that clients be given specific and adequate information about the proposed treatment procedure. This is to include the administration of the treatment, its probability of success or failure, its risks and side effects, alternative treatment procedures, and the probable consequences of not receiving treatment.

> Clients should be given specific and adequate information about their proposed treatment procedure, whether or not they request it.

It is the duty of the mental health professional to provide the necessary information whether or not the client requests it. The precise information given will depend on the nature, severity, and consequences of the proposed treatment. The mental health professional misleads the client when the beneficial effects of a treatment are exaggerated, while the dangers of the treatment are minimized or withheld. If the client is injured the mental health professional could be held responsible via malpractice or negligence claims.

The right of confidentiality-privacy

Confidentiality and privacy of information about the client must be respected at all times. The frequent necessity to exchange information about the client between health care professionals and institutions does not alter the legal requirements to protect the client's privacy. The individual revealing information about the client's condition without authorization could be subject to legal difficulties. A lawsuit for invasion of privacy, liability, or slander is possible, depending on the facts of the situation and the type of information revealed.

Statutes that pertain to the confidentiality of psychiatric hospital records vary greatly among the states. Some statutes only prohibit disclosure of infor-

The nurse has a responsibility to protect the patient's right to confidentiality and privacy.

mation about the client's diagnosis and treatment, while others prohibit disclosure of the fact of hospitalization. Most statutes permit disclosure to private physicians, welfare officials, police, and insurance companies. Some may permit disclosure to prospective employers. Other statutes prohibit disclosure to almost everyone unless the person consents to disclosure.

The client should be told of the need to share information with other persons and agencies. He should be asked to sign the appropriate consent form.

Some states consider mental health professional–client communication, including nurse-client communication, privileged. Four criteria are used for judging whether communication is privileged:

1. The communication is given with confidence in its nondisclosure.
2. Confidentiality is essential to the maintenance of the relationship.
3. The relationship is one that in the opinion of the community ought to be zealously fostered.
4. The injury that would result to the relationship by disclosure of the communication is greater than the benefit gained in winning litigation.

The unnecessary disclosure of confidential information is considered improper by law. A breach of confidence is considered to be the discussion of the client's confidential information with a third party. This type of unlawful disclosure may provide the client with a cause for action against the party revealing such information.

The right to an independent psychiatric examination

The client has a right to an independent psychiatric examination.

Fairness or due process requires that a client have an opportunity to secure a psychiatric examination by a physician of his choice. The provision of this independent judgment in commitment proceedings is designed to protect the client from the judgment of mental health professionals appointed by the court who may have motivations other than the client's interests. If the state is allowed to use such testimony, the client should have the same right. Furthermore the constitutional right to present witnesses may also necessitate that clients be allowed to choose expert witnesses. Some authorities believe that the state should provide the client with sufficient funds to retain at least one expert witness.

The right to refuse treatment

The client's constitutional right to privacy and personal autonomy forms the basis for the right to refuse treatment.

An important basis of the right to refuse treatment is the constitutional right to privacy and personal autonomy. As long as public health, safety, or morals remain unharmed, the courts will respect a client's decision to refuse treatment. Ford* states that "the constitutional origins of the right to refuse medication stem from a long-standing recognition by the courts that each person has a

---

*Ford, Maurice D.: The psychiatrist's double bind: the right to refuse medication, Am. J. Psychiatry 137(3):332-339, March, 1980.

strong interest in being free from nonconsensual invasion of his bodily integrity. . . ."

In 1976 the Third Circuit Court of Appeals found at least three constitutional deprivations that may accompany the involuntary administration of medication *(Scott vs Plante)*. The first involves the nature of psychotropic drugs, which affect mental processes and which may interfere with a person's First Amendment rights to freedom of speech and association. The second deprivation incurred when medication is administered against the client's will is the violation of his right to consent to medical treatment. In the third, the court considered that the administration of involuntary medication may raise an Eighth Amendment issue concerning cruel and unusual punishment. The nurse must be knowledgable about these issues before forcefully administering medication that the client refuses. The consequence of such an action on the nurse's part could result in a charge of assault.

The right to be free of restraints

During his hospital stay the client may become violent, and the hospital is obliged to control him so that he does not harm others or himself. If a delirious postoperative patient were left unattended by an open window and jumped from it the hospital would be considered negligent.

However, the right to restrain a client is a right limited only to the duration of real necessity. Although no one would dispute the right of hospital personnel to prevent a delirious individual from pulling out a catheter in most situations the hospital personnel cannot interfere with the actions of a client. If, for example, the client shouts obscenities but is not a threat to himself or others, hospital personnel cannot tie him down or lock him up. To commit such an act invites a suit for false imprisonment.

Some state laws have specified the type of physical restraints that may be used, including the consistency of the actual material from which the restraint is made. Nurses must be mindful of such regulations. The restraint need not be physical; threats of force are sufficient cause for legal action. One who is physically restrained may have cause to file an action for battery. Alternatives for restraining clients must be considered. One such alternative is the provision of constant observation by nursing personnel. Nurses must also be aware that understaffing is not a suitable justification for the use of chemical or physical restraints. The issue of safety is the primary concern.

Client safety should be the primary concern when the issue of patient restraints is considered.

PROFESSIONAL ACCOUNTABILITY

Negligence is defined as the omission to do something that a reasonable person guided by ordinary considerations that regulate human affairs would do, and the commission of an act as doing something that a wise and reasonable person would not do. Nursing malpractice has been defined by a California court as the nurse's neglect to apply a degree of learning and skill in treating and caring for a client that is customarily practiced in caring for and treating the sick. This definition also includes acting outside the realm of authorized nursing practice.

A *tort* is a legal wrong, injury, or damage committed on a person or property independent of a contract. A *contract* is an agreement between two or more parties, although not every agreement is a contract. In general, moral agreements, agreements of conscience, or agreements involving social obligations are not classified as contracts.

When an individual becomes a psychiatric patient he automatically contracts with licensed health care personnel, including the nurse, for treatment. In such a contract both parties implicitly agree that the nurse will provide reasonable and prudent care for the client.

If this contract is violated the client may initiate action to obtain a remedy for an injury to his rights. In this instance the client is referred to as the *plaintiff*. The nurse, or *defendant*, is then required to answer and defend her action or be judged by default. A nurse may be a defendant in a negligent tort. Under the law of negligent tort, the plaintiff must prove the following:

1. A legal duty of care existed.
2. The nurse performed her duty negligently.
3. Damages were suffered by him as a result.
4. The damages were substantial.

The majority of lawsuits in psychiatric nursing involve negligence in the observation of suicidal precautions, assistance in the administration of electroconvulsive therapy, and the reporting of information or lack of such reporting in regard to medications.

COMMUNITY ACCOUNTABILITY

By providing rules of behavioral conduct to facilitate orderly social functioning, the law not only protects the individual from society but also society from the individual. Forensic psychiatry, which is a specialty within psychiatry, is involved in the criminal justice system. Forensic psychiatrists are concerned with determinations of mental incompetency and insanity.

The doctrine of mental incompetency

Mental incompetency exists when the defendant, because of mental illness or other reasons, does not understand the object and nature of the proceedings against him. It may also mean that the defendant cannot comprehend his own condition in relation to the proceedings or for some other reason is unable to assist his lawyer in his own defense. If the defendant is deemed incompetent, all criminal proceedings are suspended and the state is denied the power to proceed against him. To prosecute an incompetent is to deny his right to due process of law. Psychiatrists are often given the responsibility for making decisions regarding competency.

Because the client is in need of nursing care, the client and the nurse have a contract in which both parties agree that the nurse will provide reasonable and prudent care for the client.

Forensic psychiatry is concerned with determinations of mental incompetency and insanity to promote orderly social functioning.

The defense of insanity

Many of the roots of the defense of insanity in use in the United States today stem from the rulings of English courts. In the seventeenth century, Sir Matthew Hale, Chief Justice of the Court of King's Bench, wrote, "Human beings are naturally endowed with these two great faculties, understanding and liberty of will. . . . The consent of the will is that which renders human actions commendable or culpable. . . ." Hale elaborated that the choice of will or liberty presupposes an act of understanding to the knowledge of a thing or an action chosen by the will. Where there is a total defect in understanding there is no free act of will. As a result judges began to charge juries that a defendant was not to be held responsible for his actions unless he had the capacity to distinguish evil from good.

In May 1800, believing that he was commanded by God to sacrifice himself for the world's salvation, Manes Hatfield fired a shot at King George III. Hatfield's counsel argued that although the defendant was not mentally ill, his delusion was truly characteristic of mental illness. The trial was stopped and the jury returned a verdict of not guilty by reason of insanity. In 1843 Daniel M'Naghten shot Daniel Drummond, Secretary to England's Prime Minister Robert Peel. The M'Naghten rule, a test of the defendant's knowledge of right and wrong, was developed as a result of the arguments and testimony in this case.

Most American jurisdictions accepted the M'Naghten rule and began to supplement it with the "irresistible impulse test." This test states that the defendant must have had a mental disease that kept him from controlling his behavior. In 1962 the American Law Institute developed the Model Penal Code, which states that "a person is not responsible for criminal conduct if at the time of such conduct, as a result of disease or defect, he lacked substantial capacity either to appreciate the wrongfulness of his conduct or to conform his conduct to the requirements of law." This modification in the M'Naghten rule is accepted in most jurisdictions. The American Psychiatric Association favors the American Law Institute test because it allows psychiatric testimony to clearly describe the history, adaptation, development, and function of patients' behavioral processes and the results of other medical tests to evaluate the clinical symptoms of mental illness in relation to alleged criminal acts.

END NOTE

This chapter discusses those aspects of the law particularly applicable to psychiatric nursing. While many segments of our society are affected by the legal system, few are as directly and frequently impacted as is the care of mentally ill persons. Since both the law and psychiatric nursing are concerned with the behavior of human beings, it is imperative that the nurse be familiar with those aspects of the law which affect her daily practice. Although this chapter discusses types of admissions, professional accountability, and community accountability, it emphasizes the rights of clients who are being treated for mental illness and urges the nurse to ensure these rights.

SUGGESTED SOURCES OF ADDITIONAL INFORMATION

Alexis A: Body searches and the right to privacy, J Psychosoc Nurs 24:5, November 1986.

Applebaum PS and Gutheil TG: Drug refusal: a study of psychiatric inpatients, Am J Psychiatr 137:340, March 1980.

Benoliel J: Ethics in nursing practice and education, Nurs Outlook 31:210, July-August 1983.

Crowder JE and Klatte EW: Involuntary admission to general hospitals: legal status is not the same issue, Hosp Commun Psychiatr 31:325, May 1980.

Garritson S and Davis A: Least restrictive alternatives: ethical considerations, J Psychosoc Nurs Ment Health Serv 21:17, December 1983.

Griffith E and Etkin K: Legal rights and involuntary transfer following a voluntary admission, Hosp Commun Psychiatr 32:319, May 1981.

Leeman C: Involuntary admissions to general hospitals: progress or threat? Hosp Commun Psychiatr 31:315, May 1980.

National Association of Mental Health Position Statement: Civil rights of mental patients, Ment Hyg 56:67, Spring 1972.

President's Commission on Mental Health: Report to the president, vol 1, Washington, DC, 1978, US Government Printing Office.

Report of the task panel on legal and ethical issues: task panel reports submitted to the President's Commission on Mental Health, vol 4, Washington, DC, 1978, US Government Printing Office.

Weiner B: Supreme Court decisions on mental health: a review, Hosp Commun Psychiatr 33:461, June 1982.

Current issues affecting the future of psychiatric nursing

3

LEARNING OBJECTIVES

After studying this chapter the student will be able to:

○ Identify one issue affecting the future of psychiatric nursing from each of the following categories: economic, social, professional, clinical, delivery system, and educational.

○ Discuss how each identified issue is likely to affect the future of psychiatric nursing.

The final years of the twentieth century will be times of challenge for psychiatric nursing. The very existence of this health care specialty is in question, while simultaneously the potential for it to make a valuable and unique contribution to the welfare of society has never been so great. Today's students of nursing will be practicing well into the twenty-first century and will be the nursing leaders of tomorrow. Since it is their nursing practice that will be affected by the way in which current issues are resolved, it is imperative that nursing students become aware of those factors which will shape the nature and scope of psychiatric nursing in the future.

This chapter is designed to highlight some of the major issues that confront psychiatric nursing. The nature of any issue is that solutions are not obvious. If they were, issues would not be present. Another characteristic of issues is the multiplicity of factors that interrelate to create them. However, whenever a discussion of issues is attempted, it becomes necessary to artificially separate each factor to facilitate discussion. Consequently, this chapter presents my view of those issues facing psychiatric nursing but does not claim to supply solutions. It is hoped that the reader's awareness of these issues will be increased whether or not the reader agrees with my analysis. As a result of an increased awareness, it is further hoped that the reader will be motivated to formulate his or her own concerns and develop a plan to address them.

ECONOMIC ISSUES

Not since the Great Depression of the 1930s has the U.S. economy been as influential a factor in shaping daily events as it is today. Unlike the Depression, when there was too little money available, we are currently living in a period where, in a sense, there is too much money available. The tragedy, however, is that despite the abundance of money, most persons are unable to attain or maintain the standard of living they desire because the cost of goods and services is also very high. Consequently, many individuals and families find themselves in a position where they have more income than ever before, but their expenses are also often higher than their income. Unfortunately, this is as true of all levels of government as it is of individuals and families and has resulted in deficit spending whereby money is borrowed to cover expenses. This practice has resulted in a level of individual, familial, and government indebtedness unprecedented in the history of this country.

Although most consumers are making more money than their parents did, they must also spread their income further to cover expenses that are often higher than their income.

The effect of the economy is all-pervasive. It is a direct or indirect factor that influences all other issues in psychiatric nursing. For example, the consumer who is faced with expenses equal to or greater than his income must establish priorities for the expenditure of the available funds. Often health care takes a low priority, particularly health care designed to promote health and prevent illness. Furthermore, health care providers are being called to ever greater accountability for the expenditure of their time. Unfortunately, it is not usually possible to demonstrate that time spent in crisis intervention with an individual or family has prevented costly mental illness. At least, this expenditure of time cannot be compared to the administration of a parenteral diuretic, the results of which are quickly visible in the improved cardiopulmonary function of the recipient.

Nurses must take responsibility for documenting the effectiveness of psychiatric nursing interventions. Quality time spent with a client has more value than meets the eye.

Nurses who care for mentally ill persons, by their very function, are highly vulnerable to the economic issue. For example, the nurse and client may interact through such activities as walking together, playing cards, or sitting silently with each other. It is understandable that the casual observer of these activities would raise questions as to their value. Nurses must assume the initiative and responsibility for engaging in research that documents the efficacy of such interactions.

Economic constraints that result in demands for increased accountability also inevitably result in increased paperwork. Unfortunately, the persons required to do this paperwork are often those who least wish to do so—people prepared to function as clinicians. In addition, events that can be quantified, that is, reduced to numbers, are more easily accounted for than events that are not quantifiable. Take, for example, the difference between health counseling, which may take 30 minutes, and changing a Foley catheter, which may take 15 minutes. The latter intervention can be easily documented as to need, action taken, and results achieved, while the former may prove difficult to justify when the same criteria are applied. Therefore the necessity for accountability has increased the value of activities that can be quantified and has devalued activities that cannot be easily translated into numerical values.

The development of Diagnosis Related Groups (DRGs) is a prominent example of the influence of the economy on health care. In the late 1960s the increasing complexity of medical care and its spiraling cost resulted in research designed to create a framework through which the quality and efficiency of institutional health care could be monitored. Continuous efforts have been mounted to refine this system, and it is now being used as a means of stabilizing health care costs through prospective payment. In other words, the amount of payment an institution receives through third-party reimbursement is determined by such variables as the patient's diagnosis, his age, and the medical procedures performed. If in a specific instance the costs exceed the coverage, these costs must be borne by the institution. The converse is true as well and provides a powerful incentive to discharge patients as quickly as possible.

It seems that the intent of the DRGs to contain health care costs is not being realized, since the cost of health care is continuing to escalate. What has occurred, however, is that the use of the DRGs as the basis for third-party reimbursement has increased the accountability of all members of the health care team. While professional accountability is long overdue, the responsibility for completion of the required paperwork unfortunately has been added to already overburdened health care professionals.

It is known that attempts to contain health care costs in many instances has led to early discharge of mentally ill clients, resulting in an increased number of acutely ill clients being treated in the community. Since only physicians and nurses are licensed to administer medication, the large number of acutely mentally ill persons in the community has led many community-based psychiatric nurses to focus much of their time administering the necessary psychotropic medications and monitoring their effects. Although these functions are certainly within the scope of nursing practice, it is feared that they will become the nurse's primary function to the neglect of other equally necessary roles such as counselor, teacher, and socializing agent.

It is also feared that hospitals will cope with decreased budgets by eliminating or curtailing inservice education programs for nurses. Although this would be a serious development for any area of nursing, it is potentially lethal for psychiatric nursing because such limited time is spent studying this subject in formal educational programs. This issue is discussed further in this chapter under the heading "Educational Issues."

DRGs are impacting all aspects of nursing: Patients are being discharged sooner and sicker from the hospital; the primary place of care is shifting from the hospital to the home.

SOCIAL ISSUES

A major social trend that has had a direct impact on psychiatric nursing is the continued, organized effort of women to achieve social and economic equality. Since nursing is primarily a women's profession, changes in the status of women are closely intertwined with changes in the profession. No longer are women content to be dependent on men; no longer are nurses willing to be handmaidens to physicians. Women are demanding more education; nurses are becoming increasingly better educated. Women are demanding wages appropriate to their preparation and responsibilities; nurses are organizing and striking to receive salaries more closely reflective of their preparation and responsibilities.

An unfortunate but, it is hoped, temporary result of the women's movement is the tendency of young women to choose careers other than those traditionally associated with women, namely, teaching and nursing. While it is certainly desirable for all young people, both men and women, to have the opportunity to pursue careers for which they are best suited, it is unfortunate that many young women are dismissing nursing as a career merely because it has been historically associated with women. Compounding this problem is the fact that the number of persons, both male and female, in the 18- to 24-year age group is dropping steadily and will continue to do so well into the twenty-first century. Consequently, the pool of persons from which students of nursing are traditionally recruited is smaller than ever before and subject to the increased recruitment efforts of other occupational groups.

An unprecedented social phenomenon is the self-help trend. Consumers no longer believe that professionals necessarily know best. Popular magazines regularly feature articles about health issues, ranging from diet to human behavior. Self-help books on a wide range of subjects are readily available, and some that deal with human emotions have been best-sellers. The result of this phenomenon is people who are well educated about health matters and who conse-

The pool of nurses will continue to dwindle as increasing numbers of young women choose to enter occupations that have traditionally been open only to males.

OF SPECIAL INTEREST

Dr. Morton Kramer, noted epidemiologist from Johns Hopkins University, projects that in the year 2005 the population of the United States will be 267,603,300. If 10% of the population, or 26,760,300 people, require only 6 hours of psychiatric nursing care that year, Dr. Kramer estimates that 107,041 psychiatric nurses will be needed.

Did you know that there are only about 52,000 RNs practicing psychiatric nursing in the United States today?

Taken from "Target-Populations for Psychiatric-Mental Health Nursing 1980-2005" by Morton Kramer, in *Psychiatric-Mental Health Nursing: Proceedings of Two Conferences on Future Directions,* U.S. Department of Health and Human Services, 1986, pp. 4-42.

quently demand quality care at reasonable cost. The field of psychiatry, which less than a century ago was scorned, has now become demystified. The implication of this trend is that all mental health care professionals, including nurses, are increasingly held accountable by consumers and cannot hide behind professional jargon and unexplained actions.

PROFESSIONAL ISSUES

A major issue is the question of whether the nurse who cares for mentally ill clients is really a nurse like any other or whether by virtue of her specialty she has forfeited her identity as a nurse. This issue affects medicine as well as nursing and stems from two factors.

One factor underlying this issue is that, despite knowledge and verbalizations to the contrary, health care professionals still practice in a manner that perpetuates a dichotomy between the mind and the body. In addition, knowledge and care of the body seem to be more valued by laypersons and professionals alike than knowledge and care of the mind. Perhaps this is the case because physiological functioning is better understood and more predictable than psychological functioning. Whatever the reason, the result is that when nurses or physicians choose to specialize in the care of mentally ill persons, they run the risk of divorcing themselves from the mainstream of health care delivery. Some persons have suggested that mental illness, as currently defined, is not an illness at all but rather a reflection of societal problems. Therefore, it is argued, preparation for the care of these persons should not be within the health care disciplines. When this issue is intensified by economic constraints, it is logical for the system to attempt to replace the nurse with less expensive attendants or aides who can be trained in a short time to focus only on behavior and engage in many of the activities performed by a nurse.

Research continues to document the fact that humans are holistic beings; the whole of the person is greater than the sum of his parts. Therefore health care directed only to the body or only to the mind is bound to be ultimately ineffective and at worst harmful. All health care professionals must have an in-depth knowledge of both the biophysical and the psychosocial sciences to practice effectively. Consequently, it is necessary for nurses who give care to mentally ill persons to remain knowledgeable about physiological as well as psychological processes and to document the difference that this knowledge makes in the nursing care they give.

Another professional issue facing psychiatric nursing is role blurring. Before the advent of the phenothiazine derivatives the roles of mental health professionals were more clearly defined. The nurse was primarily concerned with the client's activities of daily living, the psychiatrist focused on diagnosing and prescribing, the psychologist focused on testing and research, and the social worker had the client's family as her domain. Very little treatment occurred. When psychotropic drugs made clients more accessible to therapeutic interven-

Consumers are becoming more educated about health care, expect more from health care professionals, and demand more accountability from psychiatric nurses.

If the mentally ill client is a product of a "sick society," should the person who cares for him be a health care professional? Could an attendant or an aide do a better job at less cost by focusing only on the client's behavior?

Role blurring
The tendency for professional roles and functions to overlap and become indistinct.

tions all mental health disciplines began to claim these interventions within their scope of practice. The result was role blurring, where members of all disciplines engage in individual, family, and group therapy. The question then arises as to what, if anything, differentiates the nurse from the physician, the psychologist, or the social worker. Psychiatric nursing must convincingly answer this question or run the risk of extinction.

CLINICAL ISSUES

The incidence of mental illness in our society is clearly on the increase. Factors such as economic pressures, changing moral values, and an increase in violent crimes all result from and contribute to a stress-laden life-style to which individuals and families must adapt. Intervention measures designed to promote mental health and to prevent mental illness are needed in addition to measures designed to treat those who are already mentally ill. Meeting the mental health needs of its citizens presents an enormous challenge to this nation.

Most authorities acknowledge that the most cost-effective and best way to meet these needs is through programs geared to prevention. These programs are designed to alter the environment in a way that is conducive to better mental health or to helping individuals, families, and communities to increase and diversify their coping mechanisms. An example of the former is efforts directed toward decreasing violence on the streets; examples of the latter are Head Start programs, victim assistance programs, and self-help groups such as Recovery, Inc.

Although there is almost universal agreement that prevention of mental illness and promotion of mental health are the best routes in terms of long-term goals, it is exceedingly difficult to document the effects of such programs in the short term. With a scarcity of resources, government and private agencies are less likely to allocate funds to such programs, feeling a need to concentrate limited resources on short-term, obvious problems, namely, the treatment of those already mentally ill.

Most major forms of mental illness are now viewed as chronic in the sense that the individual will always need a greater or lesser degree of supervision and care. With the advent of community mental health centers there was concomitantly great hope that the bulk of those persons requiring mental health care could be maintained in and benefit from care in the community. This hope was short-lived, however, as the "revolving door" syndrome developed. This syndrome is a phenomenon whereby persons receive intensive care through hospitalization, are discharged to the community where they may or may not continue to receive care, and shortly require hospitalization again wherein the cycle is repeated. The initial response to the revolving door syndrome was a sense of failure on the part of mental health care professionals and the system. That attitude has gradually shifted from a sense of failure to an acceptance of the chronicity of mental illness.

Helping individuals to cope with a stressful lifestyle is more cost effective than treating the mental illness that can result from it.

Revolving-door syndrome
Hospitalization → discharge into community (with or without continued care) → rehospitalization.

Major changes need to take place in the mental health care delivery system. Because of the enormity and severity of the problem, there is a need for the development of treatment modalities and intervention techniques that address large population groups. Traditional one-to-one, family, and even group interpersonally based treatment modalities are no longer viable as the main forms of intervention. These techniques have proved costly and, at worst, not necessarily therapeutically effective. In addition these modalities clearly benefit only those who value feelings and thoughts, are verbally fluent, have financial resources, are highly motivated, and have the intelligence necessary to deal with the abstractions inherent in these treatment modalities. Obviously these criteria rule out large numbers of individuals as well as certain population groups such as cultural minorities, children, the elderly, and the poor. These groups have the greatest incidence of mental illness, and for them we have the least understanding of its cause and the fewest effective means of treatment. Although the need for change is well accepted by most mental health disciplines, there seem to be few ideas as to what changes can and should occur. Consequently, mental health professionals are still being educationally and experientially prepared in the traditional modes of treatment while being told that in most instances their developing skills will be to no avail in solving the larger issues of the day.

What then is required? First and foremost, research must be instituted if reliable answers to these problems are to be found. Research needs to focus on the cause, prevention, and treatment of mental illness. This is easier said than done. Research regarding human behavior is by its very nature different from pure laboratory research in a variety of ways. First, there are many variables that are difficult if not impossible to control. In a laboratory, chemical elements can be isolated and then systematically combined with other elements one by one and the effects clearly observed. When dealing with human beings it is impossible to isolate a subject's personality from his intelligence or from his culture. Second, many laboratory experiments yield results in a relatively short period, at least within the lifetime of the researcher. In contrast, much behavioral research is longitudinal, requiring the observation and study of the subjects over a generation or two. In addition to the time and money involved, longitudinal research also runs the risk of incurring environmental changes that may affect the outcome, for example, a war.

A prime concern in behavioral research, perhaps the core issue, is the necessity felt in a democratic society to protect the rights of each individual. Therefore procedures involved in research as well as treatment are subjected to vigorous scrutiny and are not approved if there is any potential for harm to the persons involved. It is clearly unethical, for example, to create situations that are believed to produce schizophrenia in an effort to determine the cause of this tragic illness. Consequently, the best that behavioral research can show is a relationship between and among variables after the fact. Despite these obstacles, however, it is essential that society continue to support behavioral research di-

As mental illness continues to grow into one of society's major health problems, treatment programs are needed that are aimed at large segments of the population: cultural minorities, children, the elderly, the poor.

Behavioral research must be conducted that focuses on the causes, prevention, and treatment of mental illness while protecting the individual rights of the patient.

rected toward understanding the cause of mental illness and developing effective treatment modalities.

DELIVERY SYSTEM ISSUES

The philosophical basis of the community mental health movement was and still is seen as desirable. Not only is it more humane, but it is also believed to be more cost effective to maintain persons outside institutions. While the society and the health care professions endorse the end result, it appears that little thought has been given to the changes that this would require in treatment methods and therefore in educational preparation of health care professionals. Unfortunately, in too many instances the community mental health movement has meant little more than a change of setting: the same treatment philosophy and methods have been moved from the institution to a decentralized center in the community.

Rather than solving any problems this short-sighted approach has in many instances compounded existent problems and created new ones. Chief among these are the revolving door syndrome, the community disorganization resulting from scores of mentally ill persons with few or no resources being thrust into the streets, and the inadequate treatment received by mentally ill persons. Another irony or paradox of the community mental health movement is the fact that the best prepared health care workers, including nurses, are slowly but steadily moving into the community as a result, in part, of a powerful attitudinal shift elevating the status of those working in the community and degrading those who choose to work in institutions. Consequently, some authorities fear that the care of institutionalized, chronically and acutely ill persons will be left to the least well-prepared health care workers. This situation, it is feared, will result in such terrible treatment that the "back wards" of the late nineteenth and early twentieth centuries will be seen as model treatment settings in comparison. This view may be an overstatement of the reality, but there is no doubt that the potential for this situation to occur is great enough to cause grave concern.

Another major delivery system issue is the geographical maldistribution of mental health care professionals and treatment centers that tend to be clustered together in large urban areas, particularly on the East and West coasts of the United States. In these areas professionals can receive not only appropriate salaries, but also the intellectual, cultural, and social stimulation they desire. As a result large groups of consumers do not have geographical access to continuous mental health care.

As previously stated, mental health professionals continue to be educationally prepared in the traditional treatment modalities, so it is understandable that they choose to work with those clients who can benefit from these techniques. Therefore, in addition to geographical maldistribution, there is also a disproportionately small number of mental health care professionals who choose to work

As more patients are discharged from the hospital to the community, followed by more nurses choosing to work in the community rather than the hospital, a major concern is that patients needing hospitalization will receive less than adequate care by underprepared personnel.

with the poor, including the inner-city poor, the educationally and culturally disadvantaged, minority groups, children, and the elderly. Since these groups represent the largest number of mentally ill persons, it should be clear that the mental health needs of this country are not being met. This situation is so serious that the U.S. Congress has directed the National Institute of Mental Health to fund only those training programs and research projects which address one or more of these target populations.

EDUCATIONAL ISSUES

The cost of higher education in this country is skyrocketing daily and therefore placing college education out of the reach of more and more people at a time when scientific and technological advances require increasingly more educational preparation for those who wish to contribute to society. This situation is particularly true for women and members of cultural minorities who are attempting to achieve equality, in part, through education. Consequently, a smaller proportion of black and Hispanic people and women are able to afford the cost of higher education, which in turn results in fewer health care professionals from those populations that require the most health care.

Of great concern is the fact that fewer and fewer nurses are choosing to work in psychiatric settings or to pursue graduate education in this field. It is believed that the reasons for this are multiple and complex. Many psychiatric nurse educators, however, believe that a major contributing factor is the trend in undergraduate nursing programs to integrate content. This trend is a result of nursing's attempt to teach in a way that helps the student view the client holistically and to move away from the medical model that tends to segment clients according to the disease or illness from which they are suffering. While these goals are commendable, one unexpected effect has been that some nursing students do not have a specific learning experience with clients who are mentally ill. Consequently, it is understandable that graduates of these programs are unlikely to choose psychiatric nursing as a field in which to work, and therefore the pool of persons who are interested in and qualified to pursue graduate education in psychiatric nursing is lessened. As with all other issues, the cyclical nature of this problem is evident in the fact that as fewer nurses become prepared at the graduate level there ultimately will be fewer psychiatric nurses prepared to teach, which in turn results in poorer preparation of beginning practitioners in psychiatric nursing, ending with fewer choosing to work in the area. Thus the cycle is complete and is set to repeat itself. Unless efforts are made to recruit qualified persons into psychiatric nursing, this health care specialty will die a natural death and need not fear extinction from external forces.

END NOTE

This chapter discusses some major issues that currently confront psychiatric nursing. Included are the economic, social, professional, clinical, delivery sys-

Populations most at risk for mental illness are receiving the least amount of time and attention from mental health professionals: those in the inner city, with little or no education/cultural advantages, minorities, children, and the elderly.

Holistic health care
A system of comprehensive or total patient care that considers the physical, emotional, social, economic, and spiritual needs of the person, the response to illness, and the impact of the illness on the person's ability to meet self-care needs.

As a result of the holistic approach to nursing education, fewer nurses are choosing the specialty area of psychiatric nursing. The cyclical effect of this trend could lead to a demise of psychiatric nursing as it is practiced today.

tem, and educational factors that are likely to negatively impact the future practice of psychiatric nursing unless they are addressed in the present. The reader is encouraged to seriously consider these and other issues to contribute to solutions that will help meet the nation's mental health needs.

SUGGESTED SOURCES OF ADDITIONAL INFORMATION

Aiken L: The impact of federal health policy on nurses. In Aiken L, editor: Nursing in the 1980's, Philadelphia, 1982, JB Lippincott Co.

Chamberlain J and Marshall S: Recruitment problems from the psychiatric nursing education perspective, Proceedings: Psychiatric Mental Health Nursing Recruitment to the Specialty, Rockville, Md, 1982, DHHS.

Fagin C: Concepts for the future: competition and substitution, J Psychosoc Nurs 21:21-31, 36-40, 1983.

Fagin C: Psychiatric nursing at the crossroads: quo vadis, Perspect Psychiatr Care 19:99, May-August 1981.

Goldman H et al: Prospective payment for psychiatric hospitalization: questions and issues, Hosp Commun Psychiatr 35:460, May 1984.

Griffith H: Nursing practice: substitute or complement according to economic theory, Nurs Economics 2:105, 1984.

Joel L: DRGs and RIMs: implications for nursing, Nurs Outlook 32:42, January-February 1984.

Lamb HR: Deinstitutionalization and the homeless mentally ill, Hosp Commun Psychiatr 35(9):899, September 1984.

Lamb HR and Peele R: The need for continuing asylum and sanctuary, Hosp Commun Psychiatr 33(8):798, August 1984.

McBride AB: Present issues and future perspectives of psychosocial nursing: theory and research, J Psychosoc Nurs 24(9):27, September 1986.

Martin EJ: A specialty in decline? Psychiatric-mental health nursing, past, present and future, J Prof Nurs 1(1):48, January-February 1985.

Pearlmutter DR: Recent trends and issues in psychiatric-mental nursing, Hosp Commun Psychiatr 36(1):56, January 1985.

Peplau H: Tomorrow's world, Nurs Times 83(1):29, January 1987.

Robinson L: The future of psychiatric/mental health nursing, Nurs Clin North Am 21(3):537, September 1986.

Ruch M: The multidisciplinary approach: when too many is too much, J Psychosoc Nurs Ment Health Serv 22:18, September 1984.

Slavinsky A: Psychiatric nursing in the year 2000: from a nonsystem of care to a caring system, Image: J Nurs Scholarship 16(1):17, Winter 1984.

Walgrove NJ: Mental health aftercare: where is nursing? Nurs Clin North Am 21(3):473, September 1986.

Self-awareness

4

LEARNING OBJECTIVES

After studying this chapter the student will be able to:

○ Explain the significance of self-awareness in the effective practice of psychiatric nursing.

○ Differentiate between self-awareness and self-understanding.

○ Discuss the nature of self-awareness.

○ Describe four commonly used methods to increase self-awareness.

In many ways mentally ill persons are the most challenging group of individuals with whom the nurse has an opportunity to work. In a very real sense the relationship the nurse and the client develop can be one of the most important factors in the client's therapeutic experience. Whether the nurse can be a force for developing a truly therapeutic situation for the client depends on her ability to provide him with new and more positive experiences in living with other people. To accomplish this the nurse continuously strives to understand the client's behavior and the emotional needs expressed by that behavior. However, since it is the relationship between the nurse and the client that has the potential for becoming a therapeutic experience for the client, it is not sufficient for the nurse to understand only the client; in addition, she must develop self-awareness.

Therapeutic
Beneficial

To practice psychiatric nursing effectively the nurse must constantly adjust and readjust her approaches to clients. To do so she gives much thought and consideration to her own behavior as it influences the behavior of others. In other words, the nurse needs to be prepared to make positive use of her own personality, her primary tool, as she works therapeutically with clients. Many nurses successfully make therapeutic use of their personality without recognizing their interpersonal effectiveness or being able to analyze how they succeed. However nurses who work with mentally ill persons cannot trust to luck in the hope of developing the self-awareness fundamental to being therapeutically effective. Although the effective practice of psychiatric nursing probably does not require particular personality attributes or attitudes, it does require a consistent, thoughtful effort directed toward developing awareness of self and others.

HISTORICAL PERSPECTIVE

The importance of self-awareness when working with emotionally ill persons was not recognized until Freud's revolutionary discovery of the unconscious mind and its role in influencing behavior. Freud demonstrated by his treatment of patients how the origins of present behavior often lay in repressed emotions and experiences of early childhood. He logically concluded that what was true of his patients was also true of all human beings, namely, that much behavior is determined by beliefs and feelings that are beyond awareness. He also believed that if one is to help others, one must have an in-depth understanding of one's own beliefs and feelings so as not to inadvertently interfere with the progress of the patient. The practice of psychoanalysis, the treatment procedure developed by Freud, therefore required the analyst to undergo much the same rigorous process of self-examination prior to being qualified to treat others.

While Freud emphasized the importance of self-understanding, it soon became apparent that most mental health professionals could not or would not avail themselves of such a lengthy, costly, and emotionally disruptive process. Nevertheless, it became evident that increasing one's self-awareness had value to all persons, not just those involved in providing human services. During the 1960s and 1970s sensitivity training and encounter groups became popular, and groups designed to enhance self-awareness abounded. The Johari window, described in this chapter, is a tool that became popular at that time. It was named for its developers, Joseph Luft and Harry Lipton.

Although the popularity of these self-awareness groups has diminished somewhat, it is now well accepted that increased self-awareness is desirable for all persons but is mandatory for those who, like nurses, work to assist others in achieving emotional growth.

THE SIGNIFICANCE OF SELF-AWARENESS

The major therapeutic tool of the nurse who works with the mentally ill is her use of self in the interpersonal context. Since behavior is largely determined by one's beliefs and feelings, the nurse's ability to use herself as a therapeutic tool depends on her adopting beliefs and feelings conducive to the effective practice of psychiatric nursing.

Beliefs are thoughts held to be true but not proven to be so. Beliefs differ from facts in that facts are truths that have been documented. Some beliefs stem

Psychoanalysis
A branch of psychiatry founded by Sigmund Freud and devoted to the study of the psychology of human development and behavior. Treatment consists of helping the individual become aware of the existence of repressed emotional conflicts, analyzing their origin, and, through the process of insight, bringing them into the consciousness so that irrational and dysfunctional behavior can be altered.

The major therapeutic tool of the psychiatric nurse is the use of self in the interpersonal context.

from ignorance of the facts. Other beliefs have their source in the prior experience of the individual or the cultural norms of the society. Some beliefs ultimately will be tested and proven to be either facts or falsehoods. Others are not amenable to testing because of their very nature. For example, a belief that stems from a value, such as the belief that human beings are basically good, does not lend itself to known methods of documentation.

Feelings are affective states or emotions. Recent research has demonstrated that feelings often arise from beliefs, rather than beliefs stemming from feelings as is commonly thought. For example, the mother of a teenage driver who is 2 hours late in arriving home often will think of all the negative events that could account for her child's delay. The belief that only a tragedy could cause her child to be late can result in the mother's feeling great amounts of anxiety. On the other hand, if the same mother thought her child was delayed because of a positive event, or because he merely had overlooked the time, her resultant feeling likely would be pleasure or annoyance, not anxiety.

It is important to understand that beliefs and feelings are inextricably related and affect each other in a cyclical fashion. It is also important to understand and appreciate the fact that the behavior of human beings, including nurses, is greatly influenced by their combined beliefs and feelings.

Many nurses hold the beliefs and feelings necessary to the effective practice of psychiatric nursing. However, unless these beliefs and feelings are brought to a level of awareness, they cannot be used purposefully. Furthermore, nurses whose beliefs and feelings are not conducive to the effective practice of psychiatric nursing cannot hope to alter them unless they can become aware of them. While it is desirable for all nurses to learn to examine their beliefs and feelings, it is imperative for the nurse who works with mentally ill persons to do so.

The reader will note that the desired goal is self-awareness, not self-understanding. Self-understanding implies a knowledge of why one believes and feels as one does; this often requires a lengthy, in-depth process of self-examination guided by a qualified professional. Not many nurses have the opportunity to engage in this process, nor is it necessary for most. However, all nurses can become aware of what they believe and feel without necessarily having to understand why they believe and feel as they do. Heightened self-awareness is within the grasp of all persons if they are willing to work at achieving it.

> Self-awareness differs from self-understanding in that self-awareness does not require a knowledge of why one believes and feels as one does.

THE NATURE OF SELF-AWARENESS

A helpful model for understanding the nature of self-awareness is the Johari window (Fig. 4-1). The upper left quadrant of the window represents a person's beliefs and feelings that are known to him and to others. This quadrant is termed "open." For example, a nurse may believe that acutely psychotic persons are very amenable to therapeutic intervention. Furthermore, she may be aware that she is the type of person who is gratified by relatively rapid changes in a client's behavior. Consequently, she often volunteers to assume the nursing care

	Known to self	Unknown to self
Known to others	Open	Blind
Unknown to others	Private	Closed

FIGURE 4-1   Johari window.

of acutely psychotic clients, allowing others to infer this particular belief and feeling from her behavior.

The upper right quadrant, the "blind" quadrant, represents those beliefs and feelings hidden from a person's awareness, usually because of their anxiety-producing nature. The person defends against awareness of such beliefs and feelings by using mental mechanisms. However, his behavior reveals these beliefs and feelings to others. For example, the nurse may believe that clients who abuse alcohol are morally degenerate and any contact with them makes her angry. This belief and feeling may be unacceptable to her and so do not exist at a level of awareness. However, her comments about these clients and her behavior when around them reveal her negative feelings to others, including the clients.

The lower left quadrant of the Johari window represents beliefs and feelings known to the person but purposefully and consciously concealed from others. This quadrant is termed "private" and usually exists because the individual fears rejection if his beliefs and feelings were known. For example, the nurse may believe that clients who seek readmission to the hospital at the end of the month when they have run out of money are really malingerers and therefore she feels they are undeserving of care. Being aware of this belief and consequent feeling but fearing she would be criticized by her peers if they were known, she extends herself to provide care for these clients in an effort to conceal her attitude toward them.

Finally, the lower right quadrant (the "closed" quadrant) represents beliefs and feelings so deeply buried in the person's unconscious mind that they are unknown both to him and to others. This does not imply that these beliefs and feelings do not affect the person's behavior but rather that behavioral manifestations are likely to be indirect and therefore not easily understood by either the person or others.

Using the Johari window as a model, the goal of self-awareness can be understood to be the decrease of the size of the blind and private quadrants, thereby enlarging the size of the open quadrant. In this way a greater number of beliefs and feelings will become known to the person and to others. Working toward this goal has two major advantages. First, it requires energy to conceal beliefs and feelings from oneself or from others. Therefore an increase in self-awareness and self-disclosure can free energy that can then be used more profitably. Second, an increase in self-awareness and self-disclosure gives the person more control over his own behavior as well as a better understanding of others' response to him.

Under usual circumstances it is unlikely that the size of the closed quadrant will be reduced, but as is true of self-understanding, the effective practice of psychiatric nursing does not require complete self-awareness.

INCREASING SELF-AWARENESS

For the nurse to increase her self-awareness, she must examine her beliefs and her feelings. Several methods can be employed to achieve this. However, all require a willingness to explore one's own behavior as a means of uncovering one's beliefs and feelings, much as the nurse who is learning a new psychomotor skill is willing to practice the technique until she has mastered it. Unfortunately, this is more easily said than done in that we are conditioned from birth to view our own behavior and that of others judgmentally. In other words, we are prone to evaluate observed behavior as either good or bad and to understandably avoid recognition of our own behavior that we deem "bad." Nevertheless, when attempting to heighten self-awareness, we need to reserve such judgment in an effort to allow the underlying beliefs and feelings to surface.

Four methods commonly used to increase self-awareness are described below.

Introspection

Introspection is the process of observing one's own behavior in various situations and identifying its themes and patterns. In a sense, introspection requires stepping out of oneself to watch oneself in interaction with others. This practice

When attempting to heighten self-awareness, the nurse needs to explore her own behavior as a means of uncovering her beliefs and feelings.

Four methods commonly used to increase self-awareness are introspection, discussion, enlarging one's experience, and role playing.

OF SPECIAL INTEREST

The pursuit of self-awareness is not recent and is not limited to health professionals. Perhaps the earliest and best known reference to self-awareness is the statement, "The life which is unexamined is not worth living." This phrase is found in Plato's *Apology* and is thought by many to have been said by Socrates, Plato's mentor.

More recently, a moving tribute to the value of self-understanding was written by Katherine Mansfield, a New Zealand short-story writer. The end of her *Journal,* written in 1922, states: "I want, by understanding myself, to understand others. I want to be all I am capable of becoming. . . .This all sounds very strenuous and serious. But now that I have wrestled with it, it's no longer so. I feel happy—deep down. *All is well.*"

Ms. Mansfield died of tuberculosis in January 1923 at the age of 34.

is aided by the use of a process recording in which the nurse writes down everything she can remember from an interaction as soon as possible after it occurs. This includes thoughts and feelings as well as overt behaviors. Once behaviors are identified, the nurse can ask herself, "What beliefs and feelings underlie what I did?" This process of discovery is aided immeasurably by a state of relaxation, as is often achieved through meditation or yoga, where the mind is cleared of focused thoughts and allowed to roam freely. In a sense, this is like free association where one thought leads to another.

The advantage of introspection is that it can be engaged in at any time and place and is not dependent upon the presence of another person. The disadvantage of introspection is that its success is dependent upon the individual's ability to overcome her own defenses and experience the potential emotional discomfort that may result from an unexpected discovery about oneself. As a result, introspection alone is a technique used most successfully by individuals who have already achieved some degree of self-awareness.

Discussion

Dyadic interpersonal communication
A process in which two people interact face to face as senders and receivers, as in a conversation.

Discussion is the process of having a focused conversation about one's behavior and can take place either in a group or with one other person—a dyad. While both contexts can be helpful, most persons find themselves more comfortable in one or the other situation. In either instance, it is important that the participants have developed a degree of mutual trust and respect. Discussion directed toward increasing self-awareness often involves the nurse and her instructor or supervisor or a small group of nurse colleagues, led by an experienced nurse. As is the case with introspection, the discussion focuses on the behavior of the nurse and attempts to discover that individual's underlying beliefs and feelings. In either dyadic or group situations, each person recounts his observations and shares conjectures about what the behavior might indicate.

The advantages of discussion are that the insights of more than one person are brought to bear on the situation and each participant is able to learn and be stimulated by hearing the perspectives of others. The disadvantage of discussion is that the observations made about another's behavior may be more reflective of what the speaker is thinking and feeling than what the subject is thinking and feeling. In addition, a skillful leader is necessary to help ensure that remarks remain nonjudgmental and that confidentiality is maintained.

Enlarging one's experience

Enlarging one's experience is the act of purposefully choosing to engage in unfamiliar activities and carefully noting one's reactions to them. This is a useful technique because one way human beings maintain their belief system is to limit their experiences to those which are familiar and known. For example, the nurse may believe that all mentally ill persons are assaultive and therefore she may fear contact with anyone diagnosed as mentally ill. However, when she seeks contact with a number of mentally ill persons, she soon discovers that the majority of these individuals are fearful, withdrawn persons. This realization may lead her to reexamine her beliefs and alter her feelings. The nurse who is committed to increasing her self-awareness will seek new experiences to test her beliefs and feelings in light of reality.

The advantage of enlarging experience as a means of increasing self-awareness is that it increases one's ability and therefore one's self-confidence and almost forces becoming aware of and examining one's beliefs and feelings. The disadvantage of this method is that some preparation is required to benefit from the new experience. For example, the nurse who is not prepared for an experience in psychiatric nursing may have her worst fears confirmed because she is so anxious that she elicits assaultive behavior from the clients.

Role playing

Role playing is an exercise where participants enact the parts of the persons involved in a real or anticipated interaction. It is seldom necessary to play out the entire interaction; often one participant acts as timekeeper and stops the interaction at a predetermined time. To be useful, role playing must be followed by discussion. However, unlike discussion where the interaction is limited to verbal and nonverbal exchanges about events in the recent past, role playing allows the participants to behaviorally experience situations in the present. Role playing can take place between two people but is more effective when enacted in a small group.

The advantage of role playing is that the reactions of the participants are likely to be spontaneous and less subject to unintentional censoring. In addition, this method is useful in developing empathy for the person whose role is enacted. The disadvantages are that many people feel uncomfortable role playing and are hesitant to try it; a skilled, experienced leader is necessary for optimum benefits.

Empathy
The ability to recognize and to some extent share the emotions and states of mind of another and to understand the meaning and significance of that person's behavior.

The nurse who is new to the practice of psychiatric nursing and who is just embarking upon enhancing her self-awareness may find herself consciously preoccupied with analyzing her own behavior and that of others. This is a perfectly normal occurrence, indicative of her attempts to master the practice of self-awareness prior to its becoming automatic. This process is similar to the preoccupation the nurse may have had with her physical health when she first studied pathophysiology. Concerns she may have about this preoccupation are appropriate topics to discuss with colleagues and experienced psychiatric nurses.

END NOTE

This chapter stresses the importance of the psychiatric nurse's developing self-awareness to most effectively use herself as a therapeutic tool in the interpersonal context. Self-awareness is differentiated from self-understanding, which is desirable but not essential. The nurse is encouraged to enhance her self-awareness by examining her own behavior through introspection, discussion, enlarging her experience, and role playing.

SUGGESTED SOURCES OF ADDITIONAL INFORMATION

Burnard P: Developing self-awareness, Nurs Mirror 158(21):30, May 1984.

Chapman N: An essay on the art of nursing, Perspect Psychiatr Care 21:66, April/June 1983.

Clark CC: Inner dialogue: a self-healing approach for nurses and clients, Am J Nurs 81:1191, June 1981.

Cohen S and McQuade K: Developing empathy with co-workers, Am J Nurs 83:1573, August 1983.

Cronin-Stubbs D and Brophy EB: Burnout: can social support save the psychiatric nurse? J Psychosoc Nurs 23(7):8, July 1985.

Duldty B: Helping nurses to cope with the anger-dismay syndrome, Nurs Outlook 30:168, March 1982.

Faugier J and Reilly S: Towards a communication breakthrough, Nurs Times 82(41):60, October 1986.

Hambrick-Butler A and Sarasin K: The 24-hour stay, J Psychosoc Nurs 24(4):23, April 1986.

Hughes CM: Supervising clinical practice in psychosocial nursing, J Psychosoc Nurs 23(2):27, February 1985.

Knowles R: Dealing with feelings: coping with lethargy, Am J Nurs 81:1465, August 1981.

Knowles R: Dealing with feelings: handling anger: responding vs reacting, Am J Nurs 81:2196, December 1981.

Knowles R: Dealing with feelings: managing guilt, Am J Nurs 81:1850, October 1981.

Knowles R: Dealing with feelings: overcoming guilt and worry, Am J Nurs 81:1663, September 1981.

Krikovian D and Paulanka B: Self-awareness—the key to a successful nurse-patient relationship, J Psychosoc Nurs Ment Health Serv 20:19, June 1982.

Luft J and Ingham H: The Johari window: a graphic model of awareness in interpersonal relations. In Luft J, editor: Group processes: an introduction to group dynamics, Palo Alto, Calif, 1963, National Press Books.

Milne D, Burdett C, and Beckett J: Assessing and reducing the stress and strain of psychiatric nursing, Nurs Times 82(7):59, May 1986.

Schoffstall C: Concerns of student nurses prior to psychiatric nursing experience: an assessment and intervention, J Psychosoc Nurs Ment Health Serv 19:11, November 1981.

Slimmer LW: Helping students to resolve conflicts between their religious beliefs and psychiatric–mental health treatment approaches, J Psychosoc Nurs Ment Health Serv 18:37, July 1980.

Principles of psychiatric nursing

5

LEARNING OBJECTIVES

After studying this chapter the student will be able to:

o State seven principles of psychiatric nursing, discussing the beliefs and feelings on which each principle is based.

o Define psychiatric nursing.

The current state of knowledge about human behavior is at best imprecise. It consists mostly of beliefs, and many of these beliefs are incompatible. For example, the medical model of health care holds the belief that aberrant behavior is a reflection of an individual illness that is hypothetically amenable to treatment by somatic means. In contrast, a sociological model of health care dictates the belief that aberrant behavior is a sign of deviance rather than illness and must be assessed and treated within the larger context of the society. These examples illustrate the diversity of currently held beliefs about human behavior and the necessity for all health professionals to develop an awareness of the beliefs that guide their professional practice.

Being aware of one's beliefs and feelings is necessary but not sufficient for the effective practice of psychiatric nursing. To be useful, the nurse's beliefs and feelings must be organized into an internally consistent statement about the nature of human beings and their behavior. When combined with the nurse's knowledge of the scope and nature of nursing practice, these statements constitute a *philosophy* that, in turn, provides direction for developing principles of psychiatric nursing. *Principles* are rules or laws that have proved applicable in most, if not all, situations. Identifying principles of psychiatric nursing allows the nurse to operationalize her beliefs and feelings in nursing care.

To be useful, the nurse's beliefs and feelings must be organized into a philosophy that in turn provides direction for the development of principles of psychiatric nursing.

HISTORICAL PERSPECTIVE

The principles that have guided the care of mentally ill persons over the centuries have been largely determined, by definition, by the prevailing societal beliefs about the nature of mental illness. As discussed in depth in Chapter 1, these have ranged from the belief that the mentally ill were possessed by the devil or other evil spirits, or that the phases of the moon influenced behavior, to the belief that mental illness is caused by biochemical imbalance. When it was believed that mentally ill persons were possessed by demons it was understandable, although not acceptable in today's views, that the principles guiding their treatment reflected the necessity to exorcise the evil spirits. When biochemical imbalance is believed to be the major determinant of mental illness, it follows that principles of care would emphasize somatic treatments, especially psychopharmacology.

In addition to principles of care being influenced by beliefs about the nature of mental illness, the economic status of the society strongly influences the principles underlying the treatment of mentally ill persons. For example, in prehistoric times primitive people had no means of accumulating or storing food beyond their daily needs and therefore did not have the ability to sustain members who were not able to care for themselves. Therefore, the "principle" that guided the treatment of those whose behavior was abberant was simply "each man for himself." An affluent society such as existed in the United States after World War II could literally afford to believe that every human being has a right to the best possible treatment, regardless of the contribution that person makes to society.

Finally, the cultural heritage of the society is a major determinant of its beliefs and therefore the principles underlying how its members are viewed and treated. The Western world is greatly influenced by its Judeo-Christian heritage, which dictates that each individual has worth and value. This belief has also helped to focus treatment efforts on the individual as opposed to the family or community. In contrast, Eastern cultures, which value the family unit above the worth of the individual, tend to view the family as the focus of treatment concern.

BELIEFS, FEELINGS, AND PRINCIPLES OF PSYCHIATRIC NURSING

This chapter discusses my beliefs about the nature of human beings and their behavior, feelings conducive to the effective practice of psychiatric nursing, and the resultant principles of psychiatric nursing to which I adhere. The chapter concludes with a definition of psychiatric nursing derived from my philosophy. The student is encouraged to examine her own beliefs and feelings about human beings and their behavior so that she may state a philosophy and definition of psychiatric nursing to guide her nursing care.

Psychopharmacology
The scientific study of the effects of drugs on behavior and normal and abnormal mental functions.

Judeo-Christian
Having historical roots in both Judaism and Christianity.

Viewing the client as a holistic being

Human beings are viewed as complex systems of interrelated parts, the whole of which is greater than the sum of the parts. This belief represents a holistic perspective, a stance that acknowledges the interdependence and interrelatedness of the parts to each other, to the person, and to the environment. Therefore alterations in any aspect of the system require responsive alterations in other aspects of the system.

Nurses new to the care of mentally ill persons sometimes believe that the slightest change in the environment of a mentally ill person will precipitate an untoward emotional response. It is also not unusual for such a nurse to believe that the mentally ill individual is so emotionally fragile that he can be traumatized by an inexpertly phrased statement. These beliefs may cause some nurses to fear that they may injure clients emotionally, and as a result they may avoid contact with them.

This fear and its resultant behavior are particularly unfortunate and unwarranted if the nurse views the client as a system. It is important to remember that emotionally ill persons are not defenseless and that they withstand the inappropriate approach of new staff remarkably well. It may be helpful to note that if clients were in fact defenseless it would be a relatively easy matter to interact with them in a manner that would result in emotionally corrective experiences. Rather, clients, like all human beings, are complex organisms who are usually able to sense the basic friendliness behind the nurse's approach even if it is not skillfully executed. Furthermore, the nurse who is new to the mental health setting has developed expertise in many other areas of nursing practice that can be brought to bear on the interaction. Consequently, the nurse can develop the *feeling that she has the potential to be helpful to the client,* even though she may not yet have developed expertise in the care specific to emotionally ill individuals.

A major principle of psychiatric nursing that stems from this belief and feeling is that *the nurse views the client as a holistic being with a multiplicity of interrelated and interdependent needs.* The implications of this principle are numerous. First, the nurse caring for the mentally ill individual must be skilled in understanding the interrelatedness of all the client's subsystems. For example, mental illness does not provide immunity to physical illness; mentally ill persons are as prone to the development of physical illness as are other members of the population. Therefore the nurse needs to be constantly alert to the possibility that a mentally ill client may develop a physical illness and thereby avoid the pitfall of assuming that all symptoms are simply manifestations of emotional stress. The individual must also be viewed as an integral part of his social system, simultaneously affecting the system and being affected by it. Therefore he cannot be assessed accurately in isolation from his family, his community, and the reference groups to which he belongs. As a result the well-prepared nurse

The belief that human beings are complex systems of interrelated parts, the whole of which is greater than the sum of its parts, combined with the nurse's feeling of being potentially helpful to the client, are the bases of the principle that the nurse views the client as a holistic being with numerous interrelated and interdependent needs.

who works in a mental health setting must have not only effective interpersonal skills but also current knowledge about pathophysiology and about the norms and practices of various subcultures and religions. This principle is often cited as the rationale for employing a nurse whose educational background includes preparation in the biophysical and psychosocial realms, instead of a nursing assistant whose on-the-job training focuses only on the psychosocial realm.

Focusing on the client's strengths and assets

Each individual has some strengths and a potential for growth, that is, a potential for developing increasingly effective adaptations to stress. I do not mean to suggest that all individuals have an equal number or the same type of strengths, or the same potential for growth, but rather that each individual has some strengths and some potential for growth, no matter how small or great.

Sometimes nurses who are new to working with mentally ill persons feel despair at the slow progress some clients are able to make. In fact, some nurses feel hopeless about effecting any improvement in them. This feeling often emanates from inexperience in working with persons who have a chronic illness and for whom there may be no specific treatment. However, as the nurse gains experience and adopts the belief that each individual has potential for growth, despair will be replaced by hope. Interestingly, *the feeling of hope is therapeutic in and of itself,* since it conveys to the client the feeling that change is possible.

The principle of psychiatric nursing that is derived from this belief and from the feeling of hope is that *the nurse focuses on the client's strengths and assets, not on his weaknesses and liabilities.* All clients have some strengths, no matter how few or insignificant they may seem. These strengths should be built on to encourage the emotional growth of the individual. For example the client who dresses himself without undue difficulty can build on this behavior by being encouraged to choose clothing appropriate to the occasion and weather. As the client learns to make these choices, he may very well develop an increasing sense of autonomy, which in turn may carry over to other areas of his daily living. This example is overly simplistic, but it is given to illustrate how this principle can be used in frequently encountered situations.

Autonomy
The quality of having the ability or tendency to function independently.

When mental health care was limited to institutional care, an illness orientation was all-pervasive. A client who was cooperative was all too often seen as being overly submissive; if the same client became assertive, he ran the risk of being labeled rebellious. The focus on illness not only tended to reinforce the condition and therefore stifle the client's growth but also may have contributed to the development of illness. A positive outcome of the community mental health movement has been the necessity to focus on the healthy aspects of the client in an effort to enable him to maintain himself in the community and outside the institution. In many instances this orientation has been even more successful than had been originally anticipated. Some authorities believe this may be due to the fact that when an individual is helped to identify and accept his strengths, he is less threatened and therefore more open to exploring and altering his dysfunctional behaviors. It should be noted, however, that a focus on the individual's strengths and growth potential does not mean that his limitations should not be taken into account when assessing his behavior. Failure to do so and subsequent misjudgments have accounted for many of the failures that have also accompanied the community mental health movement.

Accepting the client as a unique human being

I endorse the belief that *each individual, although sharing much in common with other persons, is unique and has inherent value.* This belief is consistent with the view of human beings as complex systems that transform energy and matter in a unique way. The belief that each individual has inherent value is a product of the Judeo-Christian heritage of our society and is manifested in numerous ways through societal practices.

In contrast, American culture also places great value on an individual's capacity to contribute to the society and thus covertly devalues those persons who are unable or who choose not to do so. Certainly many mentally ill persons are not able to make an identifiable contribution to the welfare of the society, and therefore some nurses have the feeling that mentally ill persons have less inherent value than do other more productive members of the population. It is important for the nurse to recognize this feeling if it exists and attempt to overcome it by focusing on the humanness of the client, regardless of his level of productivity. Valuing the client may also be difficult because of his appearance or his behavior. Once the nurse is able to view these factors as indicators of the client's ineffective adaptations, she is more likely to be able to *appreciate his uniqueness and inherent value.*

The principle of psychiatric nursing that stems from the belief in and feeling about the uniqueness and inherent value of each human being is that *the nurse accepts the client as a unique human being who has value and worth exactly as he is.* In fact, most authorities agree that this principle is the most basic to the effective practice of psychiatric nursing.

The conviction that each individual is unique implies that the nurse has a responsibility to observe and listen carefully to each person as if he were the only one to whom care has ever been given. The nurse must not "tune him out," even though his story has been told 100 times before. Psychological experiments have demonstrated that each person's perceptions of and reactions to the same situation are always different, depending on many variables such as previous experience and present state of being.

This principle guides the nurse in respecting the worth and dignity of persons at all times, without regard to the acceptability of their behavior. Thus the effective nurse treats clients with respect even though their behavior may be unacceptable. Inherent in this principle is the attitude that information about cli-

The belief that each individual has strengths and a potential for growth, combined with the nurse's feeling of hope about the client's ability to grow, is the basis of the principle that the nurse focuses on the client's strengths and assets and not on the client's weaknesses and liabilities.

ents is treated with appropriate professional confidentiality and that client problems must not become topics for social chatter. This principle also implies that the treatment methods in which health professionals engage must not in themselves be dehumanizing, even though such methods may have desirable outcomes. In other words, if all human beings have inherent worth and value, treatment modalities that are dehumanizing do not justify even desirable ends.

Although the nurse needs to convey to the client a belief in his potential to change and grow, acceptance of him must not depend on his reaching these goals. That would be conditional acceptance and may convey, "I value you only because of what you could become." Most clients have a long history of being rejected in social relationships because their behavior did not measure up to usual societal expectations. Therefore such individuals enter treatment situations understandably expecting the responses with which they are so familiar. If they do in fact receive these negative responses, they might just as well not have sought treatment because they will be receiving very little constructive help. Since the nurse spends more time with the client than any other professional person, she has the greatest opportunity to convey a feeling of acceptance to him. Calling the client by his surname, such as Mr. Smith, unless the client requests otherwise is an example of how acceptance and respect can be conveyed.

The belief that each individual is unique and has inherent value, combined with the nurse's appreciation of the client's uniqueness and inherent value, is the basis of the principle that the nurse accepts the client as a unique human being who has value and worth exactly as is.

The potential for establishing a relationship with most clients

In apparent contradiction to the belief that each individual is unique is the belief that *all human beings are sufficiently similar that there is a basis, no matter how small, for understanding and communicating with one another.* Harry Stack Sullivan has said that we are all more human than otherwise. I ascribe to this belief of similarity among human beings and further believe that differences in feelings and behavior are more likely to be differences in quantity rather than in quality. For example, all persons have experienced anxiety, although most individuals have not adapted to anxiety by withdrawing from reality. Almost everyone knows what it means to feel sad, or happy, or excited. Those who are mentally ill experience these same emotions, but to an exaggerated or diminished degree.

The very nature of this belief may elicit in the nurse a fear that she herself may become mentally ill. Not too many decades ago it was commonly believed by lay people that if a person worked with mentally ill persons for too long a period, he too would become mentally ill. This belief had its origins in the lack of understanding of the causes of mental illness and in the observation that many who did work with mentally ill persons were in fact emotionally disturbed themselves. This latter phenomenon was a result of the fact that the care of these people was seen as such an undesirable job that only socially deviant persons who could not find employment elsewhere were willing to work in the asylums.

The nurse of today brings into the mental health setting all the biases and prejudices of the society at large. When the nurse realizes that the behavior of most clients is not as bizarre as she had expected, another fear may be elicited—the fear that she has more problems than the clients appear to have. Consequently, some nurses initially believe that they require psychiatric treatment or hospitalization. Although this may be true in a very few instances, the nurse will learn that most persons enter a treatment situation because of an increasing inability to perform the usual activities of daily living in regard to both work and family life. In contrast, the nurse who is functioning despite the emotional problems she may have learns that the ability to function productively is an important criterion of mental health.

Beginning students of psychiatric nursing frequently experience anxiety about their state of mental health as they learn more about the dynamics underlying mental illness. This probably results from the fact that the student can more easily identify with the mentally ill person than with the physically ill person. All human beings have experienced emotional trauma, anxiety, guilt, anger, and other emotions, but not all have experienced appendicitis, myocardial infarction, or other forms of major physical illnesses.

Once again, it is important for the nurse to remember that none of the feelings and few of the experiences of mentally ill persons are different in kind from those she has personally known. In fact, the nurse will learn to *use her familiarity with the various emotions as a tool through which to develop empathy with the client's feelings.*

The principle of psychiatric nursing that is based on belief in the similarity of all human beings and the nurse's empathy with the client's feelings is that *the nurse has the potential for establishing a relationship with most, if not all, clients.* This principle implies that nurses who interact with mentally ill clients must continuously strive to discover the area of similarity between the person and themselves that can serve as a means of establishing communication. Nurses cannot hide behind the belief that it is useless to try to help an individual because his background, experience, and behavior are different from anything with which they are familiar. This does not suggest that a common cultural or experiential background between a client and a nurse may not be helpful in establishing communication, but rather that nurses must continue to strive to communicate with clients even if their frame of reference is not immediately understood. Furthermore, in some situations when the nurse and the client share a great deal in common the nurse may fail to recognize the client's uniqueness and inappropriately attribute to him her own feelings and reactions. This principle does not mean, however, that any one nurse should or could have a therapeutic relationship with all clients. The student will learn that to engage effectively in a therapeutic relationship with a client is very time-consuming and an emotionally and intellectually draining activity. Therefore such interventions should be undertaken with clients who are most likely to benefit

The belief that all human beings are sufficiently similar that there is ground for understanding and communicating with each other, combined with the nurse's feeling of empathy with the client's feelings, is the basis of the principle that the nurse has the potential for establishing a relationship with most, if not all, clients.

from the nurse's personality and style of interaction. However, the nurse can interact with every client in a helpful way if she continuously looks for areas of similarities between them to use as a basis for increasing her understanding of the client.

Exploring client behavior for its need or message

A belief central to the effective practice of psychiatric nursing is that *all behavior is purposeful and designed to meet a need or to communicate a message.* No behavior is accidental or occurs by chance.

Some nurses fear the clinical practice of psychiatric nursing not only because it is a new experience but also because of many preconceived ideas about the behavior of mentally ill persons. Nurses may have heard discussions about unusual and frightening behavior of such individuals. These discussions often exaggerate the behavior being described and tend to arouse fear on the part of the listener. A few nurses may have had an actual experience with a mentally ill person which they found frightening.

The nurse with these feelings can cope more readily with the situation by acknowledging any concerns about personal safety, by facing them frankly, and by examining these fears to discover what they involve. It is usually helpful to discuss such attitudes in situations in which students and teacher can help each other in examining, understanding, and coping with these feelings. This method is particularly effective when the discussion focuses on a specific individual whose behavior is causing concern.

Much of the fear of mentally ill persons grows out of cultural attitudes and beliefs handed down from one generation to another. Despite attempts to educate the public about mental illness, many persons still believe that all mentally ill individuals are dangerous and require drastic measures to control their behavior. Nurses being introduced to a mental health setting will be surprised at the large number of clients whose behavior is socially acceptable. They will be surprised to find that many mentally ill persons seem content to be inactive. Instead of requiring controls, many clients require stimulation and need to be helped to develop an interest in the available activities. Once the nurse has become familiar with the clients in the mental health setting and has gained more knowledge about human behavior, it will be possible for her to replace her fear of client behavior with a *feeling of curiosity about its meaning.*

The principle of psychiatric nursing that stems from the belief that all behavior is purposeful and the accompanying curiosity about its meaning is that *the nurse explores the client's behavior for the need it is designed to meet or the message it is communicating.* This principle does not imply that all behavior must be accepted or condoned as it is expressed. On the contrary, tolerance of all behavior, no matter how antisocial it may be, can convey to the client the idea that he is not important enough for the nurse to explore his behavior with him. The helpful nurse will make an effort to convey to the client her understanding that his behavior has meaning and her willingness to help him meet the need or communicate the message in a socially acceptable way. Some clients have never become aware that there are socially acceptable means through which their needs can be met. When the nurse helps the client to evaluate the consequences of his present behavior and test new patterns of behavior, she will do a great deal in furthering his feeling of being a worthwhile human being. By treating the client's socially unacceptable behavior in this manner the nurse communicates that she is not being punitive or judgmental but is primarily concerned about the client's welfare.

Assisting the client to learn effective adaptations

Another belief regarding the nature of human behavior is that *it was learned as an adaptation to earlier stressors,* especially those experienced during the influential years of infancy and childhood when the foundation of the personality is laid. Therefore *the individual's present behavior is believed to represent the best possible adaptation he is capable of making at the time.* It should be noted that all behavioral adaptations were effective in maintaining homeokinesis at the time they were learned. If, however, the interpersonal environment in which the behavioral adaptation was learned was unique or unhealthy, the behavior that was effective in the original situation becomes ineffective and dysfunctional when the person moves to a subsequent developmental stage or into the larger social system that functions in a more usual or healthy manner.

Even when they are seeking help, mentally ill persons may be shy, suspicious, withdrawn, and preoccupied with their own thoughts and problems. The nurse may interpret these behaviors as a dislike of her and react with the socially familiar response of disliking the client. As the nurse develops an understanding of mental illness, she will realize that some clients behave in this manner—even when they want very much to become acquainted with the nurse—because they fear that they will not be accepted by her. The nurse cannot expect to thoroughly like all clients, and she cannot expect all clients to genuinely like her. However, it is realistic to expect that she will develop some understanding and acceptance of all clients and learn not to view all their behavior as a reflection of their feelings toward her. She will also be able to develop *the ability to care about clients even though they may not reciprocate this feeling* if she works at developing a support group among her peers rather than looking to clients for approval and gratitude.

The principle of psychiatric nursing based on the above beliefs and feelings is that *the nurse views the client's behavior nonjudgmentally while assisting him to learn more effective adaptations.* This principle is central to the effective practice of psychiatric nursing because it implies that it is possible for the client to unlearn old adaptations and relearn new, more effective adaptations if provided with an environment that facilitates and supports this goal. Further, this principle also implies that the nurse is likely to accept the client's behavior, withhold-

The belief that all behavior is purposeful and designed to meet a need or to communicate a message, combined with the nurse's feeling of curiosity about the meaning of the client's behavior, is the basis of the principle that the nurse explores the client's behavior for the need it is designed to meet or the message it is communicating.

ing judgment. For example, adherence to this principle makes it inappropriate for the nurse to say that the client refuses to participate in group therapy; rather, the nurse is more likely to understand that at this time the client is not able to participate. In addition, this principle helps to dispel the aura of hopelessness that often surrounds the care of mentally ill persons. Although it is important to be realistic about the changes any one individual can make, it is inappropriate to believe that a person's behavior cannot change or that his overall adaptation to the stresses of life cannot become more effective.

The belief that behavior is learned and is the best possible adaptation the individual is capable of making at the time, combined with the nurse's caring about the client, is the basis of the principle that the nurse views the client's behavior nonjudgmentally while assisting him to learn more effective adaptations.

The quality of the nurse-client interaction

A final belief basic to the effective practice of psychiatric nursing is the understanding that *an individual learns behavioral adaptations primarily in interaction with significant people in his environment.* Human beings do not exist in a vacuum; their survival depends on interaction with other human beings. However, an individual cannot be expected to learn new behavioral adaptations if he is not given an opportunity to interact with others who provide experiences that are more positive than those he has known previously.

Nurses beginning an experience in psychiatric nursing sometimes find they have a strong desire to be helpful but simultaneously feel they are not skillful enough to assume a significant role in the treatment of the mentally ill person. These feelings present nurses with an uncomfortable personal dilemma from which they may seek to escape by becoming indifferent. To allow this feeling to develop would be unfortunate because indifference is one of the reactions that most mentally ill persons have already experienced much too often in their relations with family and friends. In contrast, nurses are encouraged to become emotionally involved with their clients. In fact, without such involvement the nurse can be of little real therapeutic help. However, it is essential to understand the meaning of involvement. *Involvement* implies that the nurse is genuinely and sincerely interested in the client, that she gives of her time and of herself without expecting anything in return, and that she interacts in a way that meets the need of the client instead of her own. Although initially the nurse may feel that her interpersonal skills are not developed to a level that makes her feel adequate in the situation, with guidance, practice, and persistent study of self, the early feelings of inadequacy will be replaced with *feelings of competency in her ability to interact therapeutically* with mentally ill persons.

The principle of psychiatric nursing derived from the belief and feeling just discussed is that *the quality of the interaction in which the nurse engages with the client is a major determinant of the degree to which the client will be able to alter his behavioral adaptations in the direction of more satisfying, satisfactory interpersonal relationships.* When the individual seeks help from a treatment setting, he has little impetus to alter his adaptive mechanisms if his characteristic behavior is met with the same negative, judgmental attitudes he has experienced from society. On the other hand, if despite his behavior the individual becomes involved with an interested, concerned nurse who values his worth and dignity, positive satisfactory behavioral adaptations are likely to be elicited. This principle is particularly germane to the practice of psychiatric nursing because the nurse is the professional person who is likely to spend the greatest amount of time with the client and therefore is the person who has the greatest opportunity to create the environment in which the client can unlearn previous ineffective adaptations and learn new, more effective adaptations.

DEFINITION OF PSYCHIATRIC NURSING

The nurse's philosophy of psychiatric nursing and the resultant principles provide direction for stating a definition of psychiatric nursing. The philosophy and principles just discussed lead me to define psychiatric nursing as a process whereby the nurse assists persons, as individuals or in groups, to develop a more positive self-concept, a more satisfying pattern of interpersonal relationships, and a more satisfactory role in society. See Table 5-1.

The belief that an individual learns behavioral adaptations in interaction with significant others, combined with the nurse's feeling of competency in her ability to interact therapeutically, is the basis of the principle that the quality of the nurse-client interaction is a major determinant of the degree to which the client will be able to alter his behavioral adaptation.

TABLE 5-1   *Beliefs, feelings, and principles conducive to the effective practice of psychiatric nursing*

Belief	Feeling	Principle
Human beings are complex systems of interrelated parts, the whole of which is greater than the sum of the parts	The nurse feels she can be helpful to the client, since she has expertise in many areas of nursing	The nurse views the client as a holistic being with a multiplicity of interrelated and interdependent needs
Each individual has some strengths and a potential for growth	The nurse is hopeful about the client's ability to grow	The nurse focuses on the client's strengths and assets, not on his weaknesses and liabilities
Each individual is unique and has inherent value	The nurse appreciates the uniqueness and inherent value of the client	The nurse accepts the client as a unique human being who has value and worth exactly as he is
All human beings are sufficiently similar that there is a basis for understanding and communicating with one another	The nurse feels empathy with the client's feelings	The nurse has the potential for establishing a relationship with most if not all clients
All behavior is purposeful and is designed to meet a need or to communicate a message	The nurse feels curious about the meaning of the client's behavior	The nurse explores the client's behavior for the need it is designed to meet or the message it is communicating
Behavior is learned as an adaptation to an earlier stressor and is the best possible adaptation the individual is capable of making at the time	The nurse cares about clients even though they may not reciprocate her feeling	The nurse views the client's behavior nonjudgmentally while assisting him to learn more effective adaptations
An individual learns behavioral adaptations primarily in interaction with significant people in his environment	The nurse feels competent in her ability to interact therapeutically with persons who are mentally ill	The quality of the interaction in which the nurse engages with the client is a major determinant of the degree to which the client will be able to alter his behavioral adaptations in the direction of more satisfying, satisfactory interpersonal relationships

END NOTE

Throughout this chapter, the student is encouraged to examine her beliefs and feelings about mentally ill persons to develop a philosophy of psychiatric nursing. To that end, those beliefs and feelings about mentally ill persons which are congruent with my philosophy of psychiatric nursing are discussed. From this philosophy, seven principles of psychiatric nursing are derived and discussed: The nurse views the client as a holistic being with a multiplicity of interrelated and interdependent needs; the nurse focuses on the client's strengths and assets, not on his weaknesses and liabilities; the nurse accepts the client as a unique human being who has value and worth exactly as he is; the nurse has the potential for establishing a relationship with most, if not all, clients; the nurse explores the client's behavior for the need it is designed to meet or the message it is communicating; the nurse views the client's behavior nonjudgmentally while assisting him to learn more effective adaptations; and the quality of the interaction in which the nurse engages with the client is a major determinant of the degree to which the client will be able to alter his behavioral adaptations in the direction of more satisfying, satisfactory interpersonal relationships.

Based upon my philosophy and the above principles, psychiatric nursing is defined as a process whereby the nurse assists persons, as individuals or in groups, to develop a more positive self-concept, a more satisfying pattern of interpersonal relationships, and a more satisfactory role in society.

SUGGESTED SOURCES OF ADDITIONAL INFORMATION

Chapman N: An essay on the art of nursing, Perspect Psychiatr Care 21:66, April/June 1983.

Dormer A: The miracle of caring, J Psychosoc Nurs Ment Health Serv 18:21, August 1980.

Flynn PAR: Holistic health: the art and science of care, Bowie, Md, 1980, Robert J. Brady Co.

Gedan S: This I believe . . . about psychiatric nursing practice, Nurs Outlook 19:534, 1971.

Peplau H: Interpersonal relations in nursing, New York, 1952, GP Putnam's Sons.

Rawnsley MM: Toward a conceptual base for effective nursing, Nurs Outlook 28:244, April 1980.

Schwartz MS and Shockley EL: The nurse and the mental patient, New York, 1956, John Wiley & Sons, Inc.

Sullivan HS: The interpersonal theory of psychiatry, New York, 1953, WW Norton & Co.

Effective communication

LEARNING OBJECTIVES

After studying this chapter the student will be able to:

o Define the communication process.

o Discuss the four modes of communication.

o Give examples of effective verbal and nonverbal communication.

o Identify special problems and their solutions in communicating with mentally ill persons.

Communication refers to the reciprocal exchange of information, ideas, beliefs, feelings, and attitudes between two persons or among a group of persons. As such it is a dynamic process requiring continual adaptations by those involved. Communication is effective when it accurately and clearly conveys the intended messages.

The communication process is basic to all nursing practice and, when effective, greatly contributes to the development of all therapeutic relationships. Knowledge of and skill in effective communication are essential for the nurse who works with mentally ill clients because her ability to be therapeutic is highly related to the effectiveness of her communication skills.

HISTORICAL PERSPECTIVE

Communication is not unique to human beings. Other species of animals communicate with each other. Only humans, however, have the ability to engage in the complex interaction evidenced by the use of language. In fact, the ability to use language is seen by many as an essential characteristic of being human. Effective communication is a major means by which people express many of their needs and subsequently have them met, thereby experiencing satisfying, satisfactory relationships with others.

The needs of primitive human beings most certainly centered around issues of physical survival. Therefore their ability to listen for and respond appropriately to sounds that warned of danger or assured safety was essential. Effective communication was achieved when verbal and nonverbal forms of communication were accurately transmitted and interpreted. Feedback about the effectiveness of the communication was likely to be immediate. During this period of human development communication was limited to face-to-face interaction between individuals and among small groups.

Feedback
Information produced by a receiver and perceived by a sender that informs the sender about the receiver's reaction to the message. Feedback is a cyclic part of the communication process that regulates and modifies the content of messages.

Although the alphabet was developed around 2000 BC, major changes in the communication process did not occur until the invention of the printing press in the fifteenth century. This invention made possible the mass production of the written word and essentially changed the culture of communication from a speaking-listening orientation to a visual orientation.

This change in orientation coincided with and contributed to a change in the standard of living wherein the peoples of the Western world could afford to be less concerned about survival issues and more concerned about higher-level needs related to interpersonal relationships. Paradoxically, as concern with these needs intensified, there was an increased dependence on the written word, which by definition is devoid of human contact. Some authorities believe that this dependence on the written word and consequently on a visual orientation to communication has diminished the ability of many contemporary human beings to engage in the effective verbal and nonverbal communication that characterizes satisfying interpersonal relationships. Whether this is the case or not, it is well documented that ineffective communication patterns are a predominant symptom of many forms of mental illness and that engaging in effective communication with clients can have therapeutic results.

Because of the complexity of the communication process and its important role in interpersonal relationships, effective and disturbed communication patterns have been the subject of much study by contemporary theorists. One of the best known, psychiatrist Jurgen Ruesch, has written that communication is therapeutic when it is helpful. The following discussion of communication is designed to provide the nurse with guidelines for the development of helpful and therefore therapeutic communication patterns.

MODES OF COMMUNICATION

Everyone is familiar with communication through the written word. When written material is read, the reciprocal aspects of communication are limited to the reader's ability to understand and react to the ideas and concepts that the author is attempting to convey. If the reader does not receive the intended message, effective communication has not been achieved.

Another mode of communication with which everyone is familiar is the spoken word, or *verbal communication*. If persons who are speaking together understand the same language, a major reciprocal element is present as they exchange, question, challenge, clarify, and enlarge on statements.

A mode of communication of which people are not always aware is *nonverbal communication*, which is closely related to verbal communication and is usually an integral part of it. Nonverbal communication refers to the messages sent and received through such means as facial expression, voice quality, physical posture, and gestures. Thus a person's behavior conveys a great deal to the astute observer. Nonverbal communication is often referred to as *body language*. Because nonverbal communication, or body language, is always present, it has been said that a person cannot *not* communicate.

Inner feelings are expressed by the manner in which an individual conducts himself in even such simple activities as walking down the hall, opening and closing doors, reclining in an easy chair, speaking to other people, and asking questions. The nonverbal aspects of communication sometimes convey general attitudes, feelings, and reactions more clearly and more accurately than do spoken words. An understanding of the implications of nonverbal communication is important for all nurses, especially those who work with mentally ill persons. Not only is it important for the nurse to be aware of the client's nonverbal communication, she must also be aware of her own nonverbal communication. Mentally ill persons are more aware of the nurse's nonverbal behavior than many nurses realize. The nurse who walks down the hall briskly, closes doors emphatically, and answers questions sharply is likely to be seen as an angry, unapproachable person. The nurse who smiles and speaks in a warm, friendly manner conveys an acceptance that may prompt the client to turn to her for help.

Another mode of communication, rarely recognized on a conscious level, is *metacommunication*. Metacommunication refers to the role expectation individuals have of each other in the context in which verbal and nonverbal communication take place. These role expectations strongly influence the nature of the verbal and nonverbal communication. For example, when a salesperson says to a customer, "May I help you?" it is understood by both individuals that she is asking whether she can be of assistance in helping the customer to make a purchase. On the other hand, when the nurse in a treatment setting asks the same question of a client it is understood by both that she is asking if there is something she might do, such as listening or helping the client with activities basic to his needs. Metacommunication and nonverbal communication are present in all situations in which there are two or more persons, although verbal communication may be absent at times.

Communication is most effective when the three previously mentioned modes of communication—verbal, nonverbal, and metacommunication—are congruent. Imagine the reaction of the previously mentioned salesperson if the customer responded: "Yes, you can help me. My child is ill and I am very wor-

Body language
A set of nonverbal signals—including body movements, postures, gestures, spatial positions, facial expressions, and bodily adornment—that give expression to various physical, mental, and emotional states.

Metacommunication
The context within which verbal and nonverbal communication takes place. It may support or contradict the verbal or nonverbal communication.

Congruent communication
A communication pattern in which the verbal, nonverbal, and metacommunication all convey the same message.

ried about her." In this situation the customer's reply indicates that she is responding only to the verbal communication of the salesperson and is ignoring the metacommunication. Therefore the customer's reply illustrates incongruency between her verbal communication and her metacommunication, which is likely to result in an increase in the anxiety levels of both persons involved.

DEVELOPING EFFECTIVE MODES OF COMMUNICATION

Developing modes of communication that are effective within the family, the culture, and the society in which one lives is an exceedingly complex learning process that begins at birth and comprises a large part of subsequent developmental stages. Although some of this learning takes place in a formal way through such societal agencies as the school, the foundation of the communication process is laid within the family long before the child is ready to attend school. In this respect the family acts as the representative of the society at large.

Much of the teaching and learning about communication within the family structure is achieved indirectly. For example, the child learns certain words by hearing them used in the home and without anyone overtly teaching him to associate the word with the object. This is illustrated by the 4-year-old child of two college professors who was asked by his nursery school teacher to identify pictures of objects. His classmates identified one as a *suitcase* or *bag,* but he identified the same object as an *attaché case.* Furthermore, he was unable to identify the object called *apron* by the rest of his classmates. The strong academic influence and lack of domestic interest in this child's home were clearly demonstrated by the nature of his vocabulary.

In the same way the meaning of nonverbal communication is learned. In some cultures a loud tone of voice signifies anger. In other cultures the opposite is true—that is, silence signifies anger, whereas loud, animated talking is indicative of nothing more than enthusiasm. To survive, children must learn the meaning of both the verbal and nonverbal communications of their family members, since they are highly dependent on these persons for having their needs met. It is a comment on the great intellectual potential of human beings to note how quickly the child does learn the meaning of highly complex messages.

It is not sufficient, however, for the child merely to learn the meaning of the messages he receives. He must also learn ways of responding that are acceptable within the family structure, and this is no simple task. Witness, for example, the child who lives within a family in which the verbal response to situations that are frustrating or anger-producing is to swear. Not infrequently the first time the child repeats a swear word in response to his anger or frustration, he is told by the adults that he is using a bad word that is forbidden and if he continues to use it, he will be punished.

Despite the complexity of learning the communication process, the majority of children are capable of doing so in a relatively short period and quickly become able to adapt that which they have learned in the home to the demands of the larger society. The previously mentioned 4-year-old quickly learned what an apron was and how it was used and that an attaché case is only one type of bag. In some instances, however, effective adaptation is not possible or becomes possible only after experiencing much stress. The stress of adapting to the communication in a different culture can be observed when adults travel rapidly between countries by jet airplane. Many travel agencies give their customers brochures describing the customs and frequently used words of the countries to be visited to lessen the communication shock experienced by the traveler.

The preceding examples illustrate communication problems that are normal from the standpoint of mental health. There are instances, however, when the learning of the communication process is accompanied by such a high level of stress that it produces a pattern of communication that is ineffective within either the family itself or society at large. *For our purposes, we can consider any communication to be ineffective if it does not accurately and clearly convey the message intended.* All persons occasionally experience ineffective communication. However, when this becomes a pattern (the rule rather than the exception), it frequently is a manifestation of mental illness and, in addition, is a factor in perpetuating the illness.

USING EFFECTIVE COMMUNICATION IN THE CARE OF MENTALLY ILL PERSONS

Mentally ill individuals need the opportunity to communicate with others who are sincerely interested in their problems and who care about them as people. It is important for the nurse to learn to communicate in such a way that her conversation will become a part of the total therapeutic environment. The ability to communicate therapeutically with clients requires that the nurse have an attitude of acceptance and genuine interest in them.

A climate of mutual trust and respect must be developed before mentally ill persons can feel safe enough to communicate with a nurse. This is not an easy climate to establish; it requires time, patience, knowledge, and skill. However, the nurse is rewarded for her efforts by the knowledge that when a client is helped to converse effectively with a professional person, an emotionally supportive experience often results.

Initiating a conversation

When the nurse joins the professional staff of a treatment facility, she and the clients are strangers to one another. They must become acquainted before therapeutic communication can take place. Most clients approach the nurse cautiously at first, as they approach other strangers. Some individuals may not approach the nurse at all. A few may insist on monopolizing her total attention.

Therapeutic communication
A process in which the nurse consciously uses verbal or nonverbal communication with the goal of helping the client.

The wise nurse will use some of the same skills in interacting with a client who is mentally ill as she has used successfully to interact with other strangers.

If the nurse has not already been introduced to the clients, she will begin by introducing herself. It will be helpful if she explains her status at the same time. This can be done by saying, "I am Miss Jones, a student nurse, and I will be here for 4 weeks." Or she might say, "I am Miss Smith, a graduate nurse, and I have come to work here for a while." If the nurse does not know the name of the person to whom she has introduced herself, she might say, "Will you please help me learn your name? I am sorry that I do not know it." With this invitation most persons will introduce themselves. Having learned the name of the client, the nurse uses it when speaking to him. This simple but important technique helps to individualize the conversation and encourages the client to focus his attention.

After the nurse and the client have been introduced, it is appropriate for the nurse to initiate a conversation. A conversation is one of the most common of the shared activities in which people engage. Just as the nurse initiates the conversational topics with other strangers, she may find it helpful with clients to introduce a neutral conversational topic appropriate for the time and place. If the time of year is right, baseball may be an appropriate topic. If the client seems interested in baseball, the nurse may choose to initiate a conversation with a question about a recent game. For example, she may begin by saying, "I did not have a chance to follow the game yesterday. What was the final score?" Other neutral topics that may be used include the headlines in the newspaper, the weather, or an approaching event. If the nurse notices that one person is holding a newspaper, she may begin a conversation by inquiring, "What interesting happenings are in the headlines today?"

Having introduced a topic, the sensitive nurse will wait for a response and will not feel compelled to avoid silences by immediately adding her own comments or opinions. After ample opportunity has been given for a response, it is suggested that she introduce a second conversational idea that logically follows the first.

Certainly the nurse should avoid approaching anyone with a barrage of words. In their desire to communicate effectively, nurses sometimes resort to asking a series of questions. Unfortunately this is too often the type of conversation that is reported when nurses are asked to tell about a recent conversation with a client. "How are you today?" is one of the usual questions with which many nurses begin a conversation. Such an opening sentence usually does little to develop a conversation.

Developing effective verbal communication

To be effective, the nurse's verbal communication must be guided by goals. The nurse's therapeutic potential will be greatly increased if a conscious effort is made to establish a goal for each conversation. The identified purpose for the conversation will provide a guide as to the appropriate approach to be used, the approximate duration of the conversation, and the manner in which it will be terminated.

Getting specific information. Frequently the nurse talks with the client to get specific information. When initiating this type of conversation the nurse should explain its purpose and the fact that she will be asking questions. Although in this instance it is appropriate that direct questions be asked, the nurse needs to understand that many mentally ill persons may feel threatened by direct questions. Therefore, it is useful to begin with questions designed to elicit answers that are likely to be seen as factual and therefore neutral, rather than questions that require responses that reflect feelings or opinions. Some examples are: "What is your name?" "Tell me your address." As a result of the exchange of factual information, the client may relax sufficiently to be able to provide more sensitive information, such as a response to the question, "What circumstances brought you to the hospital?" In most instances, questions beginning with the word "why" are ineffective in soliciting an informative response.

A conversation with the goal of getting specific information is usually brief and is terminated with an expression of thanks for the client's cooperation.

Establishing rapport with the client. The nurse often approaches the client with the goal of establishing a beginning rapport that can serve as a basis for developing a meaningful future relationship. With such a goal, attention is focused on the client in a manner that conveys a sincere interest in him and a willingness to listen. The focus of the conversation is on getting acquainted and establishing a feeling of mutual trust. In such a situation, direct questions are rarely necessary or useful. Rather, statements that reflect observations are most productive. The comment, "The color of your dress becomes you" is an example of such an observation, assuming, of course, this is the case.

The duration of a conversation with the goal of establishing rapport with the client is likely to be determined by its context. Thus, it may be a brief exchange when passing each other in the hall, or it may be quite long if the nurse and client are, for example, on a shopping trip. A conversation with this goal is most usefully terminated with a statement about when the interaction will resume. For example, the nurse might say, "I will be able to spend more time with you tomorrow at 10 AM and will meet you here. Is that time and place all right with you?" It is imperative that the nurse make only those promises she is reasonably certain she can keep if the ultimate goal of establishing a feeling of mutual trust is to be achieved.

Encouraging expression of thoughts and feelings. If the purpose of the conversation is to encourage the client to express his thoughts and feelings, a nondirective approach would undoubtedly achieve the most positive results. In such a situation the client would be encouraged to initiate the conversation. Responding to his comments by reflecting his thoughts and feelings back to him might be helpful in encouraging him to continue expressing his feelings without intro-

When the goal of the conversation is to get specific information, the nurse may appropriately ask questions that are more direct than those usually employed.

Rapport
Harmony, accord, confidence, and respect underlying a relationship between two persons; an essential bond between the nurse and the client if they are to interact therapeutically.

When the goal of the interaction is to establish a beginning rapport with the client, attention should be focused on the client in an attempt to convey a willingness to listen.

Nondirective approach
A therapeutic approach in which the nurse refrains from giving advice or interpretation as the client is helped to clarify and understand his feelings and values.

ducing new or unrelated ideas. For example, if the client speaks of his unhappy home life, the nurse might respond by saying, "It sounds to me as if you are saying that your home life is unhappy." This type of response conveys to the client that the nurse is listening to him and allows him an opportunity to either accept or reject the nurse's impression of his communication.

When the goal of the interaction is to encourage the client to express thoughts and feelings, a nondirective approach is most appropriate.

Once having encouraged the client to express his thoughts and feelings, the nurse may not be prepared to hear what he has to say and may respond judgmentally. Such an attitude is reflected in statements such as, "Don't be silly!" or "How could you possibly think that?" Responses such as these discourage the client from further divulging his thoughts and feelings. To be helpful, it is important that the nurse withhold her personal opinion about what the client is saying and avoid the use of words that connote a judgment.

The duration of conversations with the goal of encouraging clients to express their thoughts and feelings should be determined by the client's response. In other words, the conversation should be continued for as long as it remains productive; it should be terminated if the client becomes unduly anxious or resistant to continuing. It is useful for the nurse to summarize the content of the discussion as a means of ending the conversation.

Arriving at a decision. When the client is in a situation where he has to arrive at a decision, the nurse can be effective by helping him explore possible alternatives and their consequences. This often involves assisting the client to gather additional information or to validate information he believes he already has. However, this process is not the same as the nurse's giving advice. Even though she may have strong feelings about what would be the best decision, she should avoid sharing these feelings. The nurse is not the client and cannot know the choices that are best for him in most situations. She does not know all the past experiences that influence his present thinking and feeling and therefore is not qualified to give advice about what he should do. Giving advice suggests that the client is not capable of making choices among the available alternatives. Furthermore, while giving advice may result in a temporary positive response from the client because it relieves him of the responsibility for making a decision, in the long run it is likely to encourage him to remain dependent on some other person to make future decisions. Instead of offering advice, it is more helpful for the nurse and client together to explore the positive and negative aspects of the possible decisions.

Most decisions have a time frame within which an action must be taken. The nurse can be helpful to the client by assisting him in determining that time frame and helping him to become aware that not making a decision within the necessary time frame is, in effect, making a decision.

The duration of conversations with the goal of arriving at a decision is determined by when the decision needs to be made and by the client's response to the problem-solving activity. Therefore, only one brief conversation may be required, or several conversations about the same subject may be held over a period of time. This type of conversation is most effectively terminated by the nurse's encouraging the client to summarize the advantages and disadvantages of each identified alternative and the rationale for the choice he has made.

Providing reassurance. Almost all mentally ill persons have low self-esteem and have had many negative experiences. Consequently, they are likely to need reassurance about their value and worth as human beings as well as about the outcome of stressful events. Nurses make many comments that they hope will provide reassurance but actually fall short of this goal. Even though the nurse intends to be helpful, it is rarely helpful to make comments such as: "Don't worry," "Your doctor says this medicine will help you," "There are a great many people who are worse off than you are," and "Don't cry; you don't want people to see you crying." Such comments are not helpful and are likely to convince the client that the nurse is not able to understand his problems. Reassurance is never achieved by use of meaningless clichés. Instead, it is reassuring to the client if the nurse considers the problem thoughtfully and asks intelligent, reality-oriented questions about the situation. It is reassuring to the client when the nurse accepts his tears without comment or assures him that crying is a reasonable thing to do under the circumstances, provided, of course, the circumstances do warrant such expression. It is reassuring to the client when the nurse listens to his personal problems without showing surprise or disapproval when he talks about past social behavior that is unusual or below the nurse's standards. It is reassuring when the nurse agrees that the client has a problem and works with him in trying to problem solve. It is reassuring to the client if the nurse sits with him even when he does not feel like talking, thereby conveying a genuine interest in his problem and acceptance of him. Finally, it is reassuring to the client when the nurse reflects back the tone of the feeling she hears him expressing. For the nurse to say, "It sounds to me as if you are really upset," conveys to the client that his feelings as well as the content of what he is saying is being understood. Once again, it should be noted that the nurse is not imposing a feeling on the client by such a statement but rather is expressing her own response.

The duration of conversations with the goal of providing reassurance tend to be longer than many other types. If the topic or the emotional state of the client is such to warrant reassurance, it is unlikely that a brief conversation will be effective. In fact, when approached by a distraught client, nurses often employ meaningless clichés, as discussed above, because they sense the conversation will be long and they believe they do not have the time to spend. Rather than stating this and arranging for another time to talk—a desirable response—they mouth platitudes that discourage the client from continuing.

A conversation with the goal of providing reassurance is terminated by the client indicating that he has exhausted the topic, at least for the moment. At this point, the nurse is often tempted to ask, "Do you feel better?" This question is rarely appropriate in that it is designed to elicit an affirmative answer to reas-

When the goal of the interaction is to arrive at a decision, the nurse can be effective by helping the client to explore possible alternatives and their consequences.

When the goal of the interaction is to provide reassurance, approaches appropriate to the client and problem are likely to be helpful, but statements that represent meaningless cliches are rarely reassuring.

sure the nurse, not the client. Furthermore, if the client does feel better he often will say so spontaneously; if he doesn't feel reassured, the nurse's question may lead him to believe he should and therefore add to his concern.

Stimulating client interest. Many mentally ill persons avoid activities that involve other people as a means of protecting themselves from interpersonal interactions with which they believe they cannot cope. Others have so little energy and/or such low self-esteem that they do not attend to even the basic activities of daily living, such as bathing and grooming themselves. Much can be done to stimulate interest in activities and to help individuals alter social attitudes by using skillfully phrased suggestions. For instance, encouraging a client to participate in the activities offered by the occupational therapist may be accomplished by telling him about the activities available and by using suggestions such as, "You might enjoy the finger-painting class." At another time a second comment about this activity might be, "Many clients seem to have an interesting time when they go to occupational therapy; I think you might too." The client who refused to wash his hair for several weeks may do so if several people with whom he is acquainted comment about his attractive appearance when his hair was clean a few weeks before. One suggestion is usually not sufficient to alter an attitude or help a person accept a new idea. Suggestion must be used frequently and skillfully by persons whose opinion the client respects.

When the goal of the interaction is to stimulate client interest, skillfully phrased suggestions are useful.

The duration of conversations with the goal of stimulating client interest is almost always brief, although such conversations may occur frequently. If the goal is to be achieved, however, the nurse needs to resist the temptation to pressure the client, as would be the case if she approached the client frequently to talk of nothing other than the desired activity. This type of conversation is terminated when the client indicates an interest in the desired activity.

Table 6-1 summarizes the goal, nurse's approach, usual duration, and termination of common conversations with clients.

Developing effective nonverbal communication

One of the first steps the nurse can take in developing effective nonverbal communication is to examine her own feelings toward clients and, if possible, to focus her efforts on those for whom she feels genuine interest and acceptance. If the nurse attempts to work closely with clients with whom she has many negative feelings, she will surely communicate these feelings nonverbally. The nurse needs to recognize the importance of her personal feelings in developing a relationship with a client. It is also essential to recognize the role of nonverbal communication and to understand that it is impossible for every nurse to develop a therapeutic relationship with every mentally ill person. Equipped with this knowledge and understanding, the nurse can feel comfortable in admitting that she is not the appropriate person to provide care to a specific individual with whom she has not been able to establish a positive relationship.

TABLE 6-1 *Goal, nurse's approach, usual duration, and termination of common conversations with clients*

Goal	Nurse's approach	Usual duration	Terminated by
Getting specific information	Explain purpose Begin with questions designed to elicit factual responses	Brief	Thanking client for his cooperation
Establishing rapport	Focus on client Convey interest and willingness to listen	Variable, depending on context	Planning for next conversation
Encouraging expression of thoughts and feelings	Nondirective Reflect back client's thoughts and feelings	Determined by client's response	Nurse summarizing content discussed
Arriving at a decision	Assist client to explore possible alternatives and their consequences Assist client to gather additional information or to validate existent information Assist client to determine time frame within which a decision must be made	Determined by time frame of decision and client's response to problem solving	Client summarizing advantages and disadvantages of each alternative and the rationale for his choice
Providing reassurance	Ask intelligent, reality-oriented questions Listen nonjudgmentally Convey interest and acceptance	Lengthy	Client indicating he has exhausted the topic for the moment
Stimulating client interest	Use skillfully phrased suggestions	Brief but frequent	Client indicating interest in desired activity

After examining her own feelings toward clients the nurse can take a number of specific steps to engage in effective nonverbal communication. One of the most important of these steps is to sit near a client when talking to him. Some nurses hesitate to sit beside clients even when they are trying to converse with them. This hesitancy probably comes from experience in previous nursing situations in which the nurse was expected to administer physical comfort measures or therapeutic treatment procedures.

When the nurse stands during a conversation, she conveys the idea that she is in a hurry, that she expects the conversation to be short, and that she is prepared to remain for only a few minutes. In such a hurried atmosphere no one can expect a client to feel that there is interest or time enough for him to talk about anything important. Conversely, when sitting with a mentally ill person, it is important not to sit in such a way that the person feels trapped or in danger of attack. Astute observation of the client's nonverbal behavior will quickly reveal if the nurse is sitting in a position that produces the best climate for conversation. Examples of behaviors likely to indicate that the client feels uncom-

Effective nonverbal communication on the part of the nurse is essential for conveying acceptance of the client.

fortable are the movement of his body or chair away from the nurse, his focusing his eyes elsewhere, and physical signs of anxiety such as restlessness and
agitation. The nurse should not hesitate to alter her position if this seems appropriate from her observations of the client's behavior. When the nurse conveys her sincere interest in the client through her position and through the
warmth of her voice and facial expression, the first step has been taken toward
the establishment of a helpful interaction.

Another important step the nurse can take in developing effective nonverbal communication is to develop her listening skills. Listening implies silence,
but it does not imply passivity. The listener can and should be an active, alert,
and interested participant, even though she may make very few verbal
contributions. The nurse gives evidence of interest by being genuinely interested in the client and in what he is saying. This interest cannot be feigned.
Evidence of genuine, sincere interest is shown by the expression on the
listener's face, by the way the listener looks at the speaker, and by the verbal
encouragement that is given to the speaker. Nodding the head to suggest that
one understands or agrees is one way of giving encouragement. Comments
such as, "That must have been difficult for you" or "I see, go on" are
encouraging when said at an appropriate time with a friendly, interested tone.
If the listener cannot follow the logic of the client or the sequence of the
related incidents, it is best to ask the client to review that part of the story
again. The nurse might say, "Could you explain that last statement again for
me? I do not believe I understood it clearly." Or she might say, "I'm sorry, I
didn't understand what you said a minute ago. Could you go over the last point
again?" If the nurse fails to ask for clarification when it is needed, the client
will soon discover that she has lost the sequence and meaning of the
conversation and is trying to act as if she understands when she does not. This
is one way of losing the client's confidence.

Concluding a conversation

The conclusion of a conversation is as important as is the initiation of a
conversation. The conclusion of a conversation will often set the tone for
subsequent conversations between the nurse and the client. When the nurse
needs to leave, she should break off the conversation so that it can be resumed
at another time. Thus she might say, "I have been interested in what you have
been telling me, and I hope we can continue this discussion later on." Of
course, such a statement must be true. If she has promised to talk with the
client at another time, she must find time for resuming the conversation. She
might begin by saying, "I have been thinking about our conversation of
yesterday and I am wondering if we could talk some more about the last point
that you were making." The nurse would use this statement only if it were true.
If such a statement were not true, she would choose another that would be
appropriate for the conversation.

SPECIAL PROBLEMS IN COMMUNICATING WITH MENTALLY ILL PERSONS

Congruent communication is necessary when one is attempting to relate therapeutically with mentally ill persons. They have had much previous experience in interaction with significant others who have communicated incongruent messages, particularly in regard to simultaneous verbal and nonverbal modes of communication wherein the nonverbal message contradicted the verbal message. The consequence of this communication is that the receiver must decide which message he will respond to, aware that whichever choice he makes he will be incorrect. When this type of communication is usual rather than the exception it may result in the receiver's becoming unable to respond at all because he becomes immobilized by anxiety. Some theorists believe that this pattern of communication is characteristic of dysfunctional families in which one or more members become mentally ill as an adaptation to the stress of this form of disturbed communication. The technical term for this type of disturbed interaction is *double bind communication*.

> **Double-bind communication** Communication in which the sender gives one message verbally and another nonverbally. The listener does not know how to respond and is thus in a situation from which there is no escape.

    As the professional person spending the most time with the client in the treatment setting, the nurse has the greatest opportunity to create an environment in which the client can experience congruent communication. She can help the client to learn modes of adaptation that are more reality oriented and therefore more useful than his previous adaptation of retreating from reality into a psychosis.

    For the nurse to express congruent messages she must be aware of herself and her own feelings, a concept discussed in Chapter 4. A helpful suggestion is for the nurse to make clear to the client what she is feeling, that is, to bring into verbal communication her nonverbal messages rather than letting the client guess their meaning. An example of this might be the nurse who says after being purposely tripped, "Your behavior evokes irritation in me." It is important to note that this statement conveys a very different message than if the nurse were to say, "You irritate me." In the former statement the nurse is expressing and owning her own feelings and not rejecting the client, whereas in the latter statement she is blaming and rejecting the client, which is likely to end the possibility of any further communication.

    Since nonverbal aspects of communication usually convey the intended message most clearly, mentally ill persons, like all others, usually accurately sense the sincerity and kindness of the staff. Thus it has been observed that a staff member who is gruff and outspoken with clients may be respected and loved by them because he communicates nonverbally a basic attitude of kindness and a sincere interest in their welfare. A nurse who has adopted an unusually saccharine approach may be deeply resented by clients because nonverbally she conveys a feeling of rejection.

    Clients often ask new nurses personal questions such as, "Are you married?" or "What nursing school are you from?" or "Where do you live?" The

OF SPECIAL INTEREST

Incongruency among the verbal, nonverbal, and metacommunication modes of communication is not the only source of ineffective, non-therapeutic communication. Within the mode of verbal communication alone, confusion can reign when the speaker does not say what he means or mean what he says. Knowledge of this communication problem is not limited to health care professionals, as illustrated in the following excerpt from Lewis Carroll's *Alice's Adventures in Wonderland.*

"Then you should say what you mean," The March Hare went on.

"I do," Alice hastily replied; "at least - at least I mean what I say - that's the same thing, you know."

"Not the same thing a bit!" said the Hatter. "Why, you might just as well say that 'I see what I eat' is the same thing as 'I eat what I see'!"

natural curiosity of clients about the personal life of the professional staff is understandable. However, if the conversation is allowed to be focused on the personal life of the nurse, it quickly loses its original goal—to achieve communication that is therapeutic for the client. If the nurse wishes to do so, it is appropriate for her to respond to factual questions such as, "Are you married?" with a simple "Yes" or "No." If the client continues to ask personal questions she might state "It seems you are very interested in me," or ask, "I wonder if we could not find a topic other than my personal life to discuss?" Frequent personal questions directed to the nurse alert her to the need for focusing future conversation more carefully. It may suggest that the individual in question hopes to direct attention away from himself.

Many mentally ill persons struggle with the problem of not being able to trust other people. One of the ways a nurse can help such a person is to demonstrate that she can be trusted. If a client can begin to trust one person, it is possible that trust can eventually be extended to other people. When trying to help a client learn to trust her, the nurse sometimes finds herself in a dilemma. A client with whom the nurse is interacting may confide information that places her in an untenable position. On the one hand, she wishes to respect his confidences, while at the same time she hopes to carry out her responsibilities as a member of the professional staff. The following situation precipitated such a dilemma.

A client confided that he was planning to leave the city during the next weekend, ostensibly to visit his family. He told the nurse that he had stolen enough money to purchase a train ticket to a distant city where he was unknown and where he hoped to make a fresh start. The client cautioned the nurse not to tell anyone about these plans until after he was gone. The nurse had reason to be concerned about the client's safety and now was in conflict about keeping the confidence while still fulfilling her role as a member of the professional staff. She was understandably distressed about the situation.

It is important for the nurse to inform the client at the beginning of their interaction that she will share information essential to his treatment or safety with other members of the treatment team. When the client begins to confide information to the nurse that should be shared with other members of the professional staff, she has a responsibility to remind him that she must report the conversation to the appropriate people. The nurse might say to the client, "You know it will be necessary for me to share what you are telling me with the treatment team." Given this reminder, the client must then decide whether he will continue the discussion. A reasonable guide to follow is that the nurse has a responsibility to tell the client's therapist and the nurse in charge if the client tells her of plans that are dangerous to him or others or that interfere with the treatment plan.

When the nurse has established a relationship with the client that makes it possible for him to express his thoughts and feelings freely to her, she has a responsibility to listen with acceptance and understanding. The fact that the client confides in the nurse indicates that an atmosphere of trust has been established. However, at times a client confides feelings and thoughts to the nurse that may be more appropriately discussed with another member of the treatment team. The nurse may not be in a position to be most helpful to the client in the particular situation. In this instance the nurse can suggest that this information be shared with the other team member and that she could assist the client in doing so, if he desires. It is also necessary that the nurse and the other team member have an opportunity to discuss the client's behavior and his problems.

> Clients must be helped to understand that the nurse has a responsibility to share confidences with the treatment team when clients confide behavior that may be dangerous to themselves or others or may interfere with the treatment plan.

END NOTE

In this chapter, communication is defined as the reciprocal exchange of information, ideas, beliefs, feelings, and attitudes between two persons or among a group of persons. The three modes of communication—verbal, nonverbal, and metacommunication—are defined and discussed. Examples of verbal and nonverbal communication are given in situations where the nurse's goal is to: get specific information; establish a beginning rapport; encourage the client to express his thoughts and feelings; assist the client to arrive at a decision; provide reassurance; and stimulate client interest. Emphasis is placed on the necessity for congruency among the three modes of communication if the communication is to be effective.

SUGGESTED SOURCES OF ADDITIONAL INFORMATION

Gluck M: Learning a therapeutic verbal response to anger, J Psychosoc Nurs Ment Health Serv 19:9, March 1981.

Gruber LN: The no-demand, third person interview of the non-verbal patient, Perspect Psychiatr Care 15(1):38, 1977.

Harden S and Halaris A: Nonverbal communication of patients and high and low empathy nurses, J Psychosoc Nurs Ment Health Serv 21:14, January 1983.

Impey L: Art media: a means to therapeutic communication with families, Perspect Psychiatr Care 19:70, March/April 1981.

Kalisch BL: What is empathy? Am J Nurs 73:1548, 1973.

Kasch C: Interpersonal competence and communication in the delivery of nursing care, Adv Nurs Sci 6(2):71, 1984.

Kerr NJ: Discussion of "common errors in communication made by students in psychiatric nursing," Perspect Psychiatr Care 16:184, July-August 1978.

Knapp M: Nonverbal communication in human interaction, ed 2, New York, 1978, Holt, Rinehart & Winston, Inc.

Knowles RD: Building rapport through neurolinguistic programming, Am J Nurs 83:1010, July 1983.

Reusch J: Disturbed communication, New York, 1957, WW Norton & Co.

Reusch J: Therapeutic communication, New York, 1961, WW Norton & Co.

Reusch J and Bateson G: Communication: the social matrix of psychiatry, New York, 1968, WW Norton & Co.

Sayre J: Common errors in communication made by students in psychiatric nursing, Perspect Psychiatr Care 16:175, July-August 1978.

Stewart CJ and Cash WB: Interviewing principles and practices, ed 4, New York, 1985, William C. Brown.

Tobiason SJB: Touching is for everyone, Am J Nurs 81:728, April 1981.

Watzlawick P, Beavin J, and Jackson D: The pragmatics of human communication, New York, 1967, WW Norton & Co.

Nurse-client interactions

7

LEARNING OBJECTIVES

After studying this chapter the student will be able to:

- Discuss the concepts of acceptance and consistency as they relate to all nurse-client interactions.
- Discuss three types of nurse-client interactions in terms of their goals and degree of nurse-client involvement.
- Discuss the developmental phases of the nurse-client relationship.
- Describe the roles and functions the nurse may fulfill as she engages in nurse-client interactions.

Although nurse-client interactions that are therapeutic possess common elements, they are developed differently by each person, depending on the characteristics of the individuals involved. If an interaction is to become therapeutic, it is necessary for the nurse to recognize the client as a unique, important human being who experiences hopes, fears, joys, and sorrows as do all other people. It is also necessary to understand that the client has his own special set of problems and reactions to life. It is important for the nurse to interact with him so that she develops and reflects an understanding of his emotional responses and the probable meaning of his behavior. Through her sensitivity the nurse can develop a recognition of some of the client's emotional needs and an appreciation for some of the ways in which she can be helpful to him. In many instances the nurse will be most helpful to the client by interacting with him in a way that is different from the previous social interactions he has experienced. Many mentally ill persons have a long history of having failed at establishing and maintaining satisfying interpersonal relationships. To the degree that the nurse's in-

The nurse can often be most helpful to the client when relating in a way that differs from his previous social interactions.

teractions with the client reflect acceptance of him and consistency in response to him, they will be therapeutic by providing experiences that are corrective of earlier, less helpful interpersonal experiences.

HISTORICAL PERSPECTIVE

In 1947 McGraw-Hill Book Company published *Nurse Patient Relationships in Psychiatry* by Helena Willis Render. She was the first author to introduce the idea that the relationship the nurse establishes with the client has a significant therapeutic potential. This book stimulated much attention on the part of nurses concerning the potential therapeutic possibilities inherent in their role in psychiatric settings. In 1952 G.P. Putnam's Sons published the book *Interpersonal Relations in Nursing* by Dr. Hildegard E. Peplau, an active nurse clinician and educator. This book in many ways revolutionized the teaching and practice of psychiatric nursing in this country. Peplau's text focused on the therapeutic potential of the one-to-one relationship. It was not, however, until the widespread use of the psychotropic drugs rendered clients amenable to interpersonally based treatment modalities that psychiatric nursing began to take the form it has today, making use of the concepts originally proposed by Render and Peplau.

Currently it is acknowledged that the use the nurse makes of her own personality can be a great therapeutic influence in the experience of the client if she uses understanding and skill. It is the only tool that is uniquely hers and that she alone directs. Although the nurse may give dozens of daily medications and may assist with other somatic therapies, the major way in which she directly influences the care of the client is through the use she makes of herself as she deals with the client in face-to-face interactions.

The nurse possesses a unique tool that can have more influence on clients than any medication or therapy: herself.

DEVELOPING THERAPEUTIC NURSE-CLIENT INTERACTIONS

The foundation of all therapeutic interactions is *acceptance*. This is a commonly used word among nurses, although it is not universally understood or operationalized by them. Other behaviors that are equally important are those expressed by the adjectives *nonjudgmental* and *consistent*. All these concepts are basic in developing therapeutic interactions with any client. They are discussed here in the hope of helping the nurse to make effective use of them in caring for mentally ill persons.

Acceptance implies that the nurse treats the client as an important individual who has inherent worth and not as a diagnostic entity or a set of psychiatric symptoms. Actually, the use of diagnostic terms may encourage the nurse to adopt an impersonal attitude toward the client. The nurse implies that she is accepting the client by calling him by name and by recognizing that he has the same basic personal rights she herself possesses. Acceptance implies that the nurse tries to understand the meaning the client is conveying through his behavior. An accepting nurse recognizes that the client behaves as well as he is able at a given time. She encourages the client to express his feelings to her, realizing that in this way he is able to relieve emotional tensions. She does not censor him for statements and feelings that may not be conventionally acceptable, realizing that his behavior is an expression of his illness. She recognizes that his comments may not be directed toward her personally.

The word *nonjudgmental* is usually used in conjunction with the word *attitude* and is closely related to the concept of acceptance. One cannot be achieved without the other. A nonjudgmental attitude is neither condemning nor approving. Through tone of voice and manner the nurse conveys to the client a helpful attitude without morally judging his behavior. A nonjudgmental attitude toward the behavior of a mentally ill person implies that the nurse recognizes that behavior, like physical symptoms displayed by physically ill persons, is neither good or bad nor right or wrong but rather a learned adaptation to stress. As such she also realizes that the client has the potential to change his behavior by learning new adaptations to stress.

Acceptance of mentally ill persons and their behavior is often difficult to achieve, and almost everyone occasionally falls short of the ideal. The behavior of some mentally ill persons is offensive at times. This is true, for example, of the behavior of clients who are so confused that they soil themselves. It may be impossible for the nurse to avoid feeling repelled by the sight of a person grossly soiled, but it is possible for her to avoid making him feel that he is an offensive person. Joking in front of a client about his behavior or describing his shortcomings to others within his hearing is neither respecting nor accepting him.

Consistency is another important characteristic of therapeutic interactions. The consistent nurse maintains the same basic attitude toward the client so that he derives security from being able to predict her behavior. Not only should the client be able to expect the same positive attitudes and approaches from an individual nurse, but also the entire nursing staff should interact with consistency from the standpoint of basic attitudes and overall policies. Consistency helps lessen the client's anxiety by simplifying decision making and by avoiding uncertainties.

All mentally ill persons experience some loss of self-esteem and self-confidence. If an interaction is to be helpful to a client, it must assist him in reestablishing his self-confidence and restoring his self-esteem. This is a slow process that requires consistent work over a period of time. Recognizing the client as being an important human being, expressing genuine interest in him, spending time with him, conversing with him, and listening with understanding to his expressions of feeling are all ways of helping him feel worthwhile, important, and wanted. On the other hand indifference, insincerity, and an impersonal attitude toward the client reinforce his sense of unimportance and further convince him of what he may already believe—that he is lacking in value as a person.

The accepting nurse believes that a client behaves as well as he is able at any given time.

A nonjudgmental attitude is neither condemning nor approving. A client's behavior is neither good nor bad but a learned manner of adapting to stress.

A consistent manner on the part of the nurse ensures the client a feeling of security in knowing what to expect.

Increasing a client's sense of self-confidence and self-esteem is often a slow process in which the nurse uses the tool of positive reinforcement.

It is not possible for a nurse to interact in a way that has the same therapeutic potential and the same meaning for each individual client. It is possible, however, for the nurse to learn to know the names and something of the needs of all clients with whom she comes in close contact. With many of these persons the nurse can expect to develop a positive relationship. With a limited number she will be able to interact in a way that will lay the foundation for the development of a therapeutic relationship. With these individuals she will be able to carry on discussions that have therapeutic potential because she will know them well and will have developed a genuine interest in them as people.

A therapeutic relationship can begin with the nurse's knowing a client's name and develop over time to her knowing the client's needs.

TYPES AND CHARACTERISTICS OF THERAPEUTIC INTERACTIONS

The nurse is often involved in at least three types of one-to-one situations. These situations are differentiated on the basis of the degree of nurse-client involvement and whether the goal of the interaction is immediate, short-range, or long-range.

The first situation in which the nurse and client are likely to engage is one in which the nurse and the client do not know each other and the client is in immediate, severe difficulty that requires the nurse to intervene. In other words, an emergency exists. The nature of the emergency can range from a life-threatening situation, such as a suicidal attempt, to the client's being overwhelmed by a particular emotion, such as grief, and expressing this behaviorally. Ideally the person who intervenes in such situations should be one who knows the client and understands the plan of treatment for him. This however is not always possible because of the necessity for immediate action or the unavailability of the appropriate staff member or because the client is new to the treatment setting. When such situations arise, the nurse must not avoid intervening merely because she does not know the client. Rather, she must bring to bear on the situation her knowledge of the dynamics of human behavior and her skill in psychiatric nursing. In these emergency situations the nurse will do well to employ the principles of psychiatric nursing and good common sense. The client has a right to be protected from harming himself, either physically or emotionally, and from harming others.

In an emergency, the nurse must interact therapeutically with the client whether or not she knows him well.

Needless to say, once the emergency situation is resolved immediate efforts should be made to contact those mental health personnel who are involved with the client's treatment or to establish a long-range treatment plan and begin its implementation if one has not already been developed.

The second situation is one in which the nurse and client have an association. While they know each other, the nurse does not have major responsibility for the client's treatment. Unfortunately, some nurses believe that if they are not assigned to the care of a particular client they have little or no responsibility to behave in a thoughtful, goal-directed manner when interacting with him. This is not the case, and in fact the value of the interventions of other staff can be lessened by the thoughtless, offhand behavior of a particular nurse. Although it is not possible for the nurse to have in-depth knowledge of all the clients in any treatment setting, it is possible and important for her to be aware of the treatment goals for all clients with whom she is likely to come in contact, no matter how superficially. With this awareness the nurse's on-the-spot interactions with the client can be designed to support and enhance the treatment that is being implemented by other personnel.

This situation is particularly common in psychiatric nursing, since, unlike many physically ill persons, mentally ill persons usually have physical mobility and are able to approach the nurse whenever they wish. It is not uncommon for a mentally ill person to seek out a nurse other than the one to whom he is assigned to validate statements made to him by his assigned nurse or to otherwise engage the two nurses in a power struggle. The client's motivation may or may not be conscious and may be a manifestation of the stage of the relationship in which the client and his nurse are engaged. In any event, the manner in which the nurse responds is frequently an important factor in enhancing or impeding the therapeutic endeavors of others. These on-the-spot, seemingly casual interactions should have as their goal support of the overall treatment of the client.

The third one-to-one situation the nurse encounters is one in which she seeks to develop a therapeutic relationship with a client in an effort to provide corrective interpersonal experiences. Because such a relationship requires an in-depth knowledge of the client and much of the nurse's time and energy, it is possible for the nurse to have only a few such relationships in progress at any point in time. An understanding of the process of these relationships will make clear that it is inappropriate to use the term *nurse-client relationship* to describe all interactions between the nurse and all clients with whom she comes in contact. This is not to say that all nurse-client interactions should not be therapeutic, but rather that in only a few will the nurse be intensely involved in an ongoing relationship with the client that is designed to provide corrective interpersonal experiences. Since the nurse can be involved in only a few nurse-client relationships at any one time it is important that she make the best use of her time, energy, and skills by devoting them to those clients whose nursing diagnosis indicates a potential for benefiting from this type of nursing intervention. Not all nurses work equally effectively with all clients, since the nurse's own personality is the major tool she has for intervention. Therefore when the nursing care plan indicates that a nurse-client relationship is desirable, the nurse who develops such a relationship should be one whose self-awareness indicates that she would be likely to be effective with the particular client. Since both nurses and mentally ill persons are more human than otherwise and have the same wide variety of personality structures, it is unlikely that there ever would be a client for whom a suitable nurse were not available.

Sometimes it is difficult for nurses to differentiate between social and therapeutic relationships when dealing with mentally ill persons. In a social relationship the needs of both the involved individuals are considered. The needs of

Especially in the psychiatric setting, the nurse should know the treatment goals for all clients, even for those with whom she interacts only casually.

The most effective nurse-client relationship is one in which the nurse uses both her personality and self-awareness to provide a corrective interpersonal experience for the client.

both must be met in a satisfying way if the relationship is to continue. A social relationship usually develops spontaneously without a conscious plan. The goal of such a relationship is usually shared by the participants and is frequently limited to personal pleasure. The participants in a social relationship share mutual concern regarding reciprocal approval. This may develop more or less satisfactorily without conscious awareness of the emotional significance of the relationship.

In contrast, the therapeutic relationship focuses on the personal and emotional needs of the client. Such a relationship is therapeutically oriented and is planned after consideration has been given to the needs of the client and the therapeutic ability of the nurse. There is always a therapeutic goal toward which the nurse directs her interventions. When the nurse has accepted this role, she must strive to be consciously aware of the developing relationship and its meaning. She should seek help in reflecting objectively on the meaning of the interaction between herself and the client so that she will be prepared to guide the client in developing more appropriate behavior. In a therapeutic relationship the nurse does not necessarily seek the client's approval. She reevaluates the situation constantly so that she can distinguish between the client's actual needs and his demands. As the time for the relationship to be terminated approaches, the nurse releases the patient emotionally and strives to help him move forward to more appropriate relationships. See Table 7-1.

DEVELOPMENTAL PHASES OF THE NURSE-CLIENT RELATIONSHIP

A therapeutic relationship focuses on the personal and emotional needs of the client, whereas in a social relationship the needs of both the involved individuals are considered.

Every therapeutic relationship that a nurse develops between herself and a client has an initial phase, referred to as the *orientation phase* or the *getting acquainted period*. During this phase the nurse and client agree on a mutually acceptable contract that serves to establish the parameters of the relationship. The goals of this phase are the development of trust and the establishment of the nurse as a significant other to the client.

Although in some instances the client initiates the relationship, more fre-

TABLE 7-1   *Types and characteristics of nurse-client interactions*

Type of interaction	Degree of nurse-client involvement	Goal of interaction
Emergency	Minimal	Immediate—resolution of a severe difficulty
Association	Nurse and client know each other; nurse does not have major responsibility for client's treatment	Short range—support and enhance treatment efforts of others
Relationship	Great	Long range—provide corrective interpersonal experiences for client

quently it is the nurse who first approaches the client. She does so by introducing herself by name and position and suggesting that she would like to work with him on his problems by meeting with him for a specific period of time and at a specified time and place. It is also important for the nurse to ask the client how he would like to be addressed. Most clients respond positively to this approach, ironically because the nurse is not yet an important part of their life and the idea of developing a relationship with her is not threatening. Once the time and place of their conversations are agreed on, it is imperative that the nurse adhere strictly to this schedule. The nurse should also suggest a duration for each conversation, for example, 45 minutes. This period of time must be adhered to, despite the fact that the client may at various times attempt to entice the nurse to stay longer with him by bringing up highly charged emotional issues 5 minutes prior to the end of the session. The nurse can handle this by acknowledging that the issues at hand sound important and by suggesting that the client reintroduce them at the beginning of their next meeting. This approach is therapeutic because it demonstrates that the nurse will follow through on what she had promised—in this instance, sessions of a 45-minute length—and therefore can be trusted to do what she says. It is important to understand that clients sometimes unconsciously introduce highly significant issues shortly before the end of planned sessions as a means of letting the nurse know what is disturbing them without running the risk of having to discuss these issues at length because they know that the session will soon be over. If the nurse succumbs to the temptation to continue the discussion beyond the agreed time, the client will learn that he has to be more guarded with her in the future.

Some clients, rather than attempting to lengthen the sessions, try to shorten them by overt means such as walking away or covert means such as falling asleep. The nurse can effectively deal with such situations by remembering that this period is set aside solely for interaction with this client and by stating this to him. If the client then still walks away or falls asleep, the nurse should remain in the designated meeting place for the remainder of the agreed upon time. This behavior of the nurse also indicates to the client that she can be trusted to do what she has promised, despite his behavior.

As the nurse becomes more meaningful to the client, his behavior toward her often appears increasingly negative. He may not appear for the scheduled sessions, or his language may become profane or he may resist talking about himself and state a preference for discussing the nurse's personal life. At this point many nurses become discouraged and disappointed, since the earlier sessions had proceeded smoothly. In contrast, the nurse has reason to feel encouraged, since at this point in the relationship, the client's behavior most likely indicates that the nurse is becoming a significant other to him. Mentally ill persons have had much previous experience in familial and social relationships with persons who have initially accepted them but subsequently rejected them when their behavior became inappropriate. Therefore the client has a need to

In the orientation phase or getting acquainted period of the nurse-client relationship, the nurse's goals are the development of trust and establishing herself as a significant other to the client.

test the nurse's reliability before allowing himself to trust her. If the nurse does not view this change in the client's behavior as a test to determine just how much he can rely on her to be accepting and nonjudgmental of him, she might feel discouraged and decide to end the relationship. To act on this feeling would be a mistake, since it would confirm the client's view of the nurse as being no different than others who have disappointed him. More important, it would also confirm his view of himself as being unworthy and unacceptable. Rather than discontinuing the relationship the nurse must respond to the client's behavior with meticulous consistency. For example, if she has agreed to meet with him at a specified time and place, she must be there even if he does not appear. If she continues in this manner the client will soon have less need to test her, and the first phase of the relationship will be concluded.

It is important that the contract agreed upon by the nurse and the client be strictly adhered to.

The second phase in a therapeutic relationship between a nurse and a client is called the *maintenance* or *working phase*. The goal of this phase is the identification and resolution of the client's problem. Therefore the characteristics of this phase are highly individualized to the nature of the client's problems. Because each individual is unique and because the working phase of a relationship is so highly individualized to the particular client and nurse, few specific parameters can be given to guide the progress of this phase. An exception, however, is the necessity for limit setting, which often arises during this phase.

Limit setting is required when the client is threatening physical harm to himself or others, when he is destroying property or threatening to do so, and when his verbal hostility is upsetting and causing other clients or personnel to become tense and upset. If the client who requires limit setting is willing to discuss his behavior, it may be sufficient for the nurse to point out that he is causing a dangerous and disturbing situation and to request that he stop. For some persons such a request will be sufficient. However, others will require a more direct approach. In such an instance the nurse must speak firmly and explain that unless his disruptive behavior stops, he will have to be segregated from the group and placed in a room alone or will be given a medication to assist him to gain control of his behavior.

If the nurse initiates and enforces limit setting in an empathic and nonpunitive manner, the client will often feel a sense of relief from anxiety because another person has assumed the responsibility for identifying and enforcing the boundaries of his behavior. Rather than damaging the relationship, limit setting often serves to further convince the client that the nurse cares about him as a worthwhile individual.

In summary, the maintenance or working phase of the nurse-client relationship is the time to identify and address the client's problems. Unless both the nurse and the client are actively involved in this process the relationship cannot be effective. In maintaining a therapeutic relationship with a client, the nurse encourages him to express his concerns, fears, hopes, and problems. Sometimes she will be able to achieve this by asking direct and specific leading questions.

The nurse needs to recognize when she is able to intervene in the client's expressed concerns and when it is necessary to refer the client to other members of the treatment team who are prepared to cope with the specific problem. Therefore it is important for the nurse to understand how she and the other members of the team share responsibility for the client's therapy.

The third phase of the therapeutic relationship is referred to as the *termination* or *concluding phase*. It is unrealistic to expect a relationship to continue indefinitely. This fact should be recognized and planned for in the orientation phase of the nurse-client relationship.

When the nurse learns that it will be necessary for her to leave the client, she should discuss this fact with him as soon as possible. If the nurse knows at the outset of the relationship that it will be terminated at a specific time, the plans for the work of the nurse and the client should always include this fact. Terminating a relationship can be a traumatic experience for both the nurse and the client because they have shared much that is personal and important. At such a time many clients express the feeling that the nurse is forsaking them. The loss of a trusted nurse is an especially difficult problem for a client who has been unable to trust other people. It is not unusual for clients to act out their frustration at the news of the impending loss of a trusted nurse.

In view of the possible traumatic difficulties that the departure of the nurse presents to the client, the nurse must seek to understand the client's sense of loss and to help him express his feelings and cope with them. The goal of this phase of the relationship is to help the client to review what he has learned through the process of the relationship and to transfer these learnings to his interactions with other persons.

Although the client with whom the nurse has established an ongoing therapeutic relationship will require special help in accepting her departure, the entire group of clients with whom the nurse has been working will respond in a variety of ways to her expected loss. Ideally, clients in a psychiatric setting should experience a relatively constant professional staff with whom they can establish meaningful relationships and work out emotional problems. Clients, like all people, will react to an anticipated loss in a variety of ways, depending on the characteristic way in which they respond to loss, their unique emotional needs, and the relationship they have developed with the departing staff member. Some clients may become depressed and unconsciously believe that they have been personally responsible for the loss of the nurse. Other clients may not be able to accept the loss of this valued person and may repress the knowledge. They may report that no one told them that she was leaving. Other clients may respond with anger and may insist that the administrator take steps to see that the nurse does not leave.

When the nursing staff members are prepared for a variety of responses on the part of clients, they can understand, accept, and cope with their behavior. This means that they will need to spend time talking with and listening to cli-

The goal of the nurse in the maintenance or working phase is to help the client identify and resolve his problem. It is often necessary for the nurse to set limits during this phase.

The goal of the termination or concluding phase of the nurse-client relationship is to assist the client to review what he has learned from the relationship and to transfer this knowledge to his interactions with others.

ents. They will need to make themselves more available than usual to deal with the clients' many feelings about the situation and to reassure clients that they are not being abandoned. Sometimes it is helpful to encourage the clients to channel their feelings into some constructive activity. One way to redirect clients' concerns is to help them organize and carry out a party to honor the departing nurse.

It is unfortunate when clients are not given an opportunity to express their feelings about such a situation or helped to handle their feelings. When this happens, as it does when a valued staff member simply disappears without any explanation, the feelings are not avoided but appear in many unusual behavioral reactions. A group of clients who have suffered such an unexplained loss may suddenly rebel against the entire nursing staff, or the physician may find that many former symptoms that clients had previously experienced have been reactivated.

The client is not the only person who must cope with feelings of loss when the nurse-client relationship is terminated. By virtue of having established and maintained a relationship with the client the nurse has invested a great deal of time, energy, thought, and emotion in the client. As a result she also will experience a sense of loss when the relationship is terminated. If she does not allow herself to recognize these feelings she might express them indirectly by showing undue concern for the client's future welfare, by encouraging him to stay for a few more sessions, or by otherwise encouraging his dependence on her. As is true of the client, the nurse's previous experiences with and responses to loss are major determinants of her ability to effectively cope with the sense of loss she feels when a nurse-client relationship is terminated. Most nurses find it helpful at this time to seek the guidance of the professional who is supervising the relationship. The nurse must remember that if the termination phase is not handled skillfully by encouraging the client to assume the independence he is ready for, the nurse can negate the value of the work that has been done in the preceding phase. Table 7-2 summarizes the goals of and nurse behaviors in the nurse-client relationship.

ROLES AND FUNCTIONS OF THE NURSE

The three types of nurse-client interactions previously discussed provide the context within which the nurse assumes a variety of roles and functions. These shift frequently as the nurse strives to make her contacts with clients therapeutic. She is the creator of a therapeutic environment when she provides opportunities for clients to experience acceptance in the environment. Frequently she assumes the role of socializing agent when she helps individuals or groups to plan and participate in social events. The nurse finds that she must assume the role of counselor when clients need someone to listen with understanding and empathy while they talk about troublesome problems. The nurse is sometimes a teacher, especially when she helps clients learn to function in more socially ac-

TABLE 7-2 *Goals of and nurse behaviors in each phase of the nurse-client relationship*

Phase of nurse-client relationship	Goal	Nurse behaviors
Orientation	Development of trust Establishment of nurse as a significant other to client	Establishes mutually acceptable contract Responds to testing behavior of client by adhering strictly to terms of contract
Maintenance	Identification and resolution of client's problems	Highly individualized to the nature of the client's problems Empathic nonpunitive limit setting
Termination	Assist client to review what he has learned and to transfer this learning to interaction with others	Understands client's sense of loss Helps client express his feelings and cope with them Encourages client to channel feelings into constructive activity such as a farewell party Recognizes own feelings of loss

ceptable ways. Frequently she fills the role of parent surrogate when she gives emotional support and understanding or when she performs a nurturing activity such as feeding a client. Sometimes she functions in the familiar technical role of nurse as she performs such nursing duties as administering medications or treatments. Some nurses who have advanced educational preparation function in the therapist role by meeting with individuals, families, or groups at specified times and engaging them in a process designed to help them make fundamental system changes.

> Roles of the nurse in nurse-client interactions: (1) creator of a therapeutic environment, (2) socializing agent, (3) counselor, (4) teacher, (5) parent surrogate, (6) technician, and (7) therapist.

The nurse probably never functions in any single role at any given time; usually she fulfills all or several of them at once. For the sake of clarity, however, these roles will be discussed separately.

The nurse as creator of a therapeutic environment

One of the major therapeutic contributions the nurse can make is to develop a warm, accepting atmosphere. Although this atmosphere is related superficially to the furnishings and decor of the environment, these attributes are no substitute for genuine human warmth, which springs solely from other human beings. If the situation is to be therapeutic for clients, it is essential that the nursing staff who are in close daily contact with the clients be honest, sincere, friendly people who really care about others. If the nurse is able to establish a warm, accepting atmosphere, the contributions of all members of the treatment team can be of maximum effectiveness.

A feeling of security is an essential element in developing a therapeutic climate. When clients are provided with an emotionally secure climate, feelings of acceptance, friendliness, warmth, safety, and relaxation are present. Many mentally ill people enter a treatment setting because they are fearful, anxiety ridden, and insecure in their relationships with other people. A therapeutic climate should make it possible for such individuals to behave as they need to behave because of their illness, secure in the knowledge that they will not be rejected and that they do not need to fear retaliation.

Another essential element in creating a therapeutic climate is an attitude that anticipates positive change and growth. If the climate is to be therapeutic everyone working with clients must project an attitude that encourages improvement and positive change in behavior.

In the role of creator of a therapeutic environment, the nurse develops an accepting atmosphere.

The nurse as socializing agent

Another important role is that of socializing agent. In fulfilling this role the nurse helps clients participate successfully in group activities. Physical facilities in many mental health settings are ideal for organizing and directing group activities. In a residential setting, group activities are particularly needed during that period in the day after the evening meal. Many scheduled activities stop before supper, and clients are frequently faced with long, unoccupied evenings. The nurse who cares for clients during the evening hours has a significant opportunity to contribute to the mental health of these persons. Such a simple activity as an evening snack period can be the focus for group singing, group games, or group conversation. Activities organized by the clients themselves uncover and use hidden talent. In this way the group has an opportunity to recognize and encourage its own members and to contribute to developing the strengths of individuals. A dining room situation may lend itself to group activity. In such a situation the nurse has an opportunity to create an experience from which a feeling of belonging can develop. Mealtime is too often viewed solely from the standpoint of nutrition. Sometimes clients are hurried so that the staff can get on to some other activity. Conversation is sometimes discouraged because it slows up eating. The nurse who is with clients during mealtime may view her task solely from the standpoint of getting the clients fed as efficiently and quickly as possible. When the nurse ascribes to these views, she misses a valuable opportunity to facilitate positive learning experiences for clients.

In a nonresidential treatment setting, the nurse can assist clients to improve their social skills by introducing them to each other and then encouraging conversation by bringing up a neutral topic such as the weather. The community-based nurse who sits in an office waiting for the client to keep his appointment misses an important opportunity to assist clients to develop social skills in the common social setting of the waiting room.

The nurse makes a contribution to improving the social skills of clients by encouraging and developing the healthy aspects of their personalities. Many mentally ill persons have used withdrawal because of their extreme sensitivity and anxiety in relation to other people. The treatment setting provides opportunities for these individuals to learn to achieve success in social situations by creating opportunities through which they develop feelings of security with other people.

The nurse as counselor

Empathic listening is another important aspect of psychiatric nursing. There is probably no more important task than listening to a client in a positive, dynamic, empathic way without at the same time giving advice, stating opinions, or making suggestions. This type of active listening encourages the client to think through his problems and to arrive at a decision that is helpful to him. It helps the client to discharge anxiety and tension. It tells the client that the nurse really cares.

Empathic listening demands a great deal from the nurse both in time and emotional energy. It demands that she be skillful in reflecting the client's comments to him in such a manner that he will realize she is interested in the discussion and wants to hear as much as he needs to tell. Some nurses may not understand the vital importance of this kind of listening and may feel that they should stop the client's outpouring of problems. Unfortunately this is easily done by a comment such as, "You can tell all that to your therapist tomorrow. He's the one who needs to know these things." The nurse may respond with the even less helpful comment, "Things will be better tomorrow. Just keep a stiff upper lip." Clients often share their problems more freely with the nurse than with anyone else. The nurse and the other members of the mental health team need to determine their mutually therapeutic roles with the client so the nurse and client can assess which concerns may appropriately be channeled to which team member.

The role of the nurse is to help the client with problems of reality that deal with the here and now. Clients often discuss problems with the nurse that do deal with the areas that are her special concern, and it is in these situations that her role as a counselor is most frequently helpful.

Among the nurse's therapeutic responsibilities as a counselor is the giving of reassurance. Many situations in the life of a client require that someone give some reassurance. Sometimes the nurse may suggest that reassurance should more logically be provided by the psychiatrist, chaplain, or social worker. The nurse needs to learn what services are available and how she can get the assistance the client needs. However, more often than not it is up to the nurse to

In the role of socializing agent, the nurse can provide opportunities for clients to achieve greater success in social situations by helping them to develop feelings of security with other people.

provide the needed reassurance. Such needs appear in every area of the client's life. There is the client who cannot sleep because he fears the treatment scheduled for the morning; the client who is upset because her husband did not visit as he had promised and she is now sure that he does not love her; the client who believes he is doomed forever because he has committed an unpardonable sin; and the client who is afraid of everything. The list is endless, and the needs for reassurance frequently appear at 11 PM or at 3 AM when no help may be readily available. This is why many day-care centers provide staff members who are available by phone during the entire 24-hour period. Often the staff members are nurses or trained mental health aides whose prompt intervention can prevent the need for hospitalization.

Obviously no set of rules or suggestions will serve as a solution in each of these many situations. Probably the most effective reassurance for fearful, upset clients is a nursing staff that does not change frequently and whose members are consistently kind and accepting. Sitting beside a client may in itself be reassuring to him. This may help him feel that someone on whom he can depend is there, ready to help in whatever way possible. Listening is one of the better ways of offering reassurance. Although logical, reasonable answers are frequently not helpful, they may be reassuring for some clients. Effective reassurance is dependent on the situation, the nurse, her relationship with the client, and his personality. Obviously a suspicious client will require a different kind of help than will a depressed one.

Another aspect of the nurse's counseling role is in helping clients find acceptable outlets for anxiety. The client who is found sobbing hopelessly may be helped by a simple suggestion that he walk up and down the hallway with the nurse. Another client who is tense or excited may respond to the nurse's suggestion that he take a warm tub bath before going to bed. Some other ways in which the nurse may help clients find outlets for anxieties include assisting clients to participate in simple tasks, to become involved in some group activity, or to talk about their feelings.

The nurse as teacher

If purposeful therapeutic interventions can provide the individual with opportunities to learn to live a more satisfactory and satisfying life, they will make a significant contribution to the client's emotional growth. If the client is merely treated for the purpose of safeguarding his family, the community, or himself, and if he relies entirely on the judgment of professional personnel, it is questionable how worthwhile the experience can be. It is in helping the client to learn to cope in a more mature way that the nurse has a role as a teacher.

Problems of behavior manifested by mentally ill persons are as varied as life itself and encompass every aspect of living. Some clients, like children, must learn many simple tasks involved in living. They need help in learning to dress appropriately for the occasion; to assume responsibility for tasks assigned; to

In the role of counselor, the nurse performs the critical task of listening to a client in a positive, dynamic, empathic way without giving advice, stating opinions, or making suggestions.

care for physical needs so that they can be acceptable to others; to eat in socially prescribed ways; to accept a reasonably flexible schedule for eating, sleeping, and bathing; and to cope with many other aspects of group living.

The nurse may fill the role of teacher as she helps a client learn a new game, dance step, or song so that he may participate more actively in recreation. She may actually take the role of dance partner or may participate in a game to help a shy, frightened client become integrated into a group. The nurse may participate in an activity requiring only two persons to help a hostile, suspicious client learn that some people can be trusted. She may continue to participate with this client over a period of time until he is able to participate in a group activity without her supporting presence.

In her role as a teacher the nurse helps clients learn to participate in more socially acceptable and satisfying living activities.

The nurse has a role as a teacher in helping the client learn to participate in socially acceptable and satisfying living activities.

The nurse as parent surrogate

Traditionally in this culture the nurse has been a trusted person who performs personal services for sick people. Many of these services are similar to those a parent performs for children. Nurses who consistently function in mental health settings almost invariably become parent surrogates for some of the clients with whom they are closely associated. The role of parent surrogate is part of the traditional role of the nurse, and, although it does not imply becoming the client's parent, it includes many nurturing activities that may be required for some persons who are mentally ill. Although most mentally ill persons are able to bathe, dress, and feed themselves, there are a few who are too emotionally ill to carry out these simple tasks. For some of these persons the nurse may need to assume the traditional protective, supportive, parental role when she gives physical care.

Surrogate
A substitute parental figure.

The nurse, like an effective parent, realizes that it is important for clients to assume responsibility for their own physical care as soon as possible. Thus she gives physical care to mentally ill persons in an empathic and understanding way but looks for and seizes every opportunity to encourage them to assume responsibility for their own care as soon as possible. The effective nurse withdraws from the task of feeding or bathing a client just as soon as he is able to take over the responsibility for himself. In this way the nurse supports the client's increasing autonomy.

The nurse not only carries out the parental role in relation to the physical needs of clients, but she is also like a parent in relation to managing the treatment setting. It is she who develops many of the policies concerning the environment that profoundly affect the clients' lives. She is indirectly responsible for almost every aspect of the treatment setting, from housekeeping to securing emergency medical care. The nurse sets the tone of the treatment situation, much as parents set the tone of the family.

One of the most therapeutic aspects of the nurse's traditional role as parent surrogate is in assisting individuals and groups of clients to set limits for their own behavior. This aspect of the nurse's role probably overlaps the teacher role.

Clients who interact with each other over time may react toward each other as if they were members of the same family. These reactions are usually unconscious but are nonetheless real and may serve as a basis for much emotional and social unlearning and relearning. Therefore the nurse's role as parent surrogate offers her an opportunity to provide clients with healthy experiences in the area of emotional relationships.

While serving as the object of many of the angry, hostile feelings that some clients cannot otherwise admit or express, the nurse may be able to supply the warm, accepting, nurturing relationship that some persons require to move toward more mature behavior. In conjunction with other members of the mental health team, the nurse is able to provide experiences that may prove to be corrective of the client's earlier unsatisfactory interpersonal experiences.

The nurse's role as a parent surrogate offers her an opportunity to provide experiences that may correct earlier unsatisfactory interpersonal experiences.

The technical nursing role

The traditional role of the nurse includes those technical aspects involved in pouring and administering medications, monitoring vital signs, carrying out medical and surgical treatments, and observing and recording client behavior. Recently numerous nurses have become skilled in performing routine physical examinations. This activity, once limited to physicians, is becoming increasingly important for nurses to master as the inextricable relationship between the mind and body is recognized. Occasionally a mentally ill person can accept a nurse as a helpful counselor or teacher only after her ability to carry out the technical aspects of the role has been demonstrated. Therefore the nurse needs to be alert to the fact that such procedures as administering medications and taking vital signs provide her with an opportunity to enhance the therapeutic relationship with the client as well as to achieve the primary goal of the procedure.

The technical aspects of the nurse's role are of great value in themselves and also as a means of enhancing the therapeutic relationship.

The nurse's responsibilities regarding medications and charting are discussed below because they are two technical functions common to all psychiatric nurses. Most important, the way in which these functions are carried out has the potential for having a great impact on the well-being of the client.

Responsibilities of the nurse in regard to medications. Because of the widespread use of psychotropic agents in the treatment of mentally ill clients, it is not unusual for a nurse to spend a large part of her time preparing and administering medications. Unfortunately, some nurses believe that their responsibility has been fulfilled once these tasks are completed. However, such is not the case. The responsibilities of the nurse in regard to clients receiving psychotropic agents are numerous.

Before the client receives any medication, it is essential for a number of assessments to be made. Initially the client's medical history must be obtained, especially in regard to seizure disorder; pregnancy; cardiac, hepatic, or renal disease; and substance abuse. In addition, physiological baseline data about the client should be determined. These include blood pressure, both sitting and standing; pulse, both quality and rate; weight; sleep pattern; gait and movement; and blood chemistry. Many psychotropic agents affect these physiological processes, and an accurate assessment of their effect cannot be made unless baseline data are available to which a comparison can be made. In addition, the choice of drug and dosage are influenced by these factors.

As the nurse works with the client before he receives a medication, she often is in the best position to ascertain his attitude toward taking medications. Clients vary widely in their response to drug therapy, depending on such variables as their past experiences with psychotropic agents or other mind-altering drugs and their current state of orientation. Some clients are eager to receive medication and see it as the answer to all their problems. Others, particularly those who are suspicious, fear medication because of their feelings of loss of control. In most instances, both of these extreme views are not reality based. The client needs to be helped to develop a realistic picture of what a psychotropic agent can and cannot do.

Once having ascertained the client's medical history, his physiologic baseline, and his attitude toward taking medication, the nurse is in a position to collaborate with the physician in determining the most effective medication, dosage, frequency, and route of administration. Although the physician has the responsibility for prescribing psychotropic medications the assessments of a knowledgeable nurse are often relied on, especially in regard to dosage, frequency, and route of administration. If indicated by the assessment data, the nurse is wise to suggest the medication be ordered by alternate routes, as well as to obtain a *prn* order.

The specific actions of the prescribed drug should address those symptoms of the client's illness which are most distressing to him or to others. These symptoms are called *target symptoms,* and the degree to which they are ameliorated increases the likelihood of the client's continuing to cooperate with his treatment regimen. For example, a newly admitted client who is distressed by visual hallucinations and for whom an antipsychotic drug is prescribed will often be relieved by the diminution of this disturbing symptom. If he had been previously counseled by the nurse to expect this result, his trust in her and in the health care delivery system will be increased. However, it is important that the nurse make clear that it often takes as long as 6 or 8 weeks before improvement in target symptoms is seen.

After a drug has been ordered for the client, it is the nurse's responsibility to accurately prepare, administer, and record the medication and its effects. As previously stated, some nurses unfortunately see this phase of the treatment as the only aspect of their role or, if not the only aspect, the most important one. In reality the success the nurse has with this phase of the process depends

The nurse's responsibility to the client receiving psychotropic medications includes assessing him physiologically and attitudinally prior to and during this treatment.

The success the nurse has in administering the prescribed drug is highly dependent on the quality of the client assessment and the degree of physician-nurse collaboration.

greatly on the quality of the client assessment she has previously obtained and the degree of physician-nurse collaboration she has been able to establish.

Most nurses have much experience in preparing medications, and doing so in a psychiatric setting does not differ from executing this task in other settings. On the other hand, administering medications to mentally ill persons may be dramatically different than what the nurse is accustomed to. First, most mentally ill clients are ambulatory, and the nurse must use caution that the medications intended for a group of clients not be accessible while she is occupied with administering medications to one client. Some clients will try to steal medications for use as barter for items such as cigarettes. In addition, clients may take medications to save until a sufficient amount has been accumulated so they may attempt suicide. Finally, clients may accidentally knock the medications over, resulting in the potential loss of medication and the actual loss of the nurse's very valuable time. Therefore it is a desirable practice for the nurse to keep the medications inaccessible to the client group and to administer them to one client at a time.

While administering medication the nurse has a valuable opportunity to observe the client for side effects and adverse reactions as well as for changes in behavior. Of equal importance, she has the opportunity to interact with the client in such a way as to gain his acceptance of the medication. In this regard it is most often helpful for the nurse to refer to the drug as "medication" rather than using the word "drug" to prevent confusion with mind-altering street drugs. Nurses sometimes feel so rushed when administering medications that they resent the client's asking questions about his medications or otherwise lengthening the process. As a result it is not unusual for the nurse to be drawn into a power struggle with the client around the issue of whether or not he will take his medication and when he will do so. This common situation is unfortunate not only because it usually takes a great deal of time but, more important, because it sets a negative tone associated with taking medications. Rather than engaging in a power struggle with the client, the effective nurse takes the time to answer the client's questions and otherwise gives him as much control of the situation as possible. The client has the right and the need to know the name, dosage, actions, side effects, and adverse effects of the medicine he is taking.

While administering medication, the nurse has a valuable opportunity to observe the client for side effects, adverse reactions, and behavioral changes.

Clients who refuse medication present a particular challenge to the nurse. Before the nurse decides to omit the dose or to administer it parenterally she should make an assessment of why the client is refusing. Once again this takes time, but time might be saved in the long run. One chronically ill client was readmitted to the hospital because of an exacerbation of visual and auditory hallucinations probably precipitated by his having stopped his antipsychotic medication a month previously due to lack of money. Even though this client was known to the nursing staff as being cooperative, he refused to take his oral medication. Every time the nurse would extend her hand with the medication cup the client would become visibly distressed, perspire profusely, and wrap his arms tightly around himself. Although the staff were agreed that what this client needed most was the prescribed antipsychotic medication, they disagreed about how it should be administered. Some maintained that the client should be restrained and given the medication by injection. The nurse who knew him best, however, was struck by his uncharacteristic refusal of the medication and by the consistency of his behavior when offered it. She hypothesized that the client was perceiving the nurse's extended arm as an attack and consequently was experiencing massive amounts of anxiety when efforts were made to give him medication. Based on this assessment she approached the client from the side, laid the medication and water cups on the counter, slowly explained what they were, and gently directed the client to take the medication. Within a very short time the client complied. This thoughtful intervention by the nurse allowed the client to maintain control of the situation, accomplished the nurse's goal, and avoided the difficult and potentially traumatic situation of having to forcibly administer an injection.

> When a client refuses medication, the nurse should make an assessment of why he is refusing before deciding to omit the dose or to administer it parenterally.

It is important that the nurse document and otherwise communicate to other staff interpersonal interventions that have proven useful in working with clients who resist taking medications. The use of the same approaches will help to ensure consistency in treatment and increase the client's trust in the staff.

Once the client has begun a regimen of psychotropic medications it is the nurse's responsibility to monitor his physiological response to the medication. Obviously, to do so effectively, the nurse must be knowledgeable about the intended effects, side effects, and adverse effects of the drugs the client is receiving. She must observe him carefully and listen to his reports with concern. When side effects appear the nurse can reassure the client that these are anticipated and make suggestions for reducing his discomfort. For example, the dry mouth associated with the phenothiazines can be diminished by the client chewing sugarless gum or sucking on hard candy. If adverse effects occur, the nurse must notify the physician immediately and in most instances withhold the medication.

The ultimate goal of treatment with psychotropic medications is to enable the client to function at the highest level possible with the least amount of medication. To achieve this goal the nurse is most helpful when she works with the client on developing nonchemical adaptations to his symptoms such as increasing his interpersonal resources and skills. For clients who must remain on maintenance doses of medication, the nurse has the responsibility to help the client learn as much as he is able about the medication he is taking and also to learn how to administer it to himself correctly.

> To enable the client to function at the highest level possible with the least amount of medication is the treatment goal with psychotropic medications.

Responsibilities of the nurse in regard to charting. One of the nurse's most significant responsibilities is the accurate and perceptive observation and recording of the client's behavior. In carrying out this function skillfully and meaningfully the nurse contributes to the understanding that all members of the mental health team bring to bear on the client's problems. Nurses are the professional persons who are with clients for the longest period of time; as such they have a unique opportunity to help other professionals understand clients' needs through effective recording of samples of conversation, sleep patterns, interpersonal relationships, socialization activities, and descriptions of personal habits.

It is suggested that the client's behavior be described rather than labeled. Not only do labels have stereotypical meanings, they may also convey different messages to different readers. Instead of recording that a client is hallucinating, it is more meaningful to record exactly what was observed. The following is an example of this type of recording: "Stood near the ventilator for 10 minutes with hand cupped around ear as if trying to hear better. Carried on an animated conversation. Although no other person was present, the client could be heard saying, "How dare you call me those names! You are a liar!'"

Instead of recording that the client is disoriented and misidentifies people, it would be more meaningful to record the following: "Mr. J. greeted the nurse by saying, 'Good morning, Mary. Have you cooked breakfast yet?' In the afternoon he asked, 'When are we going to have breakfast?' Client believes that this nurse is his wife, and he is not able to differentiate between morning and afternoon."

By recording her observations in this manner, the nurse permits the reader to make his own interpretation of the meaning of the client's behavior.

The nurse as therapist

For a number of years some nurses who have had the benefit of an appropriate educational experience in psychiatric nursing have been developing the role of the nurse therapist. When the nurse functions in the role of nurse therapist, she uses the principles developed through the practice of psychotherapy.

Nursing therapy has developed differently in each situation, but basically it follows the same general guidelines. The role of the nurse therapist is carefully explained to all levels of the professional staff and to all clients in the clinical situation. Every attempt is made to be sure that the role is understood before any therapeutic activity is initiated. The nurse collaborates with other mental health professionals in the situation and confers regularly with those responsible for developing the treatment plans for the clients with whom she is working. The nurse's intervention becomes a part of the total treatment plan for the client.

As is the case with all therapists, it is essential that the nurse identify a skilled professional therapist to function on a regular basis as her preceptor or her supervisor while she is working as a nurse therapist. By doing so the nurse therapist enhances the effectiveness of her interactions with the client as well as increases her own knowledge and skill.

The nurse therapist should record each therapy session so that it can be used to (1) review the dynamics of the relationship, (2) analyze the problems

Nurses with advanced education often assume the role of nurse therapist and use the principles developed through the practice of psychotherapy.

that have been presented, and (3) evaluate client progress against the established treatment goals.

END NOTE

The focus of this chapter is, as its title suggests, nurse-client interactions. The importance of acceptance and consistency is emphasized throughout the discussion of the three types of nurse-client interactions. The characteristics of the developmental phases of the nurse-client relationship are discussed in depth because this form of interaction has the greatest potential for providing the client with a corrective interpersonal experience. The roles and functions the nurse fulfills as she engages in nurse-client interactions are discussed and include her role as: the creator of a therapeutic environment; a socializing agent; a counselor; a teacher; a parent surrogate; a technician; and, for some nurses, a therapist.

SUGGESTED SOURCES OF ADDITIONAL INFORMATION

Bayer M: Saying goodbye through graffiti: it all began when we were about to discharge Hilda, Am J Nurs 80:271, February 1980.

Garant C: Stalls in the therapeutic process, Am J Nurs 80:2166, 1980.

Johnson M: Self-disclosure: a variable in the nurse-client relationship, J Psychosoc Nurs Ment Health Serv 18:17, January 1980.

Kasch CR: Toward a theory of nursing action: skills and competency in nurse-patient interaction, Nurs Res 35(4):226, July/August 1986.

Lego SM: The one-to-one nurse-patient relationship, Perspect Psychiatr Care 18(2):67, March-April 1980.

Littlefield NT: Therapeutic relationship: a brief encounter, Am J Nurs 82:1395, 1982.

Loomis ME: Levels of contracting, J Psychosoc Nurs Ment Health Serv 23(3):8, 1985.

Payton R: Truth is essential for trust between nurse, patient, Am Nurse 16(6):11, 18, 1984.

Schroder PJ: Recognizing transference and countertransference, J Psychosoc Nurs 23(2):21, February 1985.

Topf M and Dambacher B: Teaching interpersonal skills: a model for facilitating optimal interpersonal relations, J Psychosoc Nurs Ment Health Serv 19:29, December 1981.

Trotter CMF: I never promised you a rose garden but I must remember to tell you about the thorns, J Psychosoc Nurs 23(3):15, March 1985.

Tudor GE: A sociopsychiatric nursing approach to intervention in a problem of mutual withdrawal on a mental hospital ward, J Psychiatr 15:193, 1952.

Yuen FKH: The nurse-client relationship: a mutual learning experience, J Adv Nurs 11:529, 1986.

The therapeutic environment

8

LEARNING OBJECTIVES

After studying this chapter the student will be able to:

○ State the goals of a therapeutic environment.

○ Discuss the characteristics of a therapeutic environment.

○ Explain the necessity for setting limits in a therapeutic environment.

○ Discuss the influence of the physical environment on the therapeutic environment.

○ State the significant aspects of a therapeutic community.

○ Discuss the implications of the therapeutic environment for the role of the nurse.

Research has documented that the environment in which the mentally ill person is treated is a major factor in enhancing or impeding the therapeutic effects of other treatment modalities. Thus, the existence of a therapeutic environment is necessary regardless of the type of setting in which a client is treated.

When the environment itself becomes a treatment modality, it is referred to as a therapeutic community, a specialized form of the therapeutic environment.

Because the nurse is with the client for a longer period of time than is any other professional and because both the nurse and the client are directly affected by the environment, it is well accepted that the major responsibility to create and maintain a therapeutic environment lies with the nursing staff.

Creating and maintaining a therapeutic environment are major responsibilities of the nursing staff.

HISTORICAL PERSPECTIVE

The archives of American psychiatry include records of early successful attempts to develop a homelike atmosphere for mentally ill persons with provision for social and recreational activities. Physicians and their families joined other staff members in initiating and directing some of these activities. Early in the nineteenth century emphasis on a homelike environment, recreational activities, and a sympathetic approach to clients was referred to as *moral treatment.* In 1842 Boston State Hospital was reported to have placed emphasis on moral treatment for mentally ill individuals. The superintendent of one psychiatric hospital in Massachusetts is reported to have invited inmates to his home for Sunday dinner. Intimate discussions of the inmates' personal problems and difficulties were part of the therapy offered in those institutions at that time.

Some authorities believe that the era of moral treatment ended because of the large numbers of immigrants who arrived in the United States after the Civil War. Many of these people could not cope with the problems of adjustment presented by the radically different environment they found in this country and were therefore deemed mentally ill. Large numbers of inmates with differing cultural backgrounds and languages swelled the census of mental institutions and made it difficult if not impossible to provide a homelike environment. Thus the era of moral treatment passed.

By 1940 large public hospitals were filled to overflowing. Because of the ever-increasing patient population the task of the hospital personnel was staggering. They were able to do little more than keep the inmates bathed, dressed, and fed.

An unprecedented national concern for the welfare of mentally ill persons after World War II and the introduction of the first of the antipsychotic drugs in the early 1950s fostered a resurgence of interest in the therapeutic potential of the hospital environment. It was within this context that *Social Psychiatry,* a small book by Dr. Maxwell Jones, was published in England in 1953.

When published in the United States Dr. Jones's book was titled *The Therapeutic Community,* and it soon became one of the motivating forces in the movement to use the hospital environment therapeutically in the treatment regimen of mentally ill persons. This influential book was a report of efforts at Belmont Hospital in England during and after World War II to rehabilitate neurotic patients through group methods. That experience in group living at Belmont Hospital came to be known as the *therapeutic community,* a specialized form of therapeutic environment. In the therapeutic community, particular attention was paid to the development of the social structure of the hospital and to communication between patients and the hospital staff. Dr. Jones dedicated his book to "The Nursing Staff who have formed a framework around which our therapeutic communities have been built." Although the nurses to whom he referred were not registered nurses, they were intelligent, capable, mature women who used the interpersonal skill and understanding required in psychiatric nursing. The dedication is appropriate. Without a nursing staff with insight, understanding, personal warmth, and skill in directing groups, the concept of a therapeutic community could not have developed into a reality.

GOALS AND CHARACTERISTICS OF A THERAPEUTIC ENVIRONMENT

As with any treatment regimen, a therapeutic environment is most likely to be successful if its implementation is consistent with the philosophy of the professional staff and if it is guided by goals derived from that philosophy. Based on the philosophy stated in Chapter 5, the goals of a therapeutic environment are to help the individual increase his self-esteem and feelings of personal worth, to improve his ability to relate to others, and to enable him to work and live more effectively in the community. The probability of these goals' being achieved is increased in a treatment setting that has the following characteristics:

1. The client's physical needs are met.
2. The client is respected as an individual with rights, needs, and opinions and is encouraged to express these.
3. Decision-making authority is clearly defined and distributed appropriately among clients and staff.
4. The client is protected from injury from self and others, but only those restrictions necessary to afford such protection are imposed.
5. The client is afforded increasing opportunities for freedom of choice, commensurate with his ability to make decisions.
6. All personnel, but particularly nursing staff, remain constant, e.g., unit and shift assignments remain stable.
7. The environment provides a testing ground for the establishment of new patterns of behavior.
8. Emphasis is placed on social interaction between and among clients and staff and the physical structure and appearance of the environment facilitate this interaction.
9. Programming is structured but flexible.

Providing for the client's physical needs

Although the majority of the characteristics of a therapeutic environment are concerned with its socioemotional climate and physical structure, it is important for the nurse to understand that no environment can be therapeutic if it does not provide for meeting the physical needs of clients. Great effort has been expended to improve the care of mentally ill persons by altering treatment settings from custodial to therapeutic environments. In the process, however, some benefits of "custodial" care have been discarded. For example, ensuring that clients have adequate diet and rest and appropriate clothing and are monitored for signs of illness may be sacrificed in the service of socioemotional interventions. The probability of focusing solely on the client's physical or emotional needs is enhanced by the dualistic manner in which the health care delivery system continues to function. The reality is that humans are holistic beings and therefore respond holistically. For example, it is not uncommon for a confused client to have nutritional deficits secondary to his inability to purchase, prepare, or eat nourishing meals. Furthermore, many of the psychotropic drugs

To help the client develop a sense of self-esteem and personal worth, to improve his ability to relate to others, to help him learn to trust others, and to enable him to return to the community better prepared to work and live are the goals of a therapeutic environment.

The characteristics of a therapeutic environment are related primarily to its socioemotional climate and physical structure.

The physical as well as emotional needs of the client are met in an environment that is truly therapeutic.

commonly used to treat mental illness have very serious potential side effects. Therefore, in an environment that is truly therapeutic the nursing staff continuously assesses and intervenes with each client in a comprehensive and holistic manner.

Socioemotional climate essential to a therapeutic environment

Once it is assured that the environment is designed to address the physical needs of the client, the socioemotional climate of the treatment setting must be addressed. To be therapeutic this climate must reflect respect for the client as a human being who has value and worth. As such, the nursing staff recognizes and respects the client's rights and opinions and sees him as an indispensable ally in the formulation and implementation of his treatment plan. While it is important that both the staff and the clients understand who is responsible for making which decisions, the nursing staff in a therapeutic environment frequently solicit the opinions of the clients about matters that affect them. For example, rules regarding television viewing are often more productively made by the clients rather than by the staff.

> Decision making in a therapeutic environment is guided by the principle that those influenced by a decision are involved in making the decision.

Obviously an environment that is therapeutic provides for the protection of the client from injury from both himself and others. Protecting the client from injury includes, but is not limited to, physical protection. It also includes safeguarding him against making significant decisions when he is not well enough to do so. Thus the nursing staff may find it necessary to help the client avoid making decisions about such matters as a pending divorce or separation or the sale of property.

Some clients want and need reassurance that the staff will establish rules of conduct within which all clients will function. The process of establishing and enforcing such guidelines is referred to as limit setting. The establishment of limits is best done by all those affected by the rule, including the clients and the entire treatment team. The basis for rules should be an anticipated positive effect on the growth of the clients.

> Limit setting in a therapeutic environment means establishing rules of conduct involving all those affected by a rule.

By involving all those affected by the rule in its establishment, the likelihood of imposing the personal standards of behavior of one person on all others is decreased. It is apparent that before any rule that regulates client activity is established, all aspects of the results of such action should be considered, including enforcing the rule once it is established. Consistency in enforcing limits is necessary if the rule is to have its desired effect. However, a rule that cannot be enforced is less therapeutic than no rule at all, in that clients can become quite anxious about the staff's apparent lack of control of the situation.

> Although making rules is necessary in a therapeutic environment, rules that exist should be both enforceable and beneficial for the clients.

The nurse can easily confuse limit setting with control of behavior. She may rationalize that many of the controls that have been imposed are limits placed on the situation for the safety and security of clients when in reality they exist because of tradition, personal idiosyncrasies of one or more staff members, or to facilitate ease of management of the setting. To be sure, when groups of people live together rules need to be established that may not be necessarily equally beneficial to all involved. Nevertheless, rules designed to make life easier for the nursing staff that have no benefit to the clients should be recognized as such and avoided.

Although appropriate limit setting is essential to the establishment and maintenance of an emotional climate conducive to a therapeutic environment, the nursing staff also strives to establish as few rules and regulations as possible for client behavior and restricts activity only when necessary. Opportunities for freedom of choice are provided. As the client demonstrates his ability to accept more responsibility for his behavior, opportunities for making choices are increased.

A nursing staff that is sensitive, friendly, and concerned about the welfare of each and every client is imperative if an environment is to be therapeutic. While it is not likely that every nurse will care deeply about every client, each client should feel that there is at least one nurse on whom he can rely as an advocate. To establish such a relationship requires that there be constancy among staff in the treatment setting. Unfortunately, the major determinants of staffing assignments are often the managerial needs of the setting and the personal preferences of the staff. Ironically, the relationship needs of the clients are the last factor to be considered, if they are considered at all.

As the client improves, he will experiment with different ways of viewing his world and the people in it. Thus, he will develop new ways of responding to others and of coping with stress. Some of these new methods of dealing with problems may not be appropriate. If the environment is truly therapeutic, these attempts at learning new patterns of behavior will be recognized as such and met with understanding by the nursing staff. Frequently, clients need encouragement to continue testing new patterns of behavior until they have achieved more satisfying and satisfactory patterns of behavior.

Learning new patterns of behavior and testing them should be encouraged by the nursing staff as clients begin to improve.

Finally, if the environment is to be therapeutic, the client needs to know what to expect there. Research has shown that mentally ill persons respond most favorably in environments in which activities are structured. On the other hand, the activities should not be so structured that their implementation becomes the goal rather than meeting the needs of the clients. For example, it is almost always useful to have a week's activities preplanned and made known to clients and staff alike. However, if an untoward event such as a client suicide occurs, or an unanticipated opportunity such as a field trip to the circus arises, the staff should be flexible enough to cancel the planned activity to deal with the event or to take advantage of the opportunity.

A structured environment, yet one that is also flexible, will provide an atmosphere in which a client knows what to expect—an important aspect of an environment that is therapeutic.

INFLUENCE OF PHYSICAL ENVIRONMENT ON THE THERAPEUTIC ENVIRONMENT

A therapeutic climate for mentally ill persons depends on the attitude of the staff toward mental illness and the needs of the clients and does not develop as

OF SPECIAL INTEREST

One of the most widely used tools to measure ward atmosphere is the Ward Atmosphere Scale (WAS) (Moos RH: Evaluating treatment environments: a social-ecological approach, London, 1974, Wiley). This instrument consists of ten subscales that both staff and clients complete in terms of their perception of ward atmosphere as it actually exists and what they believe should exist. The differences between the "real" and the "ideal" provide the basis for instituting change in the environment that is likely to be accepted by all concerned. The subscales and their definitions* are:

1. Involvement—Measures how active and energetic patients are in the day-to-day social functioning of the ward, both as members of the ward as a unit and as individuals interacting with other patients. Patient attitudes such as pride in the ward, feelings of group spirit, and general enthusiasm are also assessed.

2. Support—Measures how helpful and supportive patients are toward other patients, how well the staff understand patient needs and are willing to help and encourage patients, and how encouraging and considerate doctors are toward patients.

3. Spontaneity—Measures the extent to which the environment encourages patients to act openly and to freely express their feelings toward other patients and staff.

4. Autonomy—Assesses how self-sufficient and independent patients are encouraged to be in their personal affairs and in their relationships with staff; how much responsibility and self-direction patients are encouraged to exercise; and to what extent the staff are influenced by patient suggestions, criticism, and other initiatives.

5. Practical orientation—Assesses the extent to which the patient's environment orients him toward preparing himself for release from the hospital and for the future. Such things as training for new kinds of jobs, looking to the future, and setting and working toward practical goals are considered.

6. Personal problem orientation—Measures the extent to which patients are encouraged to be concerned with their feelings and problems and to seek to understand them through openly talking to other patients and staff about themselves and their past.

7. Anger and aggression—Measures the extent to which a patient is allowed and encouraged to argue with patients and staff, to become openly angry and to display other expressions of anger.

8. Order and organization—Measures how important order is on the ward, in terms of patients (how they look), staff (what they do to encourage order), and the ward itself (how well it is kept); also measures organization, again in terms of patients (do they follow a regular schedule, do they have carefully planned activities) and staff (do they keep appointments, do they help patients follow schedules).

9. Program clarity—Measures the extent to which the patient knows what to expect in the day-to-day routine of his ward and how explicit the ward rules and procedures are.

10. Staff control—Measures the extent to which it is necessary for the staff to restrict patients, i.e., in the strictness of rules and schedules, in the relationships between patient and staff, and in measures taken to keep patients under effective control.

*Taken from: Milne D: Planning and evaluating innovations in nursing practice by measuring the ward atmosphere, J Adv Nurs 11:206, 1986.

the result of any fixed type of architecture. It can be developed in any type of setting if the staff focuses on meeting the needs of clients. However, it is helpful if certain structural features are present. The needs of clients can be met more effectively if facilities for privacy, socialization, and planned activities are available. If such facilities are not already present, innovations must be introduced if a therapeutic environment is to be created.

If a person's self-esteem is to be raised, it is essential to provide an opportunity for privacy and a place where his personal belongings can be kept. In most settings a substitute has been found for the barrack-like dormitories and public showers with which many large psychiatric hospitals were once equipped. The mass approach to the care of human beings destroys self-esteem and the sense of individual worth. The key to a therapeutic environment is provision for the unique needs of individuals rather than dealing with clients as members of a crowd. In the past the idea that nothing should be arranged for one client unless it could be arranged for the group led many hospital staffs away from treating people as individuals. This attitude sometimes increased the client's difficulties rather than providing opportunities for him to solve problems.

If clients are to receive individualized care, and if the environment is to be therapeutic, living quarters must be attractive and inviting. In most instances no more than two or three persons should share the same bedroom. If possible, single rooms should be provided for individuals who have strong feelings about sharing a room with another person. Clothes closets and dressers or satisfactory substitutes for this equipment must be available. It is important for mentally ill persons to bring personal clothing and other equipment to the hospital so that they can be attractively and appropriately groomed. The use of hospital clothing may be necessary in rare instances, but in the past this dress helped to depersonalize the patients and reduced them to a group of human beings with a universal attitude of hopelessness. Because it is therapeutic for clients to assume responsibility for their personal cleanliness, laundry facilities should be available.

Furniture arrangement in communal areas such as day rooms is very important in facilitating social interaction between and among clients and staff. A variety of comfortable chairs and sofas should be organized in conversational groupings to encourage spontaneous discussion. Furthermore, the furniture should be light enough to be easily moved when a larger group needs to be accommodated. Although a television set is almost always present in a day room, it should not be the focal point of the room with all the furniture arranged to facilitate easy viewing. In such a setting, even the casual observer understands that the solitary activity of television viewing is more valued than is social interaction.

Dining room facilities are important in developing a therapeutic environment. Mealtime should be a leisurely experience and a time for sharing ideas

Meeting needs for privacy and an attractive environment play an important part in meeting the emotional needs of the client.

and reinforcing friendly relationships. It is not merely a time for the intake of food. Nurses can profitably assume a therapeutic role by serving as hostesses at small tables that seat groups of four to six clients. The role of hostess is more effective if the nurse shares the meal with the clients. This plan has been used successfully in some hospitals. As hostess the nurse can encourage conversation and can help make mealtime a happy, relaxed, and rewarding group experience. Such mealtime experiences cannot be initiated unless there is a dining room attached to the unit itself. Serving meals in large, noisy dining rooms where hundreds of people are fed gets food to clients but makes it impossible to accomplish other therapeutic goals.

Bathrooms should provide privacy. Although locks on doors may not be advisable, it is possible to provide toilet doors that close and shower rooms equipped with screens. The old practice of showering 10 to 15 persons at a time helped to reduce the individual to a member of a crowd and negated other attempts to help him feel like a respected human being. The therapeutic environment can develop most effectively when physical surroundings help clients to feel that they are respected and that their personal preferences are recognized, appreciated, and considered.

THE THERAPEUTIC COMMUNITY—A FORM OF THERAPEUTIC ENVIRONMENT

Therapeutic community
A treatment approach in which the entire milieu is used as treatment. The physical environment, the other clients, the staff, and the policies of the facility influence the function of the individual in the activities of daily living in the community.

The therapeutic community is a treatment modality wherein the environment itself is used as a therapeutic intervention. The therapeutic community strives to involve the client in his own therapy, to restore his self-confidence by providing many opportunities for decision making, to increase his self-awareness, and to focus his attention and concern away from self and toward the needs of others. It has been organized in various ways in different settings and has been most successful with groups of clients who are in contact with reality.

Significant aspects of a therapeutic community include the following:

1. The emphasis in a therapeutic community is placed on social and group interaction, with both individual clients and staff as important members of the community.
2. The goal of the therapeutic community is to provide a favorable climate in which clients can gain an awareness of their feelings, thoughts, impulses, and behavior; try new interpersonal skills in a relatively safe environment; increase personal self-esteem; and realistically appraise the potentially helpful and destructive aspects of their behavior.
3. The work of the therapeutic community and the maintenance of an open network of communication are achieved through a daily meeting attended by all staff members and all clients who work and live on the specific unit.
4. A successful therapeutic community requires that both staff and individual clients become fully aware of their roles, limitations, responsibilities, and authority.

5. Staff members in a therapeutic community make information openly available to clients with whom they share treatment responsibilities.
6. The treatment arena in the therapeutic community includes all relationships among the members of the community, with special attention being given to the network of communication among members.

An important feature of a therapeutic community is the establishment of a democratic environment in which those people who are affected by a decision are involved in making it. Historically, administrators and professional staffs have believed that persons who are ill enough to require hospitalization are incapable of making wise judgments and therefore must have all decisions made for them. Clients in most hospitals where this philosophy has been implemented have been reduced to a dependent state. Recently there has been a growing realization that forcing an adult person into such a dependent role is not usually necessary and is not therapeutic. Of course, there are some completely dependent persons for whom all decisions must be made. This is obviously true of acutely ill or unconscious patients. However, in spite of the reason for hospitalization a majority of adults are able to make valid decisions about many things involving their welfare. Forcing the dependent role on some mentally ill persons may be particularly unfortunate. Some of them have spent a lifetime struggling against an unconscious desire to accept a dependent role. When hospitalization forces this role on such an individual, he may never be able to relinquish it.

A therapeutic community requires that clients have an opportunity to participate in the formulation of hospital rules and regulations that affect their personal liberties. Following through with such a plan means that clients would be involved in formulating policies that regulate smoking, bedtime, late night privileges, weekend passes, social activities, control of the radio, television, and piano, check-in time when returning to the hospital from a weekend, reporting for meals, and the many other aspects of personal life that are influenced by rules in the usual psychiatric setting. Also, it is thought to be therapeutic to involve clients in making decisions about behavior and relationships among the unit population. Thus clients in a therapeutic community might be given responsibility for rendering a judgment about the infringement of unit rules, settling arguments between clients, judging the appropriateness of granting weekend privileges for certain members of the group, and many other decisions regarding the regulation of life on the unit.

Careful preparation of both the staff and the clients should be assured before a therapeutic community is initiated. The staff may have difficulty accepting the activities and responsibilities granted to clients. Before a therapeutic community is initiated, a thorough exploration of the implications of such an undertaking should be carried on through group discussions. All levels of staff from physicians to attendants, kitchen helpers, and cleaning people should be involved in these group discussions because all will be affected by the therapeutic community. All members of the staff need to have a thorough understanding of the goals and limitations of the undertaking. Clients should also have an opportunity to explore its implications through group discussions. Both clients and staff need to understand what responsibilities they can and cannot assume.

Active administrative sanction, acceptance, and interest are essential if the therapeutic community is to be successful. Involving clients in decision making represents a drastic change in the entire administrative philosophy of many hospitals. The therapeutic community cannot be expected to function smoothly at all times, and problems will undoubtedly arise. Decisions made by clients will not always be the most appropriate. Unless the entire staff believes that involving clients in decision making is therapeutically valuable and worth the struggle, dissenting forces may destroy the undertaking.

Meetings of the therapeutic community should be held regularly and at specific times if they are to be effective. Meetings should not be allowed to deteriorate into complaint sessions or to focus entirely on what the hospital should do for clients. This can be avoided if the group has some real responsibility for solving problems relating to clients' needs.

In one instance the members of a therapeutic community in a small unit of a large New York psychiatric hospital held a meeting to consider the problem of three suicide attempts made in one week by a young woman on the unit. Their decision was to institute a buddy system so that she would be accompanied at all times by one of a group of clients, each of whom would be assigned to spend a specific amount of time with her daily. Several weeks after this decision was made, the system was working well, and the woman had made no further suicide attempts. At this same meeting other problems considered were the problem of a client who did not return on time from a weekend holiday, a fight between two clients, and the request by a new client for a weekend pass.

It is far easier for the staff to make all decisions for clients, but there is little that is therapeutic in this procedure. When clients have the opportunity to make decisions about their own and other people's behavior, they are presented with a realistic learning experience.

THE IMPLICATIONS OF THE THERAPEUTIC ENVIRONMENT FOR THE NURSE

It is not possible to develop a therapeutic environment without the strong, intelligent leadership of a nurse. When many of the traditional rules and regulations of the psychiatric unit are discarded and it becomes a place that focuses on meeting the needs of the individual and the group, the nurse is forced to accept a more active therapeutic role with clients. She finds it necessary to assign the clerical work, which formerly kept her confined to the nurse's station, to a secretary to free herself to give leadership to the personnel as they participate with clients in all the planned activities. Mentally ill persons require mature help and guidance in initiating and carrying out social activities.

When clients begin to experiment with new ways of behaving, they will make use of the nurse as an understanding person with whom they can discuss daily problems and emotional stressors. The nurse needs to be more alert than ever to changes in behavior. In a therapeutic environment many of the traditional safeguards are removed, and therefore safety of clients depends more than ever on an alert nursing staff. Thus it becomes the responsibility of the nurse to recognize changes in mood and behavior of clients and to intervene at appropriate times.

Skill in understanding group behavior and in directing groups is essential in the therapeutic environment. The nurse needs to work actively with client government to solve many unit problems. Finally, active, functioning channels of communication are essential. The nurse's ability as a leader will be reflected in the total effectiveness of the psychiatric team and ultimately in the therapeutic climate of the psychiatric unit. To a large extent the effectiveness of the client's total hospital experience will depend on the level of professional leadership provided by the nurse.

> The nurse must take an active leadership role in creating a therapeutic environment, delegating tasks that formerly kept her confined to the nurse's station in a clerical capacity.

END NOTE

This chapter discusses the unique responsibility of the nurse for creating and maintaining a therapeutic environment to facilitate the therapeutic effects of other treatment modalities. Although the majority of the characteristics of a therapeutic environment are concerned with the socioemotional climate and physical structure, providing for the client's physical needs is seen as fundamental to achieving an environment that is truly therapeutic. The therapeutic community as a form of therapeutic environment is also discussed. Its value with clients who are in contact with reality is emphasized.

SUGGESTED SOURCES OF ADDITIONAL INFORMATION

Baldwin LJ and Ramos NB: Role of the health care supervisor in management of a therapeutic milieu, Health Care Supervisor 4(4):12, July 1986.

Baldwin S: Effects of furniture rearrangement on the atmosphere of wards in a maximum security hospital, Hosp Commun Psychiatr 36:525, July 1985.

Bell MD and Ryan ER: Where can therapeutic community ideals be realized? an examination of three treatment environments, Hosp Commun Psychiatr 36(12):1286, December 1985.

Carser D: Primary nursing in the milieu, J Psychosoc Nurs Ment Health Serv 19:35, February 1981.

Collins JF et al: Treatment characteristics of effective psychiatric programs, Hosp Commun Psychiatr 35(6):601, June 1984.

Corey LJ et al: Psychiatric ward atmosphere, J Psychosoc Nurs Ment Health Serv 24(10):10, October 1986.

Devine B: Therapeutic milieu/milieu therapy: an overview, J Psychosoc Nurs Ment Health Serv 19:20, March 1981.

Greenblatt M, York RH, and Brown IL: From custodial to therapeutic patient care in mental hospitals, New York, 1979, Arno Press, Inc.

Gutheil TG: The therapeutic milieu: changing themes and theories, Hosp Commun Psychiatr 36(12):1279, December 1985.

Islam A and Turner D: The therapeutic community: a critical reappraisal, Hosp Commun Psychiatr 33:651, August 1982.

Jones M: Beyond the therapeutic community, New Haven, Conn., 1968, Yale University Press.

Jones M: The therapeutic community: a new treatment method in psychiatry, New York, 1953, Basic Books, Inc.

Kruzich JM and Kruzich SJ: Milieu factors influencing patients' integration into community residential facilities, Hosp Commun Psychiatr 36(4):378, April 1985.

Lacy M: Creating a safe and supportive treatment environment, Hosp Commun Psychiatr 32:44, January 1981.

Milne D: Planning and evaluating innovations in nursing practice by measuring the ward atmosphere, J Adv Nurs 11:203, 1986.

Raskinski K, Razinshy R, and Pasulka P: Practical implications of a theory of the "therapeutic milieu" for psychiatric nursing practice, J Psychosoc Nurs Ment Health Serv 18:16, May 1980.

Warner S: Humor and self-disclosure within the milieu, J Psychosoc Nurs Ment Health Serv 22:17, April 1984.

Wilmer H: Defining and understanding the therapeutic community, Hosp Commun Psychiatr 32:95, February 1981.

The nursing process

9

LEARNING OBJECTIVES

After studying this chapter the student will be able to:

○ Describe the five phases of the nursing process.

○ Discuss the importance of an organizational schema in providing direction for a comprehensive client assessment.

○ Describe the characteristics of an effective interview.

○ Discuss observation as a means of client assessment.

○ State a nursing diagnosis that stems from the assessment data in a manner that provides direction for the development of a plan of nursing care.

○ Develop a hypothetical plan of nursing care from a nursing diagnosis.

All too often the same nurse who systematically plans, implements, and evaluates care for the physically ill individual relies on on-the-spot intuitive judgment in administering care to the mentally ill person. This practice is likely to result in therapeutic interactions that occur more by chance than by design and as a result decrease the probability of the client's attaining a more satisfactory level of emotional well-being. Therefore it is important for the nurse to understand how the *nursing process* can be applied to the care of mentally ill clients. Although the terms used to describe the nursing process vary, the process is always an adaptation of the problem-solving technique and involves the phases of assessing, diagnosing, planning, implementing, and evaluating.

The nursing process is an adaptation of the problem-solving technique and includes the phases of assessment, diagnosis, planning, implementation, and *evaluation.*

HISTORICAL PERSPECTIVE

Nursing began as more an art than a science. Prior to the nineteenth century, those who cared for the ill had little more to rely on to ease suffering than in-

111

tuitively administered comfort measures. With the explosion of medical knowledge in the late nineteenth century the nurse depended on the physician to direct her activities. It was not until the mid-twentieth century that a number of factors converged that ultimately led to the development of the nursing process.

The first of these factors was the extreme shortage of nurses during and after World War II. This shortage meant that a few nurses had to care for many patients. In attempting to care for patients in an efficient and effective manner the nursing care plan was developed. The nursing care plan not only standardized care but also was a major tool in facilitating communication between and among nurses. Much of the nursing care plan, however, consisted of an organization of physician's orders that were carried out by nurses.

At the same time a second factor emerged, namely, the development of psychiatric—mental health nursing as a specialty within the occupation of nursing. Until that time caring for mentally ill persons was not a desirable calling. Consequently, those who chose to do so were remarkably free of the strictures imposed by medicine in other areas of health care. It was, therefore these early psychiatric—mental health nurses who were able to design interventions that were within the domain of nursing practice and who documented the effectiveness of these interventions. Thus the independent role of the nurse flourished in the nursing care of mentally ill persons.

With an increasing number of independent nursing functions, especially the nurse-client relationship, the need to monitor the quality of nursing care became apparent. In response to this need an adaptation of the problem-solving approach was adopted as a means to systematically plan and evaluate nursing care. This approach became known as the nursing process.

Despite the number of refinements made in the nursing process since its inception, its original purpose of defining the problem, designing a plan to address the problem, and evaluating its effectiveness remains.

ASSESSMENT PHASE

In the *assessment* phase, the nurse collects data about the client and organizes it to plan the client's care.

The first phase of the nursing process is assessment. Since the focus of all nursing practice is the person's response to actual or potential health problems, the purpose of the assessment phase of the nursing process is to systematically collect data about these responses and to organize them so they become useful in planning care. Although psychiatric nursing is concerned primarily with the emotional and interpersonal responses of the client, i.e., his mental health, the nurse must remember that the human being is a unified, integrated whole. Consequently, the client must be assessed comprehensively, considering all client responses, if accurate information is to be available to plan nursing care.

What to assess

To assess the client comprehensively and therefore accurately, the nurse needs to adopt an organizing schema to direct her assessment. Furthermore, for the assessment data to provide direction for planning nursing care, they must not only be comprehensive but must also lead to the formulation of nursing diagnoses. While there is little agreement within the profession about the nature of the appropriate organizing schema, there is consensus about its necessity. One such schema can be inferred from the American Nurses' Association (ANA) Classification of Human Responses of Concern for Psychiatric Mental Health Nursing Practice.

The ANA Phenomena Task Force has organized human response patterns under the categories of activity processes, cognition processes, ecological processes, emotional processes, interpersonal processes, perception processes, physiological processes, and valuation processes. See Table 9-1 for the categories of human response patterns for each process.

The use of processes as an organizing schema seems particularly appropriate since human beings are dynamic, fluid organisms in constant interaction within themselves, with others, and with their environments. In contrast, the use of structural dimensions, such as body systems, as an organizational schema implies that human beings are fixed and static, a view that is inconsistent with nursing's focus on human responses. The above categories of human processes meet the test of providing direction for a comprehensive assessment of an individual client while simultaneously leading to nursing diagnoses. Therefore, it is recommended that these processes serve as the organizational schema for assessing the individual client.

How to assess

Assessment of the client is achieved by using the technique, measure, or tool appropriate to the process. For example, activity processes can be assessed through observation and interview in regard to the human responses of motor behavior, recreation patterns, self-care, and sleep/arousal patterns.

Assessment data are both subjective and objective. Subjective data often are referred to as symptoms—for example, what the client and others report and what the nurse observes; objective data are often called signs—what the nurse or others can measure—for example, blood pressure, intake and output, and results of psychometric tests. It is important to collect both subjective and objective data about the client. In addition, the nurse needs to collect data about the client from all appropriate sources. These include the client's chart, other health care workers, relevant texts and journal articles, and the client's family and friends. It is important to understand that the source of the data is not what makes nursing unique; what is done with the data—how they are analyzed and used—is what differentiates nursing from other health care professions.

Although all sources of information about the client should be utilized, the most important and significant source of information about the client is the client himself. To obtain data from the client the nurse needs to perfect her skills in interviewing and observing.

Assessment data can be both subjective (symptoms that can be observed) and objective (signs that can be measured).

TABLE 9-1   *Categories of human response patterns for each human process*

Human processes	Categories of human response patterns
Activity	Motor behavior
	Recreation patterns
	Self-care
	Sleep/arousal patterns
Cognition	Decision making
	Judgment
	Knowledge
	Learning
	Memory
	Thought processes
Ecological	Community maintenance
	Environmental integrity
	Home maintenance
Emotional	Feeling states
	Feeling processes
Interpersonal	Abuse response patterns
	Communication processes
	Conduct/impulse processes
	Family processes
	Role performance
	Sexuality
	Social interaction
Perception	Attention
	Comfort
	Self-concept
	Sensory perception
Physiological	Circulation
	Elimination
	Endocrine/metabolic processes
	Gastrointestinal processes
	Musculoskeletal processes
	Neuro/sensory processes
	Nutrition
	Oxygenation
	Physical integrity
	Physical regulation processes
Valuation	Meaningfulness
	Spirituality
	Values

An interview is conducted to obtain specific information. As such, it is not designed to be therapeutic or to convey information, although indirectly it may be helpful or informative to the client. An interview is guided by goals, and an effective interview requires that the nurse organize her goals and approaches before meeting with the client. Because an interview is structured it is likely that the nurse will be more directive and ask more questions than she would in an interaction designed to be therapeutic. Thus the nurse is wise to have planned sample questions, the answers to which will provide the data sought. Questions likely to be most effective in eliciting information are simple, concrete, and direct. For example, "What do you usually eat for breakfast?" is preferable to "Tell me about your usual diet."

On initiating an interview the nurse should tell the client the purpose of the interaction and approximately how long it will last. As with all interactions the nurse should introduce herself to the client if they have not already met and position herself on eye level with the client. Ideally both she and the client should sit in comfortable chairs. However, this is not always possible if the client is too anxious to sit. In that case the nurse may wish to remain standing as well. If the nurse intends to take notes during the interview, she should explain the purpose of her writing at the onset. By orienting the client in this manner the nurse establishes a foundation on which a future trusting relationship with the client can be built, either by her or by another nurse.

One of the most important goals of an initial interview is to ascertain the client's perception of his problems. While it is generally advisable to avoid using "why" questions, they are sometimes desirable when interviewing persons who are psychotic because "why" questions are concrete and direct. For example, a psychotic, hallucinating individual who is asked "What brought you to the hospital?" might very well respond by answering, "A car brought me." In contrast, the same client might respond to "Why did you come to the hospital?" by answering, "To get out of the cold" or "Because I see my grandmother all the time, and I know she is dead." Either of these responses answers the nurse's question, which is not the case when she avoided the use of a "why" question.

Having ascertained the client's perception of his problem, the nurse's next goal is to determine the duration of the problem, what circumstances led up to the problem, who else is involved, and in what way the client expects the hospital or clinic to be of help. A determination of these variables is essential to an accurate, comprehensive assessment and allows the nurse to compare the client's perceptions of the problem with the perceptions of others. Then she can design a plan of care which will be of the greatest help to the client.

Another major goal of the interview is to obtain information about such factual data as the client's daily activities, previous health history, educational level, and occupation. It is important, however, that the client not be bombarded with questions that can be answered by other sources. For example, if the nurse has access to a chart from the client's previous admission she ought not ask for such information as the client's date of birth unless she questions the reliability of the available information or is using the question to assess the client's memory.

The interview should be concluded as close to the time specified as possible. It is helpful to the client for the nurse to repeat what she said earlier about how she will use the information he shared. It is also important that the nurse inform the client what will happen next, such as the fact that she will take him

An effective interview obtains specific information, is guided by goals, requires the use of simple, concrete, and direct questions, and takes place during a specified time period.

Ascertaining the client's perception of his problem and obtaining factual information about him are major goals of the initial interview.

back to the unit, or that he should schedule another appointment with the receptionist.

The other skill that is integral to the assessment phase of the nursing process is that of observation. Observation is a frequently used term for an active goal-directed process that utilizes all appropriate senses. As the nurse talks or otherwise interacts with the client, she looks, hears, feels, and smells. In general, the goal of observation is to determine the appropriateness and congruence of the client's appearance, behavior, and verbalizations with each other and with the situation. This implies, then, that observations are planned. Not meant to be implied, however, is that the nurse should not observe phenomena that she had not anticipated. It is important for the nurse to attend to her own intuitive feelings about a situation. Experience has shown that more often than not these intuitive feelings are manifestations of the nurse's unconscious perceptions that are based on reality. The observer needs to be alert to the client's facial expression, voice quality, neatness and appropriateness of dress and grooming, participation in activities, response to other clients and staff, and many other aspects of his behavior while she is interviewing him and during the time he spends in the treatment setting, whether that be 1, 8, or 24 hours.

> While observing the client, the nurse's goal is to determine the appropriateness and harmony of the client's appearance, behavior, and speech patterns with each other and with the situation.

To validate the information gained from observations and to determine their significance, observations of the same or similar events need to be made repeatedly. For example, the nurse may observe that on one occasion a client who was unable to purchase his brand of cigarettes swore at the clerk and stalked out of the store. Many people occasionally feel this degree of frustration and sometimes act on it. If the client does not have a similar reaction in future situations, it is likely that this incident is relatively insignificant. On the other hand, if the nurse observes that on subsequent days the same client yells and walks away because he must wait for the elevator and then later displays the same behavior because his meal contains food he does not like, she would be correct in determining that she had identified a theme or pattern in this client's behavior likely to be most indicative of his problems. In some instances, however, behavior that is strikingly uncharacteristic of the client may be highly significant and should be recorded and communicated to other members of the professional team. As the nurse learns to understand more about the meaning of human behavior and learns to know the client as an individual, she will become more skillful in recognizing significant behavior.

Concluding the assessment phase

> Sorting and organizing the data into themes is the final step of the assessment phase.

The final step in the assessment phase of the nursing process is to sort and organize the data according to themes. Themes are recurring patterns that may have different manifestations but that stem from the same source. For example, the nurse may observe that the client has an unkempt appearance, speaks deprecatingly of himself, and refuses to join in group activities that are new to him. Even though these behaviors superficially may seem to have little or no relationship, with study the nurse will learn that they all may be manifestations of the same pattern. Identifying themes of the client's responses is a precursor to the diagnostic phase of the nursing process.

DIAGNOSTIC PHASE

The second phase of the nursing process is the diagnostic phase, in which the nurse makes a nursing diagnosis. This phase corresponds to the formulation of a hypothesis in the problem-solving technique, is based on a synthesis of all available assessment data, and provides direction for developing a plan for nursing care.

No other phase of the nursing process has elicited as much controversy as has the diagnostic phase. Some health care providers still believe that the process of diagnosing is solely within the province of the physician. The act of diagnosing, however, is not what distinguishes health care professions. Rather, the focus of the diagnosis is what makes the difference. A medical diagnosis identifies the disease or illness affecting the client, while a nursing diagnosis identifies the client's response to an actual or potential health problem.

A nursing diagnosis focuses on the client's response to an actual or potential health problem, while a medical diagnosis identifies the disease or illness affecting the client.

A classification of diagnoses of mental disorders has been available for many years. However, in 1980 the American Psychiatric Association published the *Diagnostic and Statistical Manual of Mental Disorders, Third Edition* (DSM-III), which for the first time not only defined and described mental disorders but also included physical disorders and conditions and categorized the severity of the client's psychosocial stressors and his highest level of adaptive functioning during the past year. This major revision of the psychiatric diagnostic taxonomy was a major step in viewing the client holistically. The DSM-III was revised in 1987 and is known as the DSM-III-R. Since the health care delivery system remains organized around the medical model of disease and illness, the psychiatric nurse must be conversant with the terminology and diagnoses used by psychiatrists. Therefore, the DSM-III-R classification is found in Appendix C.

Taxonomy
A system of classification based on natural relationships.

In recent years efforts have been made to develop a classification system of nursing diagnoses that reflects characteristic responses of persons to common health problems. One of the most recent systems, and perhaps the one most widely used, is that developed by the North American Nursing Diagnosis Association (NANDA). No claim is made that this system is complete and work on its development continues. The 1988 NANDA-approved nursing diagnostic categories are found in Appendix D.

As NANDA diagnoses evolved and gained acceptance by the nursing profession, psychiatric nurses became increasingly aware of their responsibility to identify nursing diagnoses that reflect the responses of individuals whose primary problem is psychosocial in nature. Consequently, the former Division of Psychiatric and Mental Health Nursing Practice of the American Nurses' Association sponsored a project to identify the phenomena of specific concern for psychiatric–mental health nursing. The resultant classification system consists of human response patterns, organized under eight processes. As with the NANDA diagnoses, no claim is made that the present classification is complete. Further, it is acknowledged that two other classes of response must be developed—the interpersonal/family and the community/environment classes. See Appendix E for the ANA Classification of Human Responses of Concern for Psychiatric Mental Health Nursing Practice.

The human response in and of itself is often referred to as the nursing diagnosis. However, to be most useful in providing direction for nursing care, a nursing diagnosis must be a statement that identifies the client's response along with a phrase indicating its probable etiology or antecedent factor. Some nursing authorities reject this format because of our limited knowledge about definitive etiologies, especially in regard to psychosocial responses. While this argument has validity, a nursing diagnosis that states only the client's response is of limited use in planning care. For example, the nursing diagnosis of "altered family role" is much less useful than the nursing diagnosis of "altered family role related to marriage of youngest child." The reader will note that this example connects the human response with its postulated etiology by the phrase "related to." This format implies a relationship between the two phenomena but does not rule out other factors, indirectly acknowledging the imprecise state of knowledge about human behavior.

Most clients have more than one nursing diagnosis. However, if the nurse identifies numerous diagnoses for the same client, she should question whether she has missed a unifying theme. In other words, as the nurse gains knowledge and experience she will learn that there is usually a high degree of interrelatedness among the various human responses within each category. She will attempt to identify those which will provide direction for planning nursing care but omit those which result in an unnecessarily repetitive plan of care.

PLANNING PHASE

The third phase of the nursing process is developing a plan for nursing intervention. The plan for nursing intervention is derived from the nursing diagnoses and includes statements indicating the objective of the care (the nursing goal), how the objective will be achieved (the nursing actions), and the anticipated results (the outcome criteria).

Much controversy exists about whether the objective of the care should be stated in terms of the nurse or the client. Regardless of the way in which the objective is stated, the intent is the same. For example, the nursing goal "To convey a sense of worth" means the same as the client objective, "To develop a sense of worth." Whichever format is chosen should be used consistently.

Once stated, objectives need to be prioritized as short-term or long-term goals. Criteria for prioritization include the urgency of the situation, the amount of time required to achieve the goal, and the anticipated length of contact with the client. Unless objectives are realistically prioritized, both the nurse

Etiology
Cause

In *planning* for nursing intervention, the nurse states the objective of the care, how the objective will be achieved, and the expected results.

and the client risk being continuously frustrated by failing to achieve the desired outcomes of nursing care. This is currently the case in many psychiatric hospitals where clients are discharged to aftercare clinics as soon as their behavior has stabilized. As a result, the nurses in the hospital may have contact with the client for only a few weeks, since there is a different nursing staff in the clinic. In these instances the hospital nursing staff is wise to limit objectives to those which can be achieved in a short time.

To be effective, nursing actions must be related to the goals of the care. In addition, they must be realistic in light of the resources available.

Outcome criteria are statements phrased in behavioral terms that enable the nurse to assess whether the goal has been achieved. Unlike objectives, outcome criteria are always stated in terms of client behavior and are most useful when they specify the conditions under which they will occur, their frequency, and the time period in which they are anticipated.

The plan for nursing intervention is highly individualized for each client. However, all plans for nursing intervention should reflect the principles of psychiatric nursing as discussed in Chapter 5 of this text. See Table 9-2 for an example of a plan for nursing intervention.

IMPLEMENTATION PHASE

The fourth phase of the nursing process is the implementation of the plan of care. In implementing the plan of care, the nurse utilizes a variety of roles. These roles are discussed in detail in Chapter 7.

The following situation depicts the way a nurse carried out the plan of care shown in Table 9-2 by fulfilling a variety of roles.

> "Please take me back to the ward, Miss S., I feel sick." Tall, dark-haired 17-year-old Sam G. had walked across the dance floor and was pleading with the nurse to be allowed to leave the regular Wednesday evening dance. The dance was part of the recreational program for clients. Both Sam and the nurse knew that clients

TABLE 9-2 *Example of a plan for nursing intervention*

NURSING DIAGNOSIS*

6.3.2.3 Altered self-esteem, related to developmental stressors of adolescence and increased familial responsibility

Nursing goal	Nursing action	Outcome criteria
To convey a sense of worth	Praise accomplishments, no matter how small When client verbally derogates self, disagree if appropriate without arguing	Within 1 month there will be: Increase in client's statements reflecting self-worth ("Yes, I did do that well.") Decrease in self-derogating remarks Well-groomed personal appearance, appropriate dress

*The NANDA diagnosis would be: 7.1.2 Self-esteem disturbance, related to developmental stressors of adolescence and increased familial responsibility.

were usually encouraged to remain at the dance until it was over. She also knew that Sam had not made such a request before, and intuitively she felt that something at the dance had been upsetting to him.

Miss S. quietly made the necessary arrangements with the staff member in charge of the dance and took Sam back to the homelike unit. Then she took his pulse, temperature, and respirations to be certain that he was not physically ill. When she found that these physical signs were within the normal range, she suggested that he help her make some sandwiches. Together they went into the kitchen where they prepared a snack for the other clients who would soon be returning from the dance. Sam seemed happy to help. He and the nurse chatted and joked together. He spoke at length about his mother's illness and his family's financial problems, but he did not mention feeling ill.

After finishing the sandwiches and cleaning the kitchen, the nurse thanked Sam for his help, remarking on the speed with which he accomplished the task. They then went together into the living room and sat down on the couch. "Do you think that my face is changing?" he asked. "I just looked in the bathroom mirror, and it seems to me that my nose is getting a lot longer and uglier."

The nurse looked carefully at his face and said, "It looks just the same to me. It seems to you that your nose is getting longer?"

Soon the other clients arrived from the dance. The unit was filled with the busy noise of 25 people discussing the dance and eating the evening snack. Sam took part in all this activity but sought the nurse several times to ask questions: "Do you think you ought to call my doctor?" "Will I be able to sleep tonight?" "You think that I am going to be all right, don't you?"

Each time Sam came to ask a question, the nurse took time to listen carefully to his questions and to answer truthfully and sincerely. She did call the doctor who was on duty that evening and told him about Sam's behavior. He agreed to come to see Sam. Because the doctor was not well acquainted with him, the nurse spent several minutes telling him briefly about Sam's family problems. She pointed out that he had been anxious and tense during the evening and had seemed to cling to her and to be asking for reassurance. The doctor talked with Sam. He felt that by allowing Sam to leave the dance the nurse had been able to help him avoid an anxiety attack. The doctor told the nurse that her empathic listening and her efforts at reassuring Sam had been partially successful. The next day Sam's regular therapist was able to help him look more objectively at the problem that had been so upsetting to him. As a result of the nurse's intervention and the doctor's help Sam was able to attend the dance the following week without experiencing undue anxiety.

In *implementing* the plan of care, the nurse may use a variety of roles to carry out the prescribed nursing actions.

This example is typical of situations that nurses who work with mentally ill individuals frequently encounter. In her interaction with Sam the nurse used the technical nursing role by taking and evaluating his vital signs. She simultaneously engaged in the role of parent surrogate and socializing agent when she worked with Sam to prepare and serve snacks for the other clients. The therapeutic effectiveness of this activity became apparent when Sam spoke about his family's problems and then became able to communicate his concern about his physical appearance. The nurse's response to this concern reflects the role of counselor, since she listened attentively and responded in a truthful and reassuring way. The nurse displayed an understanding of the necessity for professional collaboration by calling the physician and carefully sharing with him her assessment of the client. In summary, the nurse saw this clinical situation as an opportunity to implement the plan of care through the use of a variety of nursing roles, which proved to be very helpful to the client. Without an awareness of the therapeutic potential of these activities, the nurse might have insisted that Sam remain at the dance and thereby could have contributed to the exacerbation of an acute anxiety attack.

EVALUATION PHASE

The final phase of the nursing process is evaluation. The phases of the nursing process previously cited have been described as if they were discrete entities, and the phase of evaluation is frequently seen as the last step in this process. In reality, however, all phases of the nursing process may occur simultaneously, and some form of evaluation must take place continuously. Therefore it is imperative that the nurse review the assessment of the client, the nursing diagnoses, and the plan for nursing intervention, as well as the outcome of the nursing intervention. The results of the nursing care should be evaluated against the outcome criteria the nurse established as she planned for the care. As previously mentioned, outcome criteria need to be stated in behavioral terms and as specifically as possible.

Evaluation includes reviewing the assessment data, the nursing diagnoses, the plan for nursing intervention, and the results of the nursing intervention in light of the outcome criteria.

Inherent in all aspects of evaluation is the necessity for the nurse to evaluate her own behavior and to determine the degree to which it does or does not facilitate achievement of the goals of the plan for intervention. It should be noted that evaluation frequently serves the purpose of identifying those aspects of care that are indeed helpful to the client and therefore should be continued. See Table 9-3 for a summary outline of the nursing process as used in psychiatric nursing.

END NOTE

This chapter discusses the five phases of the nursing process and suggests the use of the processes inferred from the ANA Classification of Human Responses of Concern for Psychiatric Mental Health Nursing Practice as the organizational schema by which human responses of individual clients should be assessed. Emphasis is placed on the necessity for deriving nursing diagnoses from the assessment data so the diagnoses can be used as the basis for a plan of care that is relevant. The nurse is encouraged to utilize the principles of psychiatric nursing discussed in Chapter 5 in planning for nursing intervention and the roles of the nurse discussed in Chapter 7 in implementing the plan of care. An example of how the nurse fulfills various roles in implementing a plan of care is provided. Finally, guidelines for evaluation of the nursing process are included.

TABLE 9-3   *Nursing process*

Phase	Purpose	Examples of nursing action
Assessment	To collect data	Observe present behavior of the client, using all the appropriate senses
		Read client's chart and relevant texts and journals
		Interview client, his family, and other staff
	To validate data collected from observation	Make repeated observations; discuss perceptions with others
		Read relevant texts and journals to confirm observations
	To analyze data	Sort and organize data according to themes
Diagnostic	To establish a nursing diagnosis	Synthesize all available assessment data
		State human response and probable etiology
Planning	To plan for nursing intervention, using nursing diagnosis as a basis	Individualize a plan for intervention and identify the nursing goal, nursing action, and outcome criteria
		Use the principles of psychiatric nursing:
		1. The nurse views the client as a holistic being with a multiplicity of interrelated and interdependent needs
		2. The nurse focuses on the client's strengths and assets, not on his weaknesses and liabilities
		3. The nurse accepts the client as a human being who has value and worth, exactly as he is
		4. The nurse has the potential for establishing a relationship with most, if not all, clients
		5. The nurse explores the client's behavior for the need it is designed to meet or the message it is communicating
		6. The nurse views the client's behavior nonjudgmentally while assisting him to learn more effective adaptations
		7. The quality of the interaction in which the nurse engages with the client is a major determinant of the degree to which the client will be able to alter his behavior in the direction of more satisfying, satisfactory interpersonal relationships
Implementation	To implement plan for nursing intervention	Function in a variety of roles while using principles of psychiatric nursing:
		1. Creator of a therapeutic environment
		2. Socializing agent
		3. Counselor
		4. Teacher
		5. Parent surrogate
		6. Technical role
		7. Nurse therapist
Evaluation	To make planned, critical assessment of care	Review assessment data for accuracy and currency
		Review nursing diagnoses for accuracy and currency
	To revise or confirm plan of care	Review plan for nursing intervention
		Compare client's response to intervention with outcome criteria
	To make self-assessment	Evaluate own behavior
		Revise or confirm plan for nursing intervention based on overall evaluation

SUGGESTED SOURCES OF ADDITIONAL INFORMATION

Boettcher E and Alderson S: Psychotropic medications and the nursing process, J Psychosoc Nurs Ment Health Serv 20:12, November 1982.

Clement J and Boylan S: Actualizing theory into practice, Perspect Psychiatr Care 20:126, July-September, 1982.

Cohen S and Harris E: Programmed instruction:mental status assessment, Am J Nurs 81:1493, August 1981.

Galasso D: Guidelines for developing multidisciplinary treatment plans, Hosp Commun Psychiatr 38:394, April 1987.

Gordon M: Nursing diagnosis: process and application, New York, 1982, McGraw-Hill Book Co.

Johnson M: Theoretical basis for nursing diagnosis in mental health nursing, Issues Ment Health Nurs 6:53, 1984.

Lunney M: Nursing diagnosis: refining the system, Am J Nurs 82:456, 1982.

Mansfield E: A conceptual framework for psychiatric mental health nursing, J Psychosoc Nurs Ment Health Serv 18:36, June 1980.

Milne D: 'The more things change the more they stay the same': factors affecting the implementation of the nursing process, J Adv Nurs 10:39, 1985.

Moscovitz A: Orem's theory as applied to psychiatric nursing, Perspect Psychiatr Care 22:36, January–March 1984.

Newman MA: Looking at the whole, Am J Nurs 84:1496, December 1984.

Parsons PJ: Building better treatment plans, J Psychosoc Nurs 24:8, 1986.

Price M: Nursing diagnosis: making a concept come alive, Am J Nurs 80:668, 1980.

Reed PG: Constructing a conceptual framework for psychosocial nursing, J Psychosoc Nurs Ment Health Serv 25:24, 1987.

Somociuk G: Concept meets reality, Nurs Mirror 161:29, September 1985.

Whyte L and Youhill G: The nursing process in the care of the mentally ill, Nurs. Times 80:49, February 1984.

Williams J and Wilson HS: A psychiatric nursing perspective on DSM III, J Psychosoc Nurs Ment Health Serv 20:14, April 1982.

General systems theory and stress and adaptation
One conceptual framework

10

LEARNING OBJECTIVES

After studying this chapter the student will be able to:

- State the purpose of a conceptual framework.
- Discuss the concepts of general systems theory as applied to human systems.
- Discuss the concept of stress and adaptation as a process used by human systems.
- State an example of a nursing intervention utilizing the conceptual framework of systems theory and stress and adaptation.

For nurses to practice efficiently and effectively, they must do so within the context of a conceptual framework. The purpose of a conceptual framework is to provide a logical and coherent structure through which phenomena of concern can be understood and talked about. There is no right or wrong conceptual framework. Rather, a conceptual framework is more or less appropriate; its appropriateness is determined by its applicability and utility. A conceptual framework appropriate for nursing must help explain this profession's phenomena of concern—the concepts of person, their environments, and their health as these interact between and among themselves. It must also be broad enough to be applicable to most, if not all, clinical situations but not so broad that it becomes meaningless.

An appropriate conceptual framework for nursing must help explain nursing's concern for persons, their environments, and their health. It must be broad enough to be applicable to most clinical situations.

The conceptual framework chosen for this text is general systems theory and the theory of stress and adaptation.

HISTORICAL PERSPECTIVE

A *system* is a complex of elements in interaction wherein a relationship between these elements and their properties can be theoretically demonstrated.

General systems theory, as discussed in this chapter, was first discussed by Ludwig von Bertalanffy in 1968. However, other theorists, notably Kurt Lewin, had used its principles decades earlier to formulate their theories. General systems theory has been enthusiastically embraced by the helping professions because it is so useful in explaining relationships among apparently disparate entities. Nevertheless, some critics of this theory believe it is too mechanistic to apply to human systems.

In the 1930s Walter Cannon was the first theorist to mention the role of stress as a factor in causing disease. However, the foremost authority on the theory of stress and adaptation is probably Hans Selye, whose pioneering work on the subject was limited to a biochemical model of stress and adaptation. Since that time much research has demonstrated the same processes in the emotional and social realms.

GENERAL SYSTEMS THEORY

A *system* is commonly defined as a complex of elements in interaction wherein a relationship between these elements and their properties can be theoretically demonstrated. Since all elements can be theorized to ultimately have a direct or indirect interactional relationship, the only true system is the universe. For example, it is often said that the emotional problems of an individual are due in large part to problems within his family. The family's problems in turn are attributed to problems within the community, whose problems in turn result from state, regional, and national concerns. These concerns in turn are closely related to international problems.

Obviously the study of the universe as the true system is not possible or desirable because of the enormous amount of data that would have to be considered. Consequently, it is necessary to delineate a subsystem and define it as "the system" for the purposes of study.

OF SPECIAL INTEREST

Although general systems theory was first addressed by scientists in the 1960's, many thoughtful persons were undoubtedly aware of the existence of an ordered, interrelated universe long before the twentieth century. A notable example of such an individual is Nathaniel Hawthorne (1804-1864), author of *The Scarlet Letter* and one of America's greatest writers of fiction. Hawthorne was deeply involved in the perennial debate concerning the nature of man and in 1835 wrote in the short story *Wakefield:* "Amid the seeming confusion of our mysterious world, individuals are so nicely adjusted to a system, and systems to one another and to a whole, that, by stepping aside for a moment, a man exposes himself to a fearful risk of losing his place forever."

Systems are delineated by the establishment of *boundaries,* which enclose those elements determined to have the greatest interactional qualities in terms of energy, matter, or both. The aggregate of elements that fall within the boundary is referred to as the "system"; each element becomes a component or a *subsystem* of the newly defined system. For example, mental health professionals often define the family as the system of concern and the individuals who comprise the family as components or subsystems of the family system.

Each subsystem has its own elements, which are components or subsystems of that system. For example, the individual as a system is made up of a variety of subsystems such as the physiological, psychological, and social subsystems. These subsystems, when viewed as systems themselves, consist of their own subsystems. For example, the physiological system consists of the cardiovascular and gastrointestinal subsystems, among others.

Elements that lie outside the boundary serve as the system's *environment,* which is in reality composed of other systems. Therefore the community system serves as an environment for the family system, the family system serves as an environment for the individual system, the physiological system serves as an environment for the psychological system, and so on.

It cannot be overemphasized that boundary delineation is an artificial demarcation of one aspect of the whole—artificial, but necessary, to limit the focus of concern to that which is relevant and thereby increase the probability of comprehending the system. Because boundary delineation is artificial and is intended to enable the nurse to understand the system, boundaries can be enlarged or reduced as experience with the system dictates. For example, when the family is the system of concern an initial assessment might indicate that the system should be limited to those members living under the same roof. After working with this system, however, the nurse may discover that the grandparents who live in another state are integral components of this family system. The nurse would then enlarge the original system to include this subsystem, rather than viewing it as part of the environment.

The boundaries of a system have the necessary characteristic of permeability. This permeability may be greater or lesser when systems are compared; the degree of boundary permeability may also change at various times and places within any given system. The permeability of the system boundary regulates the exchange of matter and energy between the system and its environment. Matter and energy that move from the environment through the boundary into the system are referred to as *input.* Matter and energy that move from the system through the boundary into the environment are referred to as *output.*

In a system, matter and energy are an integral part of both the system and the system's environment. *Matter* is defined as anything that has mass and occupies space. *Energy* is defined as the ability to do work. There are two types of energy: potential and kinetic. *Potential energy* is that energy not currently engaged in work but is available for use. It is stored energy. In contrast, *kinetic*

Systems are delineated by the establishment of *boundaries* that enclose elements that have the greatest interactional qualities.

Each element within a system is a *subsystem.*

Elements outside the system's boundaries form the system's *environment.*

Because boundary delineation is an artificial process, boundaries can be enlarged or reduced as experience with the system dictates.

Matter and energy that move from the environment through the boundary into the system are called *input.* Matter and energy that move from the system through the boundary into the environment are called *output.*

Matter is defined as anything that has mass and occupies space. *Energy* is the ability to do work and is of two types, *potential* or stored energy and *kinetic* energy.

energy is that which is being currently utilized and is therefore unavailable for additional work.

Energy can neither be created nor destroyed; it can only be converted from one form into another or transported from one place to another. When energy is used it does not disappear but merely goes elsewhere or is changed to another form. The principle that energy can neither be created nor destroyed is the first law of thermodynamics; it is reminiscent of Freud's concept of psychic or libidinal energy as explained in Chapter 11.

Systems are in a constant state of dynamic movement as they exchange matter and energy within themselves and between themselves and their environments. Any attempt to study a system is to artificially suspend this motion and therefore run the risk of an inaccurate assessment. Nevertheless, it is necessary to take this risk if systems are to be studied, but any conclusions should take this factor into account.

Systems are characterized by the concept of *nonsummativity,* which states that the whole of the system is greater than the sum of its parts. The parts of a system are that system's subsystems, and the system in its totality cannot be understood or appreciated by a mere summation of its subsystems. Perhaps the most familiar example of this concept is the Indian folk tale of the six blind men who each felt a part of an elephant's body. Each then described that part to the others, and as a group they attempted unsuccessfully to describe the whole. The primary reason that the whole is greater than the sum of its parts is that each subsystem interacts directly or indirectly with all other subsystems by exchanging matter and energy, a concept called *wholeness.* The uniqueness of the system results from the transformations of matter and energy that take place in this exchange, a process known as *throughput.*

Because of the interactional quality of the system's components, changes in any one component will automatically effect compensatory changes in all other components. These changes are compensatory because a system continuously strives to maintain itself as it is. In other words, the system continuously regulates itself to attain a steady state. When referring to living organisms, this process is known as *homeokinesis.*

Human beings are complex systems of interrelated and interdependent subsystems in constant interaction with each other and with their environments. Therefore alterations in any aspect of the system require responsive alterations in other aspects of the system. For example, a person who is physically ill, for whatever reason and to whatever degree, has concomitant emotional reactions to this lack of physical well-being. Conversely, there are physical side effects of emotional reactions, such as the stomach upsets, the lightheadedness, and the heart palpitations that accompany severe anxiety or fear.

This holistic view of human beings also provides direction for assessing the individual as an integral part of his social system, simultaneously affecting that system and being affected by it. This view implies that an individual cannot be

Systems are characterized by the concept of *nonsummativity;* that is, the whole is greater than the sum of its parts.

The uniqueness of each system results from the transformations of matter and energy between and among the subsystems, a process known as *throughput.*

Systems constantly regulate themselves to attain a steady state, a process known as *homeokinesis.* Therefore changes in one component of the system automatically effect changes in all other components.

Human beings are complex systems of interrelated and interdependent subsystems in constant interaction with each other and with their environments.

assessed accurately in isolation from his family, his community, and the reference groups to which he belongs. Nurses new to working with mentally ill persons have had the experience of assisting an individual to achieve a higher level of emotional wellness only to be surprised by the observation that the behavior of another member of his family becomes increasingly disturbed. This common phenomenon reflects the fact that the family operates as a system and change in one member requires a compensatory reaction by the family system, often manifested by altered behavior in other family members.

Those human systems which are most successful in achieving their goal of maintaining themselves as close to their original state as possible ironically are systems whose very existence is in jeopardy. These systems are *relatively closed systems* and are likely to show signs of illness or dysfunction. The boundaries of relatively closed systems have little permeability, and there is relatively little exchange of matter or energy with the environment. However, boundaries cannot be totally closed in a living system. Some permeability is necessary to exchange matter and energy, a process necessary for life. The bulk of energy in a relatively closed system is used in maintaining a steady state, leaving little potential energy available to respond to input. Because input into the system is minimal, there is ultimate energy loss into the system's environment, leading to increased system disorganization. This situation is termed *entropy*.

The student is probably familiar with a family that does not respond to notes from school about the children's poor academic performance, initially resulting in the family system's being undisturbed by this news and thereby maintaining a steady state. Ultimately, however, this system's inability to recognize and process relevant input may lead to the children being left back and perhaps eventually dropping out of school. This in turn means that the children are poorly prepared to leave home and to function as financially independent adults, resulting in the family's financial resources becoming increasingly depleted. In the long run this fictional family does not change and grow but rather becomes increasingly ineffective in fulfilling its functions. This example, although oversimplified, illustrates the counterproductivity of a system attempting to achieve a steady state by maintaining relatively closed boundaries.

In contrast, a system that survives, grows, and develops is characterized by a semipermeable boundary that allows for exchange of matter and energy with its environment and by the availability of a sufficient amount of potential energy to utilize input in the service of system growth. This type of system is known as a *relatively open system* and is characterized by movement toward integration and growth, a situation referred to as *negentropy*.

A system in a state of negentropy is likely to manifest signs of health or to be considered functional. A discussion of the personality attributes of mentally healthy individuals is found in Chapter 11.

Finally, an understanding of systems theory must take into account the concept of *feedback,* a unique form of input derived from the system's output. In

The boundaries of *relatively closed systems* have little permeability, and the bulk of the system's energy is bound in maintaining a steady state, leading to energy loss and increased system disorganization. This situation is called *entropy*.

The boundaries of *relatively open systems* allow for adequate exchange of matter and energy, and a sufficient amount of potential energy to utilize input in the service of system growth and integrations is available. This situation is called *negentropy*.

other words, system output is transformed by the environment (in reality another system) and, in turn, becomes that system's output. Part of that output is fed back as input to the original system. This process is often referred to as the *feedback loop.* Feedback is the message that the system receives about the degree to which it is successful in attaining a steady state and is therefore essential if the system is to adjust or regulate itself. There is always a time lag between the system's perception of the feedback and its ability to utilize it in the service of self-regulation.

Feedback is a unique form of input that sends a message to the system about the degree to which it is successful in attaining a steady state.

Positive feedback reinforces the system, thereby encouraging the maintenance of a steady state and leading to entropy. *Negative feedback* is information that indicates change is necessary within the system for the system to grow. These concepts are often difficult for students to understand because of the belief that positive feedback is desirable and negative feedback is to be avoided. It is true that positive feedback reinforces behavior, encouraging people to continue those behaviors which are rewarded. However, inadvertently perhaps, positive feedback discourages growth if altered behavior is necessary for growth. Negative feedback, on the other hand, is growth-producing only if the system has the energy available to utilize the feedback and alter itself. For example, a very intelligent student is not motivated to achieve his potential if his minimal efforts are rewarded with high grades. On the other hand, a student who is not as intellectually capable and who is working to capacity but receiving low grades will not be helped to do better merely through criticism of his work. He does not have the energy available to utilize the negative feedback, whereas his highly intelligent counterpart does.

Positive feedback reinforces the system and encourages a steady state. *Negative feedback* disrupts the system, encouraging change and growth if the system has the potential energy available to utilize the input.

This brief discussion of general systems theory demonstrates its applicability to nursing practice in regard to describing the structure of human systems. However, its language and concepts only hint at explaining the process. For example, we know that energy is exchanged between systems, but systems theory alone does not allow us to describe the nature of that energy. Therefore to better understand the nature of the processes in which systems engage, we need to turn to another theory, that of stress and adaptation.

STRESS AND ADAPTATION THEORY

Human beings are continuously exposed to a wide variety and large number of stimuli. These stimuli may be physical, emotional, physiological, social, or spiritual and may take the form of matter or energy. These stimuli are input to the system and may emanate from within the system through the feedback loop or from external sources. The system's boundary screens and sorts input to protect the system from becoming overwhelmed while at the same time allowing sufficient input to transcend the boundary and ensure the system's viability.

In the terminology of stress and adaptation theory, system input is called a *stressor.* A stressor is neither positive or negative but has a positive or negative effect on the system.

In the terminology of stress and adaptation theory, system input is called a *stressor.* A stressor, in and of itself, is neither positive nor negative but rather has a positive or negative effect, depending on the way the system processes it.

This concept helps to explain why different people respond differently to the same stressor. For example, the death of a spouse is considered a negative event in our society. However, after the initial grieving period the surviving spouse may respond with more vigor and interest in life than before the spouse's death. Conversely, the birth of a baby is generally considered a positive event, but for some families an additional child to raise may strain emotional and financial resources unbearably.

Stressors may be classified as developmental or situational. The significance of this classification is that developmental stressors can be anticipated but situational stressors cannot; situational stressors are untoward events. For example, the adolescent is assaulted with physiological, emotional, and social stressors. Because these are a normal expected part of the maturation process, anticipatory guidance of the adolescent and his family can greatly strengthen the resources this system has available for dealing with these stressors. In contrast, the situational stressor of a middle-aged executive with two children in college who loses his job must be dealt with after it happens.

Regardless of whether a stressor is developmental or situational, the variables that determine a system's response to a stressor are multiple but always reflect the amount of potential energy available to deal with the stressor and the meaning of the stressor to the system. For example, a mild laryngitis would not greatly distress a dock worker but would be a major stressor to the opera singer.

When a stressor transcends the system's boundary it disturbs the system's steady state, automatically thrusting the system into a condition of stress. Therefore *stress* is defined as a condition in which the human system responds to input that has disturbed its steady state. As such, stress is necessary to life and is neither positive nor negative, although it is capable of causing either positive or negative effects. This technical view of stress differs markedly from the way the term is used in everyday language. One often hears the term "stress" used only in a negative sense and often as descriptive of an event rather than the condition of being.

Stress in human beings is a subjective phenomenon that cannot be observed directly but rather must be inferred from the person's response to the stressor. This response is called an *adaptation*. Integral to the theory of stress is the concept that the human system adapts holistically to stress. Regardless of the nature of the stressor, the human being responds in all his dimensions. A physiological stressor elicits not only a physiological adaptation, but also psychological and social adaptations. In like manner a social stressor elicits social, physiological, and psychological adaptations. In other words, the human system is not able to selectively respond to stressors. This generalized nonspecific response to stress is called the *general adaptation syndrome* and is consistent with the systems theory concept of wholism. For example, an adolescent experiencing the stress of her first date responds with fear about the appropriateness of her appearance and behavior. However, this response is not limited to the emo-

Stressors may be developmental or situational. Developmental stressors result from the normal maturational process and thus can be anticipated and dealt with through anticipatory guidance. Situational stressors are untoward events that cannot be anticipated and therefore must be dealt with after the occurrence.

Stress in human beings is defined as a condition of being wherein the human system responds to input that has disturbed its steady state. It is neither positive nor negative but is necessary to life.

The human system's response to stress is called an *adaptation*. Human systems respond holistically to stress. This generalized nonspecific response to stress is termed the *general adaptation syndrome*.

tion of fear but also affects her physiological subsystem by raising her blood pressure and decreasing the blood supply to the digestive subsystem, rendering her unable to eat. This response is actually preparing her for "fight or flight" as if the stressor were life-threatening. It is this fight or flight response that, if prolonged with no outlet, can result in the stress-related diseases that constitute major health problems in today's society.

In addition to the general adaptation syndrome, there may be a specific adaptation to the stressor. While the general adaptation syndrome is involuntary and unconscious, adaptations specific to a stressor may be either voluntary or involuntary and conscious or unconscious. When adaptations are voluntary and conscious they are called *coping mechanisms;* when they are involuntary and unconscious, they are called *defense mechanisms.* For example, a student in a state of stress because of an impending examination might adapt by voluntarily and consciously planning time to study and then adhering to the plan. Another student might respond to the same stressor by involuntarily utilizing the unconscious defense mechanism of rationalization by believing the exam is less important than attending social events, and therefore plan not to study. On the surface it would seem that the second student was more successful than the first in returning to the desirable state of homeokinesis in that this second student unlike the first is no longer under stress. It should be remembered, however, that the second student must use some of his available energy to remain unaware of the reality of the situation; he then has less energy available to deal with subsequent stressors. In either event this example is not complete until the outcome of each adaptation is examined. When the time of the examination arrives, it can be conjectured that the first student who studied would be prepared and therefore would do well on the test. The feedback he would receive is positive, thereby reinforcing the behavior of studying prior to an exam. The second student, however, would be unlikely to do well, and the feedback would be negative, thereby disrupting the system further and causing additional stress with less available energy to deal with it. If sufficient energy were available, however, the student could benefit from this negative feedback by utilizing it to alter his behavior and plan to study for exams in the future.

Once again, this example is overly simplistic in that it implies a linear cause-and-effect relationship between the stressor and the adaptation. In reality, the human system is always being affected by multiple stressors, and its adaptations reflect the system's ability to test reality, its previous adaptations, and its amount of potential energy. Human systems that cannot regain homeokinesis because of an inability to test reality, or that have had no previous experience with the stressor, or that lack sufficient energy to adapt to the number and potency of the stressors encountered are in a state of crisis. This condition is discussed fully in Chapter 24.

The student of psychiatric nursing should be aware that Axis IV of the *Diagnostic and Statistical Manual of Mental Disorders (Third Edition-Revised)* (DSM-

---

There may also be a specific adaptation to a stressor, which may be voluntary and conscious (*coping mechanism*) or involuntary and unconscious (*defense machanism*).

The adaptations of the human system reflect the system's ability to test reality, its previous adaptations, and its amount of potential energy.

Axis IV of the DSM-III-R provides for an assessment of the severity of psychosocial stressors and reflects the growing recognition that psychosocial stressors play a role in the development of mental illness.

III-R) (See Appendix C) provides for an assessment of the severity of the individual's psychosocial stressors in terms of both acute events (duration less than 6 months) and enduring circumstances (duration greater than 6 months). The fact that this parameter is included in this manual of psychiatric diagnoses reflects a growing recognition by the medical profession of the role that psychosocial stressors play in precipitating mental illness. On examination of this axis, the student will note that suggested examples of stressors include both developmental and situational events that range from those encountered by many people to highly unusual situations likely to be experienced by only a few persons. It should also be noted that the list of examples includes not only negative events but also those usually considered positive, such as graduation from school or marriage.

IMPLICATIONS FOR NURSING

The conceptual framework of systems theory and stress and adaptation provides nurses with organizing theories through which human behavior that seems arbitrary or inexplicable can be understood. It also provides a basis for conceptualizing the broad goals of all nursing interventions. Simply stated, the goal of all nursing interventions is to protect the system from noxious stressors or to increase the system's potential energy, thereby enhancing its ability to adapt to the stressor or to diminish the potency of the stressor. The following case history exemplifies how these goals can be achieved.

The goal of all nursing interventions is to protect the system from noxious (unhealthy) stressors, increase the system's potential energy, or diminish the stressor's potency.

> Mary Smith, a 16-year-old unmarried high school student, informed her parents that she was 2 months pregnant. Although this news was extremely upsetting to all, Mary's parents rallied around her and after many family discussions, often late into the night, the family made several decisions. Mary would not marry the child's father because they had little in common other than a strong sexual attraction. She would carry the baby to term and after its birth she would give it up for adoption so that she would be able to continue her education by going to college and perhaps fulfill her lifelong dream of becoming a lawyer. It was also decided that Mary would continue to attend the local high school. Mary's parents met with the school administrators who agreed to this plan. They also contacted an adoption agency to initiate plans for the adoption of the unborn child. These decisions were congruent with the values of the family, were agreeable to all, and seemed feasible to implement. Having adapted to the stressor of Mary's pregnancy, the Smith family regained its homeokinesis by devoting themselves to accomplishing the many household and business tasks left undone while its energy was focused on coping with this system change.
>
> Things went well for the Smith family until the fifth month, at which time Mary was visibly pregnant. Her fellow classmates began openly taunting her, her best friends no longer telephoned her or invited her to their homes, and the school board received a petition from irate parents demanding that Mary be suspended from school until the baby was born. Although the school board did not take this action and Mary's parents remained empathic and supportive, Mary became in-

creasingly depressed, unable to eat or sleep. Mr. and Mrs. Smith became alarmed and made an appointment at the mental health clinic. After several sessions at the clinic, it was decided that it would be best for Mary if she were to move to her grandparents' home in a different school district for the duration of her pregnancy. While she was there she would continue to receive counseling focused on helping her to cope with the birth and subsequent adoption of her child, as well as exploring responses she might use when she was questioned about her pregnancy. Finally, the mental health counselors in Mary's home town were concerned about the larger issue of the attitudes of the townspeople, not only for Mary's sake, but also because of what this attitude of intolerance meant to the mental health of her classmates. Because part of the mission of the mental health clinic was community education, the personnel organized evening seminars under the auspices of the school. These seminars were designed to assist interested students and parents to explore their interpersonal relationships and human values.

This case history depicts a family system thrust into a state of disequilibrium by changes in one of its subsystems caused by a situational stressor (Mary's pregnancy). The fact that the family system did not go into a state of massive disequilibrium on experiencing this change shows that it had potential energy available to bring to bear on the situation. It appears that the family utilized a problem-solving approach as the members engaged in many family discussions. The fact that this system's boundaries were relatively open is attested to by the parents' meeting with the school administrators and sharing their plans with them. They also were able to seek help from the mental health clinic when Mary's behavior alarmed them. A system with relatively closed boundaries would be unlikely to be able to exchange information effectively with other systems in its environment.

The decision for Mary to move out of the school district to her grandparents' home is an example of an intervention that utilized available resources to protect Mary and her family from the noxious stressor of peer rejection with which they were apparently unable to cope. Increasing Mary's potential energy, thereby enhancing her ability to adapt to future criticism, was accomplished by the reality-oriented counseling she continued to receive while at her grandparents' home. Finally, the action of the mental health clinic in conducting human relations seminars for the townspeople is an example of an intervention designed to diminish the potency of the stressor.

Although this situation does not specifically refer to the nurse as the mental health professional involved, the interventions employed are well within the scope of practice of a nurse functioning in a community mental health clinic.

END NOTE

This chapter discusses the importance of adopting a conceptual framework as a means to logically and coherently understand the phenomena of concern to nursing—namely, persons, their environments, and their health—as these interact between and among themselves. Systems theory and stress and adaptation are presented as a conceptual framework through which this understanding can be achieved. As a result, this conceptual framework is used throughout the text.

Within this framework, the goal of all nursing interventions is presented as protecting the system from noxious stressors or increasing the system's potential energy, thereby enhancing its ability to adapt to the stressor or diminishing the potency of the stressor. A family story is provided to illustrate how each goal was achieved in this particular situation.

SUGGESTED SOURCES OF ADDITIONAL INFORMATION

Blattner B: Holistic nursing, Englewood Cliffs, NJ, 1981, Prentice-Hall, Inc.

Flynn P: Holistic health: the art and science of care, Bowie, Md, 1980, Brady Communications Co., Inc.

Hagen D: The relationship between job loss and physical and mental illness, Hosp Commun Psychiatr 34:438, May 1983.

Hazzard ME, editor: A systems approach to nursing, Nurs Clin North Am 6: September 1971.

Hill M: When the patient is the family, Am J Nurs 81:536, 1981.

Murphy S: After Mt. St. Helen's: disaster stress research, J Psychosoc Nurs Ment Health Serv 22:8, July 1984.

Oleck L and Yoder S: Holism or hypocrisy? Perspect Psychiatr Care 19:65, March-April 1981.

Selye H: Stress without distress, New York, 1974, JB Lippincott Co.

Spiegel J: Transactions: the interplay between individual, family, and society, New York, 1971, Science House.

von Bertalanffy L: General systems theory: foundations, development, and applications, New York, 1968, George Braziller, Inc.

Psychosocial theories of personality development

11

LEARNING OBJECTIVES

After studying this chapter the student will be able to:

o Describe briefly the history of the study of personality development.
o Define the term *personality*.
o Discuss the personality attributes of a mentally healthy adult.
o Discuss the major concepts underlying the Piagetian theory of cognitive development and the Freudian, Eriksonian, and Sullivanian theories of personality development.
o Discuss each stage of cognitive and personality development in terms of its process and outcomes.

Understanding mental health and mental illness depends to a large extent on understanding the processes through which human beings develop, emotionally and cognitively. While it is imperative that the psychiatric nurse fully understand these theories, all nurses should be familiar with them, since nursing assessment and intervention for any client must be developmentally appropriate if they are to be accurate and effective.

HISTORICAL PERSPECTIVE

Before the beginning of the twentieth century the physical, emotional, and cognitive development of human beings was poorly understood. Children were viewed as miniature adults and, as such, were treated with little or no understanding of their developmentally related needs. Furthermore, the attainment of physical maturity was thought to signal the achievement of emotional and cognitive maturity. If growth was complete, so was development! It was not until

Children were historically viewed as miniature adults, who as they grew were thought to develop emotionally at the same rate that they developed physically.

Early childhood experiences and their effect on later emotional problems were at the core of Freud's theory of personality development, called the *psychosexual theory*.

The *Eight Ages of Man,* eight developmental stages that encompass the life span, were identified by Erikson.

the early twentieth century that the study of personality development of children began in earnest. Major strides in understanding cognitive development were not achieved until the midtwentieth century. Interest in the personality development of adults has emerged only recently and is currently the subject of much study because the number of persons of middle and older age is rapidly increasing.

The theories proposed by Sigmund Freud (1856–1939) revolutionized the way in which clinicians and laypersons alike viewed human behavior. It was Freud's writing that first stressed the crucial importance of early childhood experiences in the development of human personality and the relationship between some of the emotional problems in adult life and the negative influences that occurred during the individual's early years. Freud's theory of personality development is called the *psychosexual theory* of development.

During and after Freud's pioneering work, many other theorists addressed themselves to the study of personality development to better understand human behavior. Investigators such as Erik Erikson and Harry Stack Sullivan adapted, modified, and enlarged on Freud's basic theories; their work has resulted in theories that are seen as significantly different from those of Freud.

Erik Erikson was born in Frankfurt, Germany, in 1902 of Danish parents. His mother and father had separated before he was born, and when he was about 3 years old, his mother married a pediatrician who was a German Jew. With this mixed cultural heritage Erikson had difficulty establishing his own sense of identity. It is likely that his own personal quest for identity was a major factor in the development of his theory of personality development, referred to as the *Eight Ages of Man*. At age 25 Erikson left Germany to go to Vienna, where he studied the new discipline of psychoanalysis. He immigrated to Boston, Massachusetts, in 1933.

Harry Stack Sullivan was born in Norwich, New York, in 1892 and died in 1949. Sullivan became a psychiatrist during the early years of Freud's profound influence on American psychiatry. However, unlike many of his colleagues, he studied only in the United States, working closely with a group of psychoanalysts and social psychologists who were pulling away from the classical psychoanalytical model established by Freud. Sullivan's theories postulate that the most critical factor in personality development is the individual's relationship with other significant people. His theories emphasize the nature and the quality of these relationships. This fact is best illustrated by his reference to the *mothering one* to distinguish between the roles of the biological mother and the person (male or female) who provides nurturing experiences for the infant. Although Sullivan viewed the relationship between the infant and the mothering one as fundamental to personality development, he also placed great emphasis on the importance of relationships with significant others such as peers, spouse, and offspring as the person progresses throughout life. Therefore Sullivan's theory is called the *interpersonal theory of psychiatry*. In view of the fact that the nurse's role with mentally ill persons is almost totally focused on the relationship that is developed with them, Sullivan's theory seems to be particularly applicable to nursing practice.

The pioneering work on cognitive development was undertaken by Jean Piaget (1896–1980), a Swiss psychologist. Piaget was not alone in observing that children at various ages differed in their ability to think, remember, and problem solve. He was the first, however, to systematically study the processes by which these abilities develop. Piaget began his exploration of cognitive development by exhaustively observing his own three children; his resultant theory helps to clarify and augment what is known about the development of the personality.

DEFINITION OF PERSONALITY

Before a discussion of personality development can become meaningful, it is essential to understand the definition of the term *personality*. Unfortunately this word has been used to convey many different meanings and ideas. In ordinary conversation it usually refers to the personal response that the individual evokes from others. It is not unusual for someone to comment that an individual has a pleasing personality or that a certain person has a poor personality. When used technically, the term personality refers to *the aggregate of the physical and mental qualities of the individual as these interact in characteristic fashion with his environment.* Thus it can be seen that personality is expressed through behavior. The characteristic combinations of behavior distinguish one individual from another and endow individuals with their own unique identity.

This definition of personality includes the individual's biological and intellectual endowment, the attributes he has acquired through experience, and his conscious and unconscious reactions and feelings. Personality development is a complex and dynamic process. As such, the personality is constantly evolving from what it was to something different, yet it always retains a certain identifiable consistency. It is important to remember that from birth to death personality is ever changing and ever developing. This fact makes it possible for individuals of all ages to profit from corrective experiences and to modify behavior in a positive direction. This is the rationale underlying all psychotherapeutic endeavors.

PERSONALITY ATTRIBUTES OF THE MENTALLY HEALTHY ADULT

The first attempts to describe the personality attributes of the mentally healthy adult were based on inferences drawn from what was known about mentally ill persons, often leading to erroneous conclusions. Consequently, mental health was initially described in negative terms, such as the absence of incapacitating

The individual's relationship with other significant people, his interdependence, was the basis of Sullivan's *interpersonal theory* of personality development.

A child's ability to think, remember, and problem solve at different ages was studied by Piaget.

Personality
The aggregate of the physical and mental qualities of the individual as these interact in characteristic fashion with his environment.

anxiety. It was not until the late 1950s that psychologist Marie Jahoda identified criteria of positive mental health. This work was done under the auspices of the Joint Commission on Mental Illness and Health, whose report was published in 1961.

It is important to understand that the personality attributes of the mentally healthy adult are not amenable to precise measurement, as are many indices of physical health. Rather, these attributes are inferred from the individual's behavior, including what he says about himself and others. In general, socially acceptable behavior is considered indicative of mental health—socially unacceptable behavior is often considered a sign of mental illness. Consequently, mental health is culturally bound in the sense that the very same behavior that is acceptable in one culture may be deemed unacceptable in another. Furthermore, mental health is relative to time and place and situation. For example, an individual who would never consider harming another under usual circumstances but who is able to defend himself by hitting an assailant when attacked is displaying the ability to assess reality accurately, a major criterion of mental health.

The individual's level of self-acceptance is usually mentioned as an important reflection of his degree of mental health. All human beings have strengths and limitations—a mentally healthy adult works at maximizing his strengths and minimizing his limitations but at the same time accepts his strengths and limitations without inordinate pride or shame. In other words, the capacity to be comfortable with oneself is considered an important attribute of the mentally healthy adult.

The way a person perceives reality is another significant dimension of the degree of his mental health. The mentally healthy individual is one who views his environment realistically, not as filtered through his own unique need system. Therefore, the mentally healthy adult is unlikely to view the world either as always hostile and threatening or as always friendly and accepting. Rather, he is able to evaluate each situation and validate his perceptions with others whom he trusts.

Self-acceptance and a realistic perception of reality greatly influence the achievement of another attribute of mental health, namely, environmental mas-

---

Personality attributes of the mentally healthy adult

A mentally healthy adult:
    Accepts his strengths and limitations
    Perceives reality accurately
    Exhibits environmental mastery
    Engages in independent thinking and action
    Achieves a unifying, integrated outlook on life

tery. Environmental mastery suggests that the individual feels in control of himself and his environment and has made an investment in living that has necessitated the high-level development of his inherent abilities.

The mentally healthy or emotionally mature individual will have developed the capacity for independent thinking and action. This capacity is described by some as efficiency in problem solving and by others as autonomy or self-determination.

A final capacity usually included in a discussion of mental health is the ability of the individual to synthesize all his psychological functions and personal attributes, which, in turn, enables him to achieve a unifying, integrated outlook on life and a sense of direction in relation to his role in it.

These manifestations of mental health are consistent with those behaviors identified by another pioneer in the study of mental health, Abraham Maslow (1908–1970). Maslow believed that mental illness could be understood only within a framework of an understanding of mental health. He developed the widely used "hierarchy of needs" theory, often referred to as the theory of self-actualization (see Table 11-1). This theory states that all human beings strive to develop, but all have inherent basic needs, which are ordered hierarchically and which emerge only when lower-level needs have been satisfied. Further, the individual's behavior is directed toward meeting the need that is operative at the time. This explains the oft-quoted observation that a child who is hungry cannot learn. A mentally healthy individual, according to Maslow, is a self-actualizing person whose energy is directed toward meeting his unique potential. While the behavior of self-actualizing people differs because of their uniqueness, all share the ability and willingness to see reality as it is, a sense of humility integrated with creativity, an acceptance of self with little or no inner conflict, and, importantly, a capacity for joy in themselves, others, and the world in which they live.

TABLE 11-1   *Maslow's hierarchy of needs*

Need	Characteristics
Physiologic	Satisfying needs for oxygen, water, food, shelter, sleep, relief of sexual tension
Safety	Avoiding harm and achieving security and physical safety
Love and belonging	Giving and receiving affection, developing companionship, and gaining acceptance by a group
Esteem and recognition	Achieving recognition by others leading to self-esteem and feelings of prestige; achieving success in work
Self-actualization	Achieving one's own unique potential in all dimensions
Aesthetic and cognitive	Achieving an unbiased understanding and appreciation of the beauty and unity of the world and one's role in it

BASIC CONCEPTS OF PERSONALITY DEVELOPMENT

Although some psychiatrists feel that is is important to adhere strictly and consistently to the tenets of one school of thought, psychiatric theories currently in use in the United States are becoming increasingly eclectic. That is, concepts from various schools of thought are being used in combination to develop a useful theory of personality development. The necessity of an eclectic approach is particularly apparent in nursing practice; the role of the nurse in interaction with patients is probably more varied than in any other discipline. Consequently the following discussion will describe the basic concepts of Freud, Erikson, and Sullivan with a subsequent discussion of each stage of personality development as described by these theorists. It is hoped that this approach will enable the student to compare and contrast these theories and use that which is applicable as she plans, implements, and evaluates nursing care.

Freudian concepts

Freud's theories are often referred to as *intrapsychic* because they emphasize the internal emotional life of the individual as the most significant factor in the development of the personality. Even though Freud deviated widely from the accepted medical theories and practices of his day, his theories are largely based on a biological model. For example, Freud believed that each individual is born with a genetically determined amount of *libidinal energy,* a form of psychic energy that seeks pleasure in an attempt to avoid tension or pain. In this sense libidinal energy is viewed as sexual energy. This energy cannot increase or decrease in amount but must be shared among the various parts of the personality. Freud developed his conception of the stages of personality development largely around the concept of libidinal energy and delineated each stage of development according to the area of the body on which he believed the energy was focused. For example, the first stage of development is characterized by the libidinal energy being concentrated on the mouth. It is through the mouth that the infant expresses tension and pain and through the mouth that pleasure is perceived. As the child matures physiologically, the libidinal energy shifts from the mouth to other parts of the body until adulthood, when the libidinal energy is focused on the genital area, enabling the individual to establish a mature heterosexual relationship, which Freud saw as the hallmark of the normal development of personality. Therefore Freud delineated only five stages of personality development, seeing this process as being complete at adulthood with major personality alterations unlikely thereafter under usual circumstances. It is because of the libidinal energy theory and its relationship to the development of the personality that Freud's theory of personality development is called the *psychosexual theory.*

Freud's topographical descriptions of the psyche are important for the student to understand, since these concepts are used almost universally in the United States and contribute much to understanding human behavior.

Levels of consciousness. One way in which Freud described the mind topo-

Libido
The psychic energy or instinctual drive associated with sexual desire, pleasure, or creativity.

graphically was from the standpoint of levels of consciousness. These levels are referred to as the conscious, the preconscious or subconscious, and the unconscious parts of the mind.

The *conscious* part of the mind is aware of the here and now as it relates to the individual and his environment. It functions only when the individual is awake. The conscious mind is concerned with thoughts, feelings, and sensations. It directs the individual as he behaves in a rational, thoughtful way.

The *preconscious* or *subconscious* is that part of the mind in which ideas and reactions are stored and partially forgotten—it is not economical for human beings to burden the conscious mind with a multitude of facts that are infrequently used and currently not in demand. The preconscious also acts as a watchman; it prevents certain unacceptable, disturbing unconscious memories from reaching the conscious mind. These two functions make the preconscious an extremely valuable device. Material relegated to this handy storehouse can usually be brought into conscious awareness if the individual concentrates on recall.

The *unconscious* is by far the largest part of the mind and is sometimes compared to the large hidden part of an iceberg that floats under the water. In this comparison the small part of the iceberg that appears above the water represents the conscious mind. The unconscious is the storehouse for all the memories, feelings, and responses experienced by the individual during his entire life. The unconscious is one of Freud's most important concepts. Freudian theorists believe that the human mind never actually forgets any experience but stores in the unconscious all knowledge, information, and feeling about all experiences. These memories cannot be recalled at will. The individual is rarely aware of the unconscious mind, except as it demonstrates its presence through such means as dreams, slips of the tongue, unexplained behavioral responses, jokes, and lapses of memory. Material stored in the unconscious has a powerful influence on behavior because the accompanying feelings continue to act as motivating, dynamic forces. The individual is unaware of the ideas themselves, but he may continue to experience an emotional reaction as if the material were in the conscious mind. This theory underlies the belief that all behavior has meaning. In other words, no behavior occurs by accident or chance; rather, all behavior is an expression of feelings or needs of which the individual frequently is not aware.

Structure of the personality. The second topographical description developed by Freud is frequently referred to as the structure of the personality. This structure includes the concepts of the id, the ego, and the superego.

The *id* is part of and derived from the unconscious. It is unlearned, primitive, selfish, and the source of all libidinal energy. It contains the instinctual drives, included in which are the drive for self-preservation, the drive to reproduce, and the drive for group association. The id is without a sense of right and wrong and ruthlessly insists on immediate satisfaction of its impulses and desires.

When the individual is born, he is said to be a bundle of id, seeking only to

Freud identified the levels of consciousness as the *conscious*, the *preconscious*, and the *unconscious*.

Id
The part of the psyche that functions in the unconscious and is the source of instinctive energy, impulses, and drives. It is based on the pleasure principle and has strong tendencies toward self-preservation.

satisfy his needs and to find release for physiological tensions. By crying, the infant insists on receiving attention when tensions build up. He disregards all other factors in his environment as he demands that his needs be met.

During the individual's entire life the id persists in pushing the organism toward the achievement of its primitive, instinctual goals. It is described as operating on the basis of the *pleasure principle*. That is to say, the id presses for avoidance of pain at all costs and seeks to maintain pleasure. *Pleasure* in this sense refers to release of tension and the establishment of emotional and physiological equilibrium. *Pain* refers to tensions that are present when the infant is cold, hungry, frightened, or anxious. As the child matures, the concept of pain encompasses additional aspects of body equilibrium, including sexual tension, tensions that result from cultural pressures, and tension from physiological needs. Throughout the individual's entire life the id insists that the individual seek release of tension, regardless of the social outcome. It is the duty of other parts of the personality to censor the id and to keep it under control.

Ego
The part of the psyche that experiences and maintains conscious contact with reality and that tempers the primitive drives of the id and the demands of the superego with the social and physical needs of society.

The development of the *ego* is a result of the individual's interaction with the environment. It is initiated when the infant recognizes the breast or the bottle as part of the environment rather than as part of his own body. The ego promotes the individual's satisfactory adjustment in relation to his environment. Its main function is to effect an acceptable compromise between the crude pleasure-seeking strivings of the id and the inhibitions of the superego. The means through which the ego achieves this goal is reality testing. The ego deals with the demands of reality as it strives to control and derive satisfaction from the environment. Thus, as the individual matures the ego becomes the rational, reasonable, conscious part of the personality and strives to integrate the total personality into a smoothly functioning, unified, coherent whole. In the mature adult it is the ego that represents the self to others and individualizes him from other human beings.

Superego
That part of the psyche, functioning mostly in the unconscious, that develops when the standards of the parents and of society are incorporated.

Chronologically, the *superego* develops last. Its development is partially a result of the socialization process that the child undergoes. The superego incorporates the taboos, prohibitions, ideals, and standards of the parents and the other significant adults with whom the child associates. It operates mostly at the unconscious level and at this level is an inhibitor of the id. The superego is blindly rigid, strictly moralistic, and as unrelenting and ruthless as the id. There are two aspects of the superego. One is called the *conscience*. The conscience is the part of the superego that punishes the individual through guilt and anxiety when his behavior deviates from the strict standards of the superego. The other aspect is called the *ego ideal*. The ego ideal rewards the individual through feelings of euphoria and well-being when his behavior emulates those standards believed by the superego to be desirable. It is important to understand that neither the punishing nor the rewarding functions of the superego are based on the reality of the situation. Rather, they are based on the individual's internalized standards of right and wrong, good and bad, which were learned at an early age and which are stored for the most part in the unconscious mind.

If the individual does not develop an ego strong enough to arbitrate effectively between the id and the superego, he will surely develop intrapersonal and interpersonal conflicts. When the id is not controlled effectively, the individual functions in antisocial, lawless ways because his primitive impulses are expressed freely. If the superego is so strong that the individual's life is dominated by its restrictions on behavior, he is likely to be inhibited, repressed, unhappy, and guilt-ridden. Thus a mature, effective, stable adult life depends on the development of an ego powerful enough to adequately test reality and then to mediate successfully between the demands of the id and the superego.

Eriksonian concepts

Erikson's theories build on and include Freudian concepts. However, their emphasis is not on Freud's intrapsychic theories but rather on the ability of the ego to develop in a healthy, adaptive manner given a facilitative environment. Therefore Erikson's theories are variously referred to as neo-Freudian, ego psychology, and cultural. Erikson has also extended the stages of personality development to include the totality of the life span, introducing the very important idea that personality development does not cease at the achievement of adulthood. This belief helps to explain the fundamental changes in an individual's feelings and behavior that characteristically occur during his adult life.

A major contribution Erikson has made to the understanding of personality development is his identification of *developmental tasks* for each developmental period. These developmental tasks are age-specific achievements that are largely culturally determined. Achievement of each task increases the ego strength of the individual and enhances the probability of satisfactory achievement of subsequent tasks. Erikson sees the individual's ability to complete each developmental task satisfactorily as dependent not only on his genetic endowment and intrapsychic development, but also primarily on the quality of his interaction with the environment. It is important to understand that the developmental tasks identified by Erikson include both positive and negative outcomes. This means that the individual who has not satisfactorily achieved the developmental task for a specific stage of development will develop, as a result, a nondesirable and less healthy attribute in its stead. The most obvious example is the developmental task of the first developmental period—basic trust versus basic mistrust. The infant who is not successful, for whatever reason, in developing a sense of basic trust will not be left with an ego structure that demonstrates a mere lack of trust. The alternative is the development of an even more negative characteristic—a sense of basic mistrust. The significance of this paradigm is illustrated simply by the difference between the feelings of "I'm not sure that I can trust you" and "I'm sure that I cannot trust you." Therefore to understand Erikson's theory of personality development fully, the student must understand the negative as well as the positive outcomes of each developmental period.

Erikson's stages of personality development include the entire life span and are identified by age-specific achievements known as developmental tasks.

Sullivanian concepts

Sullivan's theories are firmly based on the belief that human beings are more basically different from than similar to all other animals. The uniqueness of human beings, according to Sullivan, lies in their interdependence; it is as a result of their interactions with others, not their physiological endowment, that the human personality is developed. As previously stated, Sullivan's theories are referred to as *interpersonal* because of their emphasis on human interaction. Sullivan believed that all human behavior is goal directed toward the fulfillment of two needs: the need for satisfaction and the need for security. The need for satisfaction represents the biological needs of the person for such things as air, food, and sex. The need for security represents the emotional needs of the individual for such feelings states as interpersonal intimacy, status, and self-esteem. When these needs are perceived, internal tension results, and the individual employs a variety of methods to meet them and thereby reduce the tension. Sullivan called these methods *dynamisms,* and it is partially around the dynamisms characteristic of each age group that he built his theory of personality development. For example, during the first stage of development the oral cavity is used almost exclusively by the infant as the method to meet his needs for satisfaction (by crying to be fed) and his needs for security (by crying to be held). Therefore the stage of infancy is characterized by the oral dynamism, and the oral cavity becomes important because it is the means through which the individual establishes interpersonal contact, which in turn is the means through which his needs are met and tension is reduced. In fact the individual not only gets his needs met through interpersonal contact but also through this contact he establishes the fact of his own existence. Sullivan believed that an individual's self-concept is developed as a result of the quality of his interpersonal relationships with significant others in his infancy and childhood. In fact Sullivan defined the self-concept as the result of the reflected appraisals of significant others.

Sullivan believes that all human behavior is directed toward fulfillment of two basic needs, satisfaction and security, requiring the approval of significant others.

The concept of anxiety is central to Sullivan's theory of personality development. He postulated that anxiety is a response to feelings of disapproval from a significant adult. It is important to understand that these feelings may or may not be based in reality, and that the adult whose disapproval is feared may be real or a symbolic representation. According to Sullivan, then, the development of the personality consists of a series of interpersonally based learnings in which dynamisms are used as the individual attempts to gain approval and avoid the anxiety associated with disapproval.

BASIC CONCEPTS OF COGNITIVE DEVELOPMENT

Although cognitive development refers specifically to the ability of the individual to think, to remember, and to problem solve, it is inextricably related to personality development and as such is included in this discussion. Piaget's theory of cognitive development places heavy emphasis on sequential interactions of the individual's genetically determined intellectual potential and his environment with the goal of adjusting to the environment. He believed that each individual has an innate knowledge structure, called *schema,* which initially allows him to mentally organize ways to behave in his environment. Each new environmental experience calls forth the necessity for *adaptation,* which entails the simultaneous processes of *assimilation* and *accommodation.* Assimilation refers to the adjustment of the experience so that knowledge of it can be incorporated into the child's existing body of knowledge; accommodation refers to the simultaneous modification of the body of knowledge based on the newly incorporated knowledge. In this way, schemata are built, refined, and organized within and among each other.

Piaget's theory describes four main, discrete stages of cognitive development: the sensorimotor stage, the preoperational stage, the stage of concrete operations, and the stage of formal operations.

STAGES OF PERSONALITY AND COGNITIVE DEVELOPMENT

It has been said that the first 6 years in a child's life contribute the most to personality development. When one considers that these years provide the foundation for future patterns of behavior, this statement appears to be true. However, the student must understand the influence of all stages of development on the personality to accurately assess the behavior of the adults for whom she provides nursing care. The following is a description and discussion of each of the developmental stages according to the theories of Freud, Erikson, Sullivan, and Piaget.

Infancy

The period of infancy roughly extends over the first year and a half of life. Freud referred to this period as the *oral stage* because the child's libidinal energy is focused on his mouth and its functions to the exclusion of all other considerations. This singular focus on self is technically referred to as *primary narcissism,* which means self-love.

In the first months of life the infant is unable to differentiate between himself and his environment. He therefore feels that all that happens to him is caused by him. This feeling of being all powerful is termed *omnipotence.* The infant's awareness of himself is in terms of comfort or discomfort, and his total being is focused on fulfilling the demands of the id, which insists on relief from hunger and cold, which are perceived as a diffused tension. He seeks relief from this tension by using his mouth, lips, and tongue to cry, suck, and swallow. These activities provide him with the greatest pleasures, since they reduce discomfort. In the earliest months the infant is dependent on a nurturing adult to supply the nipple that meets his need for sucking and through which he obtains milk to swallow, appeasing the tension caused by hunger. Accidentally the infant soon finds his thumb and discovers that he can meet his own needs for sucking. Although sucking his own thumb provides pleasure, it is experienced as being different from sucking the nipple. Through this simple realization the infant begins the complex, lengthy process of differentiating himself from the environment. In this way the ego or the recognition of the self or the "me" begins to develop.

Freud refers to infancy as the oral stage *because all the child's needs are focused on his mouth, through which he receives both food and self-gratification.*

When weaning is initiated the infant begins to receive fewer oral satisfactions from his environment. When the cup and solid food are substituted for the breast or bottle, the infant feels frustrated. With the adoption of more rigid schedules the infant is denied the complete attention of the mother. He may react to these frustrations orally in an aggressive, sometimes destructive way and may begin to bite and may seek symbolic oral gratification by sucking other objects.

Because food and love are given simultaneously during the oral period, oral needs become synonymous with protective love and security. These needs are universal and continue throughout life in one form or another. In adult life release of tension through oral gratification is achieved through chewing gum, eating, and drinking. Freud believed that these activities are residuals of the oral stage of personality development.

Erikson calls infancy the oral-sensory stage *and emphasizes the importance of the mother-child relationship in the developmental task of* basic trust versus basic mistrust.

Erikson's view of infancy is very similar to the Freudian view just described, although he terms it the *oral-sensory stage*. Unlike Freud, however, Erikson emphasizes the significance of the mother-child relationship in the achievement of the developmental task of the oral stage: *basic trust versus basic mistrust*. Erikson theorizes that if the infant's great need for love and attention is met consistently and unconditionally by a giving, loving mother, he will learn to trust her. Since the infant has no alternative but to view his mother as representing the world at large, this attitude of basic trust in her will strongly influence his perceptions of other people and the environment. Therefore a healthy resolution of this stage of personality development, according to Erikson, results in the development of a basic sense of trust in the mother, which serves as the basis for the development of future trusting relationships. On the other hand, if the infant's experiences with his mother are characterized by inconsistencies and anxiety, he will learn to mistrust her and subsequently generalize this attitude to the world at large. It does not take much imagination to appreciate the many great differences between the feelings and behaviors of adults who have achieved a sense of basic trust and those who have achieved a sense of basic mistrust.

Sullivan stresses the importance of the mothering one *during the stage of infancy, emphasizing the significance of the person who provides consistent nurturing of the infant.*

Sullivan referred to the first year and a half of life as the stage of infancy, rather than the oral stage, because he believed that the oral cavity has significance only in that it is the vehicle through which the infant establishes interpersonal contact. Sullivan introduced several very important concepts regarding the first stage of development. He coined the term *mothering one* to reflect the belief that the most important person in the infant's life is the individual who consistently nurtures him and that this person does not necessarily have to be the biological mother. In fact, whether the mothering one is the biological mother or not, Sullivan believed that this person and the infant must establish an interpersonal relationship, wherein they become highly significant to each other. This relationship is unique to the stage of infancy and is characterized by the *empathic linkage,* a symbolic emotional umbilical cord that makes the infant and the nurturing adult highly sensitive to each other's feeling states. Other theorists refer to this process as bonding. It is through the empathic linkage that both positive feelings of love and acceptance and negative feelings of anxiety and rejection are conveyed. Sullivan also believed that the development of the *self-concept* begins in the stage of infancy and is closely related to the quality of the infant's feeding experiences. Since the self-concept develops as the result of the reflected appraisals of significant others, if the infant frequently experiences satisfaction and security from the mothering one during the feeding process, he begins to see himself as being a worthwhile individual; that is, he will begin to develop a "good me" self-concept. Conversely, if the infant's experience with the mothering one is frequently fraught with tension and inconsistency, the foundation is laid for the development of a "bad me" self-concept, wherein the individual begins to see himself as being not worthwhile. If the infant is severely deprived during this stage, he will respond with massive amounts of anxiety that threaten his very life. To preserve his life the infant defends himself by disassociating the anxiety-generating experiences. As a result, he cannot develop a sense of self from reflected appraisals, so he develops a "not me" self-concept. This situation lays the foundation for the subsequent development of severe emotional problems.

Once the foundation is laid for its development, the self-concept tends to perpetuate itself. For example the child whose earlier reflected appraisals of significant others have led to the development of a "good-me" self-concept feels he is a worthwhile, valued person and tends to behave as such. This behavior, in turn, evokes further positive feedback from significant others and thereby reinforces the existing "good- me" self-concept. However, as the child grows he inevitably encounters people who do not respond to him in the accustomed manner. This unfamiliar experience evokes anxiety and is dealt with by the use of what Sullivan terms *security operations,* enabling the child to ignore this differing input. This process is just as applicable to people who have developed "bad-me" and "not-me" self-concepts and helps to explain why some persons succeed against all odds and others fail despite all advantages.

Piaget's first stage of cognitive development is called the *sensorimotor stage* and is operative between birth and 24 months of age. During the initial phase of this stage, the infant responds to his environment in an undifferentiated way. For example, when the newborn is startled by a loud noise, his entire body reacts. He is also egocentric, viewing himself as fused with his environment and at its center. By the end of this stage, however, the child learns that he is separate from his environment. He also learns that objects have permanence—that objects have not disappeared because they are out of sight. Mastering the concept

Piaget identifies the first stage of cognitive development as the *sensorimotor stage*. By the end of this stage, the infant realizes that he is separate from his environment and that objects are permanent.

of object permanence is the basis for the infant's pleasure in the game of peek-a-boo. Finally, by the end of the sensorimotor stage, the infant's behavior in familiar situations becomes goal directed. These cognitive outcomes are consistent with and related to the personality outcomes of the first stage of development as described by Freud and Sullivan.

Early childhood

All theorists agree that the successful resolution of the first stage of development greatly enhances the probability of a successful resolution of subsequent stages.

The period of early childhood is a phase of personality development that occurs roughly between the ages of 18 months and 3 years. Freud termed this period of time the *anal stage* because the libidinal energy shifts from the oral cavity to the anus and the urethra.

Freud calls early childhood the *anal stage* because the child takes pleasure in freely evacuating his bowels and bladder.

In the early part of this period the child freely gratifies his love of self with the pleasurable sensations involved in evacuating the bladder and bowels naturally and without restriction. Although the mouth remains an important zone of pleasure, the child derives his greatest pleasure from the anus and the urethra during these early years.

Ego development continues in this period as the child continuously develops a better defined concept of self. Superego development is initiated as the mother begins to insist that the child accept certain restrictions and controls regarding toileting. At this point the child experiences the first major frustration of his id drives. He is forced to come to terms with the reality of the situation. To retain the love of the mother the child must learn to postpone the immediate pleasure of urinating or evacuating until the appropriate time and place are available. The necessity for adapting to the wishes of the mother regarding toileting places the child and the mother in conflict. As the mother makes demands on the child in an attempt to force him to accept her standards in relation to toileting, the child develops *ambivalence* toward her, that is, he simultaneously loves and hates her.

Freud believed that if great stress is placed on the child's remaining clean during this period, he may grow up to be compulsively clean and meticulous. On the other hand, he may unconsciously deal with his anxiety by the use of reaction formation as a defense mechanism and become very untidy and unconcerned about cleanliness in his adult life. Other adult attitudes thought to be traceable to rigid toilet training include stubbornness, hoarding and collecting, excessive concern with bowel function, and sadistic or masochistic tendencies.

Erikson calls this stage the *muscular-anal stage* and stresses the importance of the mother's reaction to the child's interest in controlling himself.

Erikson refers to this stage of development as the *muscular-anal stage* and identifies *autonomy versus shame and doubt* as the developmental task to be addressed. Of great significance, according to Erikson, is the mother's response to the child's interest in assuming control over himself by controlling his urine and feces. If she treats the child with respect as an individual who is separate from her, he will begin to develop a sense of autonomy, or self-sufficiency. On the other hand, if his efforts to do for himself are ridiculed or interfered with, he will develop a sense of shame and doubt his capabilities.

Sullivan used the term *early childhood* to refer to this period of life. He acknowledged the shift in the child's interest from his mouth to his anus but emphasized the sense of power the child feels as he attempts to control himself and others, particularly the mothering one. This feeling of power often puts the child and the mothering one in conflict as the mothering one attempts to toilet train the child. The process and outcome of this power struggle are believed to serve as the prototypical experience for similar interpersonal conflicts in later life. Of equal importance during this stage of development is Sullivan's belief that the child sees his feces as an extension of himself, and therefore the mothering one's response to the child's pleasure in his feces is seen by the child as a reflection of her view of him. In that way the self-concept established in the stage of infancy is reinforced or altered.

Sullivan stresses the sense of power experienced by the child as he attempts to control himself and others, especially the mothering one.

The developmental stages of early and later childhood encompass the second period of cognitive development, which Piaget calls *preoperational*. The preoperational stage is divided into two periods, the *preconceptual,* which is in force between the ages of 2 to 4 years, and the *intuitive,* which occurs between the ages of 4 to 7 years. During the preconceptual period the child begins to understand symbols and can think in terms of past, present, and future. Increasing language development provides a powerful tool for environmental exploration. By the end of the intuitive period the child is able to think in terms of classes, see relationships—especially if they involve him, and handle number concepts. For example, he can recognize a variety of seats as "chairs" even though they may look quite different, he can understand that he will be punished if he breaks a rule, and he knows that eight of any object is more than two of the same object.

Piaget identifies the second stage of cognitive development as *preoperational*.

Later childhood

The period of later childhood is a phase of development that includes the ages from 3 to 6. Freud called this period the *phallic stage*. This descriptive term refers to the fact that the focus of pleasurable sensations has shifted from the mouth and the excretory organs to the genitalia and that the child begins to identify with the parent of the same sex and unconsciously wishes to replace that parent in the family situation. Thus it is not uncommon to hear a girl in this age-group speak of "marrying Daddy" or a little boy say, "Go away, Daddy, I will take care of Mommy."

Freud calls the period of later childhood the *phallic stage* because the child's focus has shifted away from his mouth and excretory organs to his genitalia. The child's interest centers on both his own body and the bodies of others.

Between the ages of 3 and 6 years children begin to examine purposefully their own bodies and the bodies of their playmates. They discover that pleasurable sensations can be aroused from manipulation of the penis or the clitoris. The difference between the genitalia of men and women is of great interest to them, and they wonder about the girl's lack of an obvious sexual organ. Children of this age may conclude that the penis can be lost in some way, since some people whose bodies they have observed have apparently lost this organ. Anxiety about the loss of the sex organ may develop among children in this age-group. Fears may be expressed by a little boy concerning the loss of his penis through punishment or an accident. These fears are referred to as *castration fears*. Unfortunately some parents reinforce these fears by threatening to cut off the penis if the child is observed fondling it. A little girl notices that she has no penis and may conclude that she lost it or that it has been taken away. She naturally wants what she observes some other children possess. Freud called this attitude on the part of a little girl *penis envy*.

It should be noted that many contemporary theorists believe that any evidence of castration anxiety or penis envy in children of this age is a result of cultural conditioning and not an inherent element in personality development. A serious student of human behavior would be wise to keep an open mind, observing for behavioral changes in children as cultural changes take place.

During this period the little boy who has always had a great deal of attention and love from his mother begins to feel very possessive toward her. He wants her for himself, and he resents the close tie that he feels exists between his mother and father. He develops competitive feelings toward his father and tries to become a rival with him for his mother's love. The father is such a large and formidable opponent that the little boy develops a good deal of resentment and fear of him. This situation is referred to as the *Oedipus complex*. It may precipitate castration fears because the little boy may begin to fear that the father will punish him for his resentment toward him and his attempt to replace him in his mother's life. Eventually the little boy concludes that being like his father is a more effective way of achieving his mother's love and attention. Thus he begins to take on the masculine behavior of his father. This is referred to as *identification*. In this way the little boy begins to learn the role of the male in the culture.

Similarly, during this period the little girl begins to identify with the feminine role. The process through which the girl passes in identifying with the parent of the same sex is not as clearly understood as is the process for little boys. The girl feels that somehow her mother is responsible for the fact that she does not have a penis. She also notices that she does not have breasts as her mother does. She may blame her mother for not having provided her with a complete body and may display a good deal of hostility and antagonism toward her. The little girl turns to her father for love and affection and frequently competes openly with the mother for his attention. She begins to imitate her mother because she feels that in this way she may be able to please her father. This is a difficult period for the little girl who must keep her mother's love and approval because she is still dependent on her. It is essential that the child maintain a positive relationship with her mother if she is to accomplish the task of identifying with the feminine role.

Oedipus complex
A boy child's desire for a sexual relationship with his mother, usually with strong negative feelings for his father.

The birth of a baby in the family at this time presents both boys and girls of this age with a particularly difficult adjustment problem. The 3- to 6-year-old uses almost all of his energy in controlling his incestuous desires toward the parent of the opposite sex and his rage toward the parent of the same sex. The necessity to compete with a helpless infant for the attention of the parents often results in a great deal of overt sibling rivalry.

Superego development is also at its height at this time, since in most societies the issues being addressed are seen as moralistic ones. Therefore unless this stage is successfully resolved, the potential exists for the child to develop long-lasting feelings of guilt because of his incestuous wishes for the parent of the opposite sex and his rage against the parent of the same sex.

Erikson refers to this stage of development as the *locomotor-genital stage* and describes it as having the developmental outcomes of *initiative versus guilt*. He agrees with Freud that children of this age desire to exclusively possess the parent of the opposite sex. To achieve this goal the child makes the first move, that is, he takes the initiative. In a healthy family environment the child inevitably fails to achieve his goal, but he learns a great deal about being assertive and is able to turn his failure into the process of learning how to become a spouse and parent in the future. If, on the other hand, he experiences a great deal of punitiveness and withdrawal of basic approval, his feelings of guilt that are already present will be reinforced and remain in subsequent stages.

> Erikson refers to early childhood as the *locomotor-genital stage,* which has the developmental tasks of *initiative versus guilt.*

Sullivan designated this period of life as *later childhood.* Sullivan believed that the major significance of this stage of personality development is that the child becomes capable of giving up his personal and private language and substitutes language that has universal meaning. The importance of the acquisition of the tool of language cannot be overemphasized, since it allows the child to begin to check out his perceptions and feelings with others. The term that describes this process is *consensual validation.* The ability to consensually validate experiences with others is a major factor in enabling the child to develop relationships with peers in the neighborhood or in the nursery school.

> Sullivan calls this stage *later childhood* and stresses the importance of language development.

Latency

The stage of personality development that occurs roughly between the ages of 6 and 12 was called *latency* by Freud. This term was chosen because Freud believed that the child's libidinal energy was not focused on any one area of the body as it had been in the previous three stages. He believed that this energy was lying dormant and therefore nothing of psychosexual significance occurred during this stage. The relatively stable behavior and even-tempered nature of most children of this stage attest to the temporary intrapsychic equilibrium established by the id, ego, and superego.

Erikson recognizes the very important role that school experiences play in the personality development of the child during this period. Although he agrees with Freud that no specific area of the body is of particular interest to children

> Freud identifies the period of 6 to 12 years as that of *latency,* in which stable behavior and even temperament are characteristics of the child.

> Erikson stresses the important role of school experiences during this period as the child develops mastery of his environment for both the present and future.

during this stage, he believes that psychic energy is being actively used in pursuit of knowledge and skills. In other words, the child is purposefully involved in acquiring tools through which he can deal with his environment both in the present and in the future. According to Erikson, if the child is successful in this endeavor, he will have achieved the developmental task of *industry*. If the child is unsuccessful, he will feel inadequate and develop a sense of *inferiority*.

Sullivan saw this period as being very critical to the development of a healthy adult personality. He divided Freud's and Erikson's 6-year span into two periods: the *juvenile era*, lasting roughly from ages 6 to 10; and *preadolescence*, lasting roughly from ages 11 to 12, or to the onset of puberty. During the juvenile era the child turns away from his parents as being the most significant people in his life and looks to peers of the same sex to fill the functions of providing him with a sense of security and companionship. This is the period of gang formation and fierce gang loyalties. The gang requires strict adherence to the rules of the group, and the child slavishly complies with them. During this period the child tries to find his place among his peers. In so doing he acquires two very important interpersonal tools: the ability to compete and the ability to compromise. As the child tests these modes of behavior with his peers, their responses help him to learn to use both appropriately.

Another very important function of the peer group is the reinforcement or alteration of the self-concept. A child who enters this stage of development with a positive or "good me" self-concept is very likely to behave in a manner that elicits responses from his peers that confirm and reinforce his view of self. In instances when the child enters this period with a negative or "bad me" self-concept, positive reflected appraisals from his peer group can do much to alter his view of self. This fact indicates what a very significant role the peer group plays in the life of the child during this period.

During preadolescence the child maintains great interest in the group but simultaneously develops an intense love relationship with a particular person of the same sex who the child perceives to be very similar to himself. Sullivan called this special relationship a *chum relationship*. Up until this time the child's love has been self-centered, but in the chum relationship the child experiences for the first time the capacity to put the needs of someone else ahead of his own. Sullivan saw this experience as a necessary prerequisite to the establishment of a satisfactory heterosexual relationship in subsequent stages of development. The emotional intimacy that the chums experience also helps them to explore and clarify their feelings in a way that builds self-esteem.

Sullivan also stressed the importance of the school experience in the development of the child's personality. It is at school that children meet significant adults who greatly influence the development of their self-concepts. In this culture success at school is rewarded with much approval, whereas lack of success often begins a series of defeats that carry over into adult life. The self-concept of children who do poorly in school may be irreparably damaged by the reactions

Sullivan emphasizes the importance of the child's relationships with peers of the same sex during the *juvenile era*. During *preadolescence*, the *chum relationship* and the school experience are particularly important.

of teachers, the significant adults in that important environment. On the other hand, understanding, helpful teachers may provide the child with a positive basis for self-evaluation and in some instances may constitute an opportunity for corrective interpersonal experiences with adults. Teachers are of tremendous importance in the lives of children and need to be aware of their potential for providing therapeutic experiences in their day-to-day contacts with children.

Sullivan's emphasis on the importance of the school experience for children in this developmental stage is validated by their stage of cognitive development. The third stage of cognitive development, according to Piaget, occurs between the ages of 7 to 12 years, is termed *concrete operations,* and is characterized by major intellectual and conceptual development. The enthusiasm and joy of learning exhibited by children of this age are well known by adults who have sustained contact with these children. During this stage the child develops the ability to handle more numbers in an increasingly complex way, to think logically, to relate external events to each other even if they don't involve him, and to classify persons or objects along more than one dimension. For example, he learns to understand that chairs are also furniture and that his mother is also a nurse and a wife.

Piaget identifies the third stage of cognitive development as that of concrete operations. During this time the child's intellectual and conceptual capacities grow markedly.

Puberty and adolescence

The stage of puberty and adolescence covers the years from age 12 to approximately age 18. Because all theorists agree that this stage of development is initiated by the active functioning of the sexual glands and because individuals mature physiologically at different rates, it is difficult to make a definite statement concerning the span of years included in adolescence.

Freud saw adolescence as the final stage of personality development characterized by a reactivation of libidinal energy and the focusing of this energy on the genital area. As such he designated this period the *genital stage.* Although Freud believed that this final stage lasted for the rest of the person's life, he emphasized that the intense work of this period was completed when the individual achieved a satisfactory heterosexual relationship with a mate and began the life cycle anew by establishing a family.

Freud views adolescence as the final stage of personality development known as the genital stage. It is characterized by the achievement of a satisfactory heterosexual relationship and the establishment of a family.

Adolescence can be a highly problematic stage of personality development. As the adolescent matures physiologically he is faced with the necessity of handling powerful sexual urges that threaten to put the influence of the id out of balance with the influences of the ego and superego. Because of this imbalance of psychic forces, unresolved conflicts and unsolved problems of earlier developmental periods often reemerge at this time. This is particularly true of the Oedipal conflict because of the similarity of the sexual urges experienced at both stages. Therefore the adolescent is simultaneously drawn toward his parents and driven away from them. This ambivalence is manifested by much conflict between the adolescent and his parents as the adolescent vacillates between behaving in a dependent, immature, childlike way and in an independent, mature, adult manner.

Erikson builds on Freud's theory by elaborating on the conflictual nature of the parent-child relationship. Erikson sees the developmental task of puberty and adolescence as the development of a sense of *identity versus role diffusion*. During this time the individual must emancipate himself from his parents, not only physically but also emotionally by establishing for himself his own sense of identity. He must answer the most fundamental questions of "Who am I?" and "What am I?" This requires many decisions regarding familial, occupational, and social roles. To be sure, the adolescent is strongly influenced by his family's norms and values as he struggles to make these decisions. However, if he is to successfully master this developmental stage, he must accept these norms and values as his own or reject them and establish new guidelines for himself. In other words, the adolescent's primary task is to develop an ego that has integrated previous learnings and experiences so that he develops a sense of continuity and sameness in his life. Unsuccessful mastery of this stage results in a diffuse, fragmented sense of self, the most problematic aspect of which is often the shifting between an adult and a child orientation.

Sullivan designated the period between 12 and 17 or 18 years of age as *early adolescence*. As the person experiences sexual urges (termed *lust* by Sullivan), he turns from the chum relationship to the task of establishing a relationship with a peer of the opposite sex. The peer group remains an important aspect of the adolescent's life during this stage because it serves the important function of providing security and consensual validation of the adolescent's feelings and behaviors. The influence of the peer group in regulating the adolescent's behavior is very strong.

Successful resolution of the stage of adolescence is greatly impeded when the child is seen as unacceptable by his peer group, perhaps because of physical handicaps or major cultural differences. The consequence of this nonacceptance may be a prolonged clinging to parents or parent figures to feel a sense of security and belongingness. Another pitfall of this stage occurs when the adolescent's peer group is composed of individuals who are antisocial and engage in delinquent behavior. Although the adolescent will avoid the anxiety of isolation by identifying with this group, it is also likely that he will develop behaviors that are antagonistic to the society at large and that will impede him in the successful achievement of subsequent developmental tasks.

The final stage of cognitive development begins during the stage of adolescence, approximately at age 12, and continues throughout adulthood. Piaget terms this last stage *formal operations* (Table 11-2). During this stage the individual develops abstract thinking and is able to see multiple, complex relationships among objects, categories, and events. This ability permits sophisticated use of problem solving as in the scientific method. With use, this cognitive ability continues to develop and be refined throughout the remainder of the person's life.

Erikson sees this time as characterized by conflicting parent-child relationships in which the developmental task is identity versus role diffusion.

Sullivan characterizes early adolescence as a period of sexual urges (lust) and strong identity with the peer group.

Piaget identifies the final stage of cognitive development as that of formal operations, in which the individual develops abstract thinking and complex relationship formation.

Young adulthood

The period of young adulthood has its onset at the end of adolescence and continues until adulthood. It is almost impossible to state a chronological age range for this period with any degree of accuracy, although many authorities state that it usually begins sometime in the person's twenties and is concluded in the late thirties or early forties. As the life span increases and the entry into the adult work world is delayed by the need for increasingly advanced education, it is obvious that the age ranges of the later developmental periods will have to be reevaluated.

As previously stated, Freud believed that the healthy young adult will have achieved psychosexual maturity. By this he meant that the individual will have integrated his libidinal drives in a manner that enables him to love a member of the opposite sex with whom he hopes to establish a home and nurture a family. At the same time the healthy young adult retains enough self-love to seek satisfaction for his own needs without being destructive to others. In addition he is able to direct positive feelings toward other people in his environment, to work effectively, to achieve creatively, and to fully use the capacities with which he has been endowed without being hampered by crippling anxieties. The ability to achieve these mature capabilities depends to a large extent on the person's heredity and constitutional endowment. However, psychosexual development is powerfully influenced by the experiences that the person has during his early formative years.

Although Freud's theory of psychosexual development does not preclude the potential influence of events on personality in the individual's adult life,

> Freud believes that the healthy young adult will achieve lifelong psychosocial maturity dependent on his heredity, physical constitution, and previous formative experiences.

TABLE 11-2   *Piaget's stages of cognitive development*

Age	Stage	Characteristics
Birth to 2 years	Sensorimotor	Initial egocentrism and undifferentiation from environment
		Learns object permanence and that he is separate from environment
2 to 4 years	Preoperational Preconceptual	Understands symbols
		Thinks in terms of past, present, and future
		Increased language development
4 to 7 years	Preoperational Intuitive	Thinks in classes
		Understands relationships that involve him
		Understands number concepts
7 to 12 years	Concrete operations	Handles more numbers in a complex way
		Thinks logically
		Understands relationships that don't involve him
		Classifies persons or objects along more than one dimension
12 years to adulthood	Formal operations	Thinks abstractly
		Sees multiple, complex relationships
		Engages in complex problem solving

Freud postulated that the early developmental stages were critical and that the final stage begins in the late teens and lasts for the remainder of the person's life, with major personality development alterations being unlikely during this time under usual circumstances.

Erikson sees the personality continuing to develop and mature during young adulthood, during which time important life decisions are made.

Erikson, on the other hand, sees the personality as continuing to develop dynamically throughout the remainder of the life span. During young adulthood Erikson sees the necessity for the individual to continue making decisions about significant aspects of life, such as choosing a mate with whom the individual can experience both physical and emotional intimacy. Erikson expresses this by stating that the task to be mastered during this period is the development of *intimacy versus isolation.* The ability to develop an intimate relationship with an adult of the opposite sex is highly dependent on satisfactory mastery of previous developmental tasks and leads to the establishment of a safe and congenial family environment in which children can be raised. Accepting the role of parent and the responsibility for nurturing, safeguarding, and rearing children is essential if the culture is to be perpetuated. Obviously the individual's ability to be successful in these activities is determined to a large extent by his experiences as a child within a family. Erikson also emphasizes the significance of successfully building one's lifework during this stage. Children cannot be effectively nurtured unless the family has a reasonable degree of social and financial security. Thus acceptance of family responsibilities requires that the young adult be reasonably effective in performing some aspect of work.

If the developmental task of intimacy and its concomitant responsibilities are not achieved, the young adult is likely to develop a sense of emotional isolation, having the sense that he "does not fit." Although the young adult who retreats into isolation often does so to avoid the emotional pain risked by the vulnerability associated with intimacy, he ironically discovers that the price of self-protection is not having his needs met, which increases the need to protect himself.

Sullivan calls young adulthood *late adolescence* when the individual incorporates intimacy with lust. He views this as the final stage of adult maturity.

Sullivan referred to young adulthood as the stage of *late adolescence.* He believed that the major task of this period is the incorporation of intimacy (which developed during preadolescence with a chum) with lust (which became the mode of relating during early adolescence) so that these are not experienced in isolation from each other. Sullivan viewed this mode of relating as the hallmark of adult maturity and therefore did not identify any subsequent stages of development.

Adulthood

As previously stated, neither Freud nor Sullivan identified developmental dynamics beyond the achievement of adolescence or early adulthood. However, both these theorists implied that it may take the remainder of the individual's life for him to develop the maturity that theoretically should have been achieved by those periods. Erikson, however, continued to elaborate on developmental tasks specific to later life.

According to Erikson, the developmental task of adulthood is the development of *generativity versus stagnation*. Erikson believed that as the emotionally healthy individual grows older, it becomes increasingly important to him that he transmit his values to the next generation, thereby helping to ensure his own immortality through the perpetuation of his culture. Therefore it is not unusual to see the adult become very involved in activities that are concerned with his community and the society at large. On the other hand, the individual who developed a sense of isolation during the previous period becomes increasingly self-absorbed and is often acutely aware of "marking time." This person gets little fulfillment from interpersonal relationships or work and has few if any meaningful goals. Hence Erikson's descriptive term, *stagnation*.

Current literature about the stage of adulthood makes it clear that this period is one about which we still need to learn more. Several authorities believe that the adult, because of physiological alterations, aging parents, an increasing awareness of community and societal needs, and grown children who lead lives independent of him, confronts his own mortality for the first time. It is believed that this confrontation results in much uneasiness about the status quo and a subsequent reevaluation of one's goals and purposes in life. Persons who have previously led relatively unexamined lives often find themselves in a state of crisis, which they may attempt to hide from others, since to them their concerns do not seem to be reality based. Societal manifestations of this turmoil are a marked increase in the divorce rate and major shifts in career patterns. For example the woman who has been relatively satisfied as a homemaker for the past 15 or 20 years feels as if she has been left out of the mainstream of life and suddenly develops a need to become involved in a career outside the home. Likewise, it is not uncommon for a husband and father at this stage of life to feel that the occupation in which he has been involved for the previous 20 years is unsatisfying, regardless of his monetary or social success.

It is understandable that such a reaction on the part of either wife, husband, or both, causes much disequilibrium in the family system. Many middle-aged persons decide they have made a mistake, not only in choice of vocation, but also in marriage partner, geographical location, and hobbies. It is unfortunate that many decisions are made precipitously and that these feelings are not recognized as being valid within the developmental context in which they occur.

Margaret Mead, world-famous anthropologist, eloquently pointed out that the needs and requirements of marital partners, like those of their children, change as the relationship matures. Thus the maintenance of a happy and successful marriage relationship requires that the partners continuously seek to relate to each other as individuals whose needs are in a process of dynamic evolution.

Erikson sees the developmental task of adulthood as *generativity versus stagnation*. The healthy individual feels the importance of transmitting his values to the next generation, thereby ensuring his own immortality.

Maturity

The role of aged individuals who have retired from an active social and economic life is unique in this culture. Unfortunately the wisdom they have accumulated through the years is not considered of value as it is in some cultures. Aging persons find it necessary to adjust to a reduced income, waning physical strength, and deteriorating health. This may be an anxiety-producing experience, since it represents a loss of power and independence. Loneliness is another experience with which elderly people must cope. Frequently their friends and marital partners die, leaving them in social isolation. Such lonely individuals who are no longer able to cope efficiently with their own physical requirements need to adjust to the establishment of living arrangements that are acceptable, while at the same time being faced with the need to accept a dependent role. Older persons need to establish social relationships with a group of interested, understanding peers. This need leads many older individuals to seek an affiliation with a "golden age" club or a similar organization.

The preceding statements about the stage of maturity are pessimistic in tone because of the current nature of the society in which we live and the ways in which elderly people are viewed. It should be clear that the older person must inevitably make many adjustments to altered physiological, social, and financial states. If his previous developmental tasks have been satisfactorily achieved, however, it is quite possible for him to make the necessary adjustments with grace, dignity, and a minimum of undue anxiety.

The major dynamic of the stage of maturity is the acceptance of the inevitability of death. To develop this acceptance the individual engages in a life review. If on the whole the aged person is able to feel satisfied with the uniqueness and achievements of his past life, Erikson believes the person will develop a sense of *ego integrity,* which in turn enables him to view death as the ultimate conclusion of life. If, on the other hand, the individual's life review finds him lacking, he will develop a sense of *despair* because time is too short for him to undo and redo his life to achieve the sense of fulfillment he lacks.

As with adulthood, maturity is a stage of life about which much more can be learned. Interest in and concern about this stage of development are increasing as the number of older persons in our society increases.

Table 11-3 outlines the age-related interpersonal experiences and behavioral outcomes experienced by human beings as they traverse the eight ages of man identified by Erikson. They are outlined here because of their comprehensiveness and applicability to nursing practice.

Erikson views the stage of maturity as that in which the individual must accept the inevitability of death. If he does so successfully, he will have achieved ego integrity. If he fails, he will develop a sense of despair.

END NOTE

This chapter discusses theories of cognitive and personality development according to Piaget, Freud, Erikson, and Sullivan within the context of the personality attributes of the mentally healthy adult. Although mastery of these concepts is imperative for the psychiatric nurse, understanding them is essential for

TABLE 11-3   *Interpersonal age-related experiences and behavioral outcomes based on Erikson's theory of personality development*

Ages of man	Interpersonal age-related experiences	Age-related behavioral outcomes	Ego qualities
ORAL-SENSORY			
Positive	Infant is held lovingly and tenderly by mother; needs met with sensitivity and consistency.	Infant sleeps and feeds easily; is usually relaxed and snuggles closely when held.	Basic trust
Negative	Infant continuously experiences anxiety in contact with mother; needs met inconsistently.	Infant generally tense and crying; not comforted by holding; rages when left by mother.	Basic mistrust
MUSCULAR-ANAL			
Positive	Toddler's efforts to stand on own feet are respected and encouraged; relaxed, unhurried toilet training.	Toddler takes pride in self-expression, whether making bowel movements or playing.	Autonomy
Negative	Toddler experiences rejection as efforts at self-sufficiency are ridiculed; cleanliness overemphasized.	Toddler is self-conscious, hiding face or self from others; is stubborn and has temper tantrums.	Shame and doubt
LOCOMOTOR-GENITAL			
Positive	Child's need to explore body is accepted matter-of-factly; sexual curiosity handled without anxiety.	Child begins to imitate parent of the same sex; approaches tasks with enthusiasm.	Initiative
Negative	Child's masturbatory activities are condemned and punished; sexual curiosity ignored or rebuked.	Child experiences nightmares, often symbolic of castration; hides masturbatory activities.	Guilt
LATENCY			
Positive	Child's efforts at learning are supported; new interests and friendships encouraged.	Child is obedient, prefers order and limits; works on projects to completion with peers.	Industry
Negative	Child is ridiculed in front of peers; friends and interests criticized.	Child fears failure and gives up; does not try to do or to learn.	Inferiority
PUBERTY AND ADOLESCENCE			
Positive	Youth's beginning emancipation from family is accepted; vocational choices supported.	Youth turns from parents to peer groups, joining cliques and clubs; develops crushes on other figures.	Identity
Negative	Youth's rapidly changing body, awkwardness, and interest in opposite sex are ridiculed; parents try to dominate.	Youth is unable to separate from parents; is embarrassed over physical changes; is unable to make job choice.	Role diffusion
YOUNG ADULTHOOD			
Positive	Young adult experiences support, interest, approval, and tenderness in love relationship; has job satisfaction.	Young adult is well-rounded; has varied interests in family, job, friends, and hobbies.	Intimacy
Negative	Young adult's choice of partner is rejected by parents; parents try to hold and control offspring.	Young adult sacrifices relatedness for work and drive to succeed; is unable to give emotionally to others.	Isolation

Continued.

TABLE 11-3 *Interpersonal age-related experiences and behavioral outcomes based on Erikson's theory of personality development*—cont'd

Ages of man	Interpersonal age-related experiences	Age-related behavioral outcomes	Ego qualities
ADULTHOOD			
Positive	Adult experiences orgasm with loved, trusted, and respected partner; experiences love and respect from offspring.	Adult is productive and creative; bears and nurtures children; teaches and gives to others.	Generativity
Negative	Adult experiences rejection and hostility in adult relationships; takes no pleasure in community affairs.	Adult experiences impotence/frigidity; becomes bored and resentful with job.	Stagnation
MATURITY			
Positive	Individual experiences love and respect from maturing offspring; has satisfying past recollections.	Individual looks forward to retirement as opportunity to try new things; recalls past with pleasure.	Ego integrity
Negative	Individual experiences alienation from family; loneliness occurs as friends, spouse, and others die.	Individual faces death with fear, preoccupied with reliving life because of dissatisfaction with the past.	Despair

Adapted from Lofstedt. *Mereness' Essentials of Psychiatric Nursing Learning and Activity Guide,* St Louis, 1982, The CV Mosby Company.

all nurses, since nursing assessments and interventions must be developmentally appropriate if they are to be accurate and effective.

SUGGESTED SOURCES OF ADDITIONAL INFORMATION

Arnold H: Snow White and the seven dwarfs: a symbolic account of human development, Perspect Psychiatr Care 117(5):218, September–October 1979.

Bowlby J: Attachment, New York, 1980, Basic Books, Inc.

Bowlby J: Developmental psychiatry comes of age, Am J Psychiatr 145:1, January 1988.

Bowlby J: Maternal care and mental health, Series No. 2, Geneva, 1952, World Health Organization.

Bowlby J: Separation, New York, 1980, Basic Books, Inc.

Cumming E and Henry W: Growing old: the process of disengagement, New York, 1979, Arno Press, Inc.

Erikson EH: Childhood and society, ed 2, New York, 1964, WW Norton & Co.

Freud S: The ego and the id, New York, 1962, WW Norton & Co. (Edited by J. Strachey).

Freud S: A general introduction to psychoanalysis, New York, 1972, Pocket Books.

Howell E and Bayes M, editors: Women and mental health, New York, 1981, Basic Books, Inc.

Maslow A: Toward a psychology of being, Princeton, NJ, 1962, D. Van Nostrand Co.

Maslow A: Motivation and personality, ed 2, New York, 1970, Harper & Row.

May R: Sex and fantasy: patterns of male and female development, New York, 1980, WW Norton & Co.

Munroe R: Schools of psychoanalytic thought, New York, 1955, The Dryden Press, Inc.

Piaget J: The growth of logical thinking from childhood to adolescence, New York, 1958, Basic Books, Inc.

Piaget J: The child's conception of the world, Ames, Ia, 1963, Littlefield, Adams & Co.

Powers M: Universal utility of psychoanalytic theory for nursing practice models, J Psychosoc Nurs Ment Health Serv 18:28, April 1980.

Sheehy G: Passages—predictable crises of adult life, New York, 1976, EP Dutton, Inc.

Sullivan HS: Interpersonal theory of psychiatry, New York, 1953, WW Norton & Co.

Woosley D: A working concept of intellectualization, J Psychosoc Nurs Ment Health Serv 18:36, January 1980.

Anxiety
One response to stress

LEARNING OBJECTIVES

After studying this chapter the student will be able to:

o Define the concept of anxiety and list its characteristics.

o Discuss the process through which anxiety originates as theorized by Freud and by Sullivan.

o Discuss how ego defense mechanisms, security operations, and coping mechanisms serve as adaptations to anxiety.

Anxiety is the most universal of human emotions and is experienced by all persons throughout their entire life span. Despite its all-pervasive nature, however, anxiety cannot be observed directly. Rather, its presence can be inferred only from behavior.

Anxiety is simultaneously an adaptation and a stressor. It functions as an adaptation in that it is a response to system disequilibrium and initially reduces the level of stress by obscuring the nature of the stressor. In the long run anxiety is a nonproductive adaptation because it prevents the system from focusing on and directly dealing with the source of the stress. Nevertheless, its existence is a signal that the system is having difficulty maintaining homeokinesis, and in that sense it serves a valuable function.

Anxiety also serves as a stressor in that it, unlike any other emotion, is always perceived as negative. Thus its presence thrusts the system into a state of stress, sometimes compounding rather than relieving the original stress. Because anxiety is always perceived as being negative, the system employs a variety of mechanisms to deal with it that are themselves adaptations.

Because anxiety is a basic factor in the development and manifestation of

Anxiety is the most universal of all emotions. It cannot be observed directly but must be inferred from behavior.

Anxiety is simultaneously an adaptation and a stressor.

165

human behavior, it is necessary for the nurse to acquire an in-depth understanding of its characteristics, origin, and the usual adaptations to it.

HISTORICAL PERSPECTIVE

It is reasonable to assume that people have experienced anxiety since the dawn of humanity. Until recently, however, human beings have had to struggle merely to survive. Consequently, it is likely they more frequently experienced fear than anxiety.

Fear and anxiety are indistinguishable to the person experiencing them. Fear is a response to a real stressor that threatens the very existence of the system. Because the stressor can be identified, it becomes possible to deal with it directly by fighting it or fleeing it. These adaptations provide a direct outlet for the physiological and psychological tension resulting from fear.

Such is not the case when the adaptation to a stressor is anxiety. In this instance the feeling perceived is the same as that experienced when fear is present but the stressor is unknown to the person. Consequently there is no direct outlet for the built-up tension; the anxiety becomes a stressor itself.

Sigmund Freud was the first theorist to emphasize the importance of anxiety in the development of human behavior. He first demonstrated the use of ego defense mechanisms as an adaptation to anxiety and believed that the necessity for their use indicated a greater or lesser degree of psychopathology. In contrast, contemporary theorists believe that psychopathology exists when the individual utilizes defense mechanisms as the predominant mode of dealing with anxiety, thereby obscuring reality, or when the individual utilizes only one or two such mechanisms to the exclusion of all others. In other words, it is acknowledged that a sparing use of a wide variety of mental mechanisms is within the range of healthy behavior. It should be noted, however, that as the society becomes more complex and therefore more stressful, anxiety and its adaptations become more frequent causes and effects of mental disorders. Mental disorders specific to anxiety and to its adaptations are discussed more fully in Chapter 17.

DEFINITION AND CHARACTERISTICS OF ANXIETY

Anxiety
A vague sense of impending doom, an apprehension, or a sense of dread.

Anxiety is defined as a vague sense of impending doom, an apprehension or sense of dread, that seemingly has no basis in reality. Laypersons refer to anxiety as "being nervous."

As observed earlier, anxiety is the only emotion that is always perceived as negative. In contrast to anxiety, emotions that are usually considered painful sometimes bring pleasure. For example, most people do not enjoy being angry. On occasion, however, it is satisfying to experience anger when one feels it is justified and shares it with others. Another characteristic of anxiety is its extreme communicability. Almost like a living organism, anxiety is transferred with amazing rapidity from one individual to another, often below a level of awareness.

When the individual experiences anxiety he cannot distinguish it from fear, a feeling state that occurs in response to a specific identifiable environmental threat. Because anxiety cannot be distinguished from fear, the physiological response is the same in that the autonomic nervous system is activated and the body becomes ready for "fight or flight." Since an identifiable environmental threat is not present, the individual cannot discharge the tension of anxiety by fighting or fleeing and consequently may experience such symptoms as a pounding heart and a dry mouth, the perception of which serves to increase anxiety. Furthermore, when an individual becomes aware of being anxious, he often frantically searches for a reason to explain this feeling in the hope of abolishing it. He is rarely successful, and his explanation often describes the result of his anxiety, not its cause. For example, a young woman who believes she is anxious because of the responsibilities she must assume in the care of her young infant may really be experiencing a conflict between a desire to be dependent and the need to be independent, which in turn creates anxiety, making her increasingly less able to care for the infant. Therefore her explanation of her anxiety is not its cause but rather its manifestation.

Anxiety occurs in degrees. Although it is never seen as desirable, mild anxiety serves the function of motivating the person and making him more physically and mentally alert. When the level of anxiety is extremely high, the individual may be incapable of action or may react with unusual behavior or what appears to be irrational behavior. This irrational behavior is referred to as a panic state.

Characteristics of anxiety
Always perceived as a negative feeling; extremely communicable; cannot be distinguished from fear by the person experiencing it; occurs in degrees.

ORIGIN OF ANXIETY

Most authorities believe that anxiety occurs most often as an adaptation to a threat to biological integrity, an unconscious symbolic conflict, or a threat to the self-concept.

Freud believed that anxiety is a response to the emergence of id impulses that are unacceptable to the superego. In other words, the ego detects a real or potential conflict between the id and the superego, which results in anxiety, thereby alerting the ego to the necessity for intervention. He believed that all persons experience anxiety initially during the birth process when the respiratory and cardiovascular systems must undergo rapid, extensive changes to support extrauterine life. He also viewed the birth process as the prototypical separation. These two factors—the threat to life and separation—are associatively linked to each other and to the experience of anxiety. In subsequent developmental stages, he theorized, unconscious conflicts are perceived as life threatening, are associated with separation, and result in anxiety.

Freud believed that anxiety results from the emergence of id impulses that are unacceptable to the superego.

Sullivan viewed anxiety as always occurring in an interpersonal context. That is, anxiety is generated when the individual anticipates or actually receives cues that signal disapproval from one or more significant others. This presents an individual with an approach-avoidance dilemma in that there is a desire to approach or please the other person because he is seen as being significant, but to do so incurs the risk of disapproval of self—a threat to the very existence of the individual as he knows himself. According to Sullivan the human being first experiences anxiety as an infant when either his need for satisfaction, which is physiologically based, or his need for security, which is interpersonally based, is not met by the mothering one. The student will remember that Sullivan's theory of personality development also emphasizes the empathic linkage between infant and mothering one through which anxiety is readily communicated. The empathic linkage makes the infant and mothering one uncommonly sensitive to discomfort in each other. Because of his inability to solve problems, the infant has no alternative but to believe that the mothering one's anxiety, which is communicated to him via the empathic linkage, is caused by him, even though the source of this discomfort may be external to him. This phenomenon, which all adults have experienced, by definition, during their infancy, is the basis for Sullivan's belief that anxiety is interpersonally based.

Some authorities distinguish between normal anxiety and pathological anxiety. In reality this distinction refers to the nature of the stressor that precipitates the response of anxiety rather than to the nature of the anxiety itself. *Normal anxiety* arises from a realistic apprehension of a previously unencountered situation that has symbolic meaning to the individual. For example, the anxiety a bridegroom experiences before his wedding very likely arises in response to his unconscious concern about his ability to assume the role of husband and therefore his view of the wedding as a symbolic threat to his identity as an adequate male.

In contrast, *pathological anxiety* is often a response to thoughts, feelings, wishes, or desires that, if conscious, would be unacceptable to the individual or that, if known, would cause the loss of approval or love from significant others. Therefore situations that evoke such unacceptable thoughts, feelings, wishes, or desires are associated with anxiety against which the individual must defend to maintain his self-concept. For example, a young man who has unconscious homosexual desires that if known to him would be repugnant might react with massive amounts of anxiety when circumstances force him to live in physical proximity with other young men.

ADAPTATIONS TO ANXIETY

Because moderate to high levels of prolonged anxiety can prove lethal to the human system, some method of relieving anxiety is essential if the system is to regain homeokinesis. The human being usually is able to relieve anxiety through a form of adaptation referred to as mental mechanisms. *Mental mechanisms* are patterns of thinking and behaving that are used to protect the individual from threatening aspects of his environment or from his own feelings of anxiety. Mental mechanisms are learned as being effective adaptations to anxiety during one of the phases of personality development. They are further de-

Sullivan viewed anxiety as occurring when the individual anticipates or actually receives cues that signal disapproval from one or more significant others.

The distinction between *normal anxiety* and *pathological anxiety* lies in the nature of the stressor rather than in the nature of the anxiety.

Mental mechanisms Specific defensive processes that are employed to seek resolution of emotional conflict and freedom from anxiety.

veloped and elaborated upon as the individual grows and struggles with stressors. Thus the use of these mechanisms is a matter of resorting to earlier patterns of thinking and behaving that have already proved helpful in relieving anxiety. Many of these methods of thinking and behaving are wholly unconscious, whereas others are partly conscious and partly unconscious. All, however, are a means of protecting the individual from situations he perceives as dangerous. In this regard they serve a very important function by helping the person to maintain biological integrity and self-esteem.

Ego defense mechanisms are one type of commonly used mental mechanism. These are utilized when the individual unconsciously experiences a basic conflict between id impulses and the demands of the superego. The ego unconsciously uses some of its energy to initiate a defense mechanism that effects a compromise between the demands of the id and the superego, thereby relieving anxiety.

Another form of mental mechanism is called *security operations*. These were identified by Sullivan and are called into play when anxiety is a response to a threat to the self-concept. Security operations, like ego defense mechanisms, operate without the awareness of the individual employing them.

Although the sparing use of mental mechanisms is considered healthy and serves the function of lowering anxiety, thereby enabling the system to regain homeokinesis, their use does exact a toll. The price of this adaptation is the use of system energy, resulting in less potential energy available for growth. Furthermore the stressor, whether it be a conflict or threat, is not directly addressed or resolved.

Another adaptation to anxiety is *coping mechanisms*. A coping mechanism, unlike an ego defense mechanism or a security operation, is based on a conscious acknowledgment that a problem exists. As a result the individual engages in reality-oriented problem-solving activities designed to reduce tension. It is for this reason that coping mechanisms are considered more healthy adaptations than ego defense mechanisms or security operations. For example, when a student unexpectedly fails an examination, he would be using the ego defense mechanisms of projection if he believed that he failed because the teacher was inadequate. Although this would reduce his anxiety, it would not be helpful in enabling him to pass the course. On the other hand, if this student were able to acknowledge his failure to himself, he would then be able to use the coping mechanism of going to the instructor for help. If he understands his errors, not only is his anxiety reduced but he is also able to learn what is necessary to pass the course.

> **Coping mechanism**
> Adaptation to anxiety based on conscious acknowledgment of a problem.

Ego defense mechanisms

The following is a discussion of commonly used ego defense mechanisms as identified by Freud. The student should remember that these defenses emanate from the unconscious and use psychic energy derived from the ego as they pro-

OF SPECIAL INTEREST

Have you ever known someone to overcome his or her anxiety about a particular situation without using a mental mechanism? People who are mentally healthy and confronted with a moderately anxiety-producing situation often do so by voluntarily repeating the anxiety-producing experience, in reality or symbolically, over and over again. What is most astounding is that they seem to enjoy this activity. Reducing anxiety by achieving mastery of a situation through repetition explains why many adults enjoy suspense movies, roller coaster rides, and the like, while simultaneously declaring how scared they are. It also explains the pleasure children experience when they repetitively play the same game in exactly the same way or hear the same story told in exactly the same words. Sometimes the meaning of the games or stories is symbolic. In other instances, it relates directly to the anxiety-producing situation. For example, in one family three sisters, 4, 5, and 8 years old, were aware of their parents' constant fighting even though their parents went to great lengths to be cordial with each other "in front of the girls." In view of this, their mother was shocked one day to overhear one of her daughters say to the other two, "Let's get out our doll house and play divorce again."

Can you think of an instance in which you successfully conquered your anxiety through enjoyable repetition?

---

tect it from anxiety. Furthermore, it should not be forgotten that an ego defense mechanism may originate in more than one stage of personality development, or it may originate in one stage and be reinforced in others. Ego defense mechanisms are not clear-cut and almost never appear as isolated phenomena.

Compensation. Compensation is a pattern of adaptive behavior by which anxiety resulting from feelings of inadequacy or weakness is relieved as the individual emphasizes some personal or social attribute that overshadows the perceived inadequacy or weakness and gains social approval.

The origins of this adaptation can be seen in the young infant who substitutes his thumb or toy for the nipple or bottle to relieve tension and compensate for some of the pleasurable sensations of sucking that may be lacking in quantity.

Obviously compensation is far more complicated in adults than in infants and is usually prompted by feelings of guilt or inferiority. It may explain much of the behavior observed in adults who work zealously to promote philanthropic enterprises. Compensation may be operating in the behavior of a man who is very small in physical stature but who is extremely successful in the business world through his aggressive practices. It may also be one of the mechanisms operating when a young person who is paralyzed as a result of a car accident is able to achieve many honors for outstanding scholarship in college.

Displacement. Displacement is a defense mechanism used when an individual unconsciously believes he would be in great danger if his feelings about an-

Compensation
(1) Mental mechanism, operating unconsciously, by which the individual attempts to make up for real or fancied deficiencies; (2) conscious process by which the individual strives to make up for real or imagined defects in such areas as physique, performance, skills, or psychological attributes—the two types frequently merge.

other person were known to that person. The adaptation to the resultant anxiety is the discharge of feelings onto a person or object entirely different from the one to which they actually belong. Displacement may be used by a teacher who is angry with an immediate supervisor and does not show these feelings in his presence but reacts with unreasonable anger when a pupil accidentally breaks a windowpane on that same day. The teacher may be displacing angry feelings by expressing them toward the student rather than toward the supervisor. Actually the teacher has unconsciously substituted the student for the supervisor and has displaced the feelings accordingly.

Denial. Denial is the adaptation often employed to defend the system against the stress of the sudden onset of massive amounts of anxiety. It is a process whereby the individual truly does not recognize the existence of an event or feeling. Although denial is a commonly used defense in severe emotional illnesses such as schizophrenia, it is often seen as a reaction of the healthy individual when he is unexpectedly confronted by a disastrous situation. For example, the wife of a policeman who has just been killed in the line of duty may calmly respond to the informant, "You must have made a mistake! I just had breakfast with him no more than 2 hours ago. I'm getting ready to shop now, so you'll have to excuse me."

It is important to understand that the mechanism of denial operates on a totally unconscious basis in response to the sudden onset of massive amounts of anxiety. Denial should not be confused with lying, which is a conscious effort to avoid responsibility in a situation.

Fixation. Fixation refers to the point in the individual's development at which certain aspects of the emotional development cease to advance. For reasons that are usually obscure, further development seems to be blocked. This blocking appears to arise from the inability of the individual to solve problems that occurred during the specific phase of development at which progress ceased. Thus the individual is unable to achieve the developmental tasks of that phase, and since it is not possible to entirely bypass a stage, he is always handicapped in proceeding to the stages that follow. For example, individuals who have not experienced the love and security required for the satisfactory resolution of the first stage of development may spend the remainder of their lives attempting to achieve gratification through the oral cavity. Some individuals fixated at this stage of personality development may drink huge quantities of alcohol or compulsively overeat because food and liquid intake are so closely allied to love and security in the unconscious emotional life.

Sublimation. In the mechanism of sublimation the energy involved in anxiety-producing primitive impulses and cravings is unconsciously redirected into constructive and socially acceptable channels. This is one of the chief mechanisms operating when a child learns to redirect the pleasurable sensations involved in expelling excrement at will into the more socially acceptable patterns of toilet training.

Displacement
Mental mechanism, operating unconsciously, by which an emotion is transferred or "displaced" from its original object to a more acceptable substitute object.

Denial
Mental mechanism, operating unconsciously, used to resolve emotional conflict and to allay consequent anxiety by denying some of the important elements; the feelings denied may be thoughts, wishes, needs, or external reality factors; what is consciously intolerable is disowned by the automatic and unconscious negation of its existence.

Fixation
Arrest of psychosexual maturation at an immature level; depending on degree, may be either normal or pathological.

Sublimation
Mental mechanism, operating unconsciously, through which consciously unacceptable instinctual drives are diverted into personally and socially acceptable channels.

Sublimation is one of the more positive adaptations to anxiety and is at least partially responsible for much of the artistic and cultural achievement of civilized people. It is operating when a woman redirects her sexual drives, which might be expected to result in a home and children, into a successful career as a nursery school teacher. It is probably operating when a young man who has lost his lover turns to writing poetry about love.

Reaction formation

Mental mechanism, operating unconsciously, wherein attitudes and behaviors are adopted that are the opposite of impulses the individual disowns either consciously or unconsciously.

Reaction formation. Reaction formation can occur when an individual experiences anxiety resulting from unconscious feelings or wishes that are unacceptable to him and relieves the anxiety by expressing an attitude or acting in a way that is directly opposite to that which he really feels. Thus the individual is denying, in a sense of the word, his true feelings or desires. People who are extremely friendly, overly polite, and very socially correct frequently have unconscious feelings of anger and hatred toward many people. These true feelings may be evident in slips of the tongue or in biting humor.

Reaction formation sometimes develops out of rigid toilet-training experiences. One evidence of reaction formation may be observed in adults who are untidy about their homes and their personal hygiene but whose mothers required meticulous conformity to rules of cleanliness and tidiness.

Identification

Mental mechanism, operating unconsciously, by which an individual endeavors to pattern himself after another.

Identification. Identification is a much used and extremely useful mechanism because it plays a large part in the development of a child's personality and in the process of acculturation. Through the process of identification the individual defends against anxiety resulting from feelings of inadequacy by unconsciously taking on desirable attributes found in people for whom he has admiration and affection. He integrates these attributes into his own personality. Thus the little boy takes on masculine attributes that he admires in his father. The student integrates into his personality makeup the attributes he admires in his professor. Another form of identification is observed when an individual develops an unreasoning sympathy for a criminal because of an unconscious sense of guilt.

Introjection

Mental mechanism, operating unconsciously, whereby loved or hated external objects are taken within oneself symbolically; may serve as a defense against conscious recognition of intolerable hostile impulses.

Introjection. The mechanism of introjection is closely related to identification. However, whereas the mechanism of identification adds to the individual's personality, introjection tends to replace all or part of the personality. This defense is based on the psychoanalytic concept of oral receptivity and refers to the unconscious symbolic swallowing of an aspect of a significant person in response to anxiety precipitated by the real or perceived loss of this person. Introjection is operating when the child develops the superego by incorporating the ideals and standards of the parents. When introjection is operating in adults, it suggests that the entire personality of a second person has been incorporated and has replaced the original personality. A psychotic patient who claimed to be Moses wore a beard, let his hair grow long, talked in biblical phrases, and acted as Moses might have acted. What he believed to be the personality of Moses had been incorporated by the patient, and he had given up his own personality. Introjection may operate in a less constructive way than identification, especially when it is observed in adults. For instance, a depressed person may have unconsciously incorporated another person and attempt to commit suicide to kill the introjected person whom he unconsciously hates.

Undoing. In the mechanism of undoing, the individual engages in certain behaviors as a means of symbolically canceling out unconscious thoughts or feelings that are unacceptable and therefore associated with anxiety. Although the individual is aware of his behavior, he is not aware of its purpose, and his behavior often seems irrational even to him. Undoing is seen as the basis of compulsive behavior. Undoing behavior is frequently highly repetitive because it does not achieve its aim of actually canceling out the anxiety-producing thought or feeling. A famous example of this defense mechanism is found in Shakespeare's play *Macbeth*. Lady Macbeth, the wife of the main character, compulsively washes her hands exclaiming, "Out, out damned spot!" after having goaded her husband into murdering the king.

Isolation. Isolation is a phenomenon where the feeling is detached from the event in the individual's memory, enabling the person to recall the event without its attendant anxiety. This mechanism is evident in situations when an individual relays a harrowing experience without any evidence of emotion.

Rationalization. Rationalization is a mental mechanism that is almost universally employed. It is an attempt to make one's behavior appear to be the result of logical thinking rather than the result of unconscious desires or cravings that are anxiety producing. It is used when the individual has a sense of guilt about something he does or believes or when he is uncertain about his behavior. It is a face-saving device that may or may not deal with the actual truth. Rationalization should not be confused with falsehoods or alibis, since the latter are conscious avoidance maneuvers. Rationalization is almost totally unconscious, and although it is used to put the individual in the best possible light, it does not have the deliberate aspect of other conscious avoidance maneuvers.

The person who does not want to keep an appointment because to do so would create anxiety and says that the appointment slipped his mind is not telling a falsehood but rather is using rationalization as a defense mechanism. Although rationalization relieves anxiety temporarily, it is not an effective mechanism of adjustment because it assists the individual to avoid facing the reality of the situation.

Repression. Repression is a widely used and completely unconscious mechanism. Painful experiences, unacceptable thoughts and impulses, and disagreeable memories are forcibly dismissed from consciousness to relieve the anxiety associated with them. The psychic energy with which they were invested becomes an active free-floating source of anxiety in the unconscious mind. Many painful experiences are repressed during early childhood and become unconscious sources of emotional conflict in later life. Selfish, hostile feelings and sexual impulses are frequently repressed. Such repression always causes internal conflict. This repressed material may find escape through conversion into phys-

---

Undoing
Primitive defense mechanism, operating unconsciously, by which something unacceptable and already done is symbolically acted out in reverse, usually repetitiously, in the hope of "undoing" it and thus relieving anxiety.

Isolation
Mental mechanism whereby the feeling is detached from the event in an individual's memory, thus enabling the event to be recalled without its attendant anxiety.

Rationalization
Mental mechanism, operating unconsciously, by which the individual attempts to justify or make consciously tolerable by plausible means those feelings, behaviors, and motives that would otherwise be intolerable.

Repression
Mental mechanism, operating unconsciously, in which there is involuntary relegation of unbearable ideas and impulses into the unconscious whence they are not ordinarily subject to voluntary recall but may emerge in disguised form through use of the various mental mechanisms.

ical symptoms or into obsessions or pathological anxiety that arises without apparent reason.

Regression. Regression occurs when an individual is faced with anxiety stemming from a conflict or problem that cannot be solved by using the adaptive mechanisms with which he customarily solves problems. In such a situation he may unconsciously resort to behavior that was successful at an earlier stage in his development but that he had presumably outgrown. Thus regression is a return to patterns of behavior appropriate to an earlier developmental stage. Any retreat into a state of dependency on others to avoid facing acute problems can be called a regressive trait. "Crying on someone's shoulder" is symbolic of the infant's seeking comfort on the maternal bosom. Although some seeking of a dependency relationship is a benign form of regression, this mechanism may become the main element in the development of a serious psychosis.

Projection. Projection is a frequently used unconscious mechanism that relieves anxiety by transferring the responsibility for unacceptable ideas, impulses, wishes, or thoughts to another person. The mechanism is used when the individual's own hostile, aggressive thoughts are unacceptable to him and thus cause anxiety. Although all people use this mechanism to some extent, it is not a healthy method of adaptation and is more frequently used by mentally ill persons than by more healthy individuals. It may be operative in such psychotic symptoms as delusions and hallucinations. In the latter, the individual hears voices saying things about him that he unconsciously fears are true. The paranoid person may project his own inner hate of others by saying that a group of people is plotting to kill him. Less pathological use of projection is evident when a worker blames the boss for his difficulties on the job or when a student blames the teacher for his failure on an examination. Paranoid persons frequently project their feelings of sexual inadequacy on others. Thus a common delusion concerns the unfaithful spouse, when the actual lack of fidelity is in the mind of the accuser.

Symbolization and condensation. A symbol is an idea or object used by the conscious mind in lieu of the actual idea or object, which if consciously perceived would be anxiety producing. Instinctual desires may appear through symbols, the meanings of which are not clear to the conscious mind. For example, a man who unconsciously harbors feelings of inadequacy about his masculinity may defend against this anxiety by owning only large automobiles despite the fact he cannot afford to purchase or operate them. The phallic symbolism of large automobiles serves to reassure this individual about his adequacy as a male.

Symbols are the language of the unconscious. Such symbols appear in dreams or in fantasies and may emerge through various rituals or obsessive behavior. Symbols may become further merged by condensation to represent a wide range of anxiety-producing ideas that become lumped together so as to lose their painful significance. When they rise to the conscious level they take

---

Regression
Partial or symbolic return to more infantile ways of gratification.

Projection
Mental mechanism, operating unconsciously, whereby that which is unacceptable in the self is unconsciously rejected and attributed (projected) to others.

Symbolization
Mental mechanism, operating unconsciously, in which a person forms an abstract representation of a particular object, idea, or constellation. The symbol carries, in more or less disguised form, the emotional feelings vested in the initial object or ideas.

the form of an apparently incoherent jumble of words, the real meaning of which is hidden in the unconscious. Such condensations of thinking are frequently noted in the apparently irrational language of the schizophrenic individual. However, these condensations have meaning and significance for him.

Conversion. Conversion refers to the expression of emotional conflicts through a physical symptom for which there is no demonstrable organic basis. The use of this mechanism is preceded by the use of repression whereby the anxiety resulting from the emotional conflict was previously adapted to by repressing the conflict into the unconscious. When the conflict reappears as a physical symptom, the individual is unaware of any connection between the two phenomena. Thus a child who is highly anxious because of chronic friction between her parents, both of whom she loves, may find herself suddenly blind. This symptom literally relieves her of the necessity of seeing such incompatibility. In like manner, a young soldier who simultaneously loves his country but abhors killing may suddenly develop a paralysis of his right hand rendering him unable to pull the trigger of a gun. Table 12-1 summarizes the ego defenses.

Although the physical symptom is symbolically related to the nature of the conflict, conversion is not always expressed in a direct and easily recognized manner. Frequently it is difficult to determine which repressed conflicts in the unconscious produce a certain physical symptom. The symptom always serves to distract attention from the individual's real problems. This mechanism is entirely unconscious and is not used by mature, well-adjusted individuals.

Security operations

The following is a discussion of the security operations identified by Sullivan as protective measures against anxiety. It should be remembered that Sullivan stressed that anxiety emanates from an interpersonal context and is highly communicable.

Apathy. The security operation of apathy is similar to the ego defense of isolation wherein the individual defends against anxiety by not allowing himself to feel the emotion associated with an anxiety-producing event. Thus the individual utilizing apathy manifests an extreme indifference to an event that would usually elicit a high degree of emotion. This security operation protected a young wife against massive amounts of anxiety when her husband was convicted of involvement in organized crime and sentenced to 15 years in prison. Although she had no previous knowledge of his business, she was able to recount to her parents the events that transpired after his arrest without any emotion, leading them to conclude that she didn't care.

Somnolent detachment. The security operation of somnolent detachment manifests itself by the individual falling asleep when confronted by a highly threatening, anxiety-producing experience. It has its origin in the developmental stage of infancy where the baby can be observed to fall asleep after his crying fails to bring the mothering one to feed him. Although somnolent detachment is

Conversion
Mental mechanism, operating unconsciously, in which emotional conflicts ordinarily resulting in anxiety are repressed and transformed into symbolic physical symptoms having no organic basis.

Apathy
Security operation whereby the individual defends against anxiety by not experiencing the emotion associated with an anxiety-producing event; there is a manifestation of extreme indifference.

Somnolent detachment
Security operation with its origin in infancy, whereby the individual falls asleep when confronted by a highly threatening, anxiety-producing experience.

TABLE 12-1   *Ego defense mechanisms*

Defense mechanism	Definition	Example
Compensation	Exaggerating one trait to make up for feelings of inadequacy or inferiority in another dimension	A physically small man verbally bullies his employees
Displacement	Attributing feelings to a person or object that are really directed at another person or object	Kicking the cat after an argument with one's boss
Denial	Failing to perceive some threatening object or event in the external world	A woman sets a place for dinner for her husband who has just been killed
Fixation	Remaining "stuck" in a developmental stage	A husband is totally dependent upon his wife for most of his activities of daily living
Sublimation	Redirecting socially unacceptable urges into socially acceptable behavior	An angry, hostile young man becomes a boxer
Reaction formation	Substituting directly opposite wishes for one's true wishes	An adult who grew up in a very messy home is compulsively neat in his home
Identification	Integrating desirable attributes of an admired person to compensate for perceived inadequacy	A shy adolescent girl styles her hair like that of a popular rock star
Introjection	Incorporating another person to avoid the threat posed by him or one's own urges	A psychotically depressed woman attempts suicide to kill her mother who she states is in her stomach
Undoing	Engaging in certain thoughts and actions so as to cancel out, or atone for, threatening thoughts or actions that have previously occurred	A business executive studies to become a nursery school teacher after having had an abortion
Isolation	Severing the connection between the thoughts and feelings associated with an event so the event can remain conscious without undue anxiety	A single parent talks unemotionally about her only child's recent diagnosis of a malignant brain tumor
Rationalization	Substituting a fictitious, socially acceptable reason for the genuine, unacceptable reason for one's wishes or actions	"I would have helped you if I could, but I had to take my cat to the vet"
Repression	Forcibly dismissing from consciousness anxiety-producing thoughts, feelings, events	A woman is totally unable to remember being raped by her brother when she was 10
Regression	Returning to patterns of behavior characteristic of a less anxiety-producing stage of development	A 6-year-old child begins to wet the bed at night after her mother's remarriage
Projection	Attributing to others an objectionable trait or feeling that really emanates from oneself	"My husband is cheating on me"
Symbolization and condensation	Using a neutral idea or object to represent an unacceptable idea or object	A 40-year-old has unconscious feelings of inadequacy as a man and spends all his money on guns and all his time polishing and cleaning them
Conversion	Expressing unconscious emotional conflicts through a physical symptom for which there is no demonstrable organic basis	A young woman wakes up paralyzed from the waist down on the morning of her wedding day

a primitive defense, it can be observed in adults who are in a state of great stress. For example, a young woman sitting for the licensure examination in nursing falls asleep less than a half hour after the exam begins and fails the exam.

Selective inattention. Selective inattention is the mechanism whereby anxiety-producing aspects of a situation are not allowed into awareness, thereby enabling the individual to maintain an adequate level of system homeokinesis. For example, the security of a woman whose husband is having an affair is threatened so she selectively inattends the many clues to his behavior and is consciously surprised when he asks for a divorce to marry his lover.

Preoccupation. The security operation of preoccupation is manifested by a consuming interest in a person, thought, or event to the exclusion of the anxiety-producing reality. Preoccupation was used as a protective measure by a devout Christian woman who routinely made home visits in her community to invite others to worship at her church. One Saturday she was severely bitten on her left leg by a large dog in the yard of the home she was approaching. The dog's attack caused her to fall on her right knee, and she became preoccupied with the bruise on this knee to the exclusion of concern about her mangled left leg. The anxiety she was experiencing was due not only to the suddenness of the dog's attack but more fundamentally to a threat to her security that was based in part on the belief that God would always protect her when she was doing His work.

Coping mechanisms

The variety and number of coping mechanisms are as great as the creativity and resources of human beings. They cannot all be listed and defined, but they can be categorized into short- and long-term adaptations. This categorization is based not only on a time factor but also on the object and effect of the adaptation. It should be remembered that all coping mechanisms are conscious, learned adaptations to anxiety based on problem solving and result in altered behavior.

Short-term coping mechanisms. Short-term coping mechanisms are conscious maneuvers focused on the anxiety itself rather than on its source and are designed to effect a relatively immediate relief from anxiety. Consequently, short-term coping mechanisms represent avoidance or escape behaviors. A commonly used short-term coping mechanism is *suppression*. Although historically considered an ego defense mechanism, suppression does not emanate from the unconscious. Rather, suppression is the conscious and intentional dismissal to the preconscious mind of impulses, feelings, and thoughts that are unpleasant or unacceptable to the individual. Suppressed material is easily recalled and is thus available to the conscious mind. Perhaps the most famous example of suppression is that used by Scarlett O'Hara in *Gone with the Wind*. When Scarlett's sense of security was repeatedly threatened, she would exclaim, "I'll think about

Selective inattention
Security operation whereby anxiety-producing aspects of a situation are not allowed into awareness.

Preoccupation
State of being self-absorbed or engrossed in one's own thoughts, typically to a degree that hinders effective contact with or relationship to external reality.

Coping mechanisms
Adaptations to anxiety based on conscious acknowledgment of a problem; the individual engages in reality-oriented problem-solving activities designed to reduce tension.

that tomorrow." Other examples of short-term coping mechanisms are the decisions to drink or eat when anxious or to avoid conflictual situations by pleading illness. Although these maneuvers are successful in relieving anxiety, they do not help the individual to effectively adapt to similar anxiety-producing situations in the future. Furthermore, the result of a frequently used short-term coping mechanism can become a stressor itself. For example, consistent overeating can lead to obesity.

Long-term coping mechanisms. Long-term coping mechanisms are characterized by efforts to address the source of anxiety. Therefore, the anxiety is not relieved immediately but rather continues while its source is being sought. Long-term mechanisms tend to represent confrontational behaviors in that the source of the anxiety is dealt with rather than avoided. An example of a long-term coping mechanism is the housewife's decision to attend college to prepare herself to become financially independent, thereby coping with the anxiety caused by being financially dependent upon her husband.

Long-term coping mechanisms are more functional than short-term mechanisms, since they provide the individual with patterns of behavior that increase self-esteem and can be built upon in future anxiety-producing situations. However, they can be used only in instances in which the individual is able to experience anxiety without too much system disequilibrium.

END NOTE

This chapter discusses the concept of anxiety as a universally experienced emotion that simultaneously serves as both a stressor and an adaptation. The process through which anxiety develops is described in terms of Freudian and Sullivanian theories, followed by a detailed discussion of ego defense mechanisms, security operations, and coping mechanisms. Understanding the concept of anxiety and the various mental mechanisms that individuals employ in their attempt to deal with this emotion is necessary if the nurse is to understand human behavior.

SUGGESTED SOURCES OF ADDITIONAL INFORMATION

Elliot SM: Denial as an effective mechanism to allay anxiety during a stressful event, J Psychosoc Nurs Ment Health Serv 18:11, October 1980.

Freud A: The ego and mechanisms of defense, New York, 1967, International Universities Press.

Kerr N: Anxiety: theoretical considerations, Perspect Psychiatr Care 16(1):36, January-February 1978.

Knowles R: Dealing with feelings: managing anxiety, Am J Nurs 81:110, January 1981.

Peplau H: A working definition of anxiety. In Burd S and Marshall M, editors: Some clinical approaches to psychiatric nursing, New York, 1963, The Macmillan Co.

Peterson MH: Understanding defense mechanisms, Am J Nurs 72:1651, 1972.

Tache J and Selye J: On stress and coping mechanisms, Issues Ment Health Nurs 7:3, 1985.

Biological factors influencing mental health and mental illness

13

LEARNING OBJECTIVES

After studying this chapter, the student will be able to:

○ Describe the field of psychiatric genetics and the findings of the four categories of research studies in this specialty.

○ Explain the dopamine hypothesis of schizophrenia.

○ Explain the catecholamine hypothesis of depressive and bi-polar disorder.

○ Name three brain imaging procedures and discuss their relevance to the study of mental health and mental illness.

○ Discuss several factors that have hampered research on the biological determinants of mental health and mental illness.

There is no question that there is a great deal of contemporary scientific and public interest in the biological factors that influence the development of mental illness. Rapid advances in the fields of genetics and biochemistry and increased sophistication in the technology associated with biological research have enabled scientists to conduct research studies that would have been impossible two decades ago. The results of these studies have led most experts to agree that biological factors are likely to be significant determinants of mental illness. However, current knowledge has not yet reached a point where definitive conclusions can be drawn. Rather, many biological theories about mental illness are stated as hypotheses to be further tested.

Understandably, the majority of biological studies focus on uncovering the causes of major mental illnesses rather than attempting to identify the biological factors contributing to mental health. As a result, most authorities agree that there is much to be learned about the biological determinants of mental health.

To be well informed, the nurse must become familiar with the growing evidence that points to biological factors as major determinants in the development of mental illness. In addition, a growing body of biological theories explains the action of some drugs used in the treatment of mental illness. Since the nurse is the professional who most often administers these medications and monitors their effects, she must be knowledgeable about their biological actions.

HISTORICAL PERSPECTIVE

The belief that biology is a determinant of mental illness has existed since ancient times. The Hippocratic physicians of ancient Greece thought that mental illness was caused by chemical disturbances in the brain. However, with the fall of the Greek and Roman civilizations, there was an accompanying decline in scientific and cultural developments. For centuries to follow, the cause of mental illness was explained by a variety of religious, mystical, and superstitious beliefs.

A return to scientific principles occurred in seventeenth-century Europe. During this time, a skeptical attitude toward superstitious and dogmatic thinking arose, partly as a result of resistance to the political authority of the church. The scientific community began to promote confidence in the use of "reason" and to popularize the scientific method. By the eighteenth century, the scientific method was established as a legitimate approach in all realms of human thought.

By the end of the eighteenth century, the scientific view had influenced the study of mental illness. However, despite a growing commitment to scientific principles, knowledge about mental disorders remained limited throughout the eighteenth and much of the nineteenth century. Formal research into the cause and nature of nervous and mental disease gained impetus through the work of French neurologist Jean Charcot (1825-1893), whose reputation attracted students from around the world. Knowledge about mental disorders began to expand further when the microscope became available to study brain tissue and when advances were made in laboratory methods.

The contributions of Sigmund Freud (1856-1939) created a revolution in the understanding of human behavior. Freud's psychosexual theory of human personality, discussed in Chapter 11, was essentially rooted in a biological model. For example, Freud believed that genetic factors predetermined a certain amount of libidinal energy for each individual. Personality development, in Freud's view, occurred as the growth process shifted libidinal energy to different parts of the body.

Although genetic theories of mental illness had been discussed and debated for many years before, the wide dissemination of Freudian theories made acceptable the idea that human behavior was greatly influenced by genetic factors. However, it was not until the first part of the twentieth century that the scientific method was used to study genetics as a determinant of mental illness. In 1938 Dr. Franz Kallman proposed that an autosomal recessive gene accounted for the inheritance of schizophrenia. Kallman had conducted a study of identical twins, the results of which indicated that if one twin developed schizophrenia, the other also developed this illness in 86% of the cases, even when reared in different environments. He also found that if one twin developed what is now called bi-polar disorder, the other developed the same disorder in 96% of all cases. Since that time, the field of psychiatric genetics has grown. While later studies have indicated that genetics plays a role in the development of mental illness, they have not confirmed that the influence of this factor is as strong as Kallman's early study indicated.

The emergence of many contemporary biochemical theories of mental illness can be traced to the advent of psychotropic medications in the 1950s. It was found that antipsychotic and antidepressant medications acted by altering the chemical processes involved in the transmission of nerve impulses in the brain. With this discovery came an increase in the study of neurotransmitters, substances necessary for the transmission of neural impulses. The dopamine hypothesis of schizophrenia, discussed later in this chapter, was first proposed in 1963 by Carlsson and Lindqvist. These scientists reported that antipsychotic medications worked by inhibiting the action of the neurotransmitter called dopamine.

A variety of biochemical hypotheses about mental illness have arisen since that time. Studies have related genetic factors and biochemical factors such as neurotransmitters and neurohormones to schizophrenia, bi-polar disorder, depression, and anxiety. Recent technological advances have enabled scientists to measure tissue and fluid levels of various neurotransmitters, related metabolites, and related metabolic enzymes in plasma, urine, cerebrospinal fluid, and in postmortem brain tissue.

Most recently, experts have turned their attention to the study of the interaction of multiple biological factors as these influence human behavior, thought, and emotions. For example, some experts have begun to use advanced technological procedures to explore the interactions between neurotransmitters and other related biochemicals such as hormones and peptides.

Recent advances in technology have also led some researchers to use sophisticated brain-imaging procedures, such as positron emission tomography (PET), to study the brains of people suffering from major psychiatric disorders. Others have made use of split-brain studies to examine how the left and right hemispheres of the brain act both independently and interactively to influence human behavior, thoughts, and emotions.

In summary, a combination of factors has historically contributed to a contemporary trend toward a biological perspective of mental health and mental illness. These factors include the emergence of the scientific view as a dominant intellectual perspective in the eighteenth century and the resultant scientific and technological advances that came with the popularization of the scientific method. In addition, there has been a recent attempt among psychiatrists to return to a research and treatment focus similar to that of their colleagues in other medical specialties, namely, genetics, biochemistry, and somatic treatments.

GENETIC FACTORS

Normal individuals inherit 23 pairs of *chromosomes*—one pair from their mothers and one pair from their fathers. Each chromosome is made up of a long deoxyribonucleic acid (DNA) molecule that resembles a twisted ladder. This DNA molecule carries the genetic messages that determine such characteristics as body shape, eye color, blood type, intelligence, and gender.

Scientists have identified certain physical diseases, such as Tay-Sach's disease and Huntington's chorea, that are genetically transmitted. Some of these diseases are carried by *recessive genes,* genes that carry messages that are not followed unless the individual inherits the same gene from both parents. Other diseases are carried by genes called *dominant genes,* whose messages are followed even if the other gene in its pair carries a different message. Scientists know the specific patterns of genetic transmission for some physical diseases, such as dominant or recessive, and in some instances have even identified the specific chromosomes that give rise to a specific defect or disease.

Psychiatric genetics is a specialty field that focuses specifically on the role of human heredity in the transmission of mental illness. Studies in psychiatric genetics have attempted to identify the specific influence of genetic factors on such illnesses as schizophrenia, bi-polar disorder, depression, and alcoholism. However, psychiatric genetics has not yet developed to a point where definitive statements can be made about the influence of heredity on the development of mental illness. Some experts have noted that progress in psychiatric genetics has been slower than the study of genetic influence on other illnesses because definitions of mental health and mental illness are more culture bound. Diagnostic categories of major mental illnesses also continue to be less precise than diagnostic categories of physical illnesses. For example, some experts maintain that there is little reason to believe that schizophrenia represents a single disease. Rather, schizophrenia may actually be a group of disorders with related symptoms, each influenced by a different gene or genes.

A combination of hereditary and environmental factors is more likely to influence the individual's response to life experiences than only a genetic predisposition.

Nevertheless, some recent studies indicate that some persons have a *genetic predisposition* for several major psychiatric disorders. This means that some individuals have inherited more of a tendency to develop a mental illness than others. While a genetic predisposition to some forms of mental illness may exist, it is not a sufficient precondition for the actual development of the illness. Rather, most experts agree that a combination of hereditary and environmental factors influences the way an individual will respond to life experiences.

Several methodologies are commonly used in the field of psychiatric genetics. These are family studies, twin studies, adoption studies, and genetic linkage analysis.

Family studies

Family studies are based on the notion that, if a disorder is genetically determined, blood relatives of mentally ill individuals are more likely to have inherited the predisposing gene or genes for the same mental illness than are family members related by marriage or adoption. Thus, the goals of family studies are to determine the frequency of mental illness among family members and the patterns of genetic transmission.

Some family studies have indicated that close relatives of individuals with such illnesses as schizophrenia, depression, bi-polar disorder, anxiety disorders, alcoholism, and eating disorders are more likely to develop the same illness than are individuals whose relatives do not have these illnesses. This finding has led some authorities to conclude that genetic factors play a major role in the development of these mental illnesses. Other authorities, however, argue that such conclusions cannot be drawn, since it is not possible to separate the effects of the familial and cultural environments from the effects of heredity. Thus, it is not clear whether the child whose parents suffer from a mental illness is likely to develop a mental illness because of genetic transmission or because of faulty parenting.

Twin studies

Twin studies have been used to compare the rates of mental illness between identical and fraternal twins. If a mental disorder is genetically transmitted, it is more likely that identical twins will share the same mental disorder than will fraternal twins or siblings, since identical twins are genetically alike. A number of studies show strong evidence that if one identical twin suffers from a mental illness such as schizophrenia, depression, and bi-polar disorder, the other twin is very likely to have the same illness. This pattern has not been found with fraternal twins or nontwin siblings. Rather, the probability of a fraternal twin's developing the same major mental illness as his twin is similar to the probability of a child's developing the same mental illness as his parent. Despite the convincing evidence of twin studies, it should be noted that, as with studies of the rate of mental illness among close family members, twin studies do not account for the role of environment in the development of mental illness.

Adoption studies

To separate the influences of heredity and environment, some experts have used *adoption studies* to examine the relationship between the incidence of mental illness among children separated from their mentally ill parent at birth and in twins separated at birth. The results of these studies have indicated that the off-spring of parents with schizophrenia and alcoholism are more likely to develop these syndromes than are other adopted individuals whose biological parents did not have these illnesses. Adoption studies have also indicated that genetics may be involved in suicide and in some mood disorders.

Many authorities maintain that the results of adoption studies offer the most compelling evidence that mental illness is genetically transmitted. However, other experts caution that the number of individuals studied is too small to allow for definitive conclusions.

Genetic linkage studies

Genetic linkage studies have received increased attention in the last decade. Recent technological advances have allowed experts to locate genes on a human chromosome map. Over 900 genes have been mapped thus far. With this information, scientists use various linkage markers to locate the genes associated with certain diseases on specific chromosomes. For example, linkage analysis has established that the gene for Huntington's chorea is located on chromosome number four. Advances in gene mapping allow for more accurate genetic counseling as well as improving the quality of genetic analysis as a whole.

Some psychiatric genetic experts have argued that the genetic influences on major psychiatric illnesses are complex, unlike some physical illnesses in which genetic transmission occurs in predictable patterns. In addition, these experts argue that syndromes such as schizophrenia are actually a group of related but separate illnesses. Recently, one group of scientists engaged in a genetic linkage study of a large number of individuals diagnosed as having schizophrenia. They reported that there appears to be a link between schizophrenia and an abnormally functioning gene or genes on chromosome number five. However, another group of scientists found no association between schizophrenia and chromosome number five, although they did not believe that their findings necessarily contradicted the findings of the first study. Rather, they proposed that the individuals in the first study may have been suffering from a form of the illness related to chromosome number five, while those in the second study may have been suffering from a different form of schizophrenia.

Summary

Family studies, twin studies, adoption studies, and genetic linkage studies indicate that there is likely to be a *genetic predisposition* to some psychiatric disorders.

There is a growing body of evidence that indicates that genetic factors may be influential in the development of several major forms of mental illness. Although the findings of psychiatric genetic research are not conclusive, experts agree that there is likely to be a genetic predisposition to some psychiatric disorders. Current research is focusing heavily on identifying symptoms and subtypes of major mental illnesses in the hope that more precise definitions of these illnesses will facilitate more definitive genetic research.

Genetic studies have focused primarily on efforts to explore the hereditary transmission of specific mental illnesses such as schizophrenia and bi-polar disorder. However, it should be understood that since genetic factors determine many individual human qualities, they also indirectly influence the mental health and the quality of life for any given individual. For example, such genetically determined factors as body type, gender, intelligence, temperament, and energy level all influence the nature and degree of the individual's adaptation to life stressors.

BIOCHEMICAL FACTORS

Most mental health professionals agree that biochemistry influences the presence and nature of several major mental illnesses. However, the specific symptoms of mental illness that are influenced by biochemical factors is not yet clear. Experts in biochemistry are now attempting to define various forms of mental illness more precisely and to identify relationships between interacting biochemical systems and definable human behaviors.

After the chance discovery of various psychotropic drugs in the 1950s, experts attempted to identify how these medications acted to relieve symptoms of mental illness. One of the earliest areas of investigation focused on discovering the action of psychotropic medications on *neurotransmitters,* natural chemicals necessary for the transmission of nerve impulses in the brain.

Scientists have identified the presence of many neurotransmitters in the brain. The central nervous system neurotransmitters can be classified into three major categories: the amino acids, the biogenic amines, and the neuropeptides. Each of these three major categories has several subcategories. For example, the biogenic amines include the catecholamines termed dopamine, norepinephrine, and epinephrine. The biogenic amines also include acetylcholine, histamine, and serotonin.

One of the most widely known hypotheses relating neurotransmitters to mental illness is the *dopamine hypothesis.* This hypothesis proposes that the symptoms of schizophrenia result from overactivity of the neurotransmitter named dopamine in the central nervous system. In 1963, Carlsson and Lindqvist were the first to suggest that antipsychotic drugs diminished dopaminergic activity through a blockage of dopamine in the mesolimbic and mesocortical tracts of the brain. The mesolimbic and mesocortical tracts are associated with intellectual and emotional functioning, and it is thought that some symptoms of schizophrenia, such as hallucinations and delusions, involve these two systems.

Recently, scientists have suggested that it is unlikely that schizophrenia results only from a single neurochemical problem. The neurotransmitter systems of the brain are interactive systems that continuously influence one another. Therefore, experts have begun to examine the role of neurotransmitters other than dopamine in determining schizophrenic symptoms, such as the biogenic amines norepinephrine and serotonin and the neuropeptides termed endorphins.

Psychopharmacological discoveries also led experts to examine the role of neurotransmitters in depression. The two major classes of antidepressant medications—the tricyclics and the monoamine oxidase (MAO) inhibitors—were both discovered in the 1950s. Some experts proposed that these drugs acted to relieve symptoms of depression through their effects on the group of neurotransmitters termed the catecholamines, including dopamine, norepinephrine, and epinephrine. Norepinephrine was identified as particularly linked to symptoms of depression.

The *catecholamine hypothesis* of depression proposes that some forms of depression are associated with catecholamine deficiency, particularly norepinephrine, in the brain. In contrast, manic states, in which the individual is highly overactive rather than depressed, may be related to an excess of catecholamines in the brain. Recent studies on the relationships among neurotransmitter systems, depression, and bi-polar disorder indicate that several neurotransmitter systems may be involved. For example, the biogenic amines termed acetylcholine and serotonin may be involved in depression. Experts also agree that several neurotransmitter systems may interact together in a complex fashion to produce the symptoms of depression and of bi-polar disorder.

Several studies have related mental illness to *neuroendocrinology*. This term refers to the study of the relationships between the nervous and endocrine systems. Scientists have recently discovered that the nervous and endocrine systems are interrelated and actually function together. Thus, the activities of the central nervous system, particularly the hypothalamus, play a role in controlling the secretion of various hormones of the endocrine system. At the same time, several hormones appear to be crucial in controlling neural function. A variety of endocrine disorders have been shown to produce symptoms of mental illness in physically ill individuals, such as a depressed mood, impaired concentration, or agitation. These symptoms are relieved when the endocrine disturbance is corrected. The relationship between neuroendocrine functioning and major forms of mental illness, however, is less clear.

Psychiatric neuroendocrine studies have explored the relationship of mental illness to a variety of hormones whose secretions are regulated by neurotransmitter systems. For example, some studies have indicated that depressed patients may show cortisol hypersecretion. The adrenocorticotropic hormone (ACTH) is responsible for the regulation of cortisol secretion. Other studies have indicated that some individuals with schizophrenia may have a blunted growth hormone response to a dopamine agonist termed apomorphine.

Many other biochemical factors have been related to mental illness. For example, schizophrenia has been related to low platelet monoamine oxidase

(MAO), to viral and immunological deficits, and to elevated serum creatine phosphokinase (CPK). Sophisticated technological methods, increased knowledge in the field of neurochemistry, and increased studies on psychopharmacological agents have all enhanced biochemical research in psychiatry.

Recently, experts have identified several areas in need of more specific research in the study of biological factors influencing mental health and mental illness. These areas include the need for more specificity in terms of the definitions of various forms of mental illness and the need to study the interaction of biological systems as they influence mental health and mental illness. Most experts agree that no mental disorder is caused by a single biological factor. Rather, multiple biological factors appear to interact in complex ways with one another and with environmental factors to determine mental health and mental illness in any given person.

BRAIN STUDIES

In recent years, highly sophisticated brain imaging procedures have been increasingly used in the study and diagnosis of mental illness. Some of these procedures are used to assess the presence of organic brain dysfunction or other physical problems. Others have been used to relate major mental illnesses to abnormalities in the brain. While knowledge has not yet reached the point where these procedures are used routinely for diagnosis or study of mental disorders, they offer much promise for the future development of these fields, since they allow the brain to be examined while the patient is alive.

For example, computed tomography (CT) scans compute thousands of x-rays of the brain, which can be combined to produce a three-dimensional brain image. Studies using CT scans have indicated a number of brain abnormalities in mentally ill individuals, such as cerebrellar atrophy and third ventricle enlargement among some patients with schizophrenia.

Another brain imaging procedure is known as PET. This procedure allows researchers to visualize several aspects of brain functioning, such as blood flow and glucose utilization. Some studies using PET have indicated that patients with schizophrenia have abnormalities of glucose utilization in the brain. Other studies have suggested that some patients with panic disorders have several abnormalities of blood flow, blood volume, and oxygen metabolism in the brain.

Another procedure known as magnetic resonance imaging (MRI) has permitted experts to examine the structure of the brain. Studies using the MRI procedure have indicated that some patients with schizophrenia have decreased frontal lobe size, smaller cerebrums, and smaller craniums than persons who do not have schizophrenia.

The state of knowledge about the structure and function of the brain as these influence the development of mental illness does not permit experts to draw any definitive conclusions. Rather, sophisticated brain imaging techniques

The specific symptoms of mental illness influenced by biochemical factors are not clear; however, no mental disorder is caused by a single biochemical or biological factor.

Advanced brain imaging procedures are being increasingly used in the study and diagnosis of mental illness. These offer hypotheses for future study and testing.

offer hypotheses for future testing. The nurse should be aware of these procedures as useful tools to assess organic brain dysfunction as well as to study some hypotheses about mental illness and the brain.

SYMPTOMS OF MENTAL ILLNESS ASSOCIATED WITH PHYSICAL PROBLEMS

No discussion of biological influences on mental illness would be complete without acknowledging that many persons suffer from symptoms of mental illness in conjunction with a variety of physical problems. For example, brain damage is one common organic problem to which the human organism reacts with abnormal mental symptoms. Brain tumor is another organic condition that may be accompanied by various symptoms of mental illness. Encephalitis, inflammation of the brain, can also cause specific mental symptoms such as lethargy, confusion, and stupor.

Mental symptoms commonly result from toxins in the blood or from a high blood level of certain drugs. For example, bromides, barbituric acid derivatives, sulfa drugs, cocaine, marijuana, morphine, thiocynates, and lead can produce mental symptoms. Cortisone and adrenocorticotropic hormone (ACTH) can also produce psychotic symptoms in some individuals.

The nurse should be aware that psychologic abnormalities are sometimes caused by either physical or organic problems.

All nurses need to be aware that a variety of psychological and behavioral abnormalities are specifically associated with temporary or permanent physical and organic problems.

END NOTE

This chapter discusses biological factors that may influence the development of mental illness and points out that, while there is much scientific and public interest in this area of research, little research has been conducted about the biological factors influencing the development of mental health. Several genetic and biochemical factors potentially involved in mental illness are reviewed, and recent developments in the study of the human brain are discussed. It is emphasized that most experts believe that advances in the study of mental health and mental illness will ultimately involve models that relate genetic, physiological, intrapersonal, interpersonal, and cultural factors. Therefore, for the nurse to enhance her awareness of the client as a complex, holistic system, it is necessary for her to combine her understanding of psychosocial factors influencing the development of mental health and illness with an understanding of recent findings about the influence of biological factors.

SUGGESTED SOURCES OF ADDITIONAL INFORMATION

Bowers MB: Biochemical processes in schizophrenia: an update, In Special report: schizophrenia 1980, National Institute of Mental Health, US Dept. of Health and Human Services, 1980, pp. 27-37.

Carlsson A: Does dopamine play a role in schizophrenia? Psycholog Med 7:583, 1977.

Carlsson A and Lindqvist M: Effects of chlorpromazine or haloperidol on formation of

3-methoxytyramine and normetanephrine in mouse brain, Acta Pharmacol Toxicol (Copenh) 20:140, 1963.

Deutsch S and Davis K: Schizophrenia: a review of diagnostic and biological issues, I, Hosp Commun Psychiatr 34(4):313, 1983.

Deutsch S and Davis K: Schizophrenia: a review of diagnostic and biological issues, II, Hosp Commun Psychiatr 34(5):423, 1983.

Field W: Physical causes of depression, J Psychosoc Nurs 23(10):7, 1985.

Garver D: Neuroendocrine findings in the schizophrenias, Endocrinol Metab Clin N Am 17(1):103, 1988.

Green A, Mooney J, and Schildkraut J: The biochemistry of affective disorders: an overview. In Nicholi A, editor: The new Harvard guide to psychiatry, Cambridge, The Belknap Press of Harvard University Press, 1988, pp. 129-138.

Kallman F: Heredity in health and mental disorder, New York, 1953, WW Norton Co.

Kendler K and Eaves L: Models for the joint effect of genotype and environment on liability to psychiatric illness, Am J Psychiatr 143(3):279, 1986.

Kessler S: The genetics of schizophrenia: a review. In Special report: schizophrenia, 1980, National Institute of Mental Health, US Dept. of Health and Human Services, 1980, pp. 14-23.

Kety S and Matthysse S: Genetic and biochemical aspects of schizophrenia. In Nicholi A, editor: The new Harvard guide to psychiatry, Cambridge, 1988, The Belknap Press of Harvard University Press, pp. 139-151.

Martin M, Owen C, and Morihisa J: An overview of neurotransmitters and neuroreceptors. In Hales R and Yudofsky S, editors, Textbook of neuropsychiatry, Washington, DC, 1987, American Psychiatric Press, Inc., pp. 55-88.

Meador-Woodrugg J and Greden J: Effects of psychotropic medications on hypothalamic-pituitary-adrenal regulation, Endocrinol Metab Clin N Am 17(1):225, 1988.

McGuffin P, Farmer A, Gottesman I, et al: Twin concordance studies for operationally defined schizophrenia, Arch Gen Psychiatr 41(1):541, 1984.

Rosenthal D: The genetics of schizophrenia. In Arieti S and Brody E, editors: American handbook of psychiatry, ed 2, vol 3, New York, 1974, Basic Books Inc., pp. 588-600.

Rosse R, Owen C, and Morihisa J: Brain imaging and laboratory testing in neuropsychiatry. In Hales R and Yudofsky S, editors: Textbook of neuropsychiatry, Washington, DC, 1987, American Psychiatric Press, Inc., pp. 17-40.

Schlesser M and Altshuler K: The genetics of affective disorder: data, theory, and clinical application, Hosp Commun Psychiatr 34(5):415, 1983.

Shaver J: A biopsychosocial view of human health, Nurs Outlook 33(4):186, 1985.

Spence M, Ritvo E, Marazita M, et al: Gene mapping studies with the syndrome of autism, Behav Gen 15(1):1, 1984.

Stuart E and McGuffin P: Can linkage and marker association resolve the genetic aetiology of psychiatric disorders? review and argument, Psycholog Med 15:455, 1985.

Usden E: Biochemistry of mental disorders, new vistas, New York, 1978, Marcel Dekker, Inc.

Weissmann M, Merikangas K, John K, et al: Family-genetic studies of psychiatric disorders, Arch Gen Psychiatr 43:1104, 1986.

Cultural factors influencing mental health and mental illness

14

LEARNING OBJECTIVES

After studying this chapter, the student will be able to:

○ Define the concepts of *culture* and *cultural norms* as these apply to human behavior.

○ Discuss the concept of *deviance* as it relates to mental health and mental illness.

○ Discuss the difference between cultural sensitivity and cultural stereotyping.

○ Discuss the relationship of ethnicity, gender, and socioeconomic status to mental health, symptoms of mental illness, and mental health treatment practices.

○ Discuss why it is essential to the effective practice of psychiatric nursing for the nurse to become culturally informed and sensitive.

All human beings live within a sociocultural environment that has a profound and continuous impact on shaping their values and behaviors. In fact, research has conclusively demonstrated that an individual's culture is one of the most significant factors in determining his health beliefs and behaviors.

To a large extent, behaviors that are believed to define mental health and mental illness are culturally bound. These behaviors have varied, sometimes widely, in different times and in different locations. For example, men who spend most of the day staring at the sun might be considered mentally ill in the United States, but in India they are considered holy. Since culture is a major determinant of those behaviors indicative of mental health and mental illness, it is understandable that culture also strongly influences the nature of mental health treatment that prevails in a society.

The profession of nursing has claimed the concepts of person, environment, and health as its phenomena of central concern. Therefore, the nurse must be aware of the factors that influence human health and the sociocultural context that impacts on the persons to whom she gives care. The quality of psychiatric nursing care cannot help but be enhanced when the nurse is aware of the cultural factors that help shape the society's definitions of mental health and mental illness and its choice of mental health treatment.

HISTORICAL PERSPECTIVE

The practice of considering culture as a significant factor in the assessment, diagnosis, and care of individuals and their families is a relatively recent development. Since the 1940s a variety of seemingly unrelated events have interacted in a way that has led mental health professionals to a heightened awareness of cultural issues. First, the country was alerted to a need for more knowledge about the prevention of mental illness and the treatment of those who were mentally ill as a result of the large number of psychiatric casualties during World War II. As one means to this end, attention was turned toward efforts to define those behaviors which constitute mental health. At the same time, there was a trend in other fields, such as biology and physics, to study an object as it interacted in its natural environment. A variety of scientists began to draw from theories of systems and stress and adaptation. These views were applied to the study of mental health as researchers and clinicians became increasingly aware that mental health involved the interactions that occur between the individual and his environment.

The 1960s saw the advent of what is now known as the community mental health movement. A central focus of this movement was the promotion of mental health and the prevention of mental illness and the provision of comprehensive mental health care in local community settings. Efforts were made to direct attention toward community factors that appeared to influence the level of mental health, such as poverty, unemployment, urban overcrowding and rural isolation, crime, and social support.

In the local community setting it became apparent that it was necessary to consider the ethnic, racial, and religious practices of the populations served if the goal of promotion of mental health and prevention of mental illness was to be achieved. At the same, the 1960s saw the emergence of the civil rights movement, and the nation was made aware of the concerns of minority groups and other historically oppressed populations. Thus, the relationship between the mental health of the individual and sociocultural factors became vividly apparent.

Psychiatric nursing developed the subspecialty of community mental health nursing in which the community is viewed as the focus of nursing interventions. More recently, transcultural nursing has arisen as a specialty that specifically bases intervention on beliefs and practices of the cultural groups receiving nursing care. Madeleine Leininger is one nurse theorist who has written extensively on the subject of transcultural nursing.

CULTURE AND CULTURAL NORMS

Sociology is a field that has identified human society as its focus of concern. Sociologists use the term *culture* to describe the sum of a given society's meanings, expectations, and understandings. Thus, culture can be defined as a way of life that a given society assumes to adapt to its environments.

Culture
A way of life that a society assumes to adapt to its environments.

The values and beliefs that characterize a given society are sometimes called *cultural norms*. Cultural norms exert a profound influence on the members of society, shaping individual identity and guiding social behavior. Cultural norms are not universal but vary with different cultural groups and in different historical times. What is valued in one culture may be ignored or disparaged in another, and what is considered appropriate behavior in one culture may be considered deviant in the next.

Cultural norms may also vary within a given society. In this country, for example, people come from Asian, Mexican, Italian, Greek, and other ethnic backgrounds. The cultural norms of these ethnic groups differ, in some ways and at some times, from those of the dominant American culture. Ethnicity is not the only factor influencing cultural norms; the culture may also assign different norms to people on the basis of such factors as gender and socioeconomic status.

Cultural norms
The values and beliefs that characterize a given society.

MENTAL HEALTH, MENTAL ILLNESS, AND THE CONCEPT OF DEVIANCE

The dominant culture determines the values, ideals, and expectations that guide cultural practices and social relations. In this sense, the definitions of mental health and mental illness are, to a large extent, culturally determined. These definitions vary across cultural groups, over time, and within a culture. Cultural norms also strongly influence the kinds of psychiatric treatment modalities that prevail in a given society. For example, in today's highly scientific and technological society, scientifically based biochemical interventions are receiving more attention than are psychosocial treatment modalities. Furthermore, cultural factors have been shown to influence the specific types of psychiatric symptoms that a vulnerable individual will exhibit. For example, somatic problems are the most common type of psychiatric symptom exhibited in China, a country that does not value psychological processes but that has a centuries-old history of successfully treating physical illness.

The concept of *deviance* is useful in understanding the interactions that occur among a person, his cultural environment, and his mental health. While social scientists differ about a precise definition of deviance, the term is generally used to describe behavior that violates the dominant cultural norms of a given society.

Deviance
Behavior that violates the dominant cultural norms of a given society.

Howard Becker is one sociologist who wrote about deviance. Becker proposed that deviance is a result of an interaction between a ruling social group and an individual member of that group. The individual who violates the cultural norms of the dominant group is given the label of deviant, which places that individual outside the group. There are no universal criteria for determining deviant behavior. Rather, deviance is determined by the dominant group.

Several social scientists have proposed that it serves a function for societies to label people deviant. Emile Durkheim, for example, has maintained that the presence of deviance allows the ruling group to join together. By defining who is different, the ruling group affirms the rightness of its own values. For example, at one time blacks who were not content with slavery were labeled mentally ill. This label served the function of maintaining slavery as a legitimate social institution. In patriarchal cultures, women have often been labeled inferior to men, overemotional, and frail. These labels reaffirm the superiority, rationality, and strength of men, the dominant power group in such societies.

Some authorities have maintained that the mental health system in the United States adheres to the cultural norms characteristic of the white, middle class, male member of Western society. The role of mental health professionals, in this view, is to enforce the cultural norms of a ruling class. Beliefs and behaviors that deviate from the norms of that ruling group are labeled indicative of mental illness.

Numerous theorists have attempted to explore the ways that certain individuals come to view themselves as deviant and to behave in ways that break the norms of a culture. Thomas Szasz is a psychiatrist who has written extensively about the practice of labeling socially deviant behavior mental illness. Szasz has also proposed that, to a certain extent, the deviant individual has chosen to violate the rules of culture. Others have argued that the individual who violates cultural norms is most often a member of an oppressed group who has been denied access to social success through legitimate behaviors. Talcott Parsons is a sociologist whose writings express this view.

An individual's level of mental health is greatly influenced by the covert, everyday cultural practices of treating certain members of the society as deviants. Deviance labeling can be seen to underlie such oppressive practices as racism, sexism, ageism, and classism. These discriminatory postures have been shown to have negative psychological consequences for members of both the dominant and the oppressed groups of a given culture.

Some authorities have argued that mental health professionals engage in discriminatory or oppressive behaviors. Cultural minorities, for example, may be labeled mentally ill for behaving in ways that are acceptable in their own cultural subgroups. While discrimination may not be overt, specific behaviors may be misdiagnosed when a professional lacks knowledge of the individual's culture or is otherwise insensitive to the impact of culture on human behavior. To the extent that mentally ill persons are seen as deviant, psychiatric labels themselves can also stigmatize an individual, marking him as defective or inferior. Among culturally oppressed groups, psychiatric labeling can further increase feelings of powerlessness common to cultural minorities in this country.

There has been a growing awareness of these issues among mental health professionals. Articles that describe the health beliefs and practices of members of a variety of cultural groups can be found in most professional journals and are particularly relevant to the practice of nursing. Because the very definitions of mental health and mental illness are so strongly influenced by cultural norms, the psychiatric nurse must be keenly aware of these factors in her assessment, diagnosis, intervention, and evaluation of clients.

CULTURAL SENSITIVITY AND CULTURAL STEREOTYPING

While it is imperative that the nurse be culturally informed and sensitive, she must exercise caution that cultural sensitivity does not become cultural stereotyping. *Cultural stereotyping* is a term used to describe the use of exaggerated beliefs about the members of a cultural group to justify behaving toward them in a prescribed, often derogating, manner. Unlike cultural sensitivity, which focuses on attempting to accurately understand the determinants of another's behavior, cultural stereotyping is focused on reducing one's own anxiety, which results from interacting with someone who is different from oneself.

Cultural stereotyping
The use of exaggerated beliefs about the members of a cultural group to justify behaving toward them in a prescribed, derogatory manner.

While it is important that the nurse become knowledgable about the cultures of the clients with whom she interacts, it is also necessary for her to view each client as an individual with a unique identity. Thus, the nurse must be careful not to overgeneralize, or to assume that all members of a cultural group adhere to the same beliefs, ideals, and practices. When providing nursing care to any client, the nurse can enhance the quality of that care by exploring his individual perception of his cultural beliefs, values, and practices and then basing her assessment and interventions upon what she learns from him. To follow this practice is consistent with a holistic view of human beings that requires an individual, his culture, and his health to be seen as inextricably related.

ETHNICITY

The word *ethnic* is derived from the Greek word *ethnos,* meaning people. An *ethnic group* is a racially, geographically, or historically related group who have a common and distinct culture. As previously stated, culture refers to the sum of the meanings, understandings, and expectations that characterize a given society's ways of life. In the broadest sense, then, an ethnic group is one that shares a national, racial, religious, or historical culture that shapes much of the perceptions and behaviors of its members.

Ethnic group
A racially, geographically, or historically related group of people who have a common and distinct culture.

The population of the United States comprises numerous ethnic minority groups, including Mexican, Hispanic, Asian, Indian, Italian, Polish, Greek, and black Americans. The populations of many other countries also comprise ethnically diverse people. Thus, the nurse practicing in any setting is likely to encounter ethnic diversity. Ethnic factors have been shown to exert a strong influence on the nature of the individual's personality, on the symptoms he will display if he becomes mentally ill, and on his responses to particular mental health treatment modalities.

The personality attributes and behaviors that are considered mentally healthy in one ethnic group are sometimes considered inappropriate, ineffective, or dysfunctional in another. For example, in this country shyness or introverted behavior is considered a problem that limits one's social interactions and therefore opportunities for emotional growth through social support. In China, in contrast, modesty, reserved behaviors, and good manners are considered virtues.

Ethnic differences are often expressed through family norms. For example, adolescents and young adults in white, Anglo-Saxon, Protestant families are encouraged to separate from the family group and to pursue an independent life and identity. The ability to separate at the appropriate time is considered a sign of mental health of both the individual and his family. In contrast, among some Italian families, separation from the family is neither encouraged nor accepted; continuous emotional involvement among all members of the extended family is the norm.

The cultural practices of particular ethnic groups can be mistakenly interpreted by others as signs of mental health problems or even as symptoms of mental illness. For example, among Puerto Ricans there is a common belief that the world is surrounded by spirits who have the power to attach to an individ-

OF SPECIAL INTEREST

How an individual uses his personal space is strongly influenced by his culture. For example, North Americans of Western European heritage usually are most comfortable when they are able to maintain a physical distance of several feet between themselves and others, particularly strangers. Individuals from Latin American cultures, on the other hand, may view this distance as an expression of rejection. To give effective nursing care, the nurse must be aware of the client's preference in regard to personal space.

One white middle-class nurse who was not aware of this principle encountered a Hispanic couple who was living with their three children in one large room. Because the nurse was concerned about the lack of privacy for the parents, she suggested that they partition the room, using a bedspread as a curtain. On her next home visit, the nurse observed that the curtain was in place and was pleased that the wife expressed effusive thanks for her suggestion. Imagine the chagrin of the nurse when she later learned that the partitioned area was now being rented to a friend of the family!

ual and to influence human life. This belief could readily be interpreted as a delusion (a fixed, false belief despite evidence to the contrary) indicative of mental illness. Mental health professionals do not always recognize the role that spiritual beliefs play in shaping the health beliefs and practices of ethnic groups. These cultural norms should be respected and not automatically interpreted as signs of pathology.

The cultural practices of particular ethnic groups can be mistakenly interpreted as signs of mental health problems or as symptoms of mental illness.

Members of ethnic minorities appear to be at risk for being misdiagnosed psychiatrically. For example, it was once believed that black Americans were more likely to become schizophrenic than were white Americans, since proportionately more black Americans were diagnosed schizophrenic than were white Americans. However, current studies indicate that blacks do not differ from whites in terms of the prevalence of most psychiatric disorders. This change is probably due to an increased sensitivity among white mental health professionals to the culture of black Americans, resulting in more accurate psychiatric diagnoses.

Misdiagnosing may also occur because blacks and other minorities appear to display different symptoms than do whites for the same psychiatric disorders. For example, black and Hispanic people with mood disorders appear to experience more hallucinations, delusions, and somatic symptoms and to display more hostility than white people, who often experience guilt and depression and display manic symptoms. Among Chinese people, mood disorders are most often expressed through somatic symptoms. Paranoia appears to occur more frequently among black individuals with schizophrenia than among white persons with the same diagnosis.

It is likely that the diversity of symptomatology among the various ethnic groups is related to the high levels of stress that these groups experience because of their minority position in the society and the differences in their culturally learned modes of adaptation. Cultural conflicts arise from the need for individuals from ethnic minorities to adjust to the different cultural norms of the majority while simultaneously attempting to maintain their own identity by adhering to the cultural norms of their ethnic group. Ethnic stereotyping, deviance labeling, and stigmatization can be viewed as major stressors confronting members of ethnic minorities who face many situations that cause them to feel inadequate, devalued, and unwanted.

Members of ethnic minorities are often denied access to the resources needed for successful social adaptation. Low income, poor housing, and limited opportunities for education compound the problems of some ethnic minority groups. For example, Mexicans, Puerto Ricans, and blacks in this country suffer from high rates of unemployment, low income, and poor education. Many authorities contend that these social problems are major elements contributing to the incidence of mental illness among these groups.

Differences in ethnicity have been documented as a factor in differences in response to particular kinds of psychiatric interventions. For example, Asian

Ethnic differences can cause differing responses to particular kinds of psychiatric interventions.

Americans appear to require lower doses of a variety of psychotropic medications than do whites; they also appear to experience serious side effects to these medications more readily than do whites. Hispanics may require less antidepressant medication than whites and often experience side effects at lower doses.

Members of ethnic minorities may not always benefit from the mental health interventions that prevail in the dominant culture, particularly those which are interpersonally based and rely heavily on verbal skills and the ability and willingness to engage in self-disclosure. For example, studies indicate that some black Americans tend to avoid self-disclosure more than do whites. Yet self-disclosure is viewed as a primary requisite of traditional psychotherapy.

The utilization of mental health services is also influenced by ethnic factors. For example, Asian and Hispanic Americans appear to seek help from mental health professionals less often than do whites. American Indians and black Americans appear to drop out of treatment more quickly than do whites. This underutilization of services may relate to a variety of factors, including cultural norms that prohibit seeking professional help as has been reported by some Polish Americans, the experience that certain mental health treatment modalities violate cultural norms, and the limited availability of services seen as relevant.

Some experts advocate the use of specific kinds of therapies with members of specific ethnic minorities. For example, in ethnic groups that place a high value on the family structure, family therapy is likely to be seen as more relevant than individual therapy and is therefore often recommended. Brief, crisis-oriented therapy and goal setting may also be most beneficial among some ethnic minority groups, such as Italian Americans, Polish Americans, and black Americans.

GENDER

The relationship between gender roles and mental health is becoming increasingly evident.

There is a growing awareness of the need to consider gender as a cultural factor that has a significant relationship to the level of an individual's mental health and to the nature of his mental health problems. The mental health system in this country has been accused of practicing from a male bias that declares traditional masculine behaviors the norm of mental health. Thus, traditional feminine behaviors have been deemed deviant, although interestingly women who engage in traditional masculine behaviors have also been labeled deviant.

Different cultural norms have historically existed for the male members of society than for its female members. Traditionally, men have been expected to be strong, rational, and successful in the public world. Women, in contrast, have been expected to be passive, emotional, and nurturing. These differing cultural norms for men and women have impacted significantly on the psychological development of the society's members. Karen Horney is a psychoanalyst who has written prolifically on this subject.

As consciousness has been raised about the relationship between gender roles and mental health, it has become evident that gender norms have impacted on both men and women. While women can be viewed as a more overtly oppressed group, gender norms also have psychological consequences for the male members of society. In addition, there has been a rapid change in gender roles in this country during the last several decades. Some authorities argue that the resultant role contradictions and role confusion will contribute to an increase in mental illness. Others, however, maintain that mental illness will decline with increased personal freedom and choice.

Gender appears to be a factor influencing the kinds of mental health problems that an individual will experience. For example, women are more inclined to suffer from major depressive illness, phobias, and eating disorders. In contrast, men tend more often to engage in alcohol abuse and violent behaviors. Although there are several explanations of these phenomena, most experts agree that cultural norms channel the actual expression of feelings and conflicts differently for men than for women.

The majority of individuals who use mental health services are women. Some authorities believe that this is because women are more inclined to seek help, while men view help-seeking behavior as an admission of weakness. Others maintain that women are members of an oppressed group who, like ethnic minorities, have been denied access to needed resources and who have been victims of sexist practices and who therefore need mental health services more than men. Interestingly, some recent studies indicate that women who work outside the home report fewer emotional problems and take less psychotropic medication than do women whose work is within the home in the traditional roles of wife and mother.

In terms of mental health treatment, studies indicate that there has been a bias toward traditional gender roles in the mental health system. For example, some evidence indicates that mental health professionals encourage adherence to traditional gender roles even when these roles negatively influence the individual's mental health and adaptation. Some evidence also indicates that physicians more readily prescribe psychotropic medication, particularly anxiolytic agents, for women than for men. Feminists believe that this practice simultaneously discourages women from engaging in potentially self-actualizing behaviors and denigrates their ability to address and cope with their problems.

In summary, gender has been documented as a significant cultural factor that interacts with the individual and his level of mental health. It is imperative that the nurse consider the impact of gender as she assesses the individual's mental health.

SOCIOECONOMIC STATUS

Another cultural factor that influences mental health and mental illness is socioeconomic status. The prevalence of mental illness among this nation's poor appears to be disproportionately high. One view of this phenomenon is that disadvantaged circumstances cause increased stress in an individual's life and con-

Socioeconomic status is another cultural factor influencing mental health and mental illness.

sequently contribute to the onset of mental disorders. On the other hand, others argue that persons who are mentally ill fall into disadvantaged circumstances by virtue of their mental illness, a phenomenon called *social drift*. It is important to understand that a disproportionate number of members of ethnic minorities comprise the socioeconomically disadvantaged. Furthermore, there is a growing awareness of the "feminization of poverty," wherein unmarried women and their children statistically constitute an increasingly large proportion of people living below the poverty level in this country. Consequently, socioeconomic factors appear to be intertwined with ethnicity and gender as cultural influences on mental health and mental illness.

Studies indicate that some psychiatric diagnoses appear more frequently in certain socioeconomic groups. For example, schizophrenia, major depression, and alcohol abuse appear to be most common among the nation's poor. Some researchers have suggested that the poor may be misdiagnosed more often than others and be assigned diagnoses indicative of more serious illnesses than members of higher socioeconomic groups.

The type of mental health treatment that an individual receives has also been shown to relate to his socioeconomic status. For example, persons from lower socioeconomic groups are more likely to be treated with medications, electroconvulsive therapy, or involuntary hospitalization than those from a higher socioeconomic group. Some authorities have argued that these findings are caused by a higher incidence of antisocial, aggressive behavior among the poor, while others have argued that the society holds negative cultural stereotypes about the poor that inaccurately define them as deviant and dangerous.

More research is needed to fully understand the nature of the relationship between socioeconomic status and mental illness. Currently, many experts suggest that the poor are limited in the material resources necessary to the achievement of mental health. Some recommend that mental health professionals focus less on helping the client who is poor to develop insight into his problems and expend more energy and money on assisting him to meet the basic human needs of food, shelter, and education. However, this assistance is not likely to be provided on a widespread scale if the poor continue to be labeled deviants who are responsible for their own problems. This common view further compounds feelings of powerlessness, low self-esteem, and hostility among the poor, while at the same time limits their access to mental health services that have the potential to assist them in coping with daily stressors.

END NOTE

This chapter discusses culture as a factor that strongly influences human behavior, shapes the society's definition of mental health and mental illness, and serves as a major determinant of the nature of its mental health system and mental health treatment. The concept of deviance is introduced as one way of understanding the relationships among a person, his culture, and his mental health.

Ethnicity, gender, and socioeconomic status are introduced as cultural factors that have been demonstrated to influence the individual's mental health, the incidence and manifestation of mental illness, and the type and effectiveness of mental health treatment. The nurse is urged to become culturally informed and sensitive to ensure comprehensive assessment, accurate diagnosis, and effective nursing care of all clients.

SUGGESTED SOURCES OF ADDITIONAL INFORMATION

Berger P and Berger B: Sociology: a biographical approach, New York, 1975, Basic Books, Inc.

Burke A: Is racism a causatory factor in mental illness? Int J Soc Psychiatr 30(1,2):1, 1984.

Campinha-Bacote J: Culturological assessment: an important factor in psychiatric consultation-liaison nursing II, Arch Psych Nurs 2(4):244, 1988.

Chesler P: Women and madness, Garden City, NY, 1973, Arno Press.

Flaskerud J: Community mental health nursing: its unique role in the delivery of services to ethnic minorities, Persp Psychiatr Care 20(1):37, 1982.

Flaskerud J and Soldevilla E: Filipino and Vietnamese clients: utilizing an Asian mental health center, J Psychosoc Nurs 24(8):32, 1986.

Goffman E: Stigma, Englewood Cliffs, NJ, 1963, Prentice-Hall.

Horney K: Feminine psychology, New York, 1967, WW Norton & Company.

Howell E and Bayes M, editors: Women and mental health, New York, 1981, Basic Books, Inc.

Kerson TS: The impact of ethnicity on community mental health, J Nurs Educ 20(3):32, 1981.

Knab S: Polish Americans, J Psychosoc Nurs 26(1):31, 1986.

Lawson W: Racial and ethnic factors in psychiatric research, Hosp Commun Psychiatr 37(1):50, 1986.

Leininger M: Transcultural nursing: concepts, theories, and practices, New York, 1978, Wiley.

Lin T: A global view of mental health, Am J Orthopsychiatr 54(3):369, 1984.

Minrath M: Breaking the race barrier: the white therapist in interracial psychotherapy, J Psychosoc Nurs 23(8):19, 1985.

Parsons T: The social system, Glencoe, Ill, 1951, The Free Press.

Reeves K: Hispanic utilization of an ethnic mental health center, J Psychosoc Nurs 24(2):23, 1986.

Rosenfield S: Race differences in involuntary hospitalization: psychiatric vs. labeling perspectives, J Health Soc Behav 25:14, 1984.

Rozendal N: Understanding Italian-American cultural norms, J Psychosoc Nurs 25(2):29, 1987.

Schwartz D: Caribbean folk beliefs and western psychiatry, J Psychosoc Nurs 23(11):26, 1985.

Szasz T: The myth of mental illness, New York, 1961, Hoeber-Harper.

Tien J: Do Asians need less medication? J Psychosoc Nurs 22(12):19, 1984.

Tripp-Reimer T: Retention of a folk-healing practice (matiasma) among four generations of urban Greek immigrants, Nurs Res 32(2):97, 1983.

Individuals with thought disorders

15

LEARNING OBJECTIVES

After studying this chapter, the student will be able to:

o Describe the symptoms exhibited by a person with the medical diagnosis of schizophrenia.

o Discuss the causative factors associated with thought disorders.

o State the desired effects, side effects, and adverse effects of the antipsychotic medications commonly prescribed for individuals with thought disorders.

o Describe the behaviors the nurse is most likely to observe in an individual with a thought disorder.

o State examples of nursing diagnoses likely to be applicable to an individual with a thought disorder.

o Develop a hypothetical plan of nursing care for an individual with a thought disorder.

The ability of an individual to deal subjectively and behaviorally with the demands of living in a highly complex society presupposes that he is capable of filtering, processing, and adapting to the immeasurable number of internal and external stimuli with which he is continuously bombarded. After engaging in these processes, the person then must test reality and consensually validate his perceptions with others whom he trusts. When, for reasons of physiological dysfunction or a consistently high level of anxiety, the individual is not able to perform these functions, a pattern of reality distortion becomes established. When an individual's distorted perceptions of reality result from and contribute to disturbed thought processes, that individual may be suffering from *schizo-phrenia.*

Although not all authorities agree that the cluster of symptoms currently labeled as schizophrenia represents the same syndrome, all are in agreement that this illness is one of the most serious forms of mental illness. For the vast majority of persons affected, it results in a chronic disability that lasts a lifetime. The personal, social, and economic tragedy of this illness can be appreciated best when one understands that the onset of schizophrenia characteristically is during late adolescence or young adulthood. Furthermore, schizophrenia is a relatively common mental illness. It is estimated that 2 million Americans suffer from schizophrenia and that 1% of the population of the Western world will be diagnosed as having schizophrenia by the time they reach age 55.

HISTORICAL PERSPECTIVE

The thought disorder known today as schizophrenia undoubtedly has existed throughout human history. However, the deviant behavior associated with this disorder was not always viewed negatively. Some primitive societies elevated those who saw visions and heard voices to a position of prominence, believing they had supernatural powers.

Not until the end of the nineteenth century was formal research into the cause and nature of nervous and mental disease conducted. The pioneer of that effort was Jean Charcot (1825-1893), the great French neurologist whose clinics attracted students from every country in the world.

In 1883 Emil Kraepelin (1856-1926), a German professor of psychiatry, published the first edition of *Psychiatrie,* which in English translation changed the whole view of classifications of mental disorders in America. Kraepelin classified human behavior on the basis of symptomatology and labeled what is now called schizophrenia *dementia praecox.* This label reflected Kraepelin's belief that the deterioration associated with the illness was inevitable, progressive, and irreversible. Eugene Blueler (1857-1939), a Swiss psychiatrist, elaborated the concept of dementia praecox by recognizing underlying disturbances in the thought processes and therefore renamed the syndrome schizophrenia in 1911. His description of schizophrenia was refined and enlarged over the years but remained essentially the same until 1980 when the American Psychiatric Association published the third edition of the *Diagnostic and Statistical Manual of Mental Disorders* (DSM-III). This manual and its most recent revision, the DSM-III-R published in 1987, describe the illness in behavioral terms, and its multi-axial approach allows, for the first time, a holistic assessment of the individual.

Although a necessary first step, descriptions of a disorder do not necessarily provide direction for treatment. Over the centuries many modalities have been adopted to treat persons with thought disorders, with varying degrees of success. For example, in 1933 Dr. Manfred Sakel developed insulin shock therapy, a procedure where a series of hypoglycemic shocks are induced by injections of insulin. This treatment, as well as other somatic therapies such as hydrotherapy, has been almost completely replaced by the use of antipsychotic medications and behaviorally oriented interventions. These treatment modalities, while not curing thought disorders, have proven sufficiently safe and effective in controlling symptoms that it was hoped many individuals with thought disorders could be maintained in the community with only infrequent and limited hospitalization.

This hope is far from being fully realized. While it is true that the average length of hospitalization of individuals with thought disorders has been drastically reduced, the number and frequency of readmissions have escalated. Furthermore, the quality of life experienced by the individual and his family when he is not hospitalized is often very poor. Currently, much research is being conducted to determine not only those factors which contribute to the development of thought disorders but also those factors which are necessary to enable individuals with thought disorders to live in a satisfying and satisfactory way in the mainstream of community life.

SCHIZOPHRENIC DISORDERS

Schizophrenia is one of the *functional psychoses*. This term describes those mental illnesses for which there is no demonstrable organic disease or intellectual deficit and where the illness is all-pervasive, affecting all dimensions of the person's existence.

To be medically diagnosed as schizophrenic, the individual must exhibit characteristic symptoms continuously for at least 6 months. In addition, he must be functioning below the highest level previously achieved, or, in the case of children and adolescents, he must have failed to achieve the expected level of social development.

The symptoms of schizophrenia are often classified as either positive or negative. *Positive symptoms reflect the presence of unusual behavior,* specifically distortions in both the content and form of thought and in perception. *Negative symptoms reflect the absence of behavior normally expected,* specifically in the dimensions of affect, definition of self, volition, interpersonal relations, and, in some cases, psychomotor behavior.

The most common symptom associated with distortions of content of thought is *delusions*. Delusions are false beliefs out of keeping with the individual's level of knowledge and his cultural group; the belief is maintained against logical argument and despite objective evidence to the contrary. Delusions characteristic of schizophrenia include delusions about one's thoughts, feelings, and activities being controlled by some external force (delusion of being controlled), delusions about one's thoughts being broadcast into the external world (thought broadcasting), inserted from the external world into one's mind (thought insertion), or removed from one's head by some external source (thought withdrawal). Persecutory, religious, and somatic delusions are not uncommon.

Functional psychosis
A severe emotional disorder characterized by personality derangement and the loss of ability to function in reality, but without evidence that the disorder is related to the physical processes of the brain.

Distortions in the form of thought are manifested by *loosening of associations* (derailment), whereby the individual's idea or trend of thought skips off one track onto another that is completely unrelated. As a result, the person's speech may be unintelligible to the listener even though individual words are understood.

Delytions, loosening of associations, and hallucinations are positive symptoms of schizophrenia.

One of the most dramatic symptoms of schizophrenia is related to distortions in perception and is called *hallucinations*. Hallucinations are false sensory perceptions in the absence of an actual external stimulus. Although any of the five senses may be involved in a hallucinatory experience, auditory hallucinations, often of a persecutory nature, are most characteristic of schizophrenia.

One of the most prominent negative symptoms of schizophrenia is a disturbance in affect. The term *affect* refers to the feeling tone of the individual. The person afflicted with schizophrenia characteristically exhibits a blunt or flat affect, in contrast to the healthy individual whose affect conveys a feeling that is indicative of his emotional state and is congruent with the content of what he is saying. In individuals with schizophrenic disorders one observes that the feeling tone conveyed by the individual does not enhance what he is saying. It is not unusual to spend a great deal of time talking with a person with schizophrenia without learning what he is feeling, despite the fact that much of the conversation was his attempt to describe his feelings. It is also not unusual for the individual to convey a feeling tone that is inappropriate to the content of what he is saying; for example he may laugh while stating how upset and sad he is because his mother just died.

The individual with schizophrenia also has a very poorly defined sense of self and experiences extreme confusion about such issues as who he is, both in relation to his environment and other people, and what his purpose and role are in the larger scheme of things. When he is acutely ill, he may not be able to differentiate literally between where he begins and ends and where others and the environment begin and end. This very frightening feeling is referred to as a loss of ego boundaries.

Disturbance in volition refers to the individual's inability to engage in self-initiated, goal-directed activity. This symptom impacts greatly on his ability to engage in self-care, recreational, and work activities. It is often accompanied by *ambivalence,* where the person exhibits approach-avoidance behavior resulting from experiencing two mutually exclusive emotions such as love and hate, at exactly the same time.

Impaired interpersonal functioning is one of the most obvious and distressing symptoms of schizophrenia. An individual with schizophrenia tends to withdraw into his own subjective world. Withdrawal is manifested behaviorally by an increasing aversion to interpersonal interactions and often is the symptom that causes the most distress to the client's family. In the extreme, this symptom develops into *autism.* Autism is a form of thinking that does not take reality factors into account and therefore makes it impossible for the person to relate to others in his environment. The individual's autistic world is unique to him and consequently difficult for others to understand. One can appreciate the nature of autistic thinking to some degree by recalling the daydreaming frequently engaged in by adolescents. The process is similar in that both autistic thinking and daydreaming are designed to meet unfulfilled needs. A major difference is that the daydreamer can easily call himself back to the world of reality, whereas the individual who is engaged in autistic thinking cannot.

Finally, the individual suffering from schizophrenia commonly displays abnormal psychomotor behavior, which is manifested as either physical and mental overactivity or inactivity.

See Table 15-1 for a summary of the positive and negative symptoms of schizophrenia.

Once the medical diagnosis of schizophrenia is made, the individual's behavior is further categorized into types of schizophrenia. Psychiatrists have sub-

Disturbance of affect, a poorly defined sense of self, disturbance in volition, impaired interpersonal functioning, and abnormal psychomotor behavior are negative symptoms of schizophrenia.

TABLE 15-1   *Positive and negative symptoms of schizophrenia*

	Symptom	Description
Positive symptoms	Delusion	False belief out of keeping with the individual's level of knowledge and his cultural group that is maintained against logical argument and despite objective evidence to the contrary
	Loosening of association	The idea or trend of thought skipping off one track onto another that is completely unrelated
	Hallucination	False sensory perception in the absence of actual external stimulus
Negative symptoms	Disturbance in affect	Blunt or flat feeling tone
	Disturbance in sense of self	Poorly defined conception of who he is and of the meaning of his life; loss of ego boundaries
	Disturbance in volition	Inability to engage in self-initiated, goal-directed activities
	Disturbance in interpersonal functioning	Withdrawal from others; autism in extreme situations
	Disturbance in psychomotor behavior	Decrease or increase in physical and mental activity (considered a positive symptom when psychomotor activity is increased)

The five major types of schizophrenia are disorganized, catatonic, paranoid, undifferentiated, and residual.

classified schizophrenia into five major types, depending on the predominant patterns of behavior displayed. These subclassifications are the disorganized, the catatonic, the paranoid, the undifferentiated, and the residual types. The *disorganized type* is characterized by severe personality disintegration, including hallucinations, inappropriate behavior (for example, silly laughter), and regression. The *catatonic type* is characterized by an acute stupor associated with a sudden loss of animation and a tendency to remain motionless in a stereotyped position; this behavior may alternate with periods of excitement and explosive overactivity. The *paranoid type* is characterized by suspiciousness and ideas of persecution or grandeur called *paranoid delusions*. The *undifferentiated type* is characterized by the prominence of psychotic symptoms that fall into more than one subtype or that do not meet the criteria for any one subtype. The *residual type* is the diagnosis used for individuals who no longer exhibit overtly psychotic symptoms but do exhibit inappropriate behavior characteristic of schizophrenia.

Whether it is possible to help an individual with schizophrenia to reestablish himself in his family and return to his work depends on several factors:

1. The character of the prepsychotic personality. The prepsychotic personality includes the effectiveness of the individual's adaptation before becoming mentally ill, the type of interests that were maintained, and the coping mechanisms that were used.
2. The nature of the onset of the illness. Did the illness develop insidiously over a long period of time as the result of progressively more unsatisfactory methods of coping with life's problems, or was the onset rapid and precipitated by a situation external to the life of the individual?
3. The timing and nature of the treatment. Was treatment sought early in the illness, and was treatment individualized and personalized?

An individual who has adapted reasonably well to the stressors of life before becoming ill will have a better chance of recovery, at least of returning to his prepsychotic level of effectiveness, than will someone who has never adapted effectively and therefore has limited system energy. It is also obvious that someone whose illness has developed slowly and insidiously has a less optimistic future than does someone whose illness was precipitated only after experiencing great stress emanating from his environment.

Persons who receive help very soon after the development of the illness and are given individualized, skilled, and highly personalized care have a good chance of making a social recovery. This is much less true of persons who receive treatment after the illness has been fullblown for a year or more.

Authorities suggest that expectations for recovery should be in terms of social recovery and not necessarily in terms of cure. During remission, these individuals may maintain a marginal adjustment, still retaining an essentially shallow affective response and shyness. They can be thought of as interpersonally fragile and may require professional help from time to time. Many require a daily maintenance dose of one of the antipsychotic medications.

Causative factors of thought disorders

If one were to ask the person with a thought disorder what caused his illness he might respond by relating a particularly stressful event that preceded the onset of his illness by days, weeks, or months. Although not all persons with schizophrenia have such events in their lives, enough experience them to make it important to distinguish between a precipitating event and causation. Although there is much ongoing debate over the cause of thought disorders, all authorities agree that the cause is likely to be a process of long standing, either physical or emotional or both. It is considered highly unlikely that a single event, either physical or emotional, no matter how catastrophic, would be sufficient to cause the drastic personality alteration seen in schizophrenia. The events reported by these persons as the possible causes of their illness are usually viewed by authorities as precipitating factors. Laypersons express this concept when they refer to the "straw that broke the camel's back." The underlying physiological and psychological structure is so fragile that the traumatic event cannot be integrated within the context of reality and the individual adapts, albeit dysfunctionally, to protect himself against total personality disintegration. It should be noted that many such individuals are unable to identify a precipitating event; instead, the onset of the syndrome is often insidious.

The cause of schizophrenia is likely to be a process of long-standing, either physical or emotional or both.

Although there is no conclusive scientific proof of the cause of thought disorders, many authorities believe that they are related to factors inherent in highly complex cultures such as that of the United States. Recent studies point to the influence of a genetic factor in schizophrenia and some authorities believe that there is likely to be a certain biochemical composition that predisposes individuals to a dysfunctional adaptation to stress. Credence is given to these theories by the number of schizophrenic individuals whose families report that, even as infants, these persons resisted attempts at cuddling, which set up a cyclically unsatisfying relationship between the infants and their parents.

ANTIPSYCHOTIC MEDICATIONS

Although natural and synthetic chemical substances had been used for centuries in an effort to normalize behavior, it was not until 1953 that relatively safe and effective psychotropic medications were developed. In 1956 the most useful of the new medications, chlorpromazine, was introduced. It was marketed under the name of Thorazine and today is only one of a number of medications that are effective in diminishing the psychotic symptoms associated with schizophrenia; thus, these medications are referred to as *antipsychotic drugs.* Over the years, clinical experience with the use of these medications has shown that they are particularly effective in reducing the positive symptoms of schizophrenia, namely, delusions, loosening of associations, and hallucinations. They are less effective and sometimes ineffective in ameliorating the negative symptoms.

Although it is known that not every individual is helped by these medications, it is not possible to determine at the time of diagnosis which clients will be helped and which will not. Therefore, an antipsychotic medication is initially prescribed for the vast majority of individuals experiencing an acute exacerbation of symptoms. Standard practice is to keep clients on moderate doses of antipsychotics for as long as possible, since relapse rates increase dramatically once medication is stopped. The nurse should be very aware, however, that the incidence of side effects increases as dosage and duration of use increase.

Drug manufacturers often make claims that a drug is specifically useful in alleviating a particular symptom, implying that there are major differences between drugs within a given chemical group. Clinicians, on the other hand, more commonly report that the effect of the drug seems to be idiosyncratic to the individual and that if a drug in one chemical group is not successful in alleviating the symptomatology without adverse effects, success can often be achieved by the administration of an antipsychotic drug from another chemical group.

TABLE 15-2 *Antipsychotic drugs*

Generic name	Trade name	Range of daily oral dosage (mg)	Comments
PHENOTHIAZINE DERIVATIVES: ALIPHATIC SUBGROUP			
Chlorpromazine	Thorazine	200-1000	
PHENOTHIAZINE DERIVATIVES: PIPERIDINE SUBGROUP			
Thioridazine	Mellaril	200-800	
Piperacetazine	Quide	20-160	
Mesoridazine	Serentil	100-400	Schizophrenia, organic mental disorders, and alcoholism are often treated with Serentil
PHENOTHIAZINE DERIVATIVES: PIPERAZINE SUBGROUP			
Fluphenazine	Prolixin	2.5-40	Prolixin decanoate often given intramuscularly, initially at 12.5-25 mg and repeated every 2-4 weeks for maintenence
Perphenazine	Trilafon	8-64	
Trifluoperazine	Stelazine	15-20	
BUTYROPHENONE DERIVATIVES			
Haloperidol	Haldol	1-100	Optimum dosage highly variable
THIOXANTHENE DERIVATIVES			
Chlorprothixene	Taractan	75-600	Specific for moderate to severe agitation, anxiety, and tension related to schizophrenia
Thiothixene	Navane	20-30	
DIHYDROINDOLONE DERIVATIVES			
Molindone	Moban	40-225	Specific for use in schizophrenia
DIBENZOXAZEPINE DERIVATIVES			
Loxapine succinate	Loxitane	20-250	

Because of this observation, Table 15-2 presents the antipsychotic drugs according to chemical group.

Although all medications are prescribed by a physician, it is the nurse who often has the responsibility for administering them and monitoring their effects. The student is encouraged to review the responsibilities of the nurse in regard to medications in Chapter 7 of this text. Tables 15-3 and 15-4 describe some of the side effects and adverse effects that can occur in some individuals when they receive antipsychotic medications. The nurse is often the first health care professional to notice the occurrence of adverse effects and therefore must differentiate them from unpleasant but benign side effects and initiate appropriate nursing and medical measures. These measures vary from reassuring the client in instances when side effects occur to withholding the medication and contacting the physician immediately when adverse effects occur.

TABLE 15-3   *Side effects of antipsychotic drugs*

Side effects	Comments
Dry mouth, blurred vision, constipation, urinary hesitance, paralytic ileus	These effects result from the drug's interference with acetylcholine. The first three should be treated symptomatically and client reassured. In instances of urinary hesitance and paralytic ileus medication should be withheld until medical evaluation is obtained.
Orthostatic hypotension	Drug used with great caution if cardiovascular disease is present and with the elderly. Individual should be warned about possible occurrences and taught to rise slowly and dangle legs before standing.
Photosensitivity	Protect client from ultraviolet light. Use sunscreen. Occurs most frequently with chlorpromazine. Examine skin frequently.
Endocrine changes	Weight gain, edema, lactation, and menstrual irregularities. Treat symptomatically. Reassure client.
Extrapyramidal reactions	Dose and duration related. Managed by adjusting dose of drug or adding antiparkinsonism drug.
Pseudoparkinsonism	Typical shuffling gait, masklike facies, tremor, muscular ridigity, slowing of movements, and other symptoms mimicking those seen in Parkinson's disease.
Akathisia, dystonia	Continuous restlessness, fidgeting, and pacing occur. Spasm of neck muscles, extensor rigidity of back muscles, carpopedal spasm, eyes rolled back, swallowing difficulties occur. There is acute onset, but condition is reversible with appropriate medication. Reassurance should be provided until symptoms subside.
Akinesia	Lethargy, feelings of fatigue and muscle weakness. Must be differentiated from withdrawal.

TABLE 15-4   *Possible adverse effects of antipsychotic drugs*

Adverse effects	Comments
Skin reactions	Urticarial, maculopapular, edematous, or petechial responses may occur 1 to 5 weeks after initiation of treatment. Withhold drug until after medical evaluation.
Jaundice	Develops in about 4% of the clients and is a dangerous complication; drug should be discontinued.
Agranulocytosis and leukopenia	Chlorpromazine depresses production of leukocytes. Initial symptoms of sore throat, high temperature, and lesions in mouth indicate that drug should be stopped immediately. Outcome may be lethal, but this is rare.
Ocular changes	Corneal and lenticular changes and pigmentary retinopathy may occur with high dosages over long periods of time. Periodic ocular examinations are recommended.
Convulsions	Antipsychotic agents lower seizure threshold, making seizure-prone persons more likely to have seizures. Persons with a history of seizures or organic conditions associated with seizures require an increased dosage of anticonvulsant medication if antipsychotics are used.
Tardive dyskinesia	Insidious onset of fine vermicular movements of tongue occurs, which is reversible if drug is discontinued at this time. Can progress to rhythmical involuntary movements of the tongue, face, mouth, or jaw with protrusion of tongue, puffing of cheeks, and chewing movements. No known treatment; often irreversible. Prevention is imperative. Females over 50 years on prolonged doses are particularly at risk. Do *not* withhold drug until after medical evaluation; symptoms will increase.

NURSING CARE OF INDIVIDUALS WITH THOUGHT DISORDERS
Nursing assessment

When assessing an individual with a thought disorder, it is important for the nurse to remember that the medical classification of schizophrenia into five types has little practical significance for designing a plan for nursing care. It is necessary for the nurse to attempt to understand the needs of the person rather than to focus on diagnostic entities.

The following discussion is organized around the human processes introduced in Chapter 9. Although behaviors in each category are presented as separate entities, it should be understood that they are highly interrelated and are adaptations to similar stressors. Further, in many instances behavior designed as an adaptation to one stressor becomes a stressor itself in another dimension. Therefore, nursing care directed at altering one behavior will inevitably have an effect on others.

Activity processes. It is unusual for an individual with a thought disorder to exhibit normal psychomotor behavior, that is, both mental and physical activity congruent with the requirements of the situation. Rather, the person frequently exhibits retardation or overactivity in the psychomotor realm. An extreme example of psychomotor retardation is seen in persons who are in a catatonic stupor. These persons move very slowly and can take hours to walk the distance of a city block or to eat a meal. Concomitantly, they speak very slowly, which reflects an extreme slowing down of mental processes. The term *retarded* as used in this context does not mean the client has an intellectual deficit. Individuals with a thought disorder do not necessarily suffer from intellectual impairment, although this may appear to be the case because of their temporarily diminished ability to comprehend and respond to mental stimuli.

Psychomotor overactivity is manifested by loud, rapid talking (pressure of speech) and frequent, rapid, gross motor movements that seem aimless. Despite the quantity of activity, fine motor movements are usually impaired. This person literally finds it impossible to sit still and frequently paces, swinging his arms and talking continuously.

When questioned about his recreational patterns, many clients with a thought disorder will report that their only recreation is listening to the radio or watching television. These passive activities are solitary and do not require much concentration. Other clients enjoy reading but not material that evokes emotional responses such as romance novels. Once again, reading is a solitary activity and nonverbally discourages social approaches from others.

Neglect of all areas of self-care is often the first sign of an impending psychosis. It is not unusual for the individual with a thought disorder to neglect his personal hygiene and become poorly groomed and inappropriately dressed. He often has many unmet physical needs because he has not attended to his basic needs for food, water, or shelter and has not sought health care. The severely ill individual may be incontinent of urine and/or feces, not due to loss of sphincter control but because of an inability to decide to go to the bathroom.

Cognition processes. Decision making and judgment are both commonly impaired in individuals with thought disorders. These persons may be observed vacillating over seemingly simple decisions such as whether to go outdoors, or what to wear if they do.

As its name indicates, the major impairment experienced by people with thought disorders is in relation to their thought processes. Their inability to think abstractly is dramatically manifested through psychological tests that require the client to explain proverbs. For example, when asked the meaning of "a rolling stone gathers no moss," the client is likely to say, "When a stone rolls down a hill it will not catch on the grass because it is moving." If asked what brought him to the hospital, he is likely to reply, "a bus."

Delusions, regardless of their nature, are another indication of altered thought processes. Many clients, especially if they have been ill for a while, have learned not to divulge their delusional thinking to an individual whom

Psychomotor retardation or overactivity, passive recreational activity, and neglect of self-care are exhibited in persons with schizophrenia.

they are meeting for the first time. Therefore, the nurse who is making the initial assessment may be unaware of their existence.

Ecological processes. As is the case with self-care, the individual with a thought disorder is unlikely to be able to engage in the activities required to maintain a home, such as cleaning, shopping, and transacting normal business activities such as paying rent.

Emotional processes. It is not unusual to hear someone describe a conversation with a client who has a thought disorder with phrases such as, "I feel there is an intangible wall between us" or "I just can't seem to get through to him." This reaction is often the result of the client's blunt or flat affect, whereby the feeling tone associated with the client's words does nothing to enhance their meaning.

Because the client's grasp on reality is tenuous and because he may be stimulated by intrapsychic phenomena such as voices or visions, the client may strike out at things or persons in the environment. Even though the nurse has learned in social situations to associate aggressive, physical behavior with the feeling of anger, this seemingly hostile behavior on the part of the client is more likely to be his adaptation to feelings of anxiety or fear.

Interpersonal processes. Social ineptitude is a prominent feature of the behavior of individuals with thought disorders. They often have not been able to learn many of the rudimentary social skills healthy adults take for granted. Such common occurrences as meeting people for the first time can precipitate overwhelming anxiety and may lead to highly inappropriate behavior. It is not uncommon for these persons to go to great lengths to avoid social situations and activities such as dating and team sports. Instead, they prefer to engage in solitary activities, which enables them to keep their anxiety at a manageable level but also increases their social ineptitude. They often report that they have few if any friends; the nurse may observe that few if any people visit or inquire about the client's welfare.

The social ineptitude of these clients stems, in part, from and is compounded by their communication problems, which, in turn, result from their thought disorder. As previously stated, these individuals think in a very concrete and personalized manner and consequently have difficulty understanding and appropriately responding to the superficial chatter present in most social situations.

Perception processes. Visual hallucinations are not uncommon in persons with a thought disorder. The individual experiencing hallucinations rarely offers this information spontaneously. Rather, he will be observed cocking his head to one side as if listening, staring into space as if watching something, and talking as if to someone, although no one is present.

Physiological processes. Behaviors related to unmet physical needs may or may not be related to the client's emotional problems. It cannot be overemphasized that emotional illness provides no immunity to physical illness. Therefore,

Marginal notes:

Impaired decision making and judgment, inability to think abstractly, delusional thinking, blunt or flat affect, and social ineptitude are common indications of altered thought processes.

Complaints of physical discomfort must be thoroughly investigated to determine whether they are related to physical illness or to the individual's emotional state.

in the initial assessment it is imperative that the nurse determine the degree of general physical health of the client. Complaints of physical discomfort must be thoroughly investigated to determine whether they are related to physical illness or to the individual's emotional state.

When making the initial assessment, it is important to determine whether the person has taken any psychotropic medications and, if so, the kind, dosage, and frequency. The purpose of these medications is to alter emotional states biochemically, which brings about altered behavior. In addition, the medications themselves may have side effects that are reflected behaviorally. It is important to differentiate between behavior induced by medications and behavior reflecting the emotional state, since the subsequent intervention differs.

Because of the nature of thought disorders, it is not uncommon to find a number of physical problems that are a consequence of the thought disorder. Malnutrition is usual, due to psychomotor retardation, suspiciousness, or generalized neglect of activities of daily living. Even though the client might not be able to tell the nurse his usual weight, the nurse can observe whether his clothing fits properly. If an individual has been taking psychotropic medications for a period of time, especially the phenothiazines, he may be overweight, since these medications have the effect of stimulating the appetite. Obesity should not be seen as evidence of a sound nutritional state; many obese people are in fact malnourished because food high in caloric value frequently has limited nutritional value.

The individual may not spontaneously report a physical condition of long standing such as diabetes or hypothyroidism caused by a thyroidectomy, either of which may require daily medication. The nurse should be alert to indications of these and other physical conditions by observing for such evidence as scars or injection marks.

Finally, because of psychomotor retardation or overactivity, the person may have circulatory problems evidenced by peripheral edema or may be verging on a state of exhaustion.

Valuation processes. Because of his thought disorder, the client is often perplexed about his existence, its meaning, and its goal. It is not unusual for him to state that he is simultaneously "at one with the universe but all alone in this world."

Nursing diagnosis

As with all nursing diagnoses, the nursing diagnoses for the individual with a thought disorder are based on the themes identified during the assessment phase of the nursing process. Categories of human responses from the ANA Classification of Human Responses of Concern for Psychiatric–Mental Health Nursing Practice that may be specifically applicable to individuals with a thought disorder include the following:

1.1.2   Altered Motor Behavior
1.2.2   Altered Recreation Patterns

1.3.4   Altered Self-Care
2.1.2   Altered Decision Making
2.2.2   Altered Judgment
2.6.2   Altered Thought Processes
3.3.2   Altered Home Maintenance
4.1.4   Flat Affect
5.2.2   Altered Communication Processes
5.4.2   Altered Family Processes
5.5.3   Ineffective Individual Coping
5.7.2   Altered Social Interaction
6.3.2   Altered Self Concept
6.4.2   Altered Sensory Perception
7.1.1   Potential for Alteration in Circulation
7.2.1   Potential for Alteration in Elimination Processes
7.7.1   Potential for Alteration in Nutrition
8.1.2   Altered Meaningfulness

NANDA nursing diagnostic categories which may be specifically applicable to the individual with a thought disorder include:

1.1.2.1   Altered Nutrition: More than body requirements
1.1.2.2   Altered Nutrition: Less than body requirements
2.1.1.1   Impaired Verbal Communication
3.1.1   Impaired Social Interaction
3.1.2   Social Isolation
3.2.1   Altered Role Performance
3.2.2   Altered Family Processes
5.1.1.1   Ineffective Individual Coping
5.3.1.1   Decisional Conflict (Specify)
6.5.2   Bathing/Hygiene Self Care Deficit
6.5.3   Dressing/Grooming Self Care Deficit
7.1.3   Personal Identity Disturbance
7.2   Sensory/Perceptual Alterations (Specify) (Visual, auditory, kinesthetic, gustatory, tactile, olfactory)
8.3   Altered Thought Processes

To develop a nursing diagnosis that fulfills its function of providing direction for planning nursing care, the nurse is encouraged to postulate and state etiologic or antecedent factors for each human response and connect the two phrases by using the term "related to." For example:

1.1.2   Altered Motor Behavior related to extreme ambivalence

Planning and implementing nursing care

The plan for nursing care is derived from the nursing diagnoses and includes the objectives of the care, the nursing actions, and outcome criteria. To be ef-

An individualized nursing care plan, based on nursing diagnoses that reflect an understanding of the assessment data, enables the nurse to select appropriate interventions that are designed to act as corrective experiences for the individual client.

fective the plan needs to be highly individualized. The suggestions that follow should be seen as general guidelines to be used if they are appropriate to the client's needs. All too often clients are required to conform to the dictates of a standardized nursing care plan rather than receiving care specifically designed for them.

In general, the objectives of all nursing care for the individual with a thought disorder should relate to helping him to increase his functional adaptations to reality, particularly in regard to activities of daily living; decrease his dysfunctional adaptations, particularly in regard to his tendency to withdraw; and learn to identify and avoid those stressors that are particularly noxious to him.

Since the client's nursing diagnoses are often interrelated, stemming as they do from similar etiologies or antecedents, the student will see that the appropriate nursing actions are also interrelated. In other words, by intervening in one dimension, the nurse will also affect other dimensions.

Activity processes. Clients with a thought disorder often have one or more nursing diagnoses in the category of activity processes. Since the client's behavior is unconsciously motivated and may have little logical relation to the immediate environmental situation, it is often difficult to understand. *Inappropriate* and *bizarre* may be accurate descriptive terms for much of his behavior. Nevertheless, the client's behavior has real meaning for him, and if it is closely studied its meaning often becomes clear. Therefore, one important aspect of the nursing care plan is to record what the nurse observes the client doing and saying.

It is often necessary for the nurse to take the initiative in stimulating the client's interest in recreational activities. It is important that she know something of the client's background so she can initiate conversations in which he can participate. When the client begins to trust the nurse, participation in some recreational activity can be encouraged. This may be accomplished by extending an invitation such as, "I need a partner for a game of table tennis; come and join me in a game." Initially, it may be best for the nurse to limit the activity to only the client she invited. As he develops more confidence, however, other participants should be added.

Some clients with a thought disorder may have difficulty in accomplishing even the most basic elements of self-care. While it is important for the nurse to help the client take responsibility for his own personal hygiene and grooming, she temporarily may have to assist him with toileting, bathing, and dressing. The therapeutic value of a client being clean, well-groomed, and appropriately and attractively dressed should not be underestimated, since this appearance is likely to elicit the sorely needed positive reflected appraisals of others. Assisting the client with these basic activities also has the potential for initiating a positive relationship with him and therefore should not be viewed as just one more task to be accomplished as quickly as possible. The services of a beautician and barber are invaluable; it may also be of great therapeutic benefit to have clients assist each other in grooming and selecting appropriate clothing.

Cognition processes. A client with a thought disorder will frequently have a nursing diagnosis related to cognition processes. While he may not necessarily experience alterations in knowledge, learning, or memory, he almost always will demonstrate altered thought processes, often manifested by delusional thinking. When the client talks about his delusions, it is not therapeutic for the nurse to try to explain them away or to argue with him about them. Such an approach will result in the client's becoming increasingly adamant about his false beliefs and perhaps hostile and suspicious. If the nurse can appreciate the necessity of the delusion to preserving the client's fragile personality organization, she will understand the futility of trying to change his ideas through logic. Generally, it is wise to listen to the client without commenting on the content of his delusions.

Emotional processes. The client's consistent affective indifference or emotional impoverishment makes it likely that he will have a nursing diagnosis related to emotional processes. The client's impairment in affect may make it difficult for the nurse to express warmth and demonstrate spontaneous interest in him. It is helpful for the nurse to understand that the client feels lonely, isolated, and hungry for human contact but is often incapable of inviting a friendly approach from another person. Only when the plan directs the nurse to approach the individual with an accepting attitude and with friendliness can she be a source of therapeutic help.

Interpersonal processes. The client's inability to initiate human contact is reflective of impairment in interpersonal processes. Therefore, interpersonal experiences must be planned for and provided. It is highly desirable for the nurse to develop a relationship with the client in which she becomes a significant other. Although the nurse-client relationship is a vehicle through which many other interventions can be implemented successfully, it has value in and of itself, since it can provide a corrective emotional experience in which the client experiences, over a period of time, the unconditional positive regard of another human being who communicates in a healthy functional way.

Meticulous honesty and fairness on the part of the nurse are of primary importance when establishing and maintaining a relationship with a client with a thought disorder. Once a promise is made, the nurse is obligated to carry it out. A response should be given to all the client's requests and questions. Should the client make a request with which it is impossible to comply, a suitable answer is, "I am sorry I am not allowed to carry out such a procedure." If no answer is possible, the client should be informed that his question will be referred to an appropriate person who can give an answer or that the answer is truly not known.

When communicating verbally with the client the nurse should avoid the use of long and involved sentences. Many persons with a thought disorder are easily confused and have a limited attention span. Short phrases are more effective and specific words more helpful than generalizations. For instance, *ice cream* is more meaningful than *dessert,* and *ham* is more specific or concrete than *meat.*

The nurse must avoid the temptation to exploit the negativism displayed by some clients. For example, she may think it helpful to request the client to walk backward when she desires the exact opposite. Similarly, making use of delusional and hallucinatory content to direct the client's behavior should be avoided. If, for instance, the client believes that he hears the voice of his mother, the nurse may be tempted to say that his mother just told him to eat his lunch. These "techniques" are never therapeutic, since they diminish whatever trust the client may have in the nurse. Their use is also likely to increase his confusion and encourage withdrawal.

Perception processes. Many clients with a thought disorder experience impairment in perception processes, manifested by hallucinations. Since these experiences are often frightening, the client may ask the nurse to confirm their existence. In such a situation, it is therapeutic to answer truthfully by saying something like, "No, Mr. Jones, I do not see the face of Christ on the wall, although I understand that you do because of your illness." Such a reply simultaneously presents reality, avoids an argument, and reassures the client that his experience is a symptom of his illness.

Physiological processes. Clients with a thought disorder often have one or more nursing diagnoses related to impairment in physiological processes. For example, a client who exhibits psychomotor retardation may be temporarily unable to plan and cook a meal, resulting in inadequate nutrition. It is perfectly appropriate for the nurse to initiate such plans by helping him to prepare lists or by arranging to have his food preparation and intake supervised by others. In the case of an overactive individual, foods that are high in caloric and protein value, that require little preparation, and that can be eaten easily are to be encouraged. Milk shakes are an example of a food that meets these criteria. The nurse's interest in the client's food intake often enhances their relationship because of the symbolic link between food and security.

Persons who are withdrawn often are unaware of or do not report symptoms of physical illness; they may offer no complaints even when the condition is a painful one. Acute mastoiditis, cystitis, lung abscess, and a broken bone in the hand or foot are examples of serious disorders that have been known to exist without complaint on the part of individuals with thought disorders. The nurse should plan to be constantly alert to the physical condition of clients so that interventions can be appropriate and timely.

Standing and sitting in one position for hours may be observed frequently among persons displaying psychomotor retardation. Edema and cyanosis of the extremities are likely to develop. To avoid this the client should be encouraged to take some exercise even if it is only to walk up and down a hall.

NURSING CARE PLAN

An individual with a severe thought disorder

CASE FORMULATION

Frances B. was 19 years of age when she was admitted to a psychiatric hospital. The only child of missionary parents, she was born in a mission station in Africa. Her father was a quiet-spoken man who was rigidly consistent in the practice of his religion. Her mother was more practical and tolerant but was frightened by her husband's anger whenever she deviated from the practices he deemed right. They were very busy with the work of the mission and had little time to spend with their daughter.

During the first 5 years of her life, Frances's only playmates were native children. She reportedly had always displayed an attitude of superiority toward them. On entering a boarding school in the United States at the age of 5, she had difficulty with her classmates. She was inclined to be too critical of them and insisted on lecturing them about personal matters. When she was 12 she had a long siege of pneumonia, after which she lost weight and was chronically anemic and undernourished. She spent many hours in prayer and wrote endless letters to her parents, most of them consisting of long quotations from the Bible. She insisted on wearing old, worn clothing to school and bitterly criticized her classmates for not doing likewise.

Although her parents returned to the United States on furlough every 5 years, they could spend only a few days with Frances because they had many church meetings to attend.

Frances's social behavior improved somewhat during high school in that she no longer offended her classmates. However, she made few friends. She adopted a stray dog to which she was greatly attached and with whom she spent most of her free time taking long walks. She showed a preference for mathematics and biblical history.

Frances entered the freshman year of college some 11 months before her admission to the hos-

pital. Although her grades in college were good, she had a reputation for being a strange girl who avoided others, smiled a great deal to herself, and showed no interest in the opposite sex. Her parents, while on furlough from Africa, visited her during the Christmas holidays, during which time her mother expressed fear that she was not emotionally well. Frances displayed little interest in her parents' visit, despite the fact that she had not seen them for over 5 years.

During the commencement activities that spring, Frances disappeared from the campus for several days; later it was learned that she had spent that time at an evangelical camp meeting. She remained on the campus during the summer months to take some advanced courses in mathematics. During this time she roomed with two other young women. Her roommates were in the habit of discussing their love interests in Frances's presence, and she suddenly displayed an unusual interest in their conversations. Among other things, she inquired about various matters of sex and how to approach boys. A few nights later she told one of the girls that she saw the face of her future husband in the light fixture. She scrutinized the fixture for several hours, during which she sat in a trancelike state with a smile on her face. Early the next morning she spoke to a 13-year-old newsboy and informed him that she would marry him. When he made light of her statement, she became upset, struck him in the face, and chased him down the street. Returning to her room, she tore out the light fixture, removed her clothing, and became unmanageable.

On being admitted to the psychiatric hospital, she refused to answer questions. She smiled to herself and identified the admitting physician as "Herbert." She insisted on having the window opened because "they are playing the wedding march." Her speech was incoherent; she was hal-

NURSING CARE PLAN—cont'd

lucinating and stated that she was hearing voices that questioned her moral standards.

For the first few days after hospitalization she talked a great deal about a fantasized courtship in which she was the central character. She carried on a dialogue, at one time representing the lover, at another time the maiden. After this she entered a long period of silence, during which she was mute, resistive, and refused food. Occasionally she said, "If thy eye offend thee, cut it out." One evening she almost succeeded in enucleating her right eye with the thumb and forefinger of her right hand. She continued to talk incoherently, laughed a great deal, and made little attempt to keep herself clean.

Nursing assessment

The history of Frances's life experiences gives us little information about her as a child. We do know that her father was perceived as an authoritarian individual who placed the welfare of the mission above all else. It is quite possible that even as an infant, Frances's care was relegated to employed native women who may not have remained in the household consistently. In the development of a sense of personal security, the first 5 years of a child's life are crucial. The type of mothering person by whom the child is nurtured is of the greatest importance, especially in developing a sense of trust.

At the age of 5 years Frances was sent to a boarding school. Although this was probably the best plan the parents could develop, it was apparently not helpful to the girl. Authorities believe that this period of time in a child's life is of great significance in the scheme of psychosexual development. During this period the child is beginning to identify with the parent of the same sex, has discovered that the sexual organ is a source of pleasurable sensations, and has recognized the structural difference between the genitalia of boys and girls. When a child in this age period is removed from the parents, he is apt to feel banished as a punishment for some

transgression. Since sexual longings and fantasies have occupied some of the child's thoughts and since the child realizes that these are frowned on by the parents, it is natural for the child to feel that the banishment is related to "bad" thoughts.

Frances undoubtedly felt banished by being sent to boarding school. Because of her father's strict and rigid attitudes, it is quite likely that Frances was convinced that she was being punished. Even when parents are not a source of comfort and security for a child, the child mourns their loss when separated from them because they are the only significant reality known. Thus it is reasonable to believe that Frances passed through a period of loneliness and bereavement at being deprived from the only mothering person she knew.

Initially, children protest this separation by crying or by other aggressive acting-out behavior. After several days of hopelessness and withdrawal from activity, the child usually becomes detached and seems unwilling to resume a close relationship with any adult, even if the lost person returns. This detached attitude could be altered if the parent returned and remained with the child consistently. However, Frances undoubtedly developed a detached attitude toward other people and attempted to isolate herself personally to avoid anxiety resulting from fear of being cast aside and abandoned a second time. Her subsequent attachment to a dog suggested that she could not trust another person with her love and therefore gave it to an animal who made no demands and gave her unconditional devotion.

After Frances had a serious illness at the age of 12, she began to spend long hours in prayer, wrote letters to her parents filled with quotes from the Bible, and wore her shoddiest clothing to school. This behavior suggests that she was seeking to gain the favor and forgiveness of herp parents, who in her fantasies may have been God's representatives on earth. Perhaps she felt

Continued.

NURSING CARE PLAN—cont'd

unworthy of anything better when she chose to wear old and shoddy clothing to school and again was seeking to atone for fantasized sin.

Her unusual interest in the sexual affairs of other girls of her age and the inappropriate proposal of marriage was a reactivation of the very early problem of failure to develop an integrated ego. This person developed a limited capacity to clearly evaluate the realities of the situation in which she found herself. In addition, her weak ego development made it difficult if not impossible to resolve the conflicts between the id drives (interest in sex and marriage) and demands of the superego (the incorporated standards of her parents). Likewise, she had never been able to effectively repress hostile aggressive drives and expressed these feelings freely by tearing out the light fixture.

When Frances saw the face of her future husband in the light fixture, she was exhibiting a severe mental symptom called visual hallucinations. Hallucinations are one example of the personality disintegration that takes place in individuals suffering from an active psychosis. Hallucinations, like all symptoms, meet a basic need. In this situation the face supplied an answer for her that was an outgrowth of her unconscious longing and her inability to find answers to her own sexual needs through adapting functionally to social situations.

Hallucinations are an example of being out of touch with reality. The person experiencing hallucinations is reacting to a stimulus from within the unconscious mind that is unrelated to the real situation. The behavior of such a person becomes extremely confusing when she reacts part of the time to stimuli from the real world and part of the time to stimuli from within her own unconscious mind.

Nursing diagnosis

The assessment data, including present behavior, past life experiences, and an understanding of the underlying dynamics, led to the development of the following three pairs of nursing diagnoses for Frances. The first of each pair is from the Classification of Human Responses of Concern for Psychiatric Mental Health Nursing Practice; the second is from the approved NANDA Diagnostic Categories.

5.7.2   Altered Social Interaction related to fear of abandonment

OR

3.1.1   Impaired Social Interaction related to fear of abandonment

6.4.2   Altered sensory perception related to hallucinations

OR

7.2   Sensory/Perceptual Alterations (Visual) related to hallucinations

1.3.4   Altered Self Care related to feelings of worthlessness

OR

6.5.1   Feeding Self Care Deficit related to feelings of worthlessness

6.5.2   Bathing/Hygiene Self Care Deficit related to feelings of worthlessness

6.5.3   Dressing/Grooming Self Care Deficit related to feelings of worthlessness

Planning and implementing nursing care

The boxed material on p. 224 is a sample nursing care plan designed for Frances. Because this client was so acutely ill on admission, all the objectives are short term.

The logical starting point in carrying out the plan was the establishment of a positive relationship with Frances. It was hoped that this relationship would lead to the development of some communication with her.

Because the nurse knew that persons with thought disturbances are highly fearful of rejection, the approach to Frances was unhurried, warm, friendly, and accepting. The nurse found it necessary to make repeated verbal overtures and to modify her own nonverbal messages to Frances before Frances was able to respond.

It was decided that the entire responsibility

NURSING CARE PLAN—cont'd

for the nursing care of Frances during the first weeks of her hospital experience would be assigned to a few carefully chosen nurses. This decision was made because the staff recognized that Frances needed to develop a feeling of security and to learn to trust other people. Security can be enhanced by limiting the number of individuals with whom such ill persons come in contact and by keeping their daily routines much the same for several months. In the beginning, few demands were made on Frances.

It is recognized that the attitude of the people with whom mentally ill persons come in contact during the early part of their illness has a significant effect on their recovery. Persons such as Frances require consistent acceptance, sincere interest, and constant encouragement from nurses and the other members of the professional staff.

Although communication with Frances was difficult because she used language in a highly personal way it was important for the nurse to spend time sitting with her and talking to her even though she rarely responded verbally. The nurse used simple, uncomplicated, direct statements when talking to her.

These nursing interventions were related to the plan for development of a satisfactory relationship with a significant other, which would in turn decrease Frances's fears of abandonment. In addition much of her behavior was symptomatic of an individual who felt unworthy and guilty, and it was obvious that Frances's self-esteem was badly shattered. Thus the nurse's efforts were focused on trying to assist Frances to develop a more positive attitude toward herself. This was partially achieved by the attention provided for her and the sincere, interested way in which it was given. Self-esteem was also enhanced through the mechanism of assisting her to improve her grooming.

Early in Frances's hospital experience it was necessary for a nurse to assume a good deal of responsibility for bathing and dressing her, but in time she was encouraged to assume more and

more responsibility for this activity herself. The nurses gently suggested that she would enjoy visiting the beauty parlor. At first they accompanied her on these trips and remained with her while she was there.

The dietary intake for persons who refuse food is always of great concern. Because Frances regressed when she was first admitted, the nurses tried to help her in feeding herself by making suggestions such as, "Pick up your fork" and "Put the food in your mouth." This plan was used because it was thought that she was unable to make the necessary decisions herself. However, it was eventually necessary to spoon-feed her. The nurses used an unhurried, relaxed manner and fed her from a tray in her own room.

During the spoon-feeding periods the nurses gave Frances many opportunities to take the spoon in her own hand and assume some of the responsibility for feeding herself during a part of the meal. After a few weeks she was encouraged to return to the dining room and take her meals with others.

The problem of self-destruction was especially distressing. Criticism and reprimands for this behavior were withheld because the nurses realized that it would confirm her opinion that she was indeed a bad person. The close personal attention Frances received when she was first admitted solved the problem of self-destruction during the early part of her hospitalization. However, she was helped to reestablish her own inner controls, and the nurse served as an external authority, until Frances was able to accept responsibility for her own safety.

Evaluation

Evaluation of the plan of nursing care and its implementation was based on outcome criteria established at the time the plan was formulated. Since the nurse knew that Frances's illness had developed slowly and insidiously, the outcome criteria she established reflected the expectation of small but significant gains. The nurse continu-

Continued.

NURSING CARE PLAN—cont'd

ously reassessed the client as she provided care. As anticipated, after 2 weeks Frances was able to accept most of the responsibility for her own grooming and ate in the dining room with the other clients. In addition, days elapsed without any evidence of hallucinations and her self-destructive behavior had stopped.

After 1 month Frances showed little evidence of accepting her assigned nurse as a significant other. Although she did call the nurse by name and seemed to recognize her at most times, she rarely appeared for their meetings at the agreed-upon time. Frances's nurse was discouraged about this and arranged to have the nursing care plan reviewed at a team meeting. In view of this client's history with significant others and her progress in other areas, the team felt that the

nurse's outcome criteria for this diagnosis were unrealistic in terms of time. As a result, the nurse revised this aspect of the care plan to indicate a 6-week time frame.

After 6 weeks, Frances's behavior did indicate a beginning level of trust in her assigned nurse. At that time the nurse reassessed the client's condition, developed revised nursing diagnoses, and designed a new plan of care that indicated long-term goals. She was careful to develop outcome criteria that were realistic in light of Frances's lifetime of dysfunctional adaptation. It was anticipated that Frances could be expected to recover sufficiently to be discharged to a sheltered living situation but it was likely she would require a maintenance dose of the prescribed antipsychotic medication.

NURSING CARE PLAN FOR *Frances B.*

Nursing diagnosis	Objective	Nursing actions	Outcome criteria

5.7.2 Altered Social Interaction related to fear of abandonment
OR
3.1.1 Impaired Social Interaction related to fear of abandonment
	To assist the client to develop a sense of trust in another human being	Assigned nurse establishes relationship with client
		  Approach client in a calm, friendly manner
		  Orient client to purpose and structure of relationship
		  Determine times and places for meeting 3 times a day for 20 minutes
		Convey consistent acceptance of client as an individual who has value and worth
		Use simple, direct statements when talking with client
			Within 1 month client will:
			  Call nurse by name
			  Show evidence of beginning trust in assigned nurse by appearing for meetings on time

NURSING CARE PLAN—cont'd

		Sit silently with client if she is hallucinating	
6.4.2 Altered sensory perception related to hallucinations OR 7.2 Sensory/Perceptual Alterations (Visual) related to hallucinations	To diminish frequency of hallucinations	Administer antipsychotic medication as prescribed Observe for side effects and adverse reactions to medications Reassure client about side effects Record medications given Observe for and record changes in behavior indicative of hallucinations	Within 2 weeks client will manifest behavior indicative of hallucinations only when exposed to numerous external stimuli, such as 2 persons talking to her at the same time
	To protect client from self-destructive acts	Restrain client as necessary Do *not* reprimand client if she attempts to injure self	Within 2 weeks client will not attempt to injure self
1.3.4 Altered Self Care related to feelings of worthlessness OR 6.5.1 Feeding Self Care Deficit related to feelings of worthlessness	To assist client to assume responsibility for bathing and dressing appropriately	Establish and implement routine for bathing and dressing Bathe client as necessary Dress client as necessary Encourage client to assist with bathing and dressing	Within 2 weeks client will show interest in activities of bathing and dressing as manifested by such statements as "I'll wash my own face."
6.5.2 Bathing/Hygiene Self Care Deficit related to feelings of worthlessness 6.5.3 Dressing/Grooming Self Care Deficit related to feelings of worthlessness	To provide adequate nutrition	Ascertain and serve, if possible, client's favorite foods Present food in small amounts Help client eat by providing simple directions Spoon feed if necessary Allow client to eat at her own pace Record amount eaten Encourage client to go to dining room, accompany if she indicates desire to go	Within 2 weeks client will eat 1800 calories among three well-balanced meals in the dining room

Other physical problems may result from the medications the client may receive. It is imperative that the nurse know which medications, if any, the client is taking and plan to purposefully observe for any adverse effects.

END NOTE

This focus of this chapter is the nursing care of individuals with thought disorders. As a means of understanding the needs of these clients, the positive and negative symptoms of schizophrenia and the behaviors these clients are likely to exhibit are discussed. A case formulation from which a hypothetical nursing care plan is derived, implemented, and evaluated is presented.

SUGGESTED SOURCES OF ADDITIONAL INFORMATION

Arieti S: Understanding and helping the schizophrenic, New York, 1980, Basic Books, Inc.

Baker AF: How families cope: living with a chronically ill schizophrenic can place great stress on individual family members and the family unit, J Psychosoc Nurs Mental Health Serv 27(1):31-36, January 1989.

Bellack A and Mueser K: A comprehensive treatment program for schizophrenia and chronic mental illness, Commun Ment Health J 22:175, Fall 1986.

Chamberlain J: Everyman's psychosis, Perspect Psychiatr Care 21:59, April-June 1983.

del Campo EJH, Carr C, and Correa E: Rehospitalized schizophrenics, J Psychosoc Nurs Ment Health Serv 21:29, June 1983.

Drake R and Sederer L: Inpatient psychosocial treatment of chronic schizophrenia: negative effects and current guidelines, Hosp Commun Psychiatr 37:897, September 1986.

Gerace L: Schizophrenia and the family: nursing implications, Arch Psychiatr Nurs 2:141, June 1988.

Kahn EM: Psychotherapy with chronic schizophrenics, J Psychosoc Nurs Ment Health Serv 22:20, July 1984.

Koontz E: Schizophrenia: current diagnostic concepts and implications for nursing care, J Psychosoc Nurs Ment Health Serv 20:44, September 1982.

McGill C, Falloon I, Boyd J, and Wood-Silverio C: Family educational intervention in the treatment of schizophrenia, Hosp Commun Psychiatr 34:934, 1983.

Middlemiss MA and Beeber LS: Update on psychopharmacology: issues in the use of depot antipsychotics, J Psychosoc Nurs Mental Health Serv 27(6):36-37, June 1989.

Plante TG: Social skills training: a program to help schizophrenic clients cope, J Psychosoc Nurs Mental Health Serv 27(3):6-10, March 1989.

Pope H: Distinguishing bipolar disorder from schizophrenia in clinical practice: guidelines and case reports, Hosp Commun Psychiatr 34:322, 1983.

Rosenthal T and McGuiness T: Dealing with delusional patients: discovering the distorted truth, Issues Ment Health Nurs 8:143, February 1986.

Sarbin T and Mancuso J: Schizophrenia, medical diagnosis or moral verdict? New York, 1980, Pergamon Press, Inc.

Schmidt C: Withdrawal behavior of schizophrenics; application of Roy's model, J Psychosoc Nurs Ment Health Serv 19:26, November 1981.

Seymour R and Dawson N: The schizophrenic at home, J Psychosoc Nurs Ment Health Serv 26:28, January 1986.

Sulliger N: Relapse, J Psychosoc Nurs Ment Health Serv 26:20, June 1988.

Individuals with mood disorders

16

LEARNING OBJECTIVES

After studying this chapter the student will be able to:

o Describe the symptoms exhibited by a person with the medical diagnosis of a mood disorder.

o Differentiate between the emotion of grief and the mood of depression.

o Discuss the causative factors associated with mood disorders.

o State the desired effects, side effects, and adverse effects of antidepressant medications, lithium carbonate, and electroconvulsive therapy.

o Describe behaviors the nurse is most likely to observe in an individual experiencing depression.

o State examples of nursing diagnoses likely to be applicable to an individual who is depressed.

o Develop a hypothetical plan of nursing care for an individual who is depressed.

o Describe those behaviors the nurse is most likely to observe in an individual who is elated and overactive.

o State examples of nursing diagnoses likely to be applicable to an individual who is elated and overactive.

o Develop a hypothetical plan of nursing care for an individual who is elated and overactive.

All human beings are familiar with the emotions of joy and sadness. Healthy adults experience these emotions in a predictable way, usually in response to an external stimulus. For example, graduating from college or achieving a promotion may cause great joy, while the death of a parent may precipitate sadness. These emotions are experienced by healthy adults to an extent and for a length of time appropriate to the situation. In contrast, individuals who suffer from mood disorders experience a great depth of joy or sadness, seemingly unrelated to external stimuli, and for a long period. Furthermore, these emotions pervade the person's entire being and may fluctuate widely from one to another.

There is great national concern about the increasing number of adults who experience mood disorders. Of particular concern is the incidence of depression, which has been accelerating rapidly since the 1970s and shows no sign of abating. A recent study by the National Institute of Mental Health indicates that 6 percent of the population of the United States suffers from depression during any 6-month period. Middle-aged females and the elderly of both sexes are particularly vulnerable to severe depression.

Mood disorders seriously interfere with the quality of life enjoyed by the affected person and his family. In addition, depression increases the risk of death by suicide. Nurses in all settings have a responsibility to recognize and appropriately intervene in situations where the individual is experiencing a mood disorder.

HISTORICAL PERSPECTIVE

Mood disorders, especially depression, have been documented since ancient times. An Egyptian papyrus of 1500 BC contains a discourse on old age and says of it that "the heart grows heavy and remembers not yesterday." The Old Testament records the erratic behavior of King Saul as his moods fluctuated between elation and depression. If he were alive today, this influential person would undoubtedly bear the medical diagnosis of bipolar disorder.

In 1896 Emil Kraepelin identified the illness known today as bipolar disorder and called it manic-depressive psychosis. He was among the first to recognize the cyclical nature of this disorder.

Hippocrates (460-375? BC), the greatest of the old Greek physicians, knew the symptoms of depression well and believed it resulted from a surplus of black bile, which is termed *melancholē* in the Greek language. The English word *melancholy* is derived from this Greek word.

Treatment of mood disorders was not effective until the development of the convulsion-producing drug pentylenetetrazol (Metrazol) by Meduna followed by the introduction of electroconvulsive therapy by Cerletti and Bini in 1938. Electroconvulsive therapy was first developed as a treatment for persons with thought disorders; however, it has been found to be most effective for persons suffering from depression. Although still in use today, electroconvulsive therapy has been supplanted as a treatment for mood disorders by the psychotropic agents, specifically the antidepressant medications and lithium carbonate.

MOOD DISORDERS

Mood disorders are subdivided into the medical diagnoses of depressive disorders and bipolar disorders.

Individuals medically diagnosed as having a depressive disorder experience an all-pervasive depressed mood or loss of interest or pleasure in all, or almost all, activities for at least a 2-week duration. Associated symptoms include appetite disturbance, resultant change in weight, sleep disturbance, psychomotor agitation or retardation, decreased energy, feelings of worthlessness and guilt, difficulty thinking or concentrating, and recurrent thoughts of death.

To be medically diagnosed as having a bipolar disorder, the individual must have a history of one or more manic episodes, usually with a history of episodes of major depression. During manic episodes, the elated mood may be so pronounced and sustained that the individual expresses the belief that every good thing is possible or will soon be consummated and every wish will be fulfilled. Ideas emerge in an easy, fluid manner; thinking seems to be effortless; memory is quickened; and the individual shows a quick but superficial wit. There is an apparent sense of self-security, and fears are pushed to the background. The individual may be aggressive, cocksure in his opinions, and ready to talk with conviction on anything and everything. The ego seems to be unrestrained, and ideas pour out so rapidly and with such ease that the tongue cannot give them full expression. Hence the individual may utter only segments of ideas and may jump from one to another in a rapid barrage. He recognizes persons and objects quickly and has a tendency to argue. The person is apt to be domineering and becomes irritable, denunciatory, and hypercritical of everything that interferes with his desire for free action. He is likely to become overactive and may extend this excessive motor excitement in every direction. When limits must be set for his behavior, he sometimes becomes noisy, belligerent, and violent. His insight is always poor. This person's interest is in the outside world rather than in himself. His ideation is concerned with his environment. In fact, the individual can almost be said to be at the mercy of his environment.

Surprising as it may seem, at another time such an aggressive, overactive individual may exhibit quite different behavior. Within a few months he may be sad, may have difficulty in thinking and expressing thoughts, and may be very slow in his physical responses, or he may exhibit agitation. Such a person may have difficulty in formulating answers, may lose his ability to concentrate, and may be unable to choose a direct line of action. The individual may be tormented by a sense of insecurity or by ideas of remorse and self-abasement or may be overcome by a sense of guilt. He may complain of a total lack of affection and of a loss of interest in the things for which he formerly had much concern. He may feel that he is lost or being punished. Such a person may have an overpowering sense of futility, a "feeling of emptiness," and a desire to retreat from everything, to seek oblivion, and to end his life. The danger of suicide is

Depressive disorders and bipolar disorder are the two types of mood disorders.

the outstanding feature of this condition, and this alone justifies the greatest caution and consideration in care and treatment.

The probability of recovery from a single episode of overactivity or depression is great. Recurrences are to be expected, although second and third attacks need not necessarily occur. An attack of overactivity in early adult life generally means more attacks later. Depressions are most likely to occur in the later years of life.

It is never safe to predict the probable duration of any given attack. There are great variations, and even the same individual may have both short and long periods of elation and depression. The average length for all untreated attacks of elation is about 6 months; for untreated depressive episodes it is generally longer. When depressive periods show a strong element of fear, anxiety, and hypochondriasis, the condition may endure for many years. Likewise, elation may become chronic, particularly in older individuals, if it is associated with organic changes in the brain such as arteriosclerosis. Current treatments, including maintenance levels of lithium carbonate as a preventive measure, have shortened the length of attacks in both elation and depression.

An outstanding feature of mood disorders is that even after repeated attacks intellectual capacities are rarely impaired. During remissions of this disorder the individual is usually able to carry on his regular occupation and live an entirely normal life.

Although a bipolar disorder is a common type of mood disorder, some individuals suffer from severe mood disturbances that do not meet the criteria for this diagnosis. However, the principles stated in the following discussion are applicable to all individuals with mood disturbances, regardless of their medical diagnosis.

DIFFERENTIATION BETWEEN THOUGHT DISORDERS AND MOOD DISORDERS

It is sometimes difficult for students of nursing to differentiate between the overactivity demonstrated by some individuals with thought disorders and the overactivity that the manic individual exhibits. Both of these individuals may be physically overactive, and at times both may talk excessively. The individual who exhibits catatonic behavior may fluctuate from being almost stuporous to exhibiting explosive overactivity. In such a situation the individual is probably responding to inner thoughts and feelings that are not related to reality but that are threatening, upsetting, and disturbing. This type of overactivity is especially difficult to understand because there is often disharmony between the mood and the ideas expressed. The person may smile inappropriately or laugh while speaking of the disturbing thoughts that are uppermost in his mind. He may experience terrifying visual or auditory hallucinations.

In contrast, the overactivity of an individual displaying manic behavior is characterized by glib argumentative speech that may be humorous but may change quickly to sarcasm and verbal abuse. Such a person may appear to have boundless energy. He is usually irrepressible, demanding, and irritable. He frequently expresses ideas of grandeur and delusions of having great power and wealth. There is a dominant tone of euphoria even though the person may demonstrate an underlying mood of sorrow. Some authorities believe that the overactivity of the manic individual is actually a defense against depression. The professional person usually finds that manic overactivity can be understood because the client maintains some contact with reality except in the most extreme examples of this illness.

Withdrawal and depression may be difficult for the beginning student of nursing to differentiate because individuals suffering from these states are usually physically inactive. However, the individual with a thought disturbance who is withdrawn demonstrates a disharmony of thought, feeling, and behavior. Although there may be a persistent mood, it has little apparent relationship to the situation in which the person finds himself or to his past experiences. In contrast, everything about the depressed individual conveys this feeling to the observer. The way the person sits, the facial expression, the voice quality, and the ideas expressed all suggest hopelessness and a sense of impending doom. Depressed individuals remain well aware of reality, and their feelings seem understandable to individuals working with them.

> Individuals with thought disorders and those with mood disorders display some of the same characteristics but with subtle differences that the experienced nurse can detect.

Some authorities believe that the attempt to differentiate these behavioral reactions is actually an artificial and unwarranted exercise. These authorities suggest that such reactions may be aspects of one broad disease entity.

DIFFERENTIATION BETWEEN GRIEF AND DEPRESSION

Although grief is a human condition characterized by a disturbance in mood, it is a normal, common, necessary reaction to the loss of a highly valued individual or object. The nurse may help the grieving person to cope with his sense of loss and guilt by encouraging him to talk about his feelings. The goal is to assist the individual to integrate this emotional reaction with similar experiences in his past and to learn from it.

Depression is a profound disturbance in mood that shares some characteristics with grief; however, it differs in many ways. Depression is not as common an expression as grief, but it occurs frequently. All nurses should be able to differentiate between the normal reaction called grieving and the pathological elaboration of grief, which is called depression. The nurse needs to recognize that normal grieving should be encouraged and that it usually terminates within a few months or a year without professional help. In contrast, depression is not self-limiting, usually does not improve without professional help, and is dangerous for the individual because of the potential for suicide.

The following listing contrasts grief and depression in terms of cause, symptoms, and outcome.

Grief (bereavement)

1. Grief is a disturbance in mood that is normal, universal, and necessary in the life experience of an individual.

2. Grief is a reaction to the *real* loss of a highly valued object that may be tangible or intangible.

3. Grief is self-limiting and gradually diminishes over a period of about a year, except in the elderly, where 2 years may be necessary. Except in the early, acute stage, grief is not incapacitating.

4. The three phases of normal grieving are:
   a. Shock and disbelief
   b. Developing awareness of the pain of the loss, which eventually results in crying
   c. Restitution, which involves the mourning experience and eventual elevation of the memory of the lost object to a degree of perfection. New objects replace the lost one at the end of this phase.

Depression

1. Depression is a disturbance in mood that is a pathological elaboration of grief. It is related to grief but is not the same.

2. Depression is a reaction to the actual, threatened, or imagined loss of a valued object, tangible or intangible. It is an overwhelming response to what the individual considers a catastrophic loss.

3. Depression is not self-limiting and goes beyond grief in duration and intensity. Depression is prolonged, severe, and increasingly incapacitating in all areas of the individual's life.

4. Depression does not enter the phase of restitution within a few weeks or months. Professional help is often required.

CAUSATIVE FACTORS OF MOOD DISORDERS

Mood deviations extreme enough to be categorized as either mania or depression have no specific causative factors that can be identified with scientific certainty. However, many scientists believe that heredity is a factor because 60% to 80% of these individuals come from families in which a history of this illness exists. Furthermore, recent biomedical research has indicated that neuroendocrine abnormalities, particularly involving the neurotransmitters of norepinephrine, serotonin, and dopamine, are associated with extreme mood deviations. For example, Seasonal affective disorder (SAD) is a form of depression that is characterized by depression that occurs annually at the same time each year. A major study of this disorder at the National Institutes of Health indicates that individuals who suffer from this "seasonal" disorder are responding biochemically to the lack of natural light during the winter months.

Psychoanalytically oriented theorists believe that extreme mood disturbances are closely related to the infant's early feeding experiences. During this period the mother who provides food and attention is both an object of love and a source of frustration for the infant. Ambivalent feelings of both love and hate for the mothering person may exist in this early period and may be carried out throughout life. In adult life ambivalent feelings are directed toward the environment and the significant persons in the environment. Individuals who develop extreme mood disturbances such as elation and depression are thought to be reacting to the unconscious loss of a real or fantasied love object that was incorporated at an early phase of personality development. The individual first responds as if mourning for the lost love object and eventually begins to express hostility because he feels abandoned. The aggressive, overactivity of mania is thought to be a defense against the real problem of depression.

In depression the individual is thought to turn his hostility toward himself. He feels that he is at fault, that he is responsible for the loss of the love object, and that he is unworthy; thus he hates himself. He is said to be at the mercy of a punishing, sadistic superego. Such an individual has many narcissistic love needs. His adult relationships are likely to be immature and dependent. The lifelong problems with which these individuals struggle are hostility and the feelings of guilt that the hostility precipitates when their security is threatened.

> Elated, overactive individuals are believed to be venting their hostility on their environment, whereas depressed individuals have turned their hostility on themselves.

ANTIDEPRESSANT MEDICATIONS

A major category of psychotropic medications is the antidepressants, which act to lift the depression of many individuals. In fact statistics show that about 70% of the depressed individuals treated with these drugs improve markedly. Unfortunately, when drugs from this category are given, there is a delay of several weeks in the therapeutic effect. This fact suggests that suicidal individuals are best hospitalized during this period, not only for their protection but also to allow the professional staff to assess the onset of the drug's effect, which clients often do not report because of their depression.

The antidepressants fall into two main chemical structures: the tricyclic antidepressants and the monoamine oxidase (MAO) inhibitors. Table 16-1 gives the generic name, trade name, range of daily oral dosage in milligrams, and comments about the specific uses for some of the most commonly used antidepressants.

Side effects of antidepressants

Dryness of the mouth is experienced by all who take any one of the antidepressants. Other side effects that may be experienced by many who take one of the antidepressants include difficulties in visual accommodation, perspiration about the head and neck, and postural hypotension that often leads to injuries. A mild degree of urinary retention or constipation may also occur. These drugs aggravate glaucoma. In addition, MAO inhibitors may also produce a variety of central nervous system symptoms that may include tremor of the upper extremities, convulsions, twitching, and ataxia. If such symptoms appear, they can be easily controlled by decreasing the dosage.

TABLE 16-1   *Antidepressant medications*

Generic name	Trade name	Range of daily oral dosage (mg)	Comments
TRICYCLIC ANTIDEPRESSANTS			
Imipramine	Tofranil	75-300	Most effective when used for depression in which there is psychomotor retardation. Helpful in severe anxiety attacks and enuresis in children.
Amitriptyline	Elavil	75-150	Hypnotic effect useful when depressed individuals have severe sleep disturbance.
Desipramine	Pertofrane, Norpramin	75-200	More quickly effective therapeutically than imipramine or amitriptyline.
Nortriptyline	Aventyl, Pamelor	75-150	
Doxepin	Sinequan, Adapin	75-300	Has antianxiety effect.
MONOAMINE OXIDASE INHIBITORS			
Isocarboxazid	Marplan	30-60	Monoamine oxidase inhibitors potentiate effects of many other drugs, including sedative, hypnotic actions of alcohol and barbiturates. When cautiously administered with appropriate dietary restrictions and careful observation of blood pressure, their therapeutic effect may outweigh their danger in individuals who have not responded to an adequate trial of tricyclic antidepressants.
Phenelzine sulfate	Nardil	45-90	
Tranylcypromine	Parnate	20-30	

Adverse effects of antidepressants

Adverse effects of the tricyclic antidepressants include exacerbation of the psychosis and cardiac arrhythmias. The most serious and potentially lethal adverse effect of the MAO inhibitors is a *hypertensive crisis*. Monoamine oxidase is essential in the metabolism of tyramine, a substance contained in many commonly eaten foods that exerts a pressor effect. When a client is taking an MAO inhibitor, particularly tranylcypromine (Parnate), and eats a food containing tyramine, the tyramine cannot be metabolized, and this can cause a hypertensive crisis. This syndrome is often referred to as the *Parnate-cheese reaction*. Foods containing tyramine that must be avoided include aged cheese, whiskey, beer, cream, chocolate, canned figs, coffee, licorice, Chianti and sherry wines, live yeast or yeast extracts such as yogurt, fava beans, soy sauce, pickled herring, pickles, chicken liver, sauerkraut, smoked salmon, snails, and raisins. These dietary restrictions should be maintained for at least 2 weeks after the medication is discontinued to allow for its complete resynthesis.

MAO inhibitors potentiate epinephrine, so clients who are taking these drugs must be warned to avoid other drugs containing ephedrine because this combination may cause extreme hypertension. Examples of commonly used over-the-counter medications that must not be taken include many cold remedies and antihistamines.

Finally, MAO inhibitors should not be administered with the tricyclic antidepressants. If a client's medication is changed from one category of antidepressant to another, a lag period of at least 2 weeks should elapse to avoid an adverse synergistic effect.

LITHIUM

Another widely used psychotropic drug is lithium. This drug is now recognized as effective in the treatment of mania and in preventing the recurrence of bipolar disorder when given on a maintenance basis. About three-fourths of the individuals who have a definite diagnosis of bipolar disorder improve remarkably when treatment with lithium is properly carried out. The optimum dose of lithium is based on both the clinical response and the serum lithium level. The usual dose for a patient in an acute manic state is 600 mg T.I.D. The desired serum lithium level is between 1.0 and 1.5 mEq/L. Maintenance doses are usually 900 to 1200 mg daily. The desired maintenance serum lithium level is between 0.6 and 1.2 mEq/L.

Lithium does not impair intellectual activity, consciousness, or range or quality of emotional life. However, the toxic levels of lithium are close to the therapeutic levels. Adverse effects of lithium, or lithium toxicity, can be monitored by measuring serum lithium levels. Thus facilities for prompt and accurate serum lithium level determinations should be readily available to the client. Clinical symptoms of an adverse reaction to lithium include nausea, abdominal cramps, vomiting, diarrhea, thirst, and polyuria. These symptoms can occur at lithium levels below 2 mEq/L. If the drug dosage is not reduced at the first sign of toxicity, serious central nervous system and cardiovascular system damage may ensue. Recent studies have shown that prolonged use of lithium even without symptoms of adverse reactions may lead to renal tubule damage, cardiac toxicity, and thyroid imbalance. Therefore, despite its effectiveness, lithium is prescribed cautiously and is unlikely to fulfill its promise of curing bipolar disorder.

ELECTROCONVULSIVE THERAPY

Electroconvulsive therapy (ECT) is sometimes prescribed for depressed persons who have not improved after an adequate trial of antidepressant medications and whose depression manifests itself in agitated behavior. It is also used for individuals who are actively suicidal and for whom no other intervention has been effective. Although very little is known about how ECT achieves its results, it seems to break through the psychotic process and make the individual more accessible to interpersonal interventions.

Electroconvulsive therapy breaks through the psychotic process and makes the individual more accessible to interpersonal interventions.

ECT is a fairly simple procedure to administer. It consists of applying controlled electric current to the individual's frontal lobes through electrodes placed on his temples. Since unconsciousness results, the client is prepared for this procedure in the same manner as a patient would be prepared for surgery.

After five or six treatments, clients frequently complain of confusion and loss of memory, particularly for recent events. This situation puzzles and perplexes the individual. He may fear that his memory will not return. Relatives are likely to express concern about this development unless the treatment has been carefully explained to them before it was undertaken. They should be prepared to expect such developments and to understand that the symptoms will clear up completely after the series of treatments has been concluded. They should be reassured that there will be no permanent untoward after effects from the treatments.

The number of treatments a client receives is largely dependent on his clinical response. ECT is often administered on an outpatient basis, especially if the client is not actively suicidal and has sufficient supervision in the community.

NURSING CARE OF INDIVIDUALS WHO ARE DEPRESSED
Nursing assessment

The following discussion is organized around the human processes introduced in Chapter 9. Although behaviors in each category are presented as separate entities, it should be understood that they are highly interrelated and are adaptations to similar stressors. Further, in many instances behavior designed as an adaptation to one stressor becomes a stressor itself in another dimension. Therefore, nursing care directed at altering one behavior will inevitably have an effect on others.

Activity processes. The depressed individual may exhibit psychomotor retardation where every word and action takes monumental effort. On the other hand, this individual may display agitation, often pacing the floor and wringing the hands. When agitation is present, it usually indicates anxiety as well as depression.

The appearance of persons who are depressed is almost always unkempt, and they often have not bathed recently, since they lack the energy required for bathing and grooming. Furthermore, their unattractive appearance is congruent with their mood.

Regardless of the severity of the depression, the individual will almost always report changes in sleep patterns. Less severely depressed persons find they sleep for longer intervals and more frequently than usual. More severely depressed persons report they have little difficulty falling asleep but awaken in the early hours of the morning, usually between 3 and 4 AM. At that time their feelings of loneliness, overwhelming anxiety, and worthlessness are most pronounced. Time seems to move very slowly, and they believe daylight will never come. Repeated episodes of early morning wakefulness may make them fearful of going to sleep in the evening. No matter how much sleep the depressed individual has had, he complains of constant fatigue. The simplest task often seems insurmountable, requiring more mental and physical energy than the person possesses.

Cognition processes. Most individuals who are depressed maintain contact with reality but view themselves and the world around them in the most pessimistic light. This symptom is more reflective of a disturbance in emotional processes than in cognition processes. However, severely depressed individuals experience difficulty in concentration and sometimes suffer from self-accusatory delusions. For example, the client may believe he is responsible for a natural disaster such as an earthquake, since he views the earthquake as evidence that God is trying to swallow him up. In such instances, the client is experiencing a disturbance in cognition processes.

Ecological processes. Just as the depressed individual's self-care suffers, so does his ability to care for his environment. Even the most basic activities associated with cleaning, washing dishes and clothes, and caring for pets and plants go unattended. The result of this lack of attention is often a dirty, cluttered environment, which, in turn, acts as a further stressor. One community mental health nurse reported making a home visit to a depressed client because he had failed to keep several clinic appointments. The nurse found the client sitting in his living room among a number of houseplants that were dead due to lack of water. The client's environment reflected his depressed mood to such an extent that the nurse had difficulty in not feeling sad herself.

Emotional processes. The individual suffering from depression expresses despair, gloom, a sense of foreboding, and feelings of guilt, sadness, and shame. These feelings are so overwhelming that the nurse can sense them even before the person describes them.

Needless to say, depressed persons report that they find no pleasure in any activity, even those they had previously enjoyed.

While laypeople often associate crying with depression, this expression of anguish may not be present in severely depressed individuals. Sometimes these persons may sob, but tearlessly. At other times, they may not cry, but their faces wear tortured expressions.

Interpersonal processes. Although not every depressed individual harbors suicidal thoughts, almost every person who attempts suicide is depressed. Consequently, every depressed client should be considered as potentially suicidal unless there is reason to believe otherwise.

Some authorities believe that all individuals who contemplate suicide give clues of their intention. Common clues include a dramatic change in behavior, giving away treasured possessions, or actually talking about their intentions. The common belief that a person who talks about suicide never attempts it is a fallacy. People usually talk about the thoughts that are uppermost in their minds. An individual alludes to suicide because he is thinking about it. The person who makes statements about life not being worth living, who suggests that he may not be around much longer, or who has actually injured himself should be considered at risk for suicide.

A person who is depressed is at the greatest risk for suicide after his depression has begun to lift. Suicide attempts at this time are common because the individual has sufficient mental and physical energy to plan and implement a self-destructive act while still being sufficiently depressed to desire death.

Another common fallacy about suicide is that questioning the depressed individual about the presence of suicidal thoughts will give him the idea that this might be a solution to his problems. Nothing could be further from the truth. If the individual were so responsive to suggestion, it would be a relatively easy matter to suggest that life is worth living. The nurse should never hesitate to ask a depressed person if he is contemplating suicide, especially if his behavior raises that suspicion in her mind.

Perception processes. Low self-esteem is a predominant characteristic of individuals who are depressed. These feelings of worthlessness are likely to be of long standing but become more severe and prominent when the individual becomes ill. As a result, the depressed individual attends to situations and reactions of others that reinforce this belief and ignores or rationalizes those which indicate he has value.

Physiological processes. Depressed individuals who are inactive are prone to develop physical disorders because of their inactivity. The most common of these are fecal impaction, peripheral edema, and pneumonia. Infections are frequent, but the depressed person tends to ignore the symptoms of these illnesses although he almost always reports a variety of physical complaints. These complaints generally include headaches, gastrointestinal problems such as "fullness" and constipation, and chest pains. These complaints prompt many depressed individuals to visit the doctor's office.

A marked change in weight over a relatively short period of time is often associated with the client's physical complaints. Some less severely depressed persons turn to food and alcoholic beverages as a coping mechanism and thus gain large amounts of weight. Although eating and drinking may provide temporary solace, the resultant overweight becomes an additional stressor, further convincing the person of his worthlessness. Severely depressed individuals are more likely to lack appetite, as well as lacking the energy to buy and prepare food. Thus it is not unusual for them to lose a large amount of weight rapidly. They may not be aware of the amount of weight loss, but the observant nurse will make note of ill-fitting clothes.

Valuation processes. The depressed individual almost always feels helpless, hopeless, and powerless to change the situation. Expressions of these feelings include statements such as, "I feel worthless, rotten, no good," "Life is a struggle," or "I don't deserve to be taken care of, I'm just a burden to everyone."

Nursing diagnosis

As with all nursing diagnoses, the nursing diagnoses for the individual who is depressed are based on the themes identified during the assessment phase of the nursing process. Categories of human responses from the ANA Classification of

Assessment of the individual who is depressed reveals psychomotor retardation, pessimism, lack of care for the environment, despair, suicidal thoughts, low self-esteem, physical disorders, and feelings of helplessness and hopelessness.

Human Responses of Concern for Psychiatric–Mental Health Nursing Practice that may be specifically applicable to individuals who are depressed include the following:

1.1.2   Altered Motor Behavior
1.3.4   Altered Self-Care
1.4.2   Altered Sleep/Arousal Patterns
3.3.2   Altered Home Maintenance
4.1.2   Altered Feeling State
5.3.2   Altered Conduct/Impulse Processes
6.3.2   Altered Self-Concept
7.1.1   Potential for Alteration in Circulation
7.2.1   Potential for Alteration in Elimination Processes
7.4.1   Potential for Alteration in Gastrointestinal Processes
7.7.1   Potential for Alteration in Nutrition
8.1.2   Altered Meaningfulness

NANDA nursing diagnostic categories that may be specifically applicable to the individual who is depressed include:

1.1.2.2   Altered Nutrition: Less than body requirements
1.2.1.1   Potential for Infection
1.3.1.1   Constipation
5.1.1.1   Ineffective Individual Coping
6.1.1.2   Activity Intolerance
6.2.1   Sleep Pattern Disturbance
6.4.1.1   Impaired Home Maintenance Management
6.5.2   Bathing/Hygiene Self-Care Deficit
6.5.3   Dressing/Grooming Self-Care Deficit
7.1.2   Self-Esteem Disturbance
7.3.1   Hopelessness
7.3.2   Powerlessness
9.2.1.1   Dysfunctional Grieving
9.2.2   Potential for Violence: Self-directed

To develop a nursing diagnosis that fulfills its function of providing direction for planning nursing care, the nurse is encouraged to postulate and state etiologic or antecedent factors for each human response and connect the two phrases by using the term "related to." For example:

1.1.2   Altered motor behavior related to lack of energy

Planning and implementing nursing care

The plan for nursing care is derived from the nursing diagnoses and includes the objectives of the care, the nursing actions, and outcome criteria. To be effective the plan needs to be highly individualized. The suggestions that follow should be seen as general guidelines to be used if they are appropriate to the client's needs.

Increasing the individual's self-esteem is the central objective of all nursing care for the individual who is depressed.

Because of their lack of energy, clients who are depressed often need assistance in all aspects of daily living.

In general, the objectives of all nursing care for the individual who is depressed should relate to helping him to increase his self-esteem.

Since the client's nursing diagnoses are often interrelated, stemming as they do from similar etiologies or antecedents, the student will see that the appropriate nursing actions are also interrelated. In other words, by intervening in one dimension, the nurse will also affect other dimensions.

Activity processes. Clients who are depressed often have one or more nursing diagnoses in the category of activity processes. Because of their lack of energy they often need assistance in all aspects of daily living. Perhaps the most effective way of caring for a depressed person is to establish with him a simple daily schedule that provides for bathing, grooming, eating, and physical activity. Much encouragement and reassurance throughout each day will be required to help him follow the schedule.

Patience is the keynote in working with depressed individuals who are so greatly retarded in the spheres of thinking, feeling, and acting that every movement or word requires great effort and much time. The same question often needs to be asked more than once, and the nurse must wait patiently for the answer. A large part of the therapeutic value of the hospital situation lies in the fact that decisions can be made for the individual. Thus the nurse should avoid asking such questions as, "Do you want to take your bath now?" A more positive approach would be, "Your bath is ready now. I will help you with it."

Encouraging depressed individuals to take pride in their personal appearance is part of their care. This is difficult to achieve because it is in opposition to their tendency toward self-depreciation. Careful supervision of personal hygiene with attention to supplying clean clothing and helping them dress neatly is important in developing pride in personal appearance. Women need to be encouraged to accept appointments at the beauty parlor and men to go to the barbershop regularly. If a depressed individual is hospitalized because he is actively suicidal, it may be safer to ask the barber or beauty operator to come to the unit where the person is hospitalized rather than to send him to the operator.

Many depressed individuals present a difficult feeding problem. It is helpful if the nurse can discover why food is being refused. It is not uncommon for these individuals to refuse to eat because they believe they are unworthy of receiving food. Some may say that they do not deserve food because they have not paid for it. Still others seek to destroy themselves through starvation. Many of these individuals have simply lost a desire for food, along with all the other interests they formerly had in life. Inactivity also contributes to a lack of interest in food.

Finding a way to combat the depressed individual's failure to eat depends on the reason for which the food is being refused. If failure to eat is caused by a feeling of unworthiness or the thought that the food has not been paid for, the person may be reassured by being told that the food is prepared for the group and all are expected to eat regardless of whether they pay or not. It might be helpful to provide an opportunity for such an individual to wash dishes or to do some other simple tasks to give him a feeling of "paying" for the food.

If the client is unable to sleep at night, warm tub baths, warm milk, and hypnotic drugs may be of benefit. However, treatment with antidepressant medications is usually most effective in alleviating the symptom of sleep disturbance.

Emotional processes. The need that many inexperienced nurses feel to "cheer up" the person who is depressed is not helpful and often actually causes him to feel more guilty and unworthy than ever. When caring for a depressed individual, such statements as, "Buck up," "Let's see you smile," or "There is a silver lining in every cloud" are not helpful. Gaiety and laughter have a tendency to make such a person feel more guilty and thus more morose. The nurse can be most helpful by being friendly in a kind, understanding, businesslike way. Attempts at changing the client's mood through logical suggestions are fruitless and should be avoided. Sometimes just sitting beside him without trying to carry on a conversation is helpful. At others times it is effective to talk to him even though he may not answer.

> When caring for a client who is depressed, the nurse can be most helpful by being friendly in a kind, understanding, businesslike way.

One of the methods by which a nurse may contribute to the care of some depressed individuals is to provide them with tasks that will help relieve feelings of guilt. Depressed individuals have been known to ask for such menial tasks as scrubbing the floor, scouring the toilets, washing dirty socks, washing windows, or scrubbing the walls. Such tasks may provide a release for the guilt of the depressed individual and a means of atonement for real or imaginary sins. Although providing such experiences is controversial and contrary to the usual recommended treatment plan, it has proved to be of great value to selected individuals. Such work assignments for depressed persons should not be carried out unless they have been approved by the treatment team.

Interpersonal processes. The potential for a depressed person to injure or destroy himself is one of the most serious problems with which the nurse must cope. The most effective methods for dealing with this problem vary, depending on the situation and the individual. However, every nurse should be fully acquainted with some basic principles concerning the care of the self-destructive individual.

Self-destructive tendencies are probably treated most effectively by developing an environment to help the individual bear the emotional pain he is suffering. Instead of removing all the potentially dangerous items from the environment, an attempt can be made to meet his emotional needs. This may be done by assigning a staff member, preferably a skillful psychiatric nurse, to remain constantly with the individual. The nurse helps him participate in occupational, social, and recreational activities. Subtly and appropriately, ways are identified to reassure the individual that he is a worthwhile, useful human being. The acutely depressed individual should be constantly supervised, but the focus of the supervision should be to help him deal with his feelings. The

> Self-destructive tendencies in the client who is depressed are probably treated most effectively by developing an environment to help the client bear the emotional pain he is suffering.

emphasis should be on supplying safe opportunities for participation in the daily routine.

Sometimes an attempt is made to ensure the client's safety by removing from his environment all the equipment with which he might injure himself. This is extremely difficult because every piece of clothing, all eating utensils, cigarettes, furniture, bathroom equipment—literally everything an individual needs in the process of daily living—could be used if the individual wished to injure or destroy himself. One client strangled herself by using a toothbrush to fashion a tourniquet from her long braided hair; another client dived headlong into the toilet and suffered a serious head wound; a third client destroyed herself by using the armholes of her knitted underwear as a noose; and a fourth client injured herself seriously by setting fire to her dress with a cigarette. If the philosophy of making the environment safe were carried to its logical conclusion, the client would be placed in an absolutely barren room with a pallet to lie on. At best this procedure of environmental control is only a preventive measure.

Depriving clients of freedom to move about may increase their self-destructive tendencies, convincing them that their worst fears are true and that they are worthless and unworthy or that they have committed an unforgivable crime and are being justly punished. An illustration of such an occurrence is an incident in which a nurse was playing cards with a young man who was actively suicidal and confined to an empty seclusion room, dressed only in trousers. As both sat cross-legged on the floor, the client over a period of hours dealt the cards a few inches to the right and the nurse unconsciously shifted her position to accommodate to the cards. This client eventually succeeded in shifting the nurse's position so that he had free access to the door through which he fled and proceeded to fling himself through a window. This incident illustrates that even with all precautions, prevention of suicide is not always possible, and its occurrence may be increased by establishing an environment that serves as a constant reminder to the client of his destructive wishes. Although there is no question that the actively suicidal client should be closely supervised, the hospital staff would be wise to emphasize the client's participation in safe activities with others rather than the environmental modifications so often unsuccessfully employed.

If individuals are able to feel that people are truly interested in them, if their needs for recognition and emotional support are being met, and if they are accompanied by staff who help them talk out their concerns, the incidence of attempts at self-destruction will be greatly lessened.

Physiological processes. Because depressed individuals tend to be very inactive, they frequently become chilled without appearing to realize it. Therefore, they need to be supplied with extra clothing and encouraged to wear it.

The inactivity of depressed individuals also makes them susceptible to infection and gastrointestinal and circulatory problems. The nurse can help prevent these problems by insuring that the client maintains adequate food and fluid intake and engages in as much physical activity as possible. This is easier said than done. The nurse most likely to be successful offers fluids on a routine basis and small amounts of food frequently rather than insisting the client eat three full meals at regularly scheduled times. With severely depressed persons, even the simple act of walking down the hall will not take place unless the client is encouraged to do so and accompanied by a member of the nursing staff. Obviously, the nurse who works with a depressed client needs to have a great deal of patience and be willing to take the time required to provide individualized care.

NURSING CARE OF INDIVIDUALS WHO ARE ELATED AND OVERACTIVE

Nursing assessment

Activity processes. The elated, overactive individual moves constantly and finds it almost impossible to sit or stand in one spot for more than a few seconds. As a result, his hygiene needs are often unmet. In addition, his appearance is often dramatically bizarre. Frequently he dresses in clothing that is not only inappropriate to the setting or the season but is also very brightly colored. Females, in particular, adorn themselves with flowers in their hair, large pieces of ornate jewelry, and an abundance of sloppily applied makeup. One client appeared for admission to a northeastern psychiatric hospital in February dressed in a long, bright yellow ball gown and a wide-brimmed straw hat. Around her shoulders she wore a foxtail stole. Her only concession to the 20-degree weather was a pair of checkered mittens. By the time she arrived at the hospital, this individual was almost suffering from hypothermia but had no sense of discomfort.

Exhaustion and death have been known to result from long-continued failure to sleep. Many of these individuals are so alert to all environmental stimuli that they sleep only 1 to 2 hours out of every 24.

Cognition processes. The elated, overactive individual characteristically shows very poor judgment. Because of his feelings of grandiosity and his impulsivity this person may bankrupt himself and his family by charging thousands of dollars for such items as clothing, cars, jewelry, and furniture despite the fact he did not need nor could he afford these items. In fact, it is this characteristic that often leads his family to seek treatment for him. One such individual sold the family clothes dryer to a visitor who admired it. His lack of judgment was displayed not only by the fact that he sold the dryer but also by the fact that he delivered it filled with a load of partially dried clothes.

Ecological processes. As is the case with any individual who has alterations in self-care, the elated, overactive individual has great difficulty in home maintenance. He is able to give little attention to maintaining his environment in a clean, safe condition.

The nurse can help prevent infection and gastrointestinal and circulatory problems in the client who is depressed by insuring that he maintains adequate food and fluid intake and engages in physical activity.

NURSING CARE PLAN

A depressed individual

CASE FORMULATION

Carol B., 29 years of age, has been married 3 years and has one child 14 months of age. Family history reveals nothing significant except that her father was stolid and slow-going. He had a reputation for being a pessimist but was otherwise a stable, sober individual.

Five years before marriage Carol had had a period of nervousness and depression, which lasted about 3 months. This was precipitated by an unfortunate love affair. At that time she was attending summer school at a local university where she met a young man. He had encouraged her to believe he was greatly interested in her, but at the school outing that ended the summer session he ignored her and danced with another girl. Carol came home, said little or nothing to her parents, and the following morning was found in bed in a stupor. She had taken 12 1-grain phenobarbital tablets. She was rushed to a hospital, given emergency treatment, and then transferred to a mental health treatment center where she remained 2 weeks.

The present attack began about 6 weeks before admission. Again the onset was rather abrupt. Her husband returned home from work one evening and found her sobbing. After much urging on his part, she confessed that she was crying because she was a bad mother and a poor housekeeper. The husband naturally assured her that she was quite the contrary, but this only brought more sobbing and self-depreciation. She worried excessively about a small scar on her baby's temple that was caused by chicken pox. She accused herself of "marking" the child. The family suspected that she was merely tired from her spring housecleaning and hired a helper to come in and care for the baby. Her sister-in-law was called in to act as a companion. For 3 weeks she remained at home. She complained of inability to concentrate and prayed a great deal of the time. The well-meaning sister-in-law attempted to encourage her by suggesting that she "snap out of

it," but this merely served to agitate her. She was finally taken to her parents' home in the country. On two occasions she was found walking along the country road, and when questioned as to her destination, she merely stated that she wanted to "run away from everything." Her husband came to visit her one Sunday afternoon and took her for a car ride back into the city. She requested him to stop at their home, since she wanted some extra clothes for the baby. She went to the kitchen and, before the husband could realize what she was about to do, cut both her wrists with a carving knife. She was admitted to a short-term treatment unit in a community mental health center after receiving emergency treatment for her wounds.

On the day of admission she was able to give a clear account of her actions but responded in a dull manner. She frequently interjected the remark that she should be dead but that she was too big a coward to take her own life. She accused herself of being a rank failure and asserted that she should never have been born. She frequently announced that there was no sense in bothering about her, since she would die the next day. She cried but did not shed many tears. She complained of a "numb" feeling in her head, of inability to sleep, and of loss of appetite. The physical examination was entirely negative.

Nursing assessment

The history provides little information about the present episode of depression. However, it does provide information about the first attack, which came as a result of the failure of an interpersonal relationship of great importance to her and the loss of a beloved object—a cherished lover. At that time she attempted suicide by taking an overdose of sleeping pills.

It is interesting to note that psychoanalytically oriented theorists believe that individuals who resort to self-destruction are frequently fixated at the oral stage of psychosexual development. Dur-

NURSING CARE PLAN—cont'd

ing the late oral period of the child's development, the loved object (the mother or the mother's breast) is unconsciously introjected. Later in life a loved object may unconsciously represent the original object that was introjected. When Carol first attempted suicide, she may have been seeking relief from suffering or punishment for herself, or she may have been attempting to kill the introjected person.

This young woman's child was in the toilet-training period. It is at this period in the child's development that he becomes more self-assertive and begins to defy the mother. It may be that this mother viewed the change in her child from a dependent, passive organism requiring constant tender guidance to a self-assertive individual as a loss. In a sense she had lost a dependent organism and gained a demanding child. She may be overwhelmed with the new responsibilities brought about by the child's development. Thus she blamed herself for being a bad mother and a poor housekeeper and having caused a small scar on the baby's temple.

Her physical symptoms were those commonly found among depressed individuals: inability to sleep, loss of appetite, complaints of a numb feeling in the head, and crying without tears. Her emotional responses were also those frequently found among depressed individuals: inability to concentrate, self-accusatory ideas, suicidal ideas, and feelings of unworthiness. Characteristically she was able to give a clear account of all the experiences relating to her illness.

Nursing diagnoses

The assessment data, including present behavior, past life experiences, and an understanding of the underlying dynamics, led to the development of the following three pairs of nursing diagnoses for Carol. The first of each pair is from the Classification of Human Responses of Concern for Psychiatric–Mental Health Nursing Practice; the second is from the approved NANDA Diagnostic Categories.

5.3.2.9	Suicide Attempt related to feelings of guilt and worthlessness
OR	
9.2.2	Potential for Violence: Self-directed related to feelings of guilt and worthlessness
1.4.2	Altered Sleep/Arousal Patterns related to depression
OR	
6.2.1	Sleep Pattern Disturbance related to depression
7.7.2	Altered Nutrition Processes related to lack of appetite
OR	
6.5.1	Feeding Self-Care Deficit related to lack of appetite

Planning and implementing nursing care for Carol B.

The boxed material on pp. 246-247 is an example of a plan of nursing care that could be designed for Carol B. Because she was actively suicidal individual nursing care was provided for her. Nurses or other staff members with proved ability to work successfully with depressed individuals were chosen to be with her at all times until she recovered from the acute phase of the depression. They recognized the importance of showing Carol that they cared about her and set about to achieve this. Their goals for her care were to protect her from her self-destructive tendencies and to encourage her to discuss her feelings about the problems that concerned her.

These staff members adopted a kind, courteous, firm, hopeful attitude toward Carol. In this way they tried to convey the impression that she was not a hopeless case as she insisted. They listened carefully to everything she said and answered her questions carefully without disputing or agreeing with her expressions of worthlessness. They accepted her silences when she did not wish to talk. They avoided using meaningless statements such as, "Cheer up," or "You know your family loves you!"

The staff members who worked closely with

Continued.

NURSING CARE PLAN—cont'd

Carol were aware of her physical needs for food, fluid intake, and rest. They found that she ate better if served food on a tray in her room rather than going to the dining room with the other clients. If at night she wanted to sit up and talk or walk up and down the corridors, the staff member who was assigned to stay with her accompanied her in these activities.

When Carol accused herself of being a rank failure, the nurse tried to help her recognize that she was improving and had demonstrated abilities and skills since coming to the treatment center. This was an attempt to improve her self-esteem.

The staff workers made decisions for Carol until she was able to make them for herself. They tried to develop a congenial pleasant living atmosphere for her. They encouraged her to become interested in some of the activities available in the occupational therapy department and accompanied her there whenever she felt well enough to go.

Evaluation

Evaluation of the plan of nursing care and its implementation was based on outcome criteria established when the plan was formulated. Since the nurse knew that the most significant factor in alleviating the symptoms of acute depression is the prescribed antidepressant medication and that this medication requires 2 to 4 weeks to have an effect, she did not expect to see changes in Carol's behavior until then.

For several days after admission Carol remained sad and indifferent. She ate only when coaxed. She never inquired about the welfare of her child and was indifferent toward her husband during visiting hours. Although she was not particularly untidy, she was rather slipshod in appearance and made no attempt to comb her hair or keep herself presentable. She took little or no interest in unit activities or in the other clients.

In the second week of Carol's hospital stay she began to show improvement. After being in the hospital for 1 month she began clamoring for discharge, insisting that she must go home to take care of her family. She was cheerful and industrious, teaching English to a small group of foreign women in occupational therapy.

Carol's nurse joined other members of the treatment team in recommending discharge to the aftercare clinic.

NURSING CARE PLAN FOR *Carol B.*

Nursing diagnosis	Objective	Nursing actions	Outcome criteria
5.3.2.9 Suicide Attempt related to feelings of guilt and worthlessness OR 9.2.2 Potential for Violence: Self-directed related to feelings of guilt and worthlessness	To protect client from self-destructive tendencies	Assigned nurse(s) remain with client at all times Administer prescribed antidepressant medication Observe and listen carefully for clues of suicidal intention; record same Encourage constructive activity, for example, O.T., R.T. Comment positively on accomplishments	Within 4 weeks client will: No longer express desire to kill self Acknowledge positive comments by nurse about her accomplishments, for example, by saying "thank you" Spontaneously attend O.T. and R.T. activities

NURSING CARE PLAN—cont'd

		To encourage client to discuss her feelings and problems	Reflect client's statements to encourage conversation Sit with client in silence if she does not wish to talk Convey interest in what client says Do not argue with expressions of worthlessness Avoid platitudes, such as "tomorrow will be a better day" Encourage problem solving technique	Within 2 weeks client will: Spontaneously approach nurse to express feelings Show evidence of attempting to problem solve
1.4.2 OR 6.2.1	Altered Sleep/Arousal Patterns related to depression Sleep Pattern Disturbance related to depression	To increase periods of sleep at night	Discourage naps during the day Remove client from environmental stimuli (for example, TV) 1 hour before bedtime Do not discuss charged issues at bedtime If client awakes at night, do not scold; be reassuring and remain with her	Within 4 weeks client will sleep from 10:00 PM to 6:00 AM without awakening
7.7.2 OR 6.5.1	Altered Nutrition Processes related to lack of appetite Feeding Self-Care Deficit related to lack of appetite	To increase food and fluid intake	Offer small amounts of easily chewed, nutritional food at meal times Offer 6 oz. water or juice in plastic cup q2h Record amount of food and fluid taken	Within 4 weeks client will eat 3 meals a day without needing to be encouraged to do so

Emotional processes. The mood expressed by the elated, overactive individual is euphoria, although many authorities believe that this mood state is a defense against an underlying depression. The jovial, good-natured euphoria the client expresses can quickly turn into irritability and anger when his desires or activities are thwarted.

Interpersonal processes. The constant movement of the elated overactive individual is accompanied by excessive talking. The content of his verbalizations may not be immediately understood by the listener, since his thoughts occur faster than he can speak and tend to fly from one topic to another. However, with concentration the listener can usually accurately guess the missing words and thus make sense of what the person is saying, unlike when conversing with an individual with a thought disorder.

When the elated individual is left alone, the content of his speech is likely to be jovial and humorous, often with many sexual references and puns. When his stream of talk is interrupted even by as simple and common an event as being asked a question, his good-natured banter may suddenly turn to biting sarcasm, pointed profanity, and vulgarity.

Elated individuals are very adept in discovering a physical or personality defect in the person with whom they are speaking, particularly one about which the person is sensitive. They seem to take delight in repeatedly calling attention to this defect.

Because of his overactivity and irritability when thwarted, the elated individual is likely to become involved in altercations with others or accidents that may result in physical injury. These injuries range from superficial bruises to broken ribs. However, he is unlikely to complain of discomfort.

Perception processes. The elated, overactive individual is hyperalert to his environment and seemingly cannot block out stimuli. Consequently, he is unable to maintain sustained attention to anything, sometimes for any longer than a few seconds.

Physiological processes. As is true with many other individuals who are mentally ill, the elated, overactive individual may be malnourished. His overactivity consumes a great deal of energy, and he cannot concentrate long enough on one task to purchase, prepare, or eat food. For the same reason he rarely consumes sufficient fluid. Consequently, an overactive individual often loses a great deal of weight and may become severely dehydrated. He is often oblivious to physical injury or pain. Constipation, fecal impaction, and bladder distention are common problems.

Valuation processes. Although the elated, overactive individual gives the impression of feeling all-powerful, in reality he feels powerless and out of control. The content of his speech and the nature of his behavior are likely to be antisocial and in conflict with the values he espouses when he is well. It is not uncommon for his family and friends to emphasize how uncharacteristic his behavior is of him.

Nursing diagnosis

Categories of human responses from the ANA Classification of Human Responses of Concern for Psychiatric–Mental Health Nursing Practice that may be specifically applicable to individuals who are elated and overactive include the following:

    1.1.2   Altered Motor Behavior
    1.3.4   Altered Self-Care

Assessment of individuals who are elated and overactive reveals constant movement, poor judgment, difficulties in maintaining a home, euphoria, excessive talking, irritability when thwarted, hyperalertness to the environment, malnourishment, and the impression of feeling all-powerful.

1.4.2   Altered Sleep/Arousal Patterns

2.2.2   Altered Judgment

3.3.2   Altered Home Maintenance

4.1.2   Altered Feeling State

4.2.1   Altered Feeling Processes

5.2.2   Altered Communication Processes

5.3.2   Altered Conduct/Impulse Processes

6.1.2   Altered Attention

7.2.1   Potential for Alteration in Elimination Processes

7.7.1   Potential for Alteration in Nutrition

7.9.1   Potential for Alteration in Physical Integrity

7.10.1   Potential for Alteration in Physical Regulation Processes

NANDA nursing diagnostic categories that may be specifically applicable to the individual who is elated and overactive include:

1.1.2.2   Altered Nutrition: Less than body requirements

1.3.1.1   Constipation

1.6.1   Potential for Injury

2.1.1.1   Impaired Verbal Communication

3.1.1   Impaired Social Interaction

5.1.1.1   Ineffective Individual Coping

6.2.1   Sleep Pattern Disturbance

6.4.1.1   Impaired Home Maintenance Management

6.5.1   Feeding Self-Care Deficit

6.5.2   Bathing/Hygiene Self-Care Deficit

6.5.3   Dressing/Grooming Self-Care Deficit

9.2.2   Potential for Violence: Directed at others

To develop a nursing diagnosis that fulfills its function of providing direction for planning nursing care, the nurse is encouraged to postulate and state etiologic or antecedent factors for each human response and connect the two phrases by using the term "related to." For example:

1.3.4   Altered self-care related to overactivity and inability to sustain attention
        to a task

Planning and implementing nursing care

The plan for nursing care is derived from the nursing diagnoses and includes the objectives of the care, the nursing actions, and outcome criteria. To be effective the plan needs to be highly individualized. The suggestions that follow should be seen as general guidelines to be used if they are appropriate to the client's needs.

Individuals who are elated and overactive require skillful and tactful nursing care. In general, the objectives of all nursing care for the individual who is elated and overactive should relate to protecting him and others from his overactive behavior until the prescribed medications take effect.

Since the client's nursing diagnoses are often interrelated, stemming as they

Protecting the individual and others from his overactive behavior is the goal of all nursing care for the person who is elated and overactive.

do from similar etiologies or antecedents, the student will see that the appropriate nursing actions are also interrelated. In other words, by intervening in one dimension, the nurse will also affect other dimensions.

Activity processes. It is useless to attempt to hurry the elated individual because such an approach will result in anger and hostility. Thus the attitude of having all the time in the world to accomplish a task will be much more effective. Quiet persuasion is one of the chief aids in getting the elated individual to cooperate.

Because all elated, overactive individuals are stimulated by environmental factors, one of the nurse's first responsibilities is to simplify their surroundings and insofar as possible provide a sedate environment for them. The client's room should be as far away from other daily activities as possible and yet easily accessible to the nurse who needs to be constantly aware of the individual and his behavior. Pictures and colorful drapes probably should be removed because they may be too stimulating and certainly may be destroyed in a burst of excitement. The same is true of unnecessary furniture such as a small table or a light chair, either of which may be used as a weapon if the client becomes extremely irritated.

Elated, overactive individuals may not take time to sit down to eat. In such an instance it is wise to serve food that can be carried about in the hands. Sandwiches, fruit, and cupcakes are dietary items that may be "eaten on the run." Elated, overactive individuals require a high caloric intake and should have between-meal nourishment. Nurses should not disregard the need for fluids even though water fountains are usually available; the overactive individual often does not take time to drink and should have water offered to him each hour.

If the individual is served food on a tray and will take time to feed himself, the equipment on the tray should be simple and unbreakable. As in every other aspect of the care of these overactive, elated persons, the nursing procedures must be individualized to meet specific needs. In some instances the elated individual may get along well in the dining room setting. However, in most instances he is so stimulated by the dining room situation that it is more helpful if he is served on a tray in his room.

Although the individual should be encouraged to carry out his own personal hygiene, he needs to be supervised closely. Some overactive, elated individuals are too ill to assume any responsibility for their physical care and may need to have much of it done by the nurse. Other less excited individuals can take a good deal of responsibility for their own cleanliness and grooming if someone skillfull directs their activities. Such individuals may become playful and mischievous in the bathroom. Because of poor judgment these individuals have been found washing their hair in the toilet bowl, throwing water about with gay abandon, or in various other ways reducing the bathroom to a shambles. For this reason such individuals should not be left alone in the bathroom.

Keeping overactive persons warmly dressed during cold weather is some-

Simplifying the environment of an elated, overactive individual to provide safe surroundings is one of the nurse's first responsibilities in providing care.

times difficult because clothing may be an irritating factor. Excited individuals may tear off clothing that impedes the movement of arms and legs. They often appear totally unaware of body temperature and must be safeguarded against becoming chilled.

The overactive individual may react with a tremendous burst of energy for which he must find some outlet. Usually such an individual is admitted to a hospital because the outlets he has chosen for his energy have been dangerous to him or to his family. The nurse is confronted with the task of controlling or redirecting this excessive energy into more acceptable channels.

An excellent outlet for the excessive energy of individuals who are only mildly elated is writing. Most of these people are eager to write their life stories or to disclose the deficiencies of the political system to the world and thus will readily put paper and pencil to use. Many mildly elated individuals will be content to spend hours over their manuscripts.

Physical activities provided for these individuals should require large sweeping movements, since they will become annoyed and lose interest in anything requiring fine, discriminative skills. Games such as table tennis, croquet, badminton, and medicine ball are often helpful as outlets for energy, provided there is no element of competition present. In competitive games the elated client becomes overly stimulated and excited.

Emotional processes. The euphoria of overactive clients can easily turn to irritability and anger, which, in turn, may result in destructive, threatening behavior. When a client begins to threaten destructive behavior, he should be assisted to a room that is away from the center of activity and should remain there until his emotions are under control. The nurse needs to be aware of and carefully follow the legal procedures and institutional policies regarding the use of restraint and seclusion as a therapeutic intervention. Fortunately, with the availability of effective psychotropic medications, the necessity to mechanically restrain or seclude overactive individuals is less common than it once was.

More important than managing destructive, threatening behavior is learning how it can be prevented. The first step in learning to prevent problem behavior is to discover situations that are upsetting to such individuals and to discover how to keep these from occurring. The nurse needs to learn to recognize the signs of an approaching emotional outburst and to employ measures that will help individuals to handle negative feelings without acting out against the environment. Destructive behavior is rare where an attempt is made to recognize and meet emotional needs and where the personnel recognize the importance of developing positive interpersonal relationships with mentally ill persons.

Interpersonal processes. Whether the nurse can help elated, overactive clients depends to a large extent on the manner with which she approaches them. The nurse's tone of voice is of primary importance. A firm, kind, low-pitched voice that carries a coaxing quality probably is most effective. The nurse who

When the euphoria of overactive clients turns to irritability and anger, it is most important for the nurse to know how to prevent destructive, threatening behavior.

NURSING CARE PLAN

An overactive individual

CASE FORMULATION

Maurice H., 48 years of age, was an unmarried real estate salesman who was an only child. His mother had a mental illness at 46 years of age, which was probably depression of midlife. He had been educated in private schools and earned a college degree in business administration. During his junior year in college he failed to win a scholarship and became morose, sleepless, and nervous for a period of 2 months. A few years after finishing college he entered an auto sales contest and won first prize, a trip to Hawaii. While on this trip he became overactive and insisted on eating every meal at the captain's table, where he told obscene stories and embarrassed the women passengers. He participated in frequent brawls with the stewards and complained to the purser on the slightest provocation. On disembarking he refused to return to his home city. He demanded the most pretentious accommodations at the hotel, and when these were unavailable he entered into a noisy altercation with the manager that resulted in his being hospitalized because of his behavior. He remained there for 3 months and then returned to his parents' home.

The present attack began about 6 weeks before he sought help. At that time he was engaged in selling real estate in a new subdivision. He became extremely active, arose early, and approached prospective clients at bus terminals, waiting rooms, and hotel corridors. He talked in such a convincing manner that he made a good sales record in the first week. He continued to send in many deposits, bragged about his sales ability, argued noisily with his fellow salesmen, and finally was arrested because he failed to pay his fare on a city bus. He then entered a damage suit against the company for $100,000. The attorney who was approached realized the absurdities of his claims and convinced him to seek help.

Immediately after going to the mental health center he demanded to see the head physician and requested permission to use the telephone. He was fairly coherent but was circumstantial in his conversation. When asked a simple question his reply was a long, rambling, and digressive account. After being continually reminded to answer the question he did so, only to return to another long digression.

Although he believed that he was being abused, he harbored no other delusional ideas and at no time was he confused or hallucinatory. His intellect was keen and his memory, particularly for trivial things, remarkable, but he had no insight into his abnormal exaltation and irritability and his judgment was poor. He made unreasonable demands of the personnel at the clinic and if refused became abusive, sarcastic, and irritable. At this time it was discovered that when a client had refused to make a down payment on a lot, he had drawn the sum out of his own bank account and had forged a signature on the sales contract. This explained his amazing sales success.

He spent much of his time while in the short-term treatment unit of the mental health clinic writing letters to the mayor, various attorneys, and influential citizens. He wrote on odd pieces of paper with pencil in a broad, sweeping hand, underlining many words and capitalizing others. Every day he met the physicians at the door of the unit and began to revile them. He particularly enjoyed arguing with the physicians, demanding evidence to prove that he was insane and consistently denying all charges of misbehavior. In a loud voice he promised to have the director of the center removed and the physicians exposed as quacks. He was suggestively lewd in his conversation with all female staff except one young woman to whom he proposed marriage.

Throughout the 4 weeks he spent in the short-term treatment unit, he was the constant focus of commotion, a chronic critic of everything and everybody about him, collecting and

NURSING CARE PLAN—cont'd

hoarding papers, combs, magazines, and all sorts of trash and getting into quarrels with others. Occasionally he was very agreeable and jolly, particularly if he was allowed to do all the talking. On these occasions he was fond of reciting parodies of famous poems in a quick, witty fashion. Some of these he had not quoted since his high school days.

Nursing assessment

This client's mother suffered from a midlife depression. Too little is known about this situation to do more than suggest that the mother was unable to give her son the sense of security he required as an infant to develop into a well-adjusted adult. The mother's depression also raises the possibility of this individual having an inherited predisposition to mood disorder.

Maurice H. first experienced a depression at about the age of 21 when he failed to win a scholarship in college. To him this failure to achieve a prized goal represented a failure in life, and he became depressed in an unconscious effort to punish himself. For 2 months he had typical symptoms of a mild depression. He was morose, sleepless, and nervous.

A few years later Maurice won a coveted prize in an auto sales contest. This award was a trip to Hawaii that eventually resulted in Maurice's hospitalization for 3 months because of his overactivity. In this instance he probably developed anxiety over his company's high expectations. He may have reasoned that they would undoubtedly expect more and bigger sales records from him now that he had been able to achieve the award of a trip. The anxiety about being able to fulfill the future expectations of his company changed into guilt feelings that in turn caused him to feel that somehow he should be punished. To guard against the depressed feelings that arose from a sense of failure and a need to be punished, he developed overactivity and elation—the defense against depression.

Several years later he once more became involved in a competitive selling activity. His need to succeed started the chain reaction again. Anx-

iety about succeeding caused him to be concerned about the possibility of failing, and this in turn led to the depressed feelings that accompany a loss. The loss was the anticipated failure in selling, which in his own mind had already occurred. Thus the unconscious defense against depressed feelings was again used. He became expansive, overactive, argumentative, sarcastic, irritable, made unreasonable demands, and became a constant center of commotion. In a sense, he did not give himself time to become depressed because he was too busy striking out against his environment.

Typically he was not delusional, and he did not experience hallucinations. Thus he was constantly in touch with reality. His intellect was as keen as ever, and his memory was intact.

Some inexperienced people might conclude that this man was not mentally ill. However, he was unreasonable and sometimes abusive when he did not get his own way. He also wrote letters to outside authorities because he believed he should not be undergoing treatment, and he constantly sought to expose the clinic personnel for their inefficient handling of the situation. He had no insight into his condition, and his judgment was impaired.

Nursing diagnoses

The assessment data, including present behavior, past experiences, and an understanding of the underlying dynamics, led to the development of the following two pairs of nursing diagnoses for Maurice H. The first of each pair is from the Classification of Human Responses of Concern for Psychiatric–Mental Health Nursing Practice; the second is from the approved NANDA Diagnostic Categories.

5.3.2.5	Physical Aggression Toward Others related to elation and overactivity
OR	
9.2.2	Potential for Violence: Directed at others related to elation and overactivity
7.7.2	Altered Nutrition Processes related to overactivity
OR	

Continued.

NURSING CARE PLAN—cont'd

6.5.1   Feeding Self Care Deficit related to overactivity

Planning and implementing nursing care for *Maurice H.*

The plan of nursing care developed for Maurice H. is summarized on pp. 255-256.

The members of the staff assigned to care for Maurice were chosen carefully because his verbally hostile and physically aggressive behavior was difficult to accept. Not all staff members were able to control their feelings about his vulgar comments or to understand objectively why it was impossible for him to control his behavior. In addition, he related more positively to some individuals than to others. Finally, some staff members enjoyed working with him and others did not. All these factors were considered in the choice of individuals to work with him.

The staff decided that it would be best for him to be cared for in a unit of the treatment center where a single room was available. In such a room it was possible to eliminate all but the essential furnishings. The single room was helpful in avoiding the overstimulation that might have resulted from sleeping accommodations where he would have been involved with other clients.

Maurice's recreational activities needed to be controlled because it was obvious that he became loud and disruptive when involved in competitive games. He became angry when he scored lower than other players in a game and accused them of cheating. These accusations usually brought on loud arguments and sometimes fights.

When it was necessary for the staff to intervene in such an altercation, they took advantage of his distractibility and subtly redirected his attention away from the argument to an activity that could be carried on in his room with another person, one who was able to tolerate his rapid conversation and accept his pointed criticism.

The members of the staff were careful to avoid scolding or threatening Maurice when he initiated fights with other individuals. They avoided

comparing his behavior with that of other better controlled individuals or even with his own behavior on a day when he was less noisy. The staff realized that his problem behavior was part of his illness.

Maurice responded negatively to any member of the staff who attempted to speak to him somewhat sharply or who commanded him to do anything. They learned that he could not be hurried and that their approach was much more effective if they were quiet, friendly, patient, and courteous to him and used a pleasant, businesslike toneof voice. On one occasion when a staff member did order him to comply with a hospital rule, he refused and did not let the individual forget the incident.

The staff discovered that it was unwise to encourage Maurice when he was reciting or singing parodies or telling jokes. When some staff members did laugh at his jokes, he became much louder and more ribald. It was necessary for them to intervene by accompanying him to his room before he became so excited that he lost control.

In talking to this man the staff avoided getting into long, complicated discussions or giving elaborate explanations. Instead, short sentences with specific, straightforward responses to his questions seemed to satisfy him and avoid arguments.

The staff members were careful when praising him. They found that he sometimes turned the words of praise around and used them in a different context to refute a point they had been trying to make with him some time previously.

They were aware of his physical needs and realized that he frequently did not eat enough. This problem arose because his attention was distracted from the food or he left the dining room early before finishing the meal. Likewise, he sometimes had dry, cracked lips because he failed to maintain his fluid intake. Maurice was weighed every week, and when his weight had dropped below a desirable point for 2 consecutive weeks, his food was served in his room on a tray. A staff member remained with him during

NURSING CARE PLAN—cont'd

the meal and encouraged him to eat. Removing him from the dining room eliminated the many distracting features present in a group. At the same time he was placed on a schedule so that fluids were offered to him every hour.

Crayons, paper, and pencils were made available to him in his room, and he was encouraged to write and sketch there in the hope that these more sedentary activities would lessen his hyperactivity. The staff members were careful to explain to him in an honest, straightforward manner why he was not encouraged to join the rest of the clients in the dining room. In like manner all other restrictions on his behavior were explained so that he could understand the reason for them and realize that he was not being rejected as a person.

Evaluation

After receiving the prescribed amount of the drug lithium carbonate for 2 weeks, he gained some control of his behavior and became quieter and more amenable to suggestion. The professional staff did not believe that he was well enough to leave the hospital permanently. However, at the request of his mother he was allowed to go home at the end of 4 weeks with the understanding that he would continue taking lithium carbonate for 1 year and have the blood levels of this drug checked weekly by a physician.

Although the nurse who had primary responsibility for this client's nursing care continuously reassessed his behavior, she did not engage in a complete evaluation because Maurice was discharged after 4 weeks.

NURSING CARE PLAN FOR **Maurice H.**

Nursing diagnosis	Objectives	Nursing actions	Outcome criteria
5.3.2.5 Physical Aggression Toward Others related to elation and overactivity OR 9.2.2 Potential for Violence: Directed toward others related to elation and overactivity	To prevent injury to client and staff To assist client to control his hostile language and physical aggressiveness	Administer prescribed medication; observe carefully for signs of lithium toxicity Arrange for daily blood work and check results against norms Carefully select 3 staff to work with client per shift Reduce all environmental stimuli by: Assigning client to single room Avoiding competitive games Providing activities for him in his room Do not interrupt when client is singing or reciting Ignore client's jokes Speak in calm, direct manner using simple short sentences Do not argue	Within 4 weeks client will: Be able to talk with one other person for 15 minutes without sarcasm or hostility Not attempt to hit other clients or staff unless provoked

Continued.

NURSING CARE PLAN—cont'd

7.7.2	Altered Nutrition Processes related to overactivity	To promote adequate nutrition and hydration	In addition to meals, provide high caloric nutritional snacks that can be eaten standing or walking, for example, malted milk, hamburgers	Within 1 week, client will: Show signs of adequate hydration Consume sufficient calories to avoid weight loss
OR 6.5.1	Feeding Self-Care Deficit related to overactivity		Offer 6 oz. water or juice every hour Weigh weekly Observe for signs of dehydration Feed in room if client is unable to stay in dining room long enough to finish meal	

uses a loud, demanding tone not only is likely to be ineffective but also is likely to provoke hostile and aggressive behavior on the part of the client.

Consistent fairness and honesty in dealing with elated, overactive clients are essential if rapport with them is to be maintained over time. Although they deserve and must have simple, honest explanations, long discussions and explanations should be avoided.

Firmness, kindness, fairness, and honesty are essential qualities the nurse should possess when dealing with elated, overactive individuals.

In dealing with overactive, elated individuals the nurse must recognize that the behavior is a result of an illness and will be replaced by socially acceptable behavior when the person is well again. The inexperienced nurse may be embarrassed by the loud talking, the vulgarity and profanity, the destructive activity, and the overt sexual behavior that is apparent. However, part of the skillful care of such a person includes understanding why he needs to behave in such a way. With understanding will come acceptance of behavior.

The nurse who is accepting of the behavior of the elated individual will not scold or shame him for his unihibited actions or become angered by his pointed, biting remarks because she will understand that they are a part of his illness.

The physical needs of the client who is elated and overactive should be of primary importance to the nurse.

Physiological processes. The nurse needs to be vigilantly aware of the physical needs of a client who is elated and overactive. In addition to ensuring adequate food and fluid intake, the nurse must monitor his elimination and intervene appropriately if indicated.

Because overactive individuals are unlikely to report an illness or injury, it is especially important for a complete physical examination to be completed as soon as possible after admission to the mental health care delivery system. Thereafter, the nurse must be alert for signs and symptoms of physical illness that may or may not be related to the client's overactivity.

END NOTE

The focus of this chapter is the nursing care of individuals with mood disorders. The symptoms and causative factors of mood disorders are discussed, as are the psychotropic medications commonly prescribed for these clients. A case formulation from which a hypothetical nursing care plan is derived, implemented, and evaluated is presented for both an individual who is depressed and an individual who is elated and overactive.

SUGGESTED SOURCES OF ADDITIONAL INFORMATION

Akiskal H and Tashjian R: Affective disorders. II. Recent advances in laboratory and pathogenic approaches, Hosp Commun Psychiatr 34(9):822, 1983.

Akiskal H and Webb W: Affective disorders. I. Recent advances in clinical conceptualization, Hosp Commun Psychiatr 34(8):695, 1983.

Assey J: The suicide prevention contract, Perspect Psychiatr Care 23(3):99, 1985.

Blythe M and Pearlmutter D: The suicide watch: a re-examination of maximum observation, Perspect Psychiatr Care 21:90, July-September 1983.

Brenners DK, Harris B, and Weston PS: Managing manic behavior, Am J Nurs 87(5):620, May 1987.

Brown G: Expressed emotion and life events in schizophrenia and depression, J Psychosoc Nurs Ment Health Serv 24(7):31, July 1986.

Bydlon-Brown B and Billman R: At risk for suicide, Am J Nurs 88(10):1358, October 1988.

Busteed E and Johnstone C: The development of suicide precautions for an inpatient psychiatric unit, J Psychosoc Nurs Ment Health Serv 21:15-19, May 1983.

Campbell L: CE depression: acute care in the hospital, Am J Nurs 86(3):288, March 1986.

Capodanno A and Targum S: Assessment of suicide risk: some limitations in the prediction of infrequent events, J Psychosoc Nurs Ment Health Serv 21:11, May 1983.

Crockett MS: CE depression: a case of anger and alienation, Am J Nurs 86(3):294, March 1986.

Field W: Physical causes of depression, J Psychosoc Nurs Ment Health Serv 23(10):6, October 1985.

Harris E: CE lithium: In a class by itself, Am J Nurs 89(2):190, February 1989.

Hensley M and Rogers S: Shedding light on "SAD"ness, Arch Psychiatr Nurs 1(4):230, August 1987.

Maurer F: Acute depression: treatment and nursing strategies for this affective disorder, Nurs Clin North Am 21(3):413, September 1986.

Minot SR: CE depression: What does it mean? Am J Nurs 86(3):284, March 1986.

Schlesser M and Altshuler K: The genetics of affective disorder: data, theory, and clinical application, Hosp Commun Psychiatr 34(5):415, 1983.

Simmons-Alling S: New approaches to managing affective disorders, Arch Psychiatr Nurs 1(4):219, August 1987.

Thomas MD, Sanger E, and Whitney JD: Nursing diagnosis of depression, J Psychosoc Nurs Ment Health Serv 24(8):6, August 1986.

Vogel P: Lithium and the thyroid, J Psychosoc Nurs Ment Health Serv 24(2):8, February 1986.

Wright J and Beck A: Cognitive therapy of depression: theory and practice, Hosp Commun Psychiatr 34(12):1119, 1983.

Individuals with anxiety disorders

17

LEARNING OBJECTIVES

After studying this chapter the student will be able to:

o Describe the symptoms exhibited by a person with the medical diagnoses of anxiety disorder, somatoform disorder, or dissociative disorders.

o Discuss the causative factors associated with anxiety disorders.

o State the desired effects, side effects, and adverse effects of anxiolytic medications.

o Discuss the treatment technique of psychotherapy.

o Describe behaviors the nurse is most likely to observe in an individual experiencing an anxiety disorder.

o State examples of nursing diagnoses likely to be applicable to an individual who is experiencing an anxiety disorder.

o Develop a hypothetical plan of nursing care for an individual who is experiencing an anxiety disorder.

The majority of people live normal, relatively anxiety-free lives by successfully adapting to stress and its resultant anxiety through the use of various strategies and compromises, both conscious and unconscious. Nevertheless, there is a large group of individuals for whom these defenses are not effective. In fact, data recently released by the National Institute of Mental Health indicate that 8.3% of the population of the United States suffers from an anxiety disorder in the course of 6 months. These persons must continuously focus on activities and behaviors designed to control intolerable anxiety in an unsuccessful effort to achieve a state of physical and emotional homeokinesis. In the past this group of individuals has been labeled "neurotic" by both the health care delivery system and the lay public. This term has been replaced by the more descriptive phrase anxiety disorders.

Because individuals suffering from anxiety disorders are in touch with reality and often recognize the inappropriateness of their behavior, many nurses have difficulty accepting them as persons in need of health care. To achieve a more understanding attitude toward these individuals, it is important to develop some knowledge about the emotional conflicts with which they struggle and the ways in which they use symptoms to cope with the anxiety that stems from these conflicts.

HISTORICAL PERSPECTIVE

Although the emotion of anxiety has been recognized since ancient Greek times, the disorders stemming directly from an inability to adapt to stress and the subsequent anxiety were not brought into focus until the early twentieth century. At that time Sigmund Freud (1856-1939) identified the role anxiety plays in the unconscious life of the individual and demonstrated how it affects his perception of reality and subsequent behavior.

During the Victorian era in which Freud practiced, many women suffered from a condition called *hysteria*. This malady manifested itself by unexplainable fatigue and weakness, "swooning," and other forms of dramatic behavior. Today these persons would be diagnosed as having a dysfunction stemming from overwhelming anxiety. Freud developed the technique of psychoanalysis through which he helped these patients to explore their unconscious minds for the emotional conflicts that were expressed in these symptoms. He discovered that the nature of these conflicts frequently centered on real or fantasized aggressive sexual acts. Given the culture of the day in which women were expected to assume a passive, dependent role, it is understandable that they had little opportunity to resolve these conflicts and that they were expressed by symptoms indicative of passivity and dependency.

The manifestations of anxiety disorders have changed over the years. It is rare today to encounter an individual who exhibits the classical symptoms of hysteria, although phobic disorders are common. This change in symptomatology has led authorities to believe that the specific behaviors unconsciously chosen by the individual to express emotional conflict are determined in part by societal sanctions. For example, fainting at the sight of blood would not be culturally acceptable today, but an inordinate and irrational fear of heights evokes sympathy in this age of skyscrapers and jet travel.

The incidence of dysfunctions related to overwhelming anxiety has also markedly increased over the last three decades. There is no question that this increase is related to the increased stress associated with the highly complex, postindustrial society in which we live. In fact, the last half of the twentieth century is often called "the age of anxiety."

Only persons with the severest forms of anxiety disorders have ever been hospitalized. Therefore until recently nurses have not had much experience in providing care for individuals with less severe forms of anxiety disorders. Since mental health care has moved into the community, however, nurses now have the opportunity and the challenge of intervening therapeutically with these individuals on an outpatient basis.

ANXIETY DISORDERS

Anxiety disorders are categorized into seven groups: panic disorders, with or without agoraphobia; agoraphobia; social phobia; simple phobia; obsessive-compulsive disorder; posttraumatic stress disorder (PTSD); and generalized anxiety disorder. These illnesses are all characterized by symptoms of extreme anxiety and avoidance behavior.

Panic disorders are characterized by recurrent attacks of intense fear or discomfort that are unexpected and are not obviously associated with a situation consciously perceived as anxiety provoking by the individual. Seemingly, these attacks occur "out of the blue." Symptoms experienced during an attack are shortness of breath or smothering sensations; dizziness, unsteady feelings, or faintness; choking; palpitations or accelerated heart rate; trembling or shaking; sweating; nausea or abdominal distress; hot flashes or chills; chest pain or discomfort; fear of dying; and fear of going crazy or of doing something uncontrolled during the attack.

A *phobia* is a specific pathological fear reaction out of proportion to the stimulus. The painful feeling has been automatically and unconsciously displaced from its original internal source and has become attached to a specific external object or situation. The phobia may be focused on anything that in some manner suggests death, disease, or disaster.

Agoraphobia is a fear of open spaces. The incidence of its occurrence is increasing. The individual manifests agoraphobia by expressing dread at being left alone or going out of his home. He avoids crowds and public places because he anticipates some dreadful form of collapse. Agoraphobia is particularly incapacitating because it markedly interferes with the individual's ability to live a normal life.

Social phobia is a persistent fear of any group situation in which the person believes he is the focus of attention and in which he fears he will act in a way that will be humiliating or embarrassing. The most common social phobia is the fear of public speaking. Individuals who suffer from this fear often are terrified that they will collapse in front of the audience or will become mute.

Simple phobia is characterized by a persistent fear of a specific object or situation. The sufferer may fear open places, narrow corridors, small rooms, run-

Anxiety disorders are characterized by symptoms of extreme anxiety and avoidance behavior.

ning water, staircases, high places, various animals, or any other specific object or situation. When exposed to the feared object or situation, the individual immediately responds with symptoms of overwhelming anxiety, which disappear just as quickly when he is removed from the object or situation. Therefore, this person goes to great lengths to avoid such exposure.

An *obsession* is an undesirable but persistent thought or idea that is forced into conscious awareness. The thought is charged with great but unconscious emotional significance. Such a thought may include repetitive doubts, wishes, fears, impulses, admonitions, and commands. A *compulsion* is an unwanted urge to perform an act or a ritual that is contrary to the individual's ordinary conscious wishes or standards. All these intrusive ideas and compelling urges and fears appear in consciousness as though independently self-created.

The individual who suffers from an *obsessive-compulsive disorder* is driven to think about or to do something that he recognizes as being inappropriate or foolish. There is an excessive preoccupation with a single idea or a compulsion to carry out and to repeat over and over again certain acts against his better judgment. Underlying these compulsive or obsessive states is a personality that is usually conscience-driven, sensitive, shy, meticulous, and precise about bodily functions, dress, religious duty, and daily routine. Obsessive-compulsive disorder is a serious emotional illness because the imperative ideas so control the individual that he becomes a slave to his morbid preoccupation and can scarcely carry on his normal work and social activity.

Posttraumatic stress disorder (PTSD) is characterized by the reexperiencing of the terror associated with a psychologically distressing event that was actually experienced at an earlier time in the person's life. The nature of this event is always one outside the range of common human experiences, such as war, natural disaster, rape, or other unusual situations that threaten the survival of the person or his loved ones. The flashbacks of the experience and the accompanying terror are often precipitated by a stimulus that is linked to the original event. For example, the backfiring of an automobile can reawaken the anxiety originally experienced when the individual served in the military. This disorder was highly publicized in the late 1970s and early 1980s, since many Vietnam veterans were afflicted with it.

Generalized anxiety disorder is characterized by unrealistic or excessive anxiety and worry about two or more life circumstances that are usually developmentally determined. For example, a middle-aged parent may be consumed with fear that he will become bankrupt and that he will not live to see his child graduate from college. In contrast, adolescents may be unrealistically anxious about their performance in sports, extracurricular activities, or academics.

Although they are not anxiety disorders, a brief description of somatoform disorders and dissociative disorders is included here because they occur as dysfunctional adaptations to anxiety.

SOMATOFORM DISORDERS

Most somatoform disorders are characterized by the presence of long-standing, generalized physical symptoms in the absence of demonstrable organic pathology. These include body dysmorphic disorder, in which a person who is normal in appearance has a preoccupation with some imagined defect in appearance, such as the shape or size of his nose; hypochondriasis, in which the individual is preoccupied with the fear of having, or the belief that he has, a serious disease, as a result of numerous vague physical symptoms; somatization disorder, in which the person seeks constant medical attention for treatment of recurrent and multiple somatic complaints not due to any physical disorder; and conversion disorder.

Conversion disorder is an example of a somatoform disorder. This is a purposeful although unconscious psychological mode of reaction in which the individual uses a physical symptom as a disguise in an attempt to solve some acute problem or fulfill some desire, the open or conscious gratification of which is unacceptable to the individual. Conversion represents a primitive instinctual mechanism to which a person resorts when he is incapable of adjusting through the usual methods of rational volitional activity.

The person who uses a conversion disorder unconsciously selects a set of symptoms that symbolizes his problems. These symptoms are dictated by suggestion or by some previous acquaintance with persons who had the actual problem. Paralysis, blindness, and epilepsy are afflictions commonly presented by the person using conversion. The symptoms are physical, but no underlying pathophysiology can be demonstrated.

No matter what form the symptoms take, a characteristic feature of conversion is the individual's attitude of indifference toward his handicaps. There seems to be an air of contentment about the individual with conversion disorder. He seems to be more relieved than distressed, an attitude that at once suggests that he is more comfortable with the physical problem than with the mental torment.

Somatoform disorders are characterized by long-standing, generalized physical symptoms in the absence of demonstrable physical disease.

DISSOCIATIVE DISORDERS

Dissociative disorders are characterized by a disturbance or alteration in the functions of identity, memory, or consciousness, all of which are normally integrated in the healthy individual. The most dramatic dissociative disorder is multiple personality disorder.

Multiple personality disorder is characterized by the existence within the person of two or more distinct personalities, each of which recurrently takes control of the person's behavior. Each personality is distinct unto itself, often representing opposite attitudes and behaviors. This disorder is believed to be caused by violent trauma in early childhood, probably sexual in nature, which resulted in massive amounts of anxiety that threatened to destroy the individual. As a defense, the individual "split off" parts of the personality.

Dissociative disorders are characterized by a disturbance in the normal integration of identity, memory, or consciousness.

Not surprisingly, multiple personality disorder occurs predominately, although not exclusively, in women and is now thought to be more common than previously believed. It is unusual for the person to have only two personalities; the typical female has thirteen to fifteen and the typical male five to eight personalities.

Each personality may or may not be aware of some or all of the other personalities. Consequently, each is likely to be unable to account for periods of time during which the other personalities were in control.

Multiple personality disorder has been brought to the attention of the public through a number of case histories published as books. The best known of these are *The Three Faces of Eve* and *Sibyl*. Unfortunately, this disorder is often incorrectly associated with schizophrenia by the layperson.

CAUSATIVE FACTORS OF ANXIETY DISORDERS

Most authorities agree that anxiety disorders represent a conflict between two divergent drives or desires that have been repressed into the unconscious mind.

Anxiety disorders probably originate in the individual's early childhood experiences. Most authorities agree that the anxiety disorder represents a conflict between two divergent drives or desires that have been repressed into the unconscious mind. It is believed that the conflict revolves around primitive impulses unacceptable to the person and his simultaneous need for acceptance by significant others.

This conflict does not necessarily cause difficulty as long as the individual has sufficient psychic energy to keep it repressed. However, when energy is diverted by the necessity to cope with other stressors, the ego can no longer effect a compromise between these clashing desires and anxiety threatens to become conscious. At this point, symptoms develop as an adaptation to the emergent anxiety. This explains why symptomatology often first appears during adolescence when the individual must adapt to potent developmental stressors. In addition, the emergent, tumultuous sexuality of adolescence activates repressed unresolved sexual conflicts.

The symptoms of anxiety disorders are designed simultaneously to alleviate the anxiety and to obscure the nature of the conflict. Thus the symptoms are socially acceptable symbols of the original conflict. For example, the compulsive handwasher is conscious of his irrational fear of germs but is totally unaware of his unconscious sexual longing for his mother. By compulsively washing his hands 10 times after toileting, he experiences relief from the anxiety caused by his conflict. Unfortunately, this relief is only temporary because his action did not directly address the source of the anxiety. Thus the ritual must be repeated at frequent intervals.

It should be understood that an increasing amount of research indicates the probability that there is a physiological or neurochemical predisposition to the development of anxiety disorders. In other words some people seem to have nervous systems that are more irritable than others, making them less able to process input to attain psychological homeokinesis. Thus a vicious cycle is established wherein the physiological manifestations of anxiety that are experienced render the individual even less able to cope with emotional conflicts. Therefore a physiological predisposition may be a necessary, although not sufficient, ingredient for the establishment of a subsequent dysfunctional adaptation to anxiety. This theory in combination with the previously described beliefs about the development of anxiety disorders illustrates the inseparability of the human system and the fallacy of seeking a singular cause for this form of emotional disturbance.

ANXIOLYTIC MEDICATIONS

The word *anxiolytic* refers to the ability to relieve anxiety or simple emotional tension. Unfortunately, anxiolytic medications are often referred to as *minor tranquilizers*. This term is misleading in that these medications do not have a tranquilizing effect and are potent chemical agents that have a major effect on the body chemistry. The false belief that anxiolytic medications are minor tranquilizers undoubtedly has led to their being inappropriately prescribed for individuals who are not mentally ill but who are experiencing the anxiety associated with crisis states. In many instances these medications are abused by individuals who seek relief from anxiety. This practice is dangerous because these medications not only create a physiological disequilibrium but may also create a false sense of well-being, decreasing the person's motivation to address and solve those problems from which the anxiety stems.

Anxiolytic medications are most appropriately used to (1) treat individuals suffering from delirium tremens, (2) relieve anxiety in individuals experiencing moderate situational stress (for example, preoperatively), (3) potentiate anticonvulsant medications, (4) relieve muscle spasm, and (5) reduce high to moderate levels of endogenous anxiety to a moderate or mild level, rendering the client able to benefit from psychotherapy.

Table 17-1 provides the generic name, trade name, range of daily oral dosage in milligrams, and comments about the specific uses for some of the most commonly used anxiolytic medications.

All anxiolytic medications have the potential for creating physical and emotional dependence. Withdrawal symptoms similar to those experienced following withdrawal from barbiturates and alcohol have occurred following abrupt discontinuance of these medications, especially diazepam. Therefore the dosage of the drug should be gradually tapered before its discontinuance, especially with clients who have taken large doses of anxiolytic medications over an extended period of time.

Anxiolytic medications have a limited number of side effects. Sedation occurs when large doses are given, and the client needs to be warned not to engage in activities that require complete mental alertness. Ataxia is occasionally observed. Adverse effects are uncommon; the most serious are those in which a paradoxical reaction in the form of acute excitement, anxiety, hallucinations, in-

TABLE 17-1   *Anxiolytic medications*

Generic name	Trade name	Range of daily oral dosage (mg)	Comments
BENZODIAZEPINE GROUP			
Diazepam	Valium	6-40	Also useful for relief of skeletal muscle spasms
Alprazolam	Xanax	.75-4	Specific for relief of symptoms of anxiety
Chlordiazepoxide	Librium	15-100	Also useful for relief of preoperative anxiety
Clorazepate dipotassium	Tranxene, Tranxene-SD	7.5-60	Also useful to potentiate anticonvulsant medications; once optimum dosage is achieved, sustained-action tablets are recommended
Halazepam	Paxipam	60-160	
Lorazepam	Ativan	2-10	Useful for relief of anxiety associated with depression
Oxazepam	Serax	30-120	Also useful for relief of anxiety associated with alcohol withdrawal
Prazepam	Centrax	20-60	

creased muscle spasticity, insomina, or rage occurs. The medication should be discontinued if these symptoms appear.

PSYCHOTHERAPY

There is no question that anxiolytic medications have been helpful in reducing tension and providing the client with a degree of emotional comfort. In addition, behavior modification and desensitization are recognized as efficient and effective intervention techniques. However, the only permanent relief for persons suffering from intolerable anxiety and fear lies in discovering the basic cause of the problem and helping the individual understand the actual source of his symptoms. This is achieved through the treatment technique of *psychotherapy*. Psychotherapy can be conducted by any prepared mental health professional. As nurses gain additional knowledge and skill in this treatment modality, they sometimes assume responsibility for its implementation.

Any procedure that promotes the development of courage, inner security, and self-confidence can be called psychotherapy. However, the traditional use of this term is limited to sustained interpersonal interactions between the psychotherapist and client where the goal is to help the client to develop behaviors that are more functional. Psychotherapy is not a fixed technique; it is more an art than a science, and its methods must be adapted and modified to fit the individual situation. In plain language, it is a form of mental exploration. It is universally acknowledged that one cannot standardize psychotherapy, that it must be individualized, and that it will vary from client to client.

Psychotherapy is a sustained interpersonal interaction between the therapist and client where the goal is to help the client develop more functional behaviors.

Psychotherapy falls into two general types: supportive psychotherapy and "uncovering" or "insight" psychotherapy. *Supportive psychotherapy* helps the individual cope with his problems and includes such techniques as diagnosis, advice, education, guidance, counseling, and assurance. *Uncovering* or *insight psychotherapy* involves exploring and bringing to consciousness the source of repressed and suppressed conflicts and experiences that operate at unconscious levels to cause anxiety. Uncovering psychotherapy gives meaning to abnormal or irrational feelings and dysfunctional behaviors.

The type of psychotherapy used is dependent on the therapist's assessment of the interrelationship of a number of variables. Chief among these variables are the extent and severity of the client's dysfunction, the client's goals, his intellectual ability, and his personal and interpersonal resources. Generally the more mentally ill the client is, the fewer resources he has, and the less intellectually capable he is, the more he will be a candidate for supportive psychotherapy. Supportive psychotherapy requires the psychotherapist to assume a direct role by offering direction and guidance. The client may not develop an understanding of the dynamics underlying his behavior, but he can learn behaviors that are more functional.

Clients who give evidence of available ego strength, a viable support system, and at least average intelligence can often benefit from uncovering or insight psychotherapy. During this type of psychotherapy, the client is encouraged to talk about his life experiences. He is encouraged to talk freely about anything that comes to his mind, as long as he relates his own ideas and concerns. This random talk allows the client to follow freely the associations that come into his mind and is accurately described as *mental ventilation.* The therapist will note that the client dismisses quickly or avoids mentioning certain occasions and events except in a superficial way. These sensitive areas are then explored more fully. The client is encouraged to talk about them freely until they no longer cause excess emotion, a process known as *desensitization.*

The client is guided to an understanding of how his repressed feelings are related to his behavior. This is done in a simple, clear style, thereby helping the client to gain insight into the exact nature of his problem. Thus begins the process of reeducation.

It should be noted that a client who initially requires supportive psychotherapy may be able to increase his self-esteem to the point where uncovering or insight psychotherapy is indicated. A skilled psychotherapist has the ability to make this assessment and to respond accordingly.

Regardless of the type of psychotherapy employed, the client is encouraged to face his distressing problems; he is urged to think of them instead of running away from them, to become familiar with them rather than to "forget" them, and to approach their solution in a candid, open manner. He is encouraged to take an active part in his own therapy. If all goes well, he should take more and more constructive steps in the management of his own treatment. He can then

The measure of therapeutic success is the degree to which the psychotherapist gradually becomes decreasingly necessary for the client.

answer some of his own questions and make his own decisions. The therapist measures therapeutic success by the degree to which she makes herself less and less necessary.

The most important element in any psychotherapeutic process is the relationship between the therapist and the client. The client must have confidence in the therapist and some respect for the therapist's knowledge and experience. A word of assurance alone may be the deciding factor in relieving many anxious clients of their fears. Such a relationship is dependent on a positive rapport between the therapist and the client.

A very important aspect of the therapist-client relationship is the unconscious attitude of the client toward his therapist. The therapist is cast into a variety of roles, including that of a parent. The client's attitude may be competitive or even erotic. This shifting toward the therapist of desires, feelings, and relations originally experienced by the client with his own parents, siblings, and other persons is known as *transference*. Hence every nuance of feeling, ranging from trustful dependence to open hostility, may be directed toward the therapist. When the client's attitude toward the therapist appears to be favorable, the transference is regarded as being positive. Resistant or antagonistic attitudes of the client toward the therapist imply a negative transference. The client's transference reaction to the therapist may elicit an unconscious counterresponse by the therapist. This attitude of the therapist toward the client is called *countertransference*.

The development of a transference reaction between the client and the psychotherapist is often viewed as a positive sign, for it indicates that the therapist has become significant to the client, thereby establishing the potential for the client to benefit from a corrective emotional experience. For example, if the client responds to the psychotherapist in the clinging, dependent manner that he learned in early life was necessary to maintain his mother's love, the psychotherapist can subtly but consistently encourage the client to make his own decisions while still conveying approval. Through this process the client can learn that it is possible for him to take steps toward independence without jeopardizing the highly valued relationship with the psychotherapist. The client may or may not be helped to become aware of his transference reaction and the process engaged in by the therapist to use the transference therapeutically.

A countertransference reaction is rarely, if ever, seen as having therapeutic potential except insofar as it provides the therapist with an understanding of the psychodynamics underlying the client's behavior. In other words, by becoming aware of her own reaction to the client, the therapist can better understand the unconscious purpose of the client's behavioral patterns. An example of a nontherapeutic countertransference is when the client behaves toward the psychotherapist as if the therapist were his parent (transference) and the psychotherapist unconsciously responds by treating the client as if he were a child for whom all decisions need to be made (countertransference). Since both transference and countertransference occur on a unconscious level, and since countertransference is not desirable, many teachers of psychotherapy require their students to undergo psychotherapy themselves as a means of discovering their own emotional vulnerabilities and increasing their own overall level of self-awareness. Whether or not a psychotherapist has undergone personal psychotherapy, supervision of psychotherapy by a skilled colleague is necessary to identify and prevent countertransference. The occurrence of the transference and countertransference phenomena is a testimony to the fundamentally human nature of the psychotherapeutic process.

In summary, the success of the psychotherapeutic process depends to a large extent on the quality of the interpersonal experience between the client and the therapist. The therapy can be a success only if the therapist succeeds in motivating the client toward promoting his own well-being on his own behalf rather than to please another person.

> The most important element in any psychotherapeutic process is the quality of the interpersonal experience between the client and the therapist.

NURSING CARE OF INDIVIDUALS WITH AN ANXIETY DISORDER
Nursing assessment

Although each anxiety disorder has its unique features, it is possible to cite some commonalities about the behavior of all persons suffering from anxiety disorders. The following discussion is organized around the human processes introduced in Chapter 9. Although behaviors in each category are presented as separate entities, it should be understood that they are highly interrelated and are adaptations to similar stressors. Further, in many instances behavior designed as an adaptation to one stressor becomes a stressor itself in another dimension.

Activity processes. The motor behavior of the individual with an anxiety disorder may or may not be altered. However, individuals who are highly anxious often exhibit motor restlessness in the forms of pacing and wringing of their hands. Persons with obsessive-compulsive disorder often display ritualistic behaviors in which an activity is repeated in exactly the same manner for a specified number of times. For example, to be at work on time one business executive arose 3 hours earlier than necessary because she was compelled to return to her house from her car ten times to check that every window was closed and locked.

The individual suffering from an anxiety disorder often does not voluntarily engage in recreational activities because of emotional and physical fatigue and an inability to control the environment in which the activity takes place. One avid baseball player who developed a phobia about dogs had to completely stop playing ball because of his fear that a dog would wander onto the field and send him into a panic.

Self-care may or may not be affected, but it is always altered when the focus of the anxiety relates to a self-care activity. For example, an individual who is phobic about running water must go to great lengths to bathe from a basin rather than taking a shower.

Regardless of the severity of the anxiety the individual experiences, he will almost always report changes in sleep patterns. Usually the anxious individual has a great deal of difficulty falling asleep but once asleep, has difficulty getting up in the morning. Regardless of the amount of sleep he has had, he reports constant fatigue.

Cognition processes. The individual suffering from an anxiety disorder maintains contact with reality. In fact, this characteristic serves as a stressor, since the person is often well aware that his fears and behavior are not based on reality and that he may appear foolish to others.

Individuals experiencing obsessive-compulsive disorder will report the existence of one or more obsessive thoughts that torment them and over which they feel they have no control.

Ecological processes. Home maintenance is often altered. Since the individual with an anxiety disorder is chronically fatigued, in some instances altered home maintenance is reflected by a disorderly, dirty environment. In other cases the person is driven to maintain an immaculately clean and tidy environment in an effort to ward off anxiety resulting from a phobia about dirt or germs.

Emotional processes. The outstanding feature of anxiety disorders is the individual's awareness of anxiety, either continuously or in response to a specific object or situation. The person will report overwhelming feelings of impending doom. These feelings are so distressing that he will go to any length to avoid or diminish them. In extreme situations, individuals have been known to attempt suicide, not for the purpose of ending their lives, but rather with the goal of relieving their anxiety.

Interpersonal processes. The interpersonal relationships of persons with anxiety disorders are frequently strained. Family and friends have had much experience in attempting to reassure the client, all to no avail. Furthermore, they may have had increasing difficulty tolerating the person's idiosyncratic ways. For example, one middle-aged secretary suffering from a fear of germs was forced to share an office with several others in a typing pool. She offended her co-workers by covering her coffee mug with plastic wrap between sips to protect its contents from germs in the air. She also scrupulously cleaned her typewriter keys with a strong disinfectant every morning in case someone had touched them in her absence. When this woman's rituals became so time-consuming that she was unable to complete her assigned work, her job was threatened and she sought help from the local mental health clinic.

Perception processes. The individual with an anxiety disorder often exhibits a hyperalertness to environmental stimuli. He is easily startled by an unexpected movement and experiences increased anxiety when he is unable to control the events in his environment.

The self-esteem of a person who suffers from an anxiety disorder is often low because he believes that he should be able to control his behavioral and emotional responses to anxiety-producing stimuli, although he is simultaneously aware that he is incapable of doing so. Consequently, he is likely to be self-critical and report that he is "weak" and has little self-control or self-discipline.

Physiological processes. The individual with an anxiety disorder almost always has many physical complaints that are generally focused on the vital organs of the body. Tightness of the stomach, fast-beating heart, a feeling that the heart may suddenly stop, no appetite, loose bowels, and a heavy feeling in the abdomen are frequent complaints offered by the individual seeking assistance. Palpitation, a feeling of shortness of breath, compression sensations in the head, tight sensations in the throat, numbness in the extremities, and a constant feeling of exhaustion are other typical experiences reported by individuals suffering from anxiety disorders. These symptoms usually frighten the person; he cannot concentrate on his work, feels depressed, and harbors fears of sudden death or insanity. Frequently many of these symptoms appear at one time and cause the individual to respond with a panic reaction or acute fear. Consequently, anxiety about the anxiety compounds the stress.

Valuation processes. Helplessness, hopelessness, and powerlessness over the symptoms associated with the anxiety disorder are often reported by the client. In instances in which the symptoms are severe, the individual may attempt to relieve his anxiety by engaging in behaviors normally outside his value system. For example, many anxious individuals attempt to self-medicate by drinking alcohol, which may provide some temporary relief from anxiety. If the person's value system dictates abstinence from alcohol, his resorting to this measure further compounds his anxiety.

Nursing diagnosis

As with all nursing diagnoses, the nursing diagnoses for the individual with an anxiety disorder are based on the themes identified during the assessment phase of the nursing process. Categories of human responses from the ANA Classification of Human Responses of Concern for Psychiatric–Mental Health Nursing Practice that may be specifically applicable to individuals with Anxiety Disorders include the following:

1.1.2 Altered Motor Behavior
1.2.2 Altered Recreation Patterns
1.3.1 Potential for Alteration in Self-Care
1.4.2 Altered Sleep/Arousal Patterns
2.6.2 Altered Thought Processes

Assessment of the person who is anxious often reveals motor restlessness; disinterest in recreational activities; changes in sleep patterns; obsessive thoughts; either a disorderly or a very clean home environment; overwhelming feelings of impending doom; strained interpersonal relationships; low self-esteem; numerous physical complaints; and a sense of helplessness, hopelessness, and powerlessness.

3.3.2   Altered Home Maintenance
4.1.2   Altered Feeling State
5.5.2   Altered Role Performance
5.5.3   Ineffective Individual Coping
5.7.2   Altered Social Interaction
6.1.2   Altered Attention
6.3.2   Altered Self-Concept
8.1.2   Altered Meaningfulness
8.3.1   Potential for Alteration in Values

NANDA nursing diagnostic categories that may be specifically applicable to the individual with an anxiety disorder include:

3.1.1   Impaired Social Interaction
3.2.1   Altered Role Performance
5.1.1.1   Ineffective Individual Coping
5.1.1.1.2   Defensive Coping
6.1.1.2.1   Fatigue
6.2.1   Sleep Pattern Disturbance
6.3.1.1   Diversional Activity Deficit
6.4.1.1   Impaired Home Maintenance Management
7.1.2   Self-Esteem Disturbance
7.3.1   Hopelessness
7.3.2   Powerlessness
8.3   Altered Thought Processes
9.3.1   Anxiety
9.3.2   Fear

To develop a nursing diagnosis that fulfills its function of providing direction for planning nursing care, the nurse is encouraged to postulate and state etiologic or antecedent factors for each human response and connect the two phrases by using the term "related to." For example:

1.2.2   Altered Recreation Patterns related to fear of going outdoors

Planning and implementing nursing care

The plan for nursing care is derived from the nursing diagnoses and includes the objectives of the care, the nursing actions, and outcome criteria. To be effective the plan needs to be highly individualized. The suggestions that follow should be seen as general guidelines to be used if they are appropriate to the client's needs.

In general, the objectives of all nursing care for the individual with an anxiety disorder should relate to helping him lower his anxiety and/or to develop functional adaptations to his anxiety.

Since the client's nursing diagnoses are often interrelated, stemming as they do from similar etiologies or antecedents, the student will see that the appropriate nursing actions are also interrelated. In other words, by intervening in one dimension, the nurse will also affect other dimensions.

Many health professionals who work skillfully and empathically with psychotic individuals find that they are not nearly so effective when giving care to those who express anxiety through physical symptoms or ritualistic behavior. A large part of the difficulty in dealing with anxious persons originates in an unconscious attitude toward persons suffering from these problems and in a failure to understand the true nature of the illness. Because such an individual is aware of his surroundings, is not carrying on a conversation with unseen people, and complains of physical symptoms that have no organic basis, some professionals may feel unsympathetic toward him and may believe that he is "an attention getter" and that he could "snap out of it" if he really tried.

It is important to realize that all symptoms stemming from anxiety disorders develop because of an overwhelming *unconscious* conflict and that the symptoms have great unconscious significance. The word unconscious has been stressed, since it is necessary to realize that the individual does not clearly understand why the symptom has developed nor what he is gaining by using the symptom repeatedly. He does realize that the symptom helps relieve unbearable anxiety and tension.

To make an intelligent and therapeutic plan of care the nurse needs to understand the nature of the person's conflict and the meaning of his symptoms. The plan for care and treatment should be developed collaboratively by the staff who will be involved with the individual. The type of treatment required and the goals to be established should be developed in conjunction with the individual himself. Whatever the treatment goals may be, the individual requires a consistent approach from all staff with whom he will be involved.

Activity processes. The individual suffering from morbid fears and compulsions usually presents a challenging nursing problem. Some nurses who have no understanding of the forces that play a part in developing such symptoms may assume the attitude that the many maneuvers of the individual are ridiculous. Nurses have been known to force a phobic person to touch a doorknob even though it was well known that he was morbidly afraid of the dirt and germs he believed he would contact by touching the object. Other nurses have made it impossible for a client to get into the bathroom to carry out the handwashing rituals that were so important to him in releasing tensions and fears.

When phobic and compulsive individuals are not allowed to carry out the procedures they feel are necessary, they have no way of releasing tension. A high level of unreleased tension may culminate in a panic state. Nurses should make it possible for the individual to carry out the anxiety-releasing rituals he has developed. The rituals carried on by these individuals are essential for them if they are to develop a feeling of security in the situation. Because such rituals are time-consuming, time must be allowed for the individual to perform his ritualistic maneuvers.

The nurse can be helpful to the anxious client by helping him to develop interests outside himself.

One of the most helpful approaches to the care of anxious clients is to assist them to develop interest outside themselves. Thus recreational and occupational therapy are significant in their treatment. Many anxiety-ridden individuals have never been able to enter into games or group activities. It is important to help them learn to play games and to participate in group activities. This provides opportunities to release tensions as well as to develop new interests. Recreational and occupational activities are usually more successful if they are focused on interests that the individual has had in the past.

In suggesting that an anxious person participate in some social activity, it is unwise to ask, "Would you like to go swimming with the group?" Such a question will often bring the flat answer *no* or a long recital about why the individual cannot possibly go. A more effective approach would be, "The group is going swimming. I hope that you will go with us." If the objective is to get the individual to participate in a game of table tennis, more positive results will be obtained if the tennis paddle is placed in the client's hand by the nurse, who might say, "We need one more person to play this game. Come and play." This approach is more apt to elicit participation than asking if he wishes to play.

Interpersonal processes. Short-term hospitalization is usually helpful for persons who exhibit severely dysfunctional behavior because the environment is neutral, they are removed from the significant members of the family who may be associated with much emotional tension, and they are able to feel more secure where the routine is simple, makes few demands, and can be fairly accurately anticipated.

Such individuals need a warm, friendly, empathic nurse who accepts them as people in need of help and who helps them feel that they are worthwhile human beings. Scolding or sarcastic remarks will serve only to reinforce their need to protect themselves by the use of their symptoms.

Encouraging the anxious individual to talk about his concerns and feelings is an important task for the nurse.

Some nurses ignore symptoms that stem from anxiety, and in many instances this becomes synonymous with ignoring the individual himself. Since the anxious person is using symptoms to make a bid for help, ignoring him increases his need to use the symptoms more frequently.

Encouraging the anxious individual to talk about his concerns and feelings is an important aspect of his care. However, the nurse should avoid asking, "How are you today?" For anxious persons this question is often an invitation for another outpouring of physical complaints. A much more helpful way to begin a conversation might be to comment on some neutral topic that is of mutual interest.

Increased self-esteem results when the anxious individual is given the opportunity to participate in activities in which he can succeed.

Perception processes. Many uniformed health care professionals, as well as the individual's relatives and friends, attempt to discuss his symptoms reasonably in the hope of altering his behavior. This kind of pressure does nothing to help the individual and may actually cause him to feel more anxious and may lower his self-esteem further.

It is helpful if the anxious individual is provided with an opportunity to

NURSING CARE PLAN

A ritualistic individual

CASE FORMULATION

Herbert B., 47 years of age, and his wife, Jane, 46 years old, came to the community mental health center to ask for help. Mr. B. was well oriented and intelligent, had good insight, and otherwise appeared to be mentally normal. He gave the following history.

An only child, Mr. B. reported that he remembers his childhood as being uneventful. However, he also stated that his mother was a meticulous housekeeper who was known in her community as fanatical about maintaining correct standards of behavior and observing religious customs.

During his college days he had become emotionally upset and had worried excessively. His pastor was consulted, and after several conferences he was able to resume his schoolwork and graduated at the age of 21 as an accountant. He stated that he had always been very conscientious, worried a great deal about body cleanliness, and was known for his concern about keeping his room and clothing in perfect order. He was always prompt in appearing at his office and never left his desk before 5 PM. His fellow workers regarded him as very fussy, and his employer always remarked about the neatness of his desk and files—a comment that greatly pleased him. At home any irregularity in household routine upset him. His wife was fully aware of his rigid regard for rules and his scrupulousness. She spoke freely about the fact that their marital relations were unsatisfactory and disturbing. She had given up any hope of improving the situation by discussing it with him because he became extremely anxious when she introduced the topic. She also stated that she was "thankful" they never had any children, since she was sure that the "mess" that children normally make in the house would be intolerable for her husband.

Four months before he came to the center, Mr. B. had been assigned the responsibility of making out the income tax report for his firm, which dealt in stocks and bonds. This assignment was made on March 1, and he realized that he had but 6 weeks before the returns were to be filed. He worked under great pressure, and almost every day he remained in the office until late at night. With a day to spare, he entered the final figures on a roll of paper from an adding machine. Badly in need of sleep and rest, he seized this roll, thrust it into his overcoat pocket, and dashed for the midnight bus. He intended to show the slip of paper to his wife as evidence that his job was completed. On reaching his home he could not find the roll. In a frenzy he searched his clothing and ran out on the street searching the sidewalk, but failed to find it. He was put to bed in an anxious, fearful state and remained under a physician's care for several weeks.

On returning to work he found that he had developed an overwhelming compulsion. He could no longer pass a piece of crumpled paper on the floor or sidewalk without picking it up and inspecting it. During rush hour he was greatly humiliated and embarassed by the necessity of bending over and picking up odd bits of paper. On several occasions he was knocked down by a hurrying passerby while carrying out this compulsion. A wastebasket full of discarded paper literally threw him into a panic. His only relief was obtained by waiting until after office hours when he could go over each item piece by piece. His physician recommended treatment in the community mental health center.

Nursing assessment

It is significant that Herbert B.'s mother was a fastidious housekeeper and fanatical about observing religious customs and maintaining correct standards of behavior. Undoubtedly such a mother would insist that a child achieve perfection in toilet training at a very early age. In addition, she would rear him to behave in a rigidly correct manner and would covertly encourage him to repress instinctual thoughts and desires.

Continued.

NURSING CARE PLAN—cont'd

A young man who at the age of 21 is known to be overly concerned about orderliness, is overly conscientious, and is worried about bodily cleanliness is already well on the road to developing compulsive symptoms to control unconscious anxiety by employing persistently repetitive acts. This behavior, like all human behavior, has purpose and meaning for the individual who employs it, even though the forces producing it are unconscious.

Despite Herbert's early tendencies to be upset by household irregularities, he married. He and his wife managed to work out a relationship that could be tolerated. However, according to his wife their sexual relationship was unsatisfactory and such an upsetting topic to her husband that she avoided discussing it. His basic problem focused, in part at least, on his unresolved conflict about his role as a marital partner. This conflict was relieved to some extent by his fastidious attitude toward his body. Such problems probably originated in the attitudes that were learned during the habit-training period.

It was not until he was 47 that Herbert's symptoms became so severe that he required treatment. This was precipitated by the loss of a scrap of paper on which was recorded a final total of a complicated accounting problem he had been assigned to complete. It is interesting that he was attempting to elicit his wife's approval for a successful task accomplished. Since he did not have her approval as a sexual partner, her approval about some other aspect of life was very necessary. The loss of the paper probably represented much more than simply the loss of a list of figures. Symbolically it must have represented the loss of love and approval. This would account for his extreme fear and anxiety. The tax report had been completed before he left the office. Thus there is little doubt that a duplicate of the figures could have been found. The loss must have been symbolic of the loss of something more important and irreplaceable.

In compulsive individuals the repetitive act has a symbolic significance reminiscent of a magic ritual that is designed to eradicate the possible effect of unacceptable instinctual impulses. It also represents a type of self-punishment, since compulsive acts are recognized by the individual as being unreasonable and ridiculous. Despite the individual's partial insight, the tension and anxiety mount until the urge to repeat the act to control the tension becomes irresistible.

Like most severely anxious individuals, Mr. B. was well oriented, intelligent, and intellectually normal except for his compulsive behavior. This is an example of an individual whose personality is intact except in the one area that is involved with the compulsive behavior. However, despite the normal aspects of his personality, he was almost totally incapacitated by the need to examine every scrap of paper.

Nursing diagnoses

The assessment data, including present behavior, past life experiences, and an understanding of the underlying dynamics, led to the development of the following two pairs of nursing diagnoses for Herbert B. The first of each pair is from the Classification of Human Responses of Concern for Psychiatric–Mental Health Nursing Practice; the second is from the approved NANDA Diagnostic Categories.

5.5.3	Ineffective Individual Coping related to anxiety stemming from unconscious conflicts
OR	
5.1.1.1	Ineffective Individual Coping related to anxiety stemming from unconscious conflicts
5.5.2	Altered Role Performance related to client's inability to discuss the couple's sexual relationship
OR	
3.2.1	Altered Role Performance related to client's inability to discuss the couple's sexual relationship

NURSING CARE PLAN—cont'd

Planning and implementing nursing care for *Herbert B.*

The boxed material on p. 278 illustrates a nursing care plan for Herbert B. After assessing his needs and formulating nursing diagnoses, the nurse participated in a meeting of the mental health team that discussed Mr. B. As a result of this discussion, a collaborative decision was made not to hospitalize him. Rather, the psychiatrist prescribed diazepam, and the nurse made an appointment for him to see a staff psychologist for psychotherapy three times a week. In addition, she made an appointment with him for 1 hour twice a month after one of his therapy sessions. Although the nurse's goal was not to engage in psychotherapy with this client, she did have the goal of monitoring his reaction to his medication and to the family system. She was aware that as Herbert B. was able to change his behavior, his relationship with his wife would also be altered.

The nurse maintained close communication with the psychologist who was engaged in psychotherapy with the client to be able to reinforce the direction he was taking and not inadvertently interfere with their relationship.

Evaluation

After 4 weeks of biweekly appointments with Herbert B. the nurse was assured that he was taking his medication regularly and was not experiencing adverse reactions. Although he reported that he still felt a mild degree of anxiety almost continuously, he was able to overcome the urge to examine every scrap of paper he saw.

As Herbert B.'s behavior changed as a result of increased insight, family disequilibrium ensued. By the end of 4 months of psychotherapy Herbert B. had developed a beginning awareness of the relationship between his compulsion and his early childhood experiences, especially those with his mother. Although he still maintained his fastidious behavior, he grew to understand that his fear of sexual relations with his wife was related to his unconscious association of her with his mother. He became able to consider initiating a conversation with his wife about their sexual relationship. However, the first time he introduced the subject, his wife rejected his attempt by saying she did not have time to talk that evening. The nurse understood this behavior as a signal of family disequilibrium and communicated this to the mental health team. At this time the decision was made to offer this couple conjoint therapy in addition to continuing individual psychotherapy for Herbert B. It was also decided that there was no longer any reason for him to continue meeting with the nurse.

As a result of these decisions, the nurse made an appointment for Mr. and Mrs. B. with the staff social worker and made plans to discontinue her routine appointments with Mr. B. in four more visits. Even though she was not engaged in psychotherapy with this client, the nurse understood that their relationship was meaningful to him and must not be terminated abruptly or thoughtlessly.

Continued.

NURSING CARE PLAN—cont'd

NURSING CARE PLAN FOR *Herbert B.*

Nursing diagnosis	Objective	Nursing actions	Outcome criteria
5.5.3 Ineffective Individual Coping related to anxiety stemming from unconscious conflicts OR 5.1.1.1 Ineffective Individual Coping related to anxiety stemming from unconscious conflicts	To decrease anxiety	Teach client about actions and side effects of prescribed antianxiety medication Meet twice a month with client to monitor his response to medication Keep wastebaskets out of room in which nurse and client meet Listen attentively to client's complaints	Within 1 month client will give evidence of taking medication regularly and will not experience incapacitating side effects Within 4 months client will give evidence of decreased anxiety by: Reporting a decrease in anxiety Being able to resist urge to examine scraps of paper Not developing a new compulsion
	To assist client to develop insight into underlying unconscious conflicts	Refer to staff psychologist for psychotherapy Meet twice a month with client's psychotherapist	Client meets regularly with psychotherapist Psychotherapist keeps nurse apprised of process of his relationship with client
5.5.2 Altered Role Performance related to client's inability to discuss the couple's sexual relationship OR 3.2.1 Altered Role Performance related to client's inability to discuss the couple's sexual relationship	To increase meaningful communication between client and his wife	View family as a system Understand that as client alters his behavior system will enter disequilibrium Monitor degree of family equilibrium and report to mental health team Rehearse with client ways he might initiate conversations with his wife using techniques such as role playing	Within 4 months the client will report attempts to communicate meaningfully with his wife

succeed in the activities in which he participates. This is important because these individuals need help in building self-esteem and self-confidence. Giving deserved praise and recognition for activities performed well is one way of reassuring and encouraging them.

Physiological processes. It is usually wise to listen completely and with an accepting attitude when the anxious person describes his physical symptoms. Comments should be directed toward eliciting more information about the complaints. It is important to remember that these individuals can and do become physically ill and deserve medical attention if there is any reasonable doubt about the cause of the complaint. However, hospitalization on a medical unit may be unfortunate for some persons who have already focused most of their attention on physical symptoms that have no organic basis. Such individuals may become more tense, anxious, and fearful in a setting that emphasizes physical problems.

It is important to realize that the discomfort and pain of which the individual complains is actually present even though there is no organic basis that can explain the existence of the symptoms. Experts are beginning to recognize that fear plays a significant role in causing pain. Since fear is prominent in the symptomatology of many anxiety-ridden people, it is not difficult to realize that they actually feel the pain of which they complain. It is important to understand that emotionally conditioned pain is as distressing to bear as is pain that results from true physical disease.

> Listening completely and with an accepting attitude is important when assisting an anxious individual to deal with his pain.

END NOTE

This chapter focuses on the nursing care of individuals with anxiety disorders. In addition to a desription of the symptoms exhibited by individuals with anxiety disorders, a brief discussion of the symptoms associated with somatoform disorders and dissociative disorders is included because these disorders also represent dysfunctional adaptations to anxiety. Anxiolytic medications commonly used to treat these clients are discussed, as is the treatment technique of psychotherapy. A case formulation from which a hypothetical nursing care plan is derived, implemented, and evaluated is presented for an individual who displays ritualistic behavior.

SUGGESTED SOURCES OF ADDITIONAL INFORMATION

Calarco MM: Managing Myra's madness, Am J Nurs 89(3):346, March 1989.

Curtis GC and Glitz DA: Neuroendocrine findings in anxiety disorders, Endocrinol Metabol Clin North Am 17(1):131, March 1988.

Davis J: Treatment of a medical phobia including desensitization administered by a significant other, J Psychosoc Nurs Ment Health Serv 20:6, August 1982.

DiMotto JW: Relaxation, Am J Nurs 84:754, 1984.

Gagan J: Imagery: an overview with suggested application for nursing, Perspect Psychiatr Care 22:20, January-March 1984.

Greenberg W: The multiple personality, Perspect Psychiatr Care 20:100, July-September 1982.

Hagerty BK: Obsessive-compulsive behavior: an overview of four psychological frameworks, J Psychosoc Nurs Ment Health Serv 19:37, January 1981.

Jorn N: Repression in a case of multiple personality disorder, Perspect Psychiatr Care 20:105, July-September 1982.

Karl GT: Survival skills for psychic trauma, J Psychosoc Nurs Ment Health Serv 27(4):15, April 1989.

Kent F: Coping with phobias, New York, 1980, Harper & Row, Publishers.

Knowles R: Dealing with feelings: managing anxiety, Am J Nurs 81:110, 1981.

Moores A: Frightened of fear, Nurs Times 83(13):34, April 1, 1987.

Peplau HE: The power of the dissociative state, J Psychosoc Nurs Ment Health Serv 23(8):31, August 1985.

Tilley S and Weighill VE: How nurse therapists assess and contribute to the management of alcohol and sedative drug use among anxious patients, J Adv Nurs 11(5):499, September 1986.

Individuals with psychophysiological disorders

18

LEARNING OBJECTIVES

After studying this chapter the student will be able to:

○ Describe the characteristics of psychophysiological disorders.

○ Discuss the causative factors associated with psychophysiological disorders.

○ Describe behaviors the nurse is most likely to observe in an individual experiencing a psychophysiological disorder.

○ State examples of nursing diagnoses likely to be applicable to an individual who is experiencing a psychophysiological disorder.

○ Develop a hypothetical plan of nursing care for an individual who is experiencing a psychophysiological disorder.

The phenomenon referred to as *somatization* is a process whereby an individual's feelings, emotional needs, or conflicts are manifested physiologically. When the need, feeling, or conflict is on a conscious level, the somatization process occurs as an adaptation to the stress of the emotion. When the emotion is on an unconscious level, somatization also serves the function of defending the individual against conscious awareness of the nature of the emotion. In either instance the process of somatization supports the widely accepted belief that the functions and reactions of the mind and body are inextricably related.

When the somatization process is sustained and organic changes occur, the individual is said to have a psychophysiological disorder. Although it is important for the nurse to be aware of the emotional concomitants of all physical illnesses, it is imperative that she have some understanding of the etiological dynamics of those physical illnesses believed to be psychophysiological disorders.

Only with this understanding will the nurse be able to provide care likely to meet the individual's needs.

HISTORICAL PERSPECTIVE

Medical historians have found evidence that from the earliest times human beings have known that there is a relationship between the mind and the body. Beliefs about the nature of this relationship have changed over time, however. For example, some primitive people believed that deviant behavior and physical illnesses were caused by the invasion of the individual by evil spirits. This belief led to the practice of trephination, in which holes were bored into the skull of the afflicted person to facilitate departure of the evil spirit. Accompanying this surgical procedure were elaborate rituals performed by a revered member of the community known as a priest, a witch doctor, or a shaman. This procedure was sufficiently successful to justify its continued use over many centuries. Modern authorities believe that the socially sanctioned unconditional trust in the healer was the primary factor in reversing the disease process. The importance of this factor in the healing process is still seen as basic to effective intervention, whether it be physical or psychological.

Other beliefs that have supported the mind-body relationship were that deviant behavior and some forms of physical illness were caused by the individual's sinning and that a physical imbalance of body fluids or humors caused emotional problems.

Early beliefs about the mind-body relationship attempted to postulate a singular cause of either physical or behavioral dysfunction. None of these early theories took a holistic view of humans as interrelated systems in which alterations in one component inevitably result in compensatory alterations throughout the entire system, which, in turn, affect the entire system. Such is the case with psychophysiological disorders.

In the past psychophysiological disorders were referred to as *psychosomatic illnesses*. Unfortunately, this term has been incorrectly incorporated into the language as meaning that the physical illness is not real but rather is a product of the person's imagination designed to elicit attention and sympathy. No belief could be farther from the truth, and the health care team must never assume that persons with these disorders are not really sick or are merely looking for attention through their physical symptoms.

PSYCHOPHYSIOLOGICAL DISORDERS

Psychophysiological disorders are believed to have an emotional cause, to affect one body system, and to involve innervation of the autonomic nervous system. Affected individuals present a physical illness in which there is evidence of organic alteration. They are often acutely ill and in fact may have life-threatening exacerbations of the illness.

The individual often has little or no insight into the emotional conflicts un-

Psychophysiological disorders are believed to have an emotional cause, to affect one body system, and to involve the autonomic nervous system.

derlying his illness and may resent any implication that such is present. Understandably he is very distressed by his physical symptoms and seeks medical treatment of them, unlike those individuals suffering from a conversion disorder. Because his symptoms interfere markedly with his ability to function and may be life-threatening, he is often highly motivated to diminish or erase them. Consequently, he can be helped to identify the relationship between stressors and exacerbations of the illness even without gaining an awareness of the unconscious emotional conflict.

It is beyond the scope of this text to discuss each of the psychophysiological disorders in depth. The student should be aware that there are many excellent references available from which much may be learned about each of these disease entities. Discussion in this chapter will be limited to the ones most commonly encountered in general nursing practice and illustrative of different body system involvement.

Gastrointestinal system

Peptic ulcer is a very common syndrome in a highly industrialized society such as the United States. The diagnosis of peptic ulcer encompasses both gastric ulcers and duodenal ulcers, although there is evidence that emotional factors play a larger role in the development of duodenal ulcers, which tend to occur more in men than in women and in younger age groups. Duodenal ulcers stem from sustained gastric hypermotility and marked increase in gastric secretions, which eventually erode the lining of the stomach. Clinically the individual complains of epigastric pain that occurs within 1 to 4 hours after the last meal and is relieved by eating or by taking antacids. If alterations in diet and taking nonprescription remedies do not help, the person is likely to seek medical help, since the pain becomes severe enough that it cannot be ignored. Hospitalization may be necessary, either to establish the diagnosis through testing or for treatment. Although medical treatment is always conservative if possible, the presence of bleeding or intractable pain may indicate the need for surgical removal of the affected part of the stomach or severance of a branch of the vagus nerve. Unfortunately, when this occurs it is not uncommon for the individual to subsequently develop another even more severe form of psychophysiological disorder.

The personality characteristics of a person who develops a peptic ulcer are those of a person who sees himself and is seen by others as strong, independent, hard working, and unemotional. Despite their occupational successes, these persons are tormented by feelings of not having done well enough and constantly strive to achieve even higher goals. Authorities believe that underlying these behaviors are strong dependency needs in conflict with the individual's self-image that therefore cannot be directly expressed. If these needs are met, it is a result of fortuitous accident rather than goal-directed behavior.

The initial onset of the illness as well as subsequent exacerbations tend to

The diagnosis of peptic ulcer includes both gastric ulcers and duodenal ulcers, although emotional factors play a considerable role in the development of duodenal ulcers.

be precipitated by stressful life events that bring the dependency-independency conflict closer to the surface of consciousness. One man experienced his first episode of duodenal ulcer attack at the time of his marriage when he left his parents' home to establish with his wife a home of their own. Despite the fact that he married an attractive, caring woman whom he loved very much, the very act of marriage abruptly changed his role from that of son to that of husband, or symbolically from child to adult. The first gastrointestinal episode was successfully treated through diet modification and medication, and the symptoms subsided. The second attack occurred after the birth of their first child, a son, 4 years later. Once again, it can be seen that the birth of a child, particularly a son with whose infantile dependency the father may have identified, put increased pressure on this man to act as a strong, responsible adult while simultaneously decreasing direct opportunities to have his dependency needs met. As in the previous attack conservative medical treatment was successful in alleviating the ulcer symptoms, although they were more severe and took longer to disappear than in the initial episode. It is interesting to note that when their second child, a daughter, was born 4 years later, no exacerbation of ulcer symptoms occurred. The third and most severe episode of ulcer symptoms took place about a year after this man's father died. The father died as a result of bowel cancer, which was treated by colostomy and radiation but nevertheless metastasized. During the course of his illness, the father moved in with his son and daughter-in-law because of his increased need for physical care and supervision. Although the daughter-in-law provided most of the care, the son frequently willingly helped, especially with more personal tasks such as bathing. The father died in the home, and during the following year the son was deeply involved in settling his father's complex estate. After this task was completed he once again experienced ulcer symptoms so severe that surgical removal of two thirds of his stomach was ultimately required. It can be conjectured that the death of this man's father was unconsciously seen by him as the ultimate proof of his adulthood, which he was not able to withstand because he maintained a large reservoir of unmet dependency needs, and his father's death symbolically cut off all hope of having these needs met.

Although peptic ulcer is a common form of gastrointestinal psychophysiological disorder, other illnesses such as ulcerative colitis and chronic constipation also fall into this category.

Cardiovascular system

The complications of essential hypertension often occur in conjunction with life crises and are thought to be the result of repressed rage.

A health problem of increasing incidence particularly among black Americans is essential hypertension. Essential hypertension is a sustained elevation of systolic and diastolic arterial blood pressure in the absence of any of the demonstrable known causes of arterial hypertension. Although persons suffering from essential hypertension may remain asymptomatic for years, if the syndrome is sustained organic alterations, particularly renal damage, may occur. Often the acceleration of the disease with resultant complications occurs in conjunction with life crises. It is believed that huge amounts of repressed rage that have no acceptable outlet are the emotional dynamics underlying the development of essential hypertension. The mental mechanism used by the individual is usually denial, since the person also has a need to conform with the expectations of others, especially authority figures, as a means of meeting his dependency needs. Feeling and expressing rage is therefore highly anxiety producing, and the individual often has a calm, placid exterior. The frequency of occurrence of essential hypertension in the black population has led investigators to explore genetic factors simultaneously with cultural factors as major etiological predeterminants.

Respiratory system

A major psychophysiological disorder affecting the respiratory system is bronchial asthma. Bronchial asthma is caused by bronchial obstruction that does not interfere with inspiration but causes difficulty in expiration. This results in the characteristic asthmatic wheeze that sounds so similar in all patients that it is almost diagnostic. The underlying cause of the bronchial obstruction may be an infectious process, an allergic reaction, or an idiopathic bronchospasm. When an underlying disease process such as a bacterial infection is present, other symptoms such as an elevated temperature and white blood count are also present and require treatment if the asthmatic episode is to be alleviated. There are some instances, however, when there is no demonstrable physiological cause for the asthmatic episode, and here emotional factors are believed to play a major etiological role in the occurrence of the illness.

When there is no demonstrable physiological cause for episodes of bronchial asthma, emotional factors are believed to play a major role.

The personality characteristics of the individual who suffers from asthma seem to include strong dependency needs directed toward the mother or mother figure, with simultaneous anger toward this individual, which elicits unconscious fears of abandonment. In fact, some psychoanalytically oriented authorities claim that the characteristic asthmatic wheeze is a symbolic cry for the mother. During an acute asthmatic attack the individual is a clinging, dependent person whose behavior is justified to himself and others on the basis of the life-threatening symptoms. Therefore it is not uncommon for the dependency needs of the person to be met during the acute episode, but unfortunately these temporary episodes of need fulfillment do little to alter the underlying personality dynamics, and thus future episodes are not prevented. Continued episodes of asthma result in pulmonary changes that may not be reversible and may affect the vital capacity of the person's respiratory system.

Integumentary system

The integumentary system serves a unique function in the ego psychology of an individual in that it is the only body system equally visible both to the person and to others. Because of this the skin represents the self to others in the environment. An awareness of this fact is reflected in such sayings as, "He's too thick- [or thin-] skinned" or "You can't tell a book by its cover."

Because the skin is endowed with sense receptors for pain, pressure, and temperature, many emotional states are reflected in skin changes.

The skin is richly endowed with sense receptors for pain, pressure, and temperature sensations. As a result, many emotional states are reflected in skin changes—the blush of embarrassment and the paling that accompany fear are examples. These common skin changes are received by others as nonverbal clues to the emotional state of the individual, frequently despite verbal reassurances to the contrary. In healthy interpersonal relationships, the skin acts as a friendly ally in communicating to others what is being felt and therefore enhances the probability of having the individual's needs met. When the skin is involved in a psychophysiological disorder, however, it becomes a means of self-disclosure representing the individual's unconscious conflict between a repressed emotion and the simultaneous need to have this emotion known and responded to.

Numerous dermatological conditions can cause a person severe discomfort, in the form of itching, pain, or disfigurement. Although in many instances their exact cause is unknown, an amazing number of these maladies respond well to the treatment of a dermatologist who may try a number of remedies before finding one that seems to help. Although not denying the positive benefits of the physical treatment received, many authorities believe that the major benefit is achieved from the sustained, concerned interest in the individual and his illness that is frequently shown by dermatologists and that indirectly helps to meet the person's immediate needs. Exacerbations of skin rashes and severe itching are closely related to occurrences of stressful life events to which these persons seem to respond without undue emotional upset but rather react by somatization on which they and others can focus their concern. Many psychiatrists believe that skin somatization is one of the most primitive ego defenses available and therefore are very cautious in pursuing aggressive physical and psychological treatment unless the individual is in great pain or unable to carry out activities of daily living. The rationale underlying this conservative approach is that if the person is enabled to give up this defense without a considerable increase in ego strength, he might be forced to resort to the more serious and incapacitating defense of mental illness.

Musculoskeletal system

Rheumatoid arthritis is the most common and severe form of psychophysiological disorders affecting the musculoskeletal system.

The most common and severe form of psychophysiological disorder that affects the musculoskeletal system is rheumatoid arthritis. This disease results in marked organic damage and affects not only the joints but also other tissues. Its onset may occur at any age, and it affects females more frequently than males. The personality characteristics of persons affected by this disease almost universally include masochistic, self-sacrificing behavior, which is in response to a rigid, punitive superego and a weak ego organization. Their family background frequently gives evidence of maternal deprivation, leaving them with a great many unmet dependency needs. Prior to becoming ill, these individuals indirectly express their emotional needs by being helpful and kind and willing to do almost anything for others, thereby receiving positive feedback from their social system. Under usual circumstances therefore their dependency needs are minimally met through environmental and interpersonal support, allowing them to remain healthy until such time as this support is withdrawn. Many individuals report that an event such as the death of a spouse or the loss of a job immediately preceded the initial onset of the illness.

Treatment of these persons is exceedingly complex. Many of them reflect their emotional conflict by denying the severity of their illness and either refuse treatment or are unreliable in following the treatment regimen. Conversely, there are some who quickly become highly dependent on family, friends, and health care personnel despite the fact that their symptoms may be only mildly debilitating.

CAUSATIVE FACTORS OF PSYCHOPHYSIOLOGICAL DISORDERS

Although there seems to be consensus among authorities regarding the major role a person's emotions play in the development of certain physical illnesses, the exact nature of that role is not yet determined. One widely accepted theory postulates that repressed conflicts are stimulated by intrapsychic or interpersonal events and lead to an overall increase in the individual's level of anxiety. An automatic physical concomitant to an increase in anxiety is innervation of the autonomic nervous system. In other words, the person who is anxious becomes physically ready to engage in flight or fight. However, since the emotional conflict that is the basis for the anxiety and the subsequent physical response is unconscious, the individual has no outlet for the physical response, as would be possible if the conflict were conscious or if the danger were external. Consequently the state of physical readiness for flight or fight does nothing to resolve the underlying emotional conflict. Should this phenomenon be sustained, a cyclical pattern is established. This pattern results in physiological alterations such as a peptic ulcer, which is caused by increased gastric acid secretion and gastric hypermotility as compensatory to the initial decreased gastric acid secretion and hypomotility caused by the flight-fight reaction. As the individual perceives physical discomfort, it is not unlikely that his anxiety will further increase, thereby compounding the problem. The originator of this theory is a physician named Franz Alexander, whose works on the subject remain classics in the field.

A second theory postulates that certain personality types are particularly prone to the development of certain physical illnesses. An example of this theory is the designation of a specific personality type that is considered to place the individual in a high-risk category for myocardial infarction. These persons are seen to be highly competitive and overly ambitious, and they deny any need for dependency. This personality syndrome is manifested by hard work, aggressive behavior, and a great deal of risk taking as a means of getting ahead. These persons frequently have many individuals dependent on them but no one on whom they feel they can depend.

A third theory places emphasis on the symbolism of the illness. For example a person who unconsciously feels a great deal of rage at significant others and the environment in general but for whom expression of this rage is not acceptable may develop ulcerative colitis. Since ulcerative colitis is an illness in which the person has frequent bowel movements requiring, at the very least, alterations in his and others' activities, one might say that he is symbolically defecating on those around him, a very hostile act indeed.

Several widely recognized theories related to the development of psychophysiological illness suggest (1) repressed conflicts are stimulated and lead to increased anxiety, thereby innervating the autonomic nervous system, (2) certain personality types are more prone to illness, (3) the nature of the illness is symbolic, and (4) everyone has one body system that is weaker than the others.

A fourth theory is referred to as organ weakness. This theory postulates that all humans have one body system that is relatively less healthy than the others. If a person has underlying unconscious problems that interfere with his effective functioning but at the same time has sufficient ego strength so that a flight from reality is not necessary, this person may develop a physical illness as a means of coping with the unconscious problem. The type of physical illness developed will be determined by the body system that is most physiologically vulnerable.

Regardless of which theory or combination of theories proves to be correct, they all have several concepts in common, the understanding of which will prove invaluable to the nurse in caring for persons with psychophysiological disorders. Following are these concepts:

1. Persons who develop psychophysiological disorders have *unconscious* emotional conflicts that increase their anxiety and interfere with their effectively meeting their needs.
2. The physical illness is a result of or an expression of this unconscious conflict and serves as a means of lowering the anxiety level.
3. The physical illness is real in that there are demonstrable organic changes that may be life threatening.

It is also generally accepted that the onset of the psychophysiological illness is associated with a real or perceived stressful life event. The physical symptoms occur as a response to this stress and mask the emotional turmoil with which the person cannot cope, thereby achieving the purpose of lowering anxiety. This benefit is termed the *primary gain.* In our society, however, the individual also may experience unexpected and unintended benefits from the illness. These benefits may be such things as having one's dependency needs indirectly met, receiving attention and special consideration, or being relieved of responsibility. These benefits are *secondary gains,* which tend to reinforce the pattern of somatization.

NURSING CARE OF INDIVIDUALS WITH A
PSYCHOPHYSIOLOGICAL DISORDER
Nursing assessment

Although each psychophysiological disorder has its unique features, it is possible to cite some commonalities about all persons suffering from psychophysiological disorders. The following discussion is organized around the human processes introduced in Chapter 9. Although behaviors in each category are presented as separate entities, it should be understood that they are highly interrelated and are adaptations to similar stressors. Further, in many instances behavior designed as an adaptation to one stressor becomes a stressor itself in another dimension.

Activity processes. The motor behavior of the individual with a psychophysiological disorder may or may not be altered. However, in instances where the musculoskeletal system is involved, as in rheumatoid arthritis, alterations in motor behavior due to pain may be the major symptom. In disorders affecting the respiratory system, activity intolerance may be present due to decreased vital capacity.

Recreation patterns are frequently altered as an adaptation to the actual or potential limitations caused by the illness. For example, one individual who was an avid outdoorsman stopped going on camping trips after developing ulcerative colitis. This psychophysiological disorder required him to have a special diet and be close to toilet facilities, neither of which was easily achieved in the woods.

Self-care behaviors obviously are always altered when the person is acutely ill. They may or may not be altered at other times, depending upon the nature of the disorder.

Cognition processes. Cognition processes are not affected by psychophysiological disorders. However, this does not mean that individuals with psychophysiological disorders may not also have alterations in these processes related to other factors.

Ecological processes. Home maintenance may or may not be altered depending upon the nature of and symptomatology associated with the psychophysiological disorder. Understandably, individuals who are acutely ill are likely to be unconcerned about their environments. At other times, many persons are able to adjust their environments to accommodate their needs in regard to safety and hygiene.

Emotional processes. Even though psychophysiological disorders are believed to have an emotional cause, it is unlikely that the nurse will observe behaviors indicative of alterations in emotional processes, since the physical symptoms associated with the disorder serve the purpose of symbolically expressing the person's underlying emotions. At the same time, however, the individual is likely to express great anxiety about the nature of the treatment for his illness and its outcome. These expressions of anxiety tend to focus on physical symptoms and divert attention from any underlying emotional conflict.

Interpersonal processes. Interpersonal processes are almost always affected in the domains of family processes, role performance, and social interaction. An individual with a psychophysiological disorder often becomes the focus of attention within his family because of the dramatic, disabling, and long-term nature of his physical symptoms. It is not unusual for him and his family both to

Assessment of the individual suffering from a psychophysiological illness is likely to reveal changes in motor activity due to pain, adaptations in recreation patterns, lack of concern for the home environment, anxiety about the nature of treatment for the illness, frustration due to inability to continue working, and a change in self-concept due to surfacing of unmet dependency needs.

report that he "is not the same person" he was prior to the onset of the illness. For example, an individual who previously had been generous and outgoing may become demanding and intolerant of others' needs after becoming ill. If the illness is disabling, the person is unlikely to be able to fulfill his work role. This may be a major source of frustration to all concerned as well as create an economic stressor on the family.

Perception processes. There is no question that an individual who is physically ill for a period of time suffers from a change in self-concept. When the illness is psychophysiological, the problem of maintaining one's self-concept is often compounded. Many persons with a psychophysiological disorder have unmet dependency needs, which they deny because these needs are not reflective of their view of themselves. In fact, they often appear to be fiercely independent persons. When their illness thrusts them into an unavoidable position of dependency, they may become quite anxious, further compounding their symptomatology. Medical dramas on television occasionally depict a successful business man or politician who is hospitalized for a psychophysiological disorder such as a duodonal ulcer but who attempts to continue working by dictating letters and carrying on business over the telephone.

Physiological processes. The very nature of psychophysiological disorders implies that there is always an alteration in at least one physiological process. The nature and severity of the alteration are determined by the body system affected and the degree of organic change that has occurred.

Valuation processes. Whether valuation processes are affected is determined by a number of factors, including the extent to which the illness either relieves or creates anxiety, the degree to which the organic changes are life threatening, the extent to which the illness is disabling in ways meaningful to the individual, and the number and type of secondary gains the individual experiences. Obviously, if the illness creates more anxiety than it relieves, is life threatening, causes disability that is stressful, and does not elicit secondary gains, the individual is likely to express feelings of helplessness, hopelessness, and powerlessness. However, because psychophysiological disorders are thought to shield the person from awareness of unconscious emotional conflicts, it is more common for these persons to experience a deeper sense of purpose and meaning, and perhaps spirituality, than they had prior to their illness.

Nursing diagnosis

As with all nursing diagnoses, the nursing diagnoses for the individual with a psychophysiological disorder are based on the themes identified during the assessment phase of the nursing process. Categories of human responses from the ANA Classification of Human Responses of Concern for Psychiatric–Mental Health Nursing Practice that may be specifically applicable to individuals with a psychophysiological disorder include the following:

1.1.2   Altered Motor Behavior
1.2.2   Altered Recreation Patterns
1.3.4   Altered Self-Care
3.3.1   Potential for Alteration in Home Maintenance
5.4.2   Altered Family Processes
5.5.2   Altered Role Performance
6.3.2   Altered Self-Concept
7.1.2   Altered Circulation
7.4.2   Altered Gastrointestinal Processes
7.5.2   Altered Musculoskeletal Processes
7.8.2   Altered Oxygenation Processes
7.9.2   Altered Physical Integrity

NANDA nursing diagnostic categories that may be specifically applicable to the individual with a psychophysiological disorder include:

1.3.1.2   Diarrhea
1.5.1.3   Ineffective Breathing Pattern
1.6.2.1.2.1   Impaired Skin Integrity
3.2.1   Altered Role Performance
3.2.2   Altered Family Processes
5.1.1.1   Ineffective Individual Coping
6.1.1.1   Impaired Physical Mobility
6.1.1.2   Activity Intolerance
6.3.1.1   Diversional Activity Deficit
6.4.1.1   Impaired Home Maintenance Management
6.5.2   Bathing/Hygiene Self-Care Deficit
6.5.3   Dressing/Grooming Self-Care Deficit
7.1.1   Body-Image Disturbance
7.1.2.2   Situational Low Self-Esteem
9.1.1   Pain
9.3.1   Anxiety
9.3.2   Fear

To develop a nursing diagnosis that fulfills its function of providing direction for planning nursing care, the nurse is encouraged to postulate and state etiologic or antecedent factors for each human response and connect the two phrases by using the term "related to." For example:

> 5.5.2   Altered Role Performance related to inability to work as a typist because of severe pain in fingers

Planning and implementing nursing care

The plan for nursing care is derived from the nursing diagnoses and includes the objectives of the care, the nursing actions, and outcome criteria. To be effective the plan needs to be highly individualized. The suggestions that follow should be seen as general guidelines to be used if they are appropriate to the client's needs.

In general, the objectives of all nursing care for the individual with a psychophysiological disorder should relate to assisting the client to regain physiological homeokinesis and to develop alternative methods of coping with stress.

Since the client's nursing diagnoses are often interrelated, stemming as they do from similar etiologies or antecedents, the student will see that the appropriate nursing actions are also interrelated; in other words, by intervening in one dimension, the nurse will also affect other dimensions.

The care of persons suffering from psychophysiological disorders is usually directed by a physician whose emphasis is on the reduction of physical symptoms and the prevention of further organic damage. However, because of the nature of the illness, close collaboration with a psychiatrist is often necessary. Once the acute physical symptoms have abated, the psychiatrist may continue to treat the individual on an outpatient basis in an attempt to help the person deal with underlying emotional problems. The nurse is usually involved in providing care during those times when the person is hospitalized for an exacerbation of the illness or in follow-up care in the home.

Emotional processes. The nurse has many opportunities to engage in conversation with the hospitalized person. She can be of emotional assistance to him if she encourages him to talk about his feelings. It must be understood, however, that many of the client's feelings are unacceptable to him, and therefore acceptance of him and his feelings by the nurse is of primary importance. As in communicating with any client, the nurse is most helpful when she is accepting and nonjudgmental. Reflecting or restating what the client has said is an appropriate communication technique to employ, since a direct interpretation may be very threatening and raise the client's anxiety level and perhaps thereby increase the severity of his physical symptoms.

The nurse can be most helpful to the client experiencing a psychophysiological illness by encouraging the client to talk about his feelings and listening in an accepting and nonjudgmental manner.

As is true of any client, the person suffering from a psychophysiological disorder can be helped to feel in control of his situation by adequate explanations of what he can expect to experience during diagnostic and treatment procedures. Some clients, however, become increasingly anxious if they are given too much information, and their dependency needs are best met by trusting in the judgment of their physician and nurse. Therefore the amount and nature of information offered to the client should be primarily determined by an assessment of his anxiety level. Certainly the client's questions should be answered, but the degree of elaboration should be gauged by his response to the answer rather than by the nurse's need to engage in health teaching.

The nurse is helpful when she works with the client's family to help them understand the complexity of the illness and its treatment.

Interpersonal processes. Working with the client's family is necessary to aid them in understanding the complexity of his illness and its treatment. The effect of the family on the client and the effect the client and his illness have on the family is a process that is often explored in family therapy under the guidance of a skilled therapist.

Many persons are not aware of the interpersonal resources available to them within their social system. Persons with psychophysiological disorders can often benefit from help in identifying already existent interpersonal resources and in enlarging their social network, thereby increasing the possibility of having their emotional needs met by a larger variety of people.

Perception processes. Most physical illnesses, regardless of cause, present a potential threat to the person's perception of himself as an independent adult. In the case of persons with psychophysiological disorders, there often are underlying conflicts between dependency and independency needs, and the imposed dependence that results from the illness may stimulate a high degree of anxiety in the client. In such instances the nurse can be helpful if she meets the individual's needs for dependence in an indirect way while simultaneously acknowledging his status as a responsible adult. An example of such an intervention is the nurse who wisely addresses the client with a peptic ulcer as Mr. Smith instead of John. At the same time, Mr. Smith's dependency needs can be indirectly met by the nurse's administering the prescribed antacid instead of leaving it at the bedside or asking the client to ring his call light every half hour so that she can bring the medicine. By spontaneously making frequent contact with the client the nurse is indirectly saying that she is willing to take care of him without his having to assume the responsibility of asking for help. It should be noted that the administration of oral medication or food, especially milk, has great symbolic significance, since eating is the vehicle through which people have their dependency needs first met.

> Meeting the client's dependency needs while also acknowledging the individual's status as a responsible adult is a primary task of the nurse.

Physiological processes. During her involvement, the methods the nurse uses in carrying out physical care are often pivotal factors in enhancing or impeding the overall treatment goals. The nurse must fully understand and accept the fact that persons with a psychophysiological disorder are physically ill and that their symptoms may reach life-threatening proportions. The nurse must not convey the attitude that she believes the individual would get better if he merely exerted more control over his emotions.

> Meeting the physical needs of the client is very important during acute episodes of the illness.

During acute episodes of the illness, meeting the physical needs of the client is of primary importance, even if in so doing the nurse is supporting a dysfunctional emotional adaptation. For example, a couple whose tension-laden relationship exacerbates the wife's physical symptoms should not be encouraged to discuss their relationship during the acute episode of the wife's illness.

The secondary gains achieved by the individual as the result of his being physically ill need to be minimized once the acute episode has passed. The nurse can be instrumental in working with him to strengthen or develop coping mechanisms that do not involve somatization.

END NOTE

This chapter focuses on the nursing care of individuals with psychophysiological disorders. An example of a psychophysiological disorder is given for each of

NURSING CARE PLAN

An individual with asthma

CASE FORMULATION

Martha B. is a 25-year-old single woman who has suffered from asthma since the age of 2. Although respiratory infections have always precipitated an asthmatic attack, there have been many instances of asthmatic episodes unaccompanied by an infectious process. Martha is the only child of an attractive 45-year-old woman who has never married and who is not sure who Martha's father is. Martha and her mother live together in a well-furnished two-bedroom apartment in a middle-class neighborhood of a large city.

Since the age of 16 Martha's mother has engaged in prostitution and became pregnant several times. For reasons that are not clear, at the time she was pregnant with Martha she decided not to have an abortion as she had done on previous occasions. After Martha was born the mother set up housekeeping in an apartment that she furnished with the child's needs in mind.

By the time Martha was 5 years old her mother had become so successful in her occupation that she no longer was a streetwalker but rather made appointments with her customers by telephone and therefore had advance notice as to when she would not be home. At those times she left Martha with her grandmother, a warm, kind woman who seemed unaware of her daughter's activities. Martha's grandmother lived alone, and she was always delighted to have Martha visit. When Martha and her mother were together they seemed to enjoy each other and have a mutually satisfying relationship.

After Martha graduated from high school she took a position as a clerk in a large plastics company located in the heart of the city. She has remained with this company but has never accepted offers of promotion. Therefore her salary is essentially at the same level as it was when she was hired because the only raises she has received were several cost-of-living increments. For this reason she feels unable to leave her mother's home and rent her own apartment.

The event preceding Martha's latest and most severe asthmatic attack was the death and burial of her grandmother. When notified of her grandmother's death, Martha responded quite stoically and, in fact, made all the funeral arrangements because her mother was out of town. On the day of the funeral Martha began to cry softly. However, by the time the family assembled at the cemetery she was severely dyspneic and had to be rushed from the gravesite to the emergency room of the local hospital. The emergency room staff were very familiar with Martha and her family situation, although they did not know of her grandmother's death.

By the time Martha arrived at the emergency room she was in acute physiological distress, gasping for air and wheezing so loudly that she could be heard throughout the waiting room. Her mother expressed genuine concern but also stated that "this couldn't have happened at a worse time since I have to leave town tonight." She begged the hospital personnel to admit Martha so she wouldn't have to worry while she was away.

Nursing assessment

Martha's family situation contained all the elements sufficient for the development of idiopathic asthma. It can be conjectured that Martha's mother was in fact a very immature person lacking in self-esteem who engaged in prostitution as one means of reinforcing her feelings of worthlessness. If this were true, it is likely that her decision not to terminate her pregnancy with Martha was an unconscious attempt to provide herself with a consistent person who would need and value her. Unfortunately, this rarely succeeds, since children require more attention and love than they can give during their formative developmental periods. Martha undoubtedly felt that her mother's frequent absences were a result of some failing on her part, while at the same time she experienced much anger at her mother for not providing her with the emotional support

NURSING CARE PLAN—cont'd

she needed. This issue could not be openly confronted, since to do so would incur the risk of abandonment, thereby dooming forever the possibility of having her needs met by her mother. On the other hand the grandmother seemed able to meet some of Martha's needs, although her relationship with her own daughter was not growth-producing, as evidenced by their lack of communication.

Although she was 25 years old, it appears that Martha's developmental maturity was not congruent with her chronological maturity. Rather than struggling with age-appropriate developmental tasks, Martha's inability to establish herself in her own apartment indicates she was still struggling with dependency issues characteristic of the developmental phases of childhood. To the extent that Martha's grandmother was able to meet some of Martha's dependency needs, Martha was able to function. When the grandmother died, Martha lost the only stable, consistent person in her life and was unequipped to successfully cope with this developmental stressor. Therefore her wheezing was interpreted as a desperate cry to be cared for.

Nursing diagnosis

Based on the nursing assessment that included prior knowledge of the family dynamics, and an understanding of the dynamics underlying psychophysiological disorders, the nurse formulated the following pair of nursing diagnoses for Martha B. The first is from the Classification of Human Responses of Concern for Psychiatric–Mental Health Nursing Practice; the second is from the approved NANDA Diagnostic Categories.

7.8.2   Altered Oxygenation Processes related to unconscious feelings of anger at being abandoned by grandmother dying

OR

1.5.1.3   Ineffective Breathing Pattern related to unconscious feelings of anger at being abandoned by grandmother dying

Planning and implementing nursing care for *Martha B.*

A sample nursing care plan for Martha B. is found in the boxed material on p. 296.

The immediate objective was to restore physiological homeokinesis, so Martha was given the prescribed bronchodilator by intramuscular injection. Within 10 minutes she was breathing more easily and was noticeably more comfortable. This could have been accomplished in the emergency room, but in view of the family situation, the physician had decided to hospitalize her.

After her immediate physical needs were met, it was decided that Martha could benefit from constant attention from a member of the nursing staff. Therefore a student nurse who was studying the nursing care of individuals with psychophysiological disorders was assigned to stay with Martha. While it could be argued that this intervention would result in secondary gains, it was believed appropriate during this crisis.

Under supervision of her instructor the student nurse encouraged Martha to express her feelings and was careful to respond in an empathic way even though she knew that Martha's grandmother had not intentionally abandoned her. She also attempted to meet Martha's dependency needs through such interventions as offering her liquids to drink without waiting to be asked. Although Martha was allowed out of bed, the student brought her a basin of water and a towel so she could bathe in bed if she wished.

Evaluation

Martha responded so well to the interventions of medications and consistent attention that the health care team decided that she would be a good candidate for psychotherapy. This treatment option had never been offered to Martha on any previous admission, but with the loss of her grandmother it was feared that Martha would not have the resources to cope with her situation if she were not given more assistance. Martha's mother would also be invited to begin family

Continued.

NURSING CARE PLAN—cont'd

therapy with her daughter. Although the staff were not optimistic about her agreeing to participate, they felt it was important that she be of fered this help not only for Martha's well-being but for hers as well.

NURSING CARE PLAN FOR *Martha B.*

Nursing diagnosis	Objective	Nursing actions	Outcome criteria
7.8.2 Altered Oxygenation Processes related to unconscious feelings of anger at being abandoned by grandmother dying	Restore physiological homeokinesis	Administer prescribed bronchodilator Observe for respiratory distress Plan physical care to conserve client's energy	Within 20 minutes of receiving medication dyspnea will decrease
OR 1.5.1.3 Ineffective Breathing Pattern related to unconscious feelings of anger at being abandoned by grandmother dying	Meet client's dependency needs in a fashion appropriate to her chronological age Encourage client to express her feelings	Establish relationship with client by giving undivided attention Anticipate client's needs, for example, offer juice at regular intervals Listen attentively and nonjudgmentally to client's expressions of loss	Within 48 hours client will be symptom free

the following body systems: gastrointestinal, cardiovascular, respiratory, integumentary, and musculoskeletal. The nurse is encouraged to appreciate the potential life-threatening nature of these disorders, as well as to understand the complex emotional dynamics believed to underlie their development. The chapter concludes with a hypothetical plan of nursing care for a young adult who is experiencing an acute episode of idiopathic asthma.

SUGGESTED SOURCES OF ADDITIONAL INFORMATION

Alexander F: Psychosomatic medicine, New York, 1954, WW Norton & Co., Inc.

Dunbar F: Emotions and bodily changes, New York, 1954, Columbia University Press.

Byrne DG: Personal determinants of life event stress and myocardial infarction, Psychother Psychosom 40(1-4):106, 1985.

Deter HC and Allert G: Group therapy for asthma patients: a concept for the psychosomatic treatment of patients in a medical clinic, Psychother Psychosom 40(1-4):95, 1983.

Haggarty J: The psychosomatic family: an overview, Psychosomatics 24:615, July 1983.

Haggarty J and Drossman D: Use of psychotropic drugs in patients with peptic ulcer, Psychosomatics 26:277, February 1985.

Krishnan K, France R, and Houpt J: Chronic low back pain and depression, Psychosomatics 26:299, February 1985.

Matussek P, Agerer D, and Seibt G: Aggression in depressives and psoriatics, Psychother Psychosom 43:120, March 1985.

Rimon R and Laakso RL: Life stress and rheumatoid arthritis, Psychother Psychosom 43:38, January 1985.

Santonastaso R, Canton G, Giovanni BA, and Zamboni S: Hypertension and neuroticism, Psychother Psychosom 41:7, January 1984.

Sarason I, Sarason B, Potter E, and Antoni M: Life events, social support, and illness, Psychosom Med 47:156, March/April 1985.

Starkman M and Appleblatt N: Functional upper airway obstruction: a possible somatization disorder, Psychosomatics 25:327, April 1984.

Weiner H: What the future holds for psychosomatic medicine, Psychother Psychosom 42(1-4):15, 1984.

Wolf S: Peptic ulcer, Psychosomatics 23:1101, November 1982.

Individuals with substance abuse and dependence

19

LEARNING OBJECTIVES

After studying this chapter the student will be able to:

○ Differentiate between substance abuse and substance dependence.

○ Describe the effects of abuse of or dependence on narcotics, sedative hypnotics, central nervous system stimulants, hallucinogens, phencyclidine (PCP), and marijuana.

○ Discuss the causative factors associated with substance abuse and dependence.

○ Discuss the long-term treatment of substance dependent individuals.

○ Describe behaviors the nurse is most likely to observe in an individual experiencing substance dependence.

○ State examples of nursing diagnoses likely to be applicable to an individual who is experiencing substance dependence.

○ Develop a hypothetical plan of nursing care for an individual who is experiencing substance dependence.

Very few human behaviors have consequences as far reaching as do those of the substance-dependent individual. In addition to affecting his own physical, emotional, and social well-being, the behavior of the substance-dependent individual affects the well-being of his family and that of the society at large. For example, industry has documented that alcoholism is one of the primary reasons for the loss of time and productivity both on the assembly line and in the executive suite. Therefore alcohol dependence has become a significant factor in the economic health of the nation.

Criminal activity is an integral aspect of drug dependence. Hard drugs must be procured from an illegal source, thereby contributing to the maintenance of organized crime. In addition, the price they command often causes the individual to resort to criminal activity to obtain sufficient funds to maintain his dependence. Even when the drug-dependent individual does not have to engage in criminal activity to support his dependence, he most certainly must spend money better used for other purposes. As a result, it is not unusual for his family to have inadequate food, clothing, and shelter. As the substance dependence increases, the source of legally gained income inevitably is cut off, usually because of the individual's inability to maintain his job.

Another complexity surrounding substance dependence is the inevitable involvement of the individual with both the legal and health care systems. This overlap in social systems is not unique to these disorders, but the nature of the overlap is problematic, since the goals of the legal and health care systems are diametrically opposed. The goal of the legal system is to punish the offender, while the health care system views the individual as a person in need of help. This conflicting view of the same behavior developed, in part, because of lack of definitive information about the nature of substance dependence. Until research documents these behaviors as an illness or society is willing to legalize dependence, the substance-dependent individual will remain caught between the divergent purposes of these two systems.

HISTORICAL PERSPECTIVE

The nontherapeutic use of mind-altering substances is as old as the history of humanity. The Old Testament gives an account of Noah who became drunk on wine and apparently collapsed. The New Testament abounds with cautions against intemperance in many activities, including the drinking of alcoholic beverages. Thus it must be concluded that alcohol abuse was common in those days.

Historical reference to substance abuse is not limited to alcohol. Southwestern Plains Indians used hallucinogenic substances as an integral aspect of religious rituals. In the nineteenth century cocaine was widely used throughout the civilized world, as was opium.

It was not until the twentieth century, however, that the incidence of substance dependence became great enough to cause national concern. The Harrison Act of 1914 regulated drug traffic for the first time and provided for the licensing of certain groups such as physicians who could legally dispense these drugs for medicinal purposes. In the early 1920s the Volstead Act was passed, which made the sale of alcoholic beverages illegal. This law was ultimately repealed because it did little to curb the consumption of alcoholic beverages, but it did contribute to the development of crime syndicates that trafficked in the illegal manufacture and sale of liquor. The effect of the Harrison Act was similar to that of the Volstead Act, namely, addicts were forced to turn to illegal sources to obtain drugs. Governmental response has not been the same, however. Rather than legalizing mind-altering drugs as had been done with alcohol, stricter laws aimed at both the user and the supplier continue to be passed.

The number of alcohol-dependent persons in this country has always been great. Alcoholism has existed in most ethnic groups at all socioeconomic levels. In contrast, prior to World War II heroin addiction was most prevalent among Caucasians in the southern United States. Since the war the highest incidence of this type of drug dependence is found in northern urban areas among the Black and Hispanic cultures. In fact, almost 50% of the heroin addicts today are in New York City.

The use of mind-altering drugs reached epidemic proportions in the 1960s and 1970s among lower- and middle-class adolescents and young adults in urban and suburban areas throughout the entire country. It appears that the level of drug usage among this group reached its peak in the 1970s. However, there has been a concomitant rise in alcohol usage among adolescents and young adults. In fact, epidemiological data recently reported by the National Institute of Mental Health indicate that alcohol abuse or dependence is the most frequent psychiatric disorder among males from 18 to 65 years of age.

Of most recent concern is the increased use of cocaine. Prior to the 1980s cocaine was used primarily by those in the entertainment industry and young, upwardly mobile, middle-class, highly educated white males. Because of its current availability in the form of "crack," its price has dropped markedly, now making it within the economic reach of even lower income wage earners. Its availability, relatively low cost, and association with celebrities combine to make cocaine a fashionable drug.

SUBSTANCE ABUSE AND DEPENDENCE

The Diagnostic and Statistical Manual of Mental Disorders (Third Edition–Revised) (DSM-III-R) differentiates between abuse of psychoactive substances and dependence on these substances. The diagnostic criteria for substance dependence are:

A. At least three of the following:
  1. Substance often taken in larger amounts or over a longer period than the person intended
  2. Persistent desire or one or more unsuccessful efforts to cut down or control substance use
  3. A great deal of time spent in activities necessary to get the substance (e.g., theft), taking the substance (e.g., chain smoking), or recovering from its effects
  4. Frequent intoxication or withdrawal symptoms when expected to fulfill major role obligations at work, school, or home (e.g., does not go to work because hung over, goes to school or work "high," intoxicated while taking care of his or her children), or when substance

use is physically hazardous (e.g., drives when intoxicated)

5. Important social, occupational, or recreational activities given up or reduced because of substance use

6. Continued substance use despite knowledge of having a persistent or recurrent social, psychological, or physical problem that is caused or exacerbated by the use of the substance (e.g., keeps on using heroin despite family arguments about it, cocaine-induced depression, or having an ulcer made worse by drinking)

7. Marked tolerance: need for markedly increased amounts of the substance (i.e., at least a 50% increase) to achieve intoxication or desired effect, or markedly diminished effect with continued use of the same amount

NOTE: The following items may not apply to cannabis, hallucinogens, or phencyclidine (PCP):

8. Characteristic withdrawal symptoms

9. Substance often taken to relieve or avoid withdrawal symptoms

B. Some symptoms of the disturbance have persisted for at least 1 month or have occurred repeatedly over a longer period of time.

The diagnostic criteria for substance abuse are:

A. At least one of the following:

1. Continued use despite knowledge of having a persistent or recurrent social, occupational, psychological, or physical problem that is caused or exacerbated by use of the psychoactive substance

2. Recurrent use in situations in which use is physically hazardous (e.g., driving while intoxicated)

B. Some symptoms of the disturbance have persisted for at least 1 month or have occurred repeatedly over a longer period of time.

C. Never met the criteria for substance dependence for this substance.

Both substance abuse and substance dependence are deleterious to the physical, emotional, and social functioning of the individual and, as previously stated, often bring the person to the attention of the health care and legal systems.

Following is a discussion of the effects, and where applicable the short-term treatment of substance dependence, of six categories of commonly abused drugs.

NARCOTICS

Narcotics are general depressants of the central nervous system and are used medically to relieve moderate and severe pain. Most narcotics are in the chemical class termed *opiates*. Morphine, heroin, and codeine are derivatives of opium; demerol and methadone are synthetic substitutes. Although some opiate-dependent persons use morphine or demerol, most do not have access to these drugs and use heroin, which is readily available on the streets of large cities.

These drugs are parenterally administered and produce a temporary state of well-being; troubles appear to be trifling and remote and there is a comfortable sense of complete relaxation. The individual feels "normal," which means he feels as if his basic needs have been met. He feels sexually satisfied, full of food, free from anxiety and pain, and is not concerned with aggressive feelings. Whenever a heroin-dependent individual obtains an adequate dose, he may expose his addiction with an abnormal euphoria and contentment or even a sleepy languor. The pupils may show a telltale "pinpoint" constriction, and in most instances the arms and thighs are scarred or pigmented by the hypodermic needle.

Ever-increasing amounts are necessary to produce this exhilaration, so that the heroin user may require as much as 15 to 20 grains daily. Unfortunately, when the effects wear off and sufficient amounts are not immediately available, certain *withdrawal symptoms* promptly appear. Tears, sneezing, coryza, yawning, great irritability, and restlessness become quickly evident. Within 24 hours this is followed by abdominal cramps, vomiting, and diarrhea. To these distressing symptoms are added headache, sweating, and pains in the muscles and joints of the lower extremities. Finally, on the third day of abstinence the nervous irritability is so pronounced that the individual becomes hysterical, noisy, and threatening; he frequently throws and destroys objects within his reach. Within a week, however, all these painful withdrawal reactions disappear.

Heroin dependence does not cause mental deterioration, but the treatment that addicts receive from society causes them to deteriorate socially. It is important to understand that the reality with which these individuals must cope contains few elements conducive to positive mental health. They are often members of a cultural minority and live in ghetto-type surroundings with little realistic hope of changing their circumstances. They become easy prey to drug pushers as early adolescents or sooner. Once "hooked" they must continue to live close to the source of drug supply, which means that the heroin-dependent individual is compelled to associate with the people who smuggle the drug into the country and the pushers who sell it. It should be noted that few, if any, smugglers or pushers are themselves dependent on heroin but actively support its use by others.

In addition to the heroin users found in the slums of big cities, a growing number of physicians and nurses are dependent on morphine and demerol, which they illegally obtain from hospitals or fraudently written prescriptions. State licensing authorities and professional organizations are actively involved in not only punishing these persons but also in facilitating their treatment.

Withdrawal from opium derivatives has been made more humane through the use of methadone, which is a substitute for the opiate on which the individ-

> Heroin dependence does not cause mental deterioration, but the treatment that addicts receive from society causes them to deteriorate socially.

ual is dependent. The use of methadone has been a somewhat controversial method of treating narcotic addiction. This is partly because methadone has been declared to be a narcotic by the Federal Bureau of Narcotics. However, some authorities believe that the use of methadone in treating heroin addicts holds the best hope for halting their criminal activities and for making them self-supporting citizens. It has been used more or less successfully with large groups of heroin addicts in several large cities.

In the use of methadone the individual loses his heroin dependency by becoming addicted to the "substitute," methadone. The user then requires regular doses of methadone daily.

This treatment has at least two advantages: (1) it is relatively inexpensive—an individual can be maintained on methadone for a few cents a day and (2) an individual who is on methadone does not lose his ability to function normally—he can usually hold a job and function as a responsible citizen. Today most large cities have methadone clinics where several hundred individuals go to receive the daily dose of methadone. Most clinics require proof that the individual is not continuing to use heroin by requiring him to produce a urine specimen free of the drug.

SEDATIVE HYPNOTICS

This category of abused drugs includes alcohol, barbiturates, antipsychotic agents, and anxiolytic agents. Antipsychotic agents are discussed in Chapter 15; anxiolytic agents are discussed in Chapter 17.

Alcohol dependence

Alcohol is a central nervous system depressant. The amount required to produce a demonstrable effect varies according to the interrelationship of such variables as the percentage of alcohol in the beverage, the tolerance the individual has developed to the substance, his physical and emotional state of health, and the nature of the environment in which he is drinking. In addition, the amount and type of food in the stomach constitute a major factor that affects the rate of absorption. Hard liquor drunk by a person unaccustomed to alcohol who is emotionally upset, has not eaten all day, and is in the company of persons who are accepting of intoxication is certain to produce a very rapid effect.

Once alcohol is absorbed into the bloodstream it affects all body tissues, but its immediate effects are caused by its action on the brain. At a level of 0.05 percent of alcohol in the blood, inhibitions are diminished and the individual is likely to say and do things that would be unacceptable to him if he were sober. Interestingly, there is a societal norm that, to a point, excuses the behavior of an individual who has been drinking on the grounds that he has been drinking. This cyclical thinking is based on the belief that the behavior of a person when drunk is not a reflection of him but rather a manifestation of the alcohol. The reality is that the impulses acted on emanate from the person and the alcohol merely removes the barriers to their implementation.

At a level of 0.10 percent of alcohol in the blood, motor and speech activity is impaired. It is for this reason that there is a continuing national campaign against driving a motor vehicle when drinking.

Alcohol dependence may take many forms. One individual may be a *chronic alcoholic,* which means that he drinks excessively and is incapacitated most of the time. Another person may be referred to as a *periodic* or *cyclic alcoholic,* which means that he drinks excessively during certain periods of his life but during other periods may not drink at all. A third type of alcoholism is exhibited by an individual who drinks large quantities of alcohol daily over a period of years. At first he may not seem to be seriously affected by this overindulgence. Slowly and insidiously, physical, mental, and emotional deterioration occurs. Eventually this person may be described as suffering from alcoholic deterioration.

> An alcohol-dependent individual may drink excessively all the time, may drink to excess only periodically, or may drink large quantities of alcohol daily over a period of years.

Short-term, immediate treatment of the alcohol-dependent individual is focused on withdrawing him from this substance and assisting him to attain or regain physical health. This is accomplished by symptomatic treatment of the anxiety, tremors, nausea, and diaphoresis that accompany withdrawal. Seizures and delirium tremens are serious, life-threatening conditions that may occur during detoxification.

Delirium tremens is an acute reaction to the withdrawal from a heavy and consistent intake of alcohol for a period of several weeks without an adequate intake of food. In an individual who has been a chronic alcoholic for several years, delirium tremens may be precipitated by a head injury or a surgical procedure without the individual's having taken alcohol at the time of its appearance. Delirium tremens consists of confusion, excitement, and delirium. It is usually of relatively short duration and does not cause a profound and permanent change in the personality.

The delirium is preceded by loss of appetite, restlessness, and insomnia. Slight noises cause the patient to jerk with fear, and moving objects lead to great excitement and agitation. Gradually, consciousness becomes clouded, friends are no longer recognized, and shadows on the wall appear as insects or crawling animals. The person becomes terrified, picks imaginary threads off the bedclothing, feels and sees nonexistent insects on his skin. There is a ceaseless fumbling and picking movement of his fingers and hands. The person's face has an anxious or terrified expression, and his eyes are bloodshot. His skin is moist with perspiration; his tongue and lips are tremorous. His pulse is rapid and weak, and there is always some elevation of temperature.

Anticonvulsant and sedative medications, along with high-potency vitamins and copious amounts of clear liquids, are employed during this phase of treatment, to both prevent and treat seizures and delirium tremens. Because of the serious physiological disequilibrium the person experiences as he goes through withdrawal from alcohol, this procedure is best carried out in a hospital by staff who are knowledgeable about the varied problems involved.

Barbiturate dependence

Barbiturates are central
nervous system depres-
sants that have an effect
very similar to that of
alcohol. Dependence can
be dangerous because of
the possibility of lethal
overdose.

Barbiturates are central nervous system depressants and include phenobarbital, pentobarbital (Nembutal), and secobarbital (Seconal). They are legally prescribed treatments for insomnia and epilepsy. Their effect is similar to that achieved by drinking alcohol. In some respects barbiturate dependence is more dangerous than dependence on alcohol because large numbers of pills can be and are taken at the same time by suicidal people, although it is unlikely that a sufficient amount of alcohol could be consumed at one time to result in death. In addition, the mental confusion caused by both alcohol and barbiturates often leads to these substances being used together, resulting in accidental death.

Early stages of intoxication are manifested by muscular incoordination with ataxia, dizziness, nystagmus, slurred speech, and sluggish mentality. The person acquires many bruises and perhaps fractures by falling or stumbling against walls and furniture. In more profound barbiturate intoxication, there are varying degrees of stupor, speech is incoherent, memory is defective, and hallucinations may appear. When aroused, the person is usually very irritable and resistive. He presents the symptoms of a person suffering from delirium. Recovery may be slow and may leave in its wake a mild degree of permanent brain damage.

Treatment of persons dependent on barbiturates must begin with *gradual* withdrawal of the drug. Sudden, complete withdrawal is often fatal. Individuals who present themselves voluntarily for detoxification are also treated with a high-calorie, high-vitamin diet. Persons who are in a coma caused by barbiturate overdose must be treated aggressively with dialysis to lower the level of barbiturates in the blood.

CENTRAL NERVOUS SYSTEM STIMULANTS

The most frequently abused drugs in this category are cocaine and crack and amphetamines, with cocaine and crack use increasing more rapidly than amphetamines over the last few years.

Cocaine and crack

Cocaine was used for medical purposes in the late 1800s. It acts directly on the cerebral cortex and initially increases the sensation of mental and physical well-being.

Crack, a derivative of cocaine, was first seen in urban areas of the United States in the early 1980s. Unlike cocaine, crack is generally smoked, rather than snorted or injected. Its use has become widespread throughout the nation, very likely because its effects are more intense than those of cocaine and its price is lower.

Cocaine is absorbed very rapidly—3 minutes when snorted, 15 seconds when injected, and 7 seconds when smoked. It metabolizes so quickly that users may take the drug every 20 to 30 minutes to maintain their high. Crack has an even shorter period of effect than cocaine, its high lasting only 5 to 7 minutes. The intensity of the euphoria created by crack, combined with the shortness of its duration, is largely responsible for the fast and intense dependency on this drug that users frequently report.

Cocaine and crack are commonly believed to be "safe" drugs because they do not produce definitive withdrawal syndromes. However, depression is common following withdrawal and may be severe enough to precipitate a suicidal attempt. This phenomenon is called *crashing* by users. In 1983, the National Institute on Drug Abuse declared cocaine to be a "powerfully addictive" substance linked to cardiac arrests, seizures, and respiratory ailments. This agency has received reports of cocaine-related illnesses that have doubled since 1980. Cocaine-related deaths have tripled since that time, very likely due to the fact that cocaine is "cut" with other substances by the dealer, and the user can inadvertently overdose by unknowingly purchasing cocaine that is more pure than that which he has previously used.

Short-term treatment of cocaine and crack dependence is focused on treating any symptoms supportively. Long-term abstinence is difficult to achieve for the individual who has experienced the euphoria associated with the use of this drug unless he develops other coping mechanisms and support systems.

> Long-term treatment of cocaine and crack dependence is difficult to achieve unless the individual develops other coping mechanisms and support systems.

Amphetamines

Numerous chemical compounds fall in this category, the most common of which are racemic amphetamine sulfate (Benzedrine) and methamphetamine (Desoxyn). In the past these drugs have been legitimately used in small doses under medical supervision to treat depression and curb appetite. Individuals who take these drugs solely to become "high" take from 6 to 200 times the daily dose usually prescribed by a physician. Intravenous amphetamines are called "speed" in street language.

The physiological effect of these drugs is to raise the blood pressure, sometimes to dangerous levels. Large doses have been known to cause immediate death, accounting for the saying among drug users that "speed kills."

Individuals who use amphetamines think these drugs increase their physical energy, sharpen their physical and sexual reactions, and increase their confidence. Thus a period of frantic activity results from the ingestion of large amounts of amphetamines. This is followed by a great letdown in which the fatigue and depression are so tremendous that the addict is apt to seek release by taking the drug again. Chronic use of amphetamines can lead to a schizophrenic-like psychosis with paranoid features. This reaction is a result of the drug and is not related to the premorbid personality. In addition, prolonged use at high dosages can lead to massive, irreversible brain damage that may result in death. The use of amphetamines today is not as great as it was in the 1970s, probably because of the drug's deserved reputation as highly dangerous.

HALLUCINOGENS

Individuals under the influence of hallucinogens may believe they have supernatural powers and may attempt such feats as flying.

Lysergic acid diethylamide (LSD or acid) is the most commonly abused hallucinogen. It was first used in research studies in an attempt to discover the cause of schizophrenia. Ingestion of reasonably small doses produces temporary hallucinations and other schizophrenic-like symptoms. The user experiences waves of color, and vibrations seem to pass through the head. Individuals believe that they have had an almost mystical experience in which the nature of emotional conflicts becomes clear.

Although there is little evidence that the use of LSD causes physical dependence, it is dangerous for several reasons. First, this substance causes some individuals to believe they have supernatural powers, and more than one person has been killed in an attempt to fly. Second, although there is no hallucinogen withdrawal reaction even after prolonged high-dose use, a panic reaction can occur, particularly in the first-time user. This reaction is referred to as a *bad trip* and may last as long as a week. In such instances, the user can be helped by being "talked down" by a trusted friend who remains with him and points out reality. Third, "flashbacks" in which the user experiences hallucinations days or weeks after using a hallucinogen can also occur.

PHENCYCLIDINE (PCP)

Phencyclidine (PCP) has historically been classified as a hallucinogen; however, it does not have hallucinogenic effects at low to moderate doses. Rather, low doses produce mild depression and then stimulation. High doses, however, can produce a schizophrenic-like psychosis with paranoid delusions and hallucinations.

MARIJUANA

Until recently marijuana was an easily obtained and relatively inexpensive drug. It is a crude preparation from the whole *Cannabis sativa* plant, which grows wild in Mexico and is easily cultivated in the United States. It is usually absorbed into the body through the smoking of cigarettes called *reefers*. Hashish is prepared by scraping resin from the tops of the hemp plant. The active ingredient in both marijuana and hashish is tetrahydrocannabinol, with hashish being much more potent.

Inhalation of marijuana causes a state of exhilaration or euphoria. Under its influence the user feels light in body, as if he were floating through space, and his general behavior is not unlike a mild mania. Marijuana is not an aphrodisiac, but it can lower inhibitions and intensify sexual pleasure. It seems to make many users temporarily passive, in contrast to alcohol, which frequently releases aggression. Marijuana affects the individual's sense of time but not necessarily his motor and perceptual skills. Users become psychologically dependent on marijuana but may not become physically addicted as with morphine.

Currently a great deal of attention is being given to marijuana by the government because its use has risen dramatically. Official arguments have been carried on in the press concerning the relative dangers of marijuana and the appropriate penalties that should be or should not be levied against people who use it. Unfortunately, there is a limited amount of research on which to base a scientific, unbiased judgment concerning the immediate dangers of smoking marijuana or the eventual outcome of long-term use of this drug. Many of the research findings have been contradictory. Certainly the present laws controlling its use are inequitable, as well as widely unenforceable.

Inhalation of marijuana causes a state of exhilaration or euphoria. Many research findings about this drug are contradictory.

CAUSATIVE FACTORS OF SUBSTANCE ABUSE AND DEPENDENCE

Although many persons are highly critical of governmental policies concerning alcohol and other drugs, the ineffectiveness of the government in controlling the availability of these substances does not explain their appeal to such a large segment of society. The latest research indicates substance abuse and dependence cannot be explained by a single phenomenon such as availability of drugs but rather results from multiple interacting and overlapping factors.

Individual factors

Research has clearly demonstrated that the incidence of alcoholism varies significantly among ethnic groups and among families within these groups. Therefore, it is currently believed that there is likely to be a genetic predisposition to the development of this form of dependence. In addition, much current research is exploring the physiological factors that differentiate the alcoholic from others who are able to drink alcohol without deleterious effects or a subsequent craving. One theory states there is a physiological inability to absorb and/or eliminate the substance. Another theory has postulated an allergic type of reaction among some people. Although there are fewer research studies concerning the influence of genetic and biochemical factors on the development of dependence on nonalcohol drugs, the idiosyncratic responses of some people to all other drugs are well known by clinicians.

Substance abuse and dependence can only be explained by multiple interacting and overlapping individual and environmental factors.

The individual factor contributing to substance abuse or dependence that has been explored most fully is the role of the person's personality. For example, it is believed that many persons who use depressant drugs, such as alcohol, barbiturates, or heroin have not developed the ego defense mechanisms that would enable them to function as independent adults who can successfully cope with the stresses of daily living. Their use of these drugs enables them to blunt reality and withdraw from environmental and intrapsychic stressors.

In contrast, users of stimulant drugs such as amphetamines and cocaine are thought to have a personality bordering on grandiosity simultaneous with a need to consistently defend against fears of helplessness. The use of stimulant drugs allows such a person to feel active and potent in the face of an environment perceived as hostile and threatening.

Individuals who use hallucinogens and marijuana are believed to be struggling with huge amounts of repressed rage along with fears of annihilation and interpersonal isolation. It is hypothesized that they attempt to cope with these feelings through the use of drugs that alter perception and cognition, often allowing them to feel "a cosmic unity."

Environmental factors

Environmental factors include the family of the individual as well as the sociocultural environment in which the person exists.

Recently, much attention has been focused on the structure and rules of families of individuals who are substance dependent, particularly those who are alcohol dependent. The structure of such families has been found to be either enmeshed, where the boundaries are so diffuse that its members are unclear about their roles and relationships, or disengaged, where the boundaries are so rigid that there is little interdependence and family identity.

Regardless of their structure, all families have rules that set the guidelines for how they will function both within the family and with the environment. Sharon Wegscheider identifies three important characteristics of rules in the substance dependent family.

1. Inhuman—Rules often are unrealistic and impossible to keep. They encourage one to be dishonest and manipulative with others to avoid punishment or rejection. They encourage one to be dishonest with oneself to avoid feelings of guilt.
2. Rigid—Rules make no allowance for differences in people or circumstances. They discourage change, seeing it as a potential threat to the status quo (especially that of the rule-maker).
3. Closed—Certain areas of life are closed to communication. Information and feelings about these areas stay bottled up inside for each family member to handle alone.

Even this superficial discussion of the characteristics of the substance-dependent family makes clear the difficulty, if not impossibility, of a child in such a family being able to mature in a developmentally appropriate way. Thus, it should not be surprising to learn that many substance-dependent persons come from families in which one or both parents were substance dependent.

The sociocultural environment of the substance-dependent individual is known to be a major determinant in the development and maintenance of his dependence. Societal norms that condone substance use and intoxication, peer group use of such substances, and the availability of licit and illicit drugs all combine to predict a high rate of substance dependence. When these factors exist in an environment fraught with continuous stress, such as is present in urban ghettos, the likelihood of escaping substance abuse, if not dependence, is small.

LONG-TERM TREATMENT OF SUBSTANCE-DEPENDENT INDIVIDUALS

Despite the magnitude of the problem of alcohol dependency in the United States, few specific long-term measures of helping these individuals refrain from drinking have been developed. The only potentially effective long-term treatment of the alcohol-dependent individual requires that he accept the fact he is an alcoholic. This step is often the most difficult to achieve, since the defense mechanism of denial is universally employed by the alcohol-dependent person.

Mental health professionals have had less success in treating the alcohol-dependent individual than has the lay organization known as Alcoholics Anonymous. Alcoholics Anonymous was founded in 1935 by two alcoholics and usually admits to membership only individuals who have a desire to stop drinking. It has had a dramatic development and today numbers more than one million members throughout the world. Alcoholics Anonymous offers the alcoholic answers to his emotional needs because it uses psychological principles that have been recognized as being effective in helping troubled people. Alcoholics Anonymous also has affiliated groups. One is for their spouses and the other for their children.

Because membership is limited to individuals who themselves have been unable to control the problem of alcohol, members have a good deal of sympathy, patience, and understanding for each other. They work in teams of two or three and call on known alcoholics who are in need of help. Through the program of the organization they are able to meet the alcoholic's dependency needs by seeking him out, encouraging him, helping him find a job, accompanying him to meetings of the organization, and helping him develop a sense of personal value and worth. Each member is encouraged to admit that he is powerless over alcohol and is in need of help from a power greater than himself. He searches out his own past errors and, having admitted them to another human being, undertakes to make amends for them. He strives to follow a simple code of living that eventually becomes a philosophy of life. The organizational meetings include testimonials by the members concerning their struggles with alcohol and their eventual triumph.

Alcoholics Anonymous offers an experience in group participation and the use of group support. This organization is able to assist its members to develop a new emotional orientation toward life and to begin to meet the problems of life without the aid of alcohol. Many physicians refer alcoholic patients to this organization for help. Most social agencies work closely with Alcoholics Anonymous, and it is generally accepted as the most helpful approach to the problem of alcoholism available at this time.

Alcoholics Anonymous is a lay organization that assists alcoholics in developing a sense of personal value and worth through individual and group support.

In the past the United States government maintained one treatment center for drug-dependent individuals at Lexington, Kentucky. It was called the National Institute of Mental Health Clinical Research Center. In such a specialized hospital everything possible was done to help drug-dependent individuals break their habit and become useful, productive citizens. Many individuals were treated at Lexington several times. Unfortunately, many were not able to function without the emotional support the drug provides. When the programs at this facility proved ineffective, the hospital was closed.

Many communities have organized facilities for treating individuals who suffer from drug dependence. As in all situations that involve the emotions, it is necessary to discover why this kind of unusual emotional support is needed and then attempt to supply the support in more positive ways while at the same time helping the individual to give up the drug.

Some authorities believe that a more realistic approach to the problem of drug dependence would be to supply each drug-dependent individual with a minimum weekly supply of the drug on which he is dependent. This practice, it is argued, would make the illegal traffic in drugs unprofitable. It is thought that this practice of supplying a small amount of the drug to the addict each week would aid in cutting down the crimes that addicts now commit to obtain drugs. It would make it possible for the addict to purchase adequate food and maintain his physical health at an optimum level instead of denying himself food to purchase the drug, as he frequently has done in the past.

No effective means of long-term treatment of drug-dependent individuals has been developed, although Synanon, an organization similar to Alcoholics Anonymous, is having the most success.

As is true with the treatment of alcohol-dependent persons, the most effective long-term treatment for drug-dependent individuals is conducted by a self-help group called Synanon. This organization sponsors residential centers in many large cities. These centers are usually under the direction of a trained professional worker, who may have one to two other professionally trained people to assist him. Most of the therapy as well as the work required to maintain the center is done by the drug-dependent individuals who are there to be helped or by those who have been helped and who stay on to make a contribution to the work.

In these situations, drug-dependent individuals who sincerely want to stop the drug habit live with other people struggling with similar problems. The house is usually organized along the lines of communal living, with each person accepting a share of the work necessary to keep the house livable and to prepare the meals. Several group sessions are carried on each week, during which members of the group are supportive to each other but are very straightforward in demanding that the group members face their rationalizations, evasions, personal problems, and social deceptions. If a member returns to drugs, he is expected to leave the group. This realistic but supportive approach has apparently helped many drug-dependent individuals to give up drugs and return to school or to a job.

NURSING CARE OF INDIVIDUALS WITH SUBSTANCE ABUSE AND DEPENDENCE

Nursing assessment

Although abuse of or dependence on each substance has its unique features, it is possible to cite some commonalities about all persons suffering from substance abuse or dependence. The following discussion is organized around the human processes introduced in Chapter 9. Although behaviors in each category are presented as separate entities, it should be understood that they are highly interrelated and are adaptations to similar stressors. Further, in many instances behavior designed as an adaptation to one stressor becomes a stressor itself in another dimension.

Activity processes. The motor behavior of a substance dependent individual is always affected when the substance affects the central nervous system, as with opiates, alcohol, barbiturates, and amphetamines. In the case of intoxication with opioids, alcohol, and barbiturates, psychomotor retardation will be observed. Even small amounts of alcohol and low doses of barbiturates will produce incoordination and an unsteady gait in most users. Because of this fact, the individual often has bruises or fractures resulting from falls and bumping into furniture.

In contrast, intoxication with amphetamines results in psychomotor hyperactivity.

Recreation patterns are almost always altered in individuals who are substance dependent. Individuals who are dependent upon large amounts of a substance must forego recreational activities because all their time is spent obtaining the drug, using it, or engaging in activities to secure money to buy it.

Self-care ultimately is affected in all individuals who are substance dependent. Hygiene and grooming become poor as the person's judgment becomes impaired.

Sleep and arousal patterns are always impaired when the individual abuses or is dependent upon substances affecting the central nervous system. Central nervous system depressants allow the person to fall into a stuporous sleep but cause a "rebound effect" about four hours later when the person awakens with a start, often with tachycardia. Obviously, central nervous system stimulants cause insomnia and initially are often taken to achieve this effect.

Cognition processes. Cognition processes are almost always altered by substance abuse. Therefore, in the stage of acute intoxication the nurse will observe alterations in decision making, judgment, memory, and thought processes. Whether these changes will remain after withdrawal from the substance depends on whether the drug has destroyed brain tissue. Long-term alcohol abusers, for example, show evidence of diminution of cognitive capacities even after they have been abstinent for years. The long-term effect of marijuana use on cognitive processes is the subject of much current research.

Assessment of the substance-dependent individual usually reveals either psychomotor retardation or hyperactivity, altered recreation patterns, poor hygiene and grooming, impaired sleep and arousal patterns, altered cognition processes, impaired home maintenance, altered feeling states, impaired interpersonal processes, altered sexuality, poor attention or hyperalertness, malnutrition, and powerlessness and hopelessness.

Ecological processes. Needless to say, home maintenance is always altered when a person is dependent upon a substance.

Emotional processes. Feeling states are always altered during the stage of acute intoxication, and, in fact, this alteration is the conscious goal of initial substance use. As previously stated, individuals use narcotics to create a feeling of "normalcy," sedative hypnotics to create a feeling of calm, and central nervous system stimulants to create a feeling of euphoria. Withdrawal from any substance often creates anxiety, often to the degree of panic. Furthermore, during those periods when they are not using the drug, many individuals experience guilt, sadness, and shame about their behavior when they were "high."

Interpersonal processes. Interpersonal processes are always affected in the domains of conduct/impulse processes, family processes, role performance, sexuality, and social interaction.

Conduct/impulse processes are altered because the dependent individual has no choice but to go to any length to obtain the substance if he is to avoid withdrawal symptoms. This may mean that he engages in behaviors such as lying, stealing, physical aggression, or prostitution even though these behaviors may be otherwise abhorrent to him. Furthermore, when acutely intoxicated with a substance that affects the central nervous system, the individual becomes accident prone and a potential danger to himself and others.

As previously explained, family processes are always altered. Since the family operates as a system, the existence of a substance-dependent member precipitates responsive family adaptations that hinder the development of family members and the family as a unit.

The substance-dependent individual ultimately suffers severe alterations in his role performance, often losing his job or failing out of school.

Sexuality is frequently altered, especially with abuse of substances that affect the central nervous system. Social interaction with individuals who do not use the substance upon which the individual is dependent is often curtailed, and social isolation or withdrawal is common.

Perception processes. Alteration in attention is common in individuals who use drugs that affect the central nervous system. Central nervous system depressants cause inattention, while stimulants cause hyperalertness.

There is much debate about whether a poor self-concept contributes to substance dependence. Regardless of the eventual answer to this question, there is no doubt that continued substance abuse and dependence leads to altered self-esteem.

Alterations in sensory perception are always present in individuals who use hallucinogens. They are also present in individuals suffering from delirium tremens after withdrawal from large quantities of alcohol imbibed over long periods of time.

Physiological processes. All physiological processes are affected or potentially affected by substance abuse and dependence. Chief among these are alterations in nutrition. Almost every individual who abuses or is dependent upon a substance for any length of time suffers from malnutrition. This, in turn, makes him exceptionally susceptible to alterations in other physiological processes.

Examples of physiological alterations for each category of substance abuse are:

- Narcotics—Physical integrity is altered by the intravenous injection of the drug, leaving "track marks" and often causing local or systemic infections.
- Sedative hypnotics—Not only is malnutrition common, gastric ulcers may occur from large amounts of alcohol taken over long periods of time.
- Central Nervous System Stimulants—Because cocaine is often snorted, it is not uncommon for heavy users to have necrotic perforation of the nasal septum.
- Hallucinogens and PCP—There is some evidence that continued use of LSD and PCP creates chromosomal damage and teratogenicity (the production of abnormal organisms or monsters).
- Marijuana—Although this drug is considered by many to be among the most safe, the fact that it is smoked contributes to decreased vital capacity and perhaps even lung cancer among heavy users.

Valuation processes. There is no question that individuals who are substance dependent feel powerless over their addiction and hopeless about release from the vicious cycle of obtaining the drug, taking the drug, experiencing its effect, coming down from the effect, obtaining the drug, etc. They often report that life has lost all meaning other than that related to the drug.

Nursing diagnosis

As with all nursing diagnoses, the nursing diagnoses for the individual with substance abuse or dependence are based on the themes identified during the assessment phase of the nursing process. Categories of human responses from the ANA Classification of Human Responses of Concern for Psychiatric–Mental Health Nursing Practice that may be specifically applicable to individuals with substance abuse and dependence include the following:

1.1.2	Altered Motor Behavior
1.2.2	Altered Recreation Patterns
1.3.4	Altered Self-Care
1.4.2	Altered Sleep/Arousal Patterns
2.1.2	Altered Decision Making
2.2.2	Altered Judgment
2.4.2	Altered Learning Processes
2.5.2	Altered Memory
2.6.2	Altered Thought Processes
3.3.2	Altered Home Maintenance
4.1.2	Altered Feeling State

4.2.2   Altered Feeling Processes
5.3.2   Altered Conduct/Impulse Processes
5.4.2   Altered Family Processes
5.5.2   Altered Role Processes
5.6.9   Sexual Dysfunction
5.7.2   Altered Social Interaction
6.1.2   Altered Attention
6.3.2   Altered Self-Concept
6.4.2   Altered Sensory Perception
7.1.1   Potential for Alteration in Circulation
7.2.1   Potential for Alteration in Elimination
7.3.1   Potential for Alteration in Endocrine/Metabolic Processes
7.4.1   Potential for Alteration in Gastrointestinal Processes
7.5.1   Potential for Alteration in Musculoskeletal Processes
7.6.1   Potential for Alteration in Neuro/Sensory Processes
7.7.2   Altered Nutrition Processes
7.8.1   Potential of Alteration in Oxygenation
7.9.1   Potential for Alteration in Physical Integrity
7.10.1   Potential for Alteration in Physical Regulation Processes
8.1.2   Altered Meaningfulness
8.3.2   Altered Values

NANDA nursing diagnostic categories that may be specifically applicable to the individual with substance abuse and dependence include:

1.1.2.2   Altered Nutrition: Less than body requirements
1.2.1.1   Potential for Infection
1.2.2.1   Potential Altered Body Temperature
1.3.1.1   Constipation
1.3.1.2   Diarrhea
1.3.2   Altered Patterns of Urinary Elimination
1.5.1.3   Ineffective Breathing Pattern
1.6.1   Potential for Injury
1.6.1.2   Potential for Poisoning
1.6.1.3   Potential for Trauma
1.6.1.4   Potential for Aspiration
1.6.2.1   Impaired Tissue Integrity
1.6.2.1.2.2 Potential Impaired Skin Integrity
3.1.1   Impaired Social Interaction
3.1.2   Social Isolation
3.2.1   Altered Role Performance
3.2.1.1.1   Altered Parenting
3.2.1.2.1   Sexual Dysfunction
3.2.2   Altered Family Processes
3.2.3.1   Parental Role Conflict

4.1.1	Spiritual Distress
5.1.1.1	Ineffective Individual Coping
5.1.2.1.1.	Ineffective Family Coping: Disabling
6.1.1.3	Potential Activity Intolerance
6.2.1	Sleep Pattern Disturbance
6.3.1.1	Diversional Activity Deficit
6.4.1.1	Impaired Home Maintenance
6.4.2	Altered Health Maintenance
6.5.2	Bathing/Hygiene Self-Care Deficit
6.5.3	Dressing/Grooming Self-Care Deficit
7.1.2	Self-Esteem Disturbance
7.2	Sensory/Perceptual Alterations (Specify)
7.3.1	Hopelessness
7.3.2	Powerlessness
8.3	Altered Thought Processes
9.2.2	Potential for Violence: Self-directed or directed at others
9.3.1	Anxiety
9.3.2	Fear

To develop a nursing diagnosis that fulfills its function of providing direction for planning nursing care, the nurse is encouraged to postulate and state etiologic or antecedent factors for each human response and connect the two phrases by using the term "related to." For example:

> 5.5.2 Altered Role Performance related to inability to work because of dependence on heroin

Planning and implementing nursing care

The plan for nursing care is derived from the nursing diagnoses and includes the objectives of the care, the nursing actions, and outcome criteria. To be effective the plan needs to be highly individualized. The suggestions that follow should be seen as general guidelines to be used if they are appropriate to the client's needs.

In general, the objectives of all nursing care for the individual with substance abuse or dependence should relate to assisting the client to regain physiological homeokinesis, to increase his self-esteem, and to develop functional methods of coping with stress.

Until recently, the nurse was likely to be in a position to give care to an individual with substance abuse or dependence only when he was admitted to an acute care hospital because of serious physiological alterations due either to his drug abuse or dependence or to another unrelated illness. There is an increasing awareness, however, that some seriously mentally ill persons, particularly young adult chronically ill clients, present themselves as substance-dependent individuals, when in reality their substance dependence is an adaptation to

In caring for the individual with substance abuse or dependence, the nurse should assist him to regain physiological well-being, increase self-esteem, and develop functional methods of coping with stress.

the symptoms of their mental illness. Consequently, these individuals are now being treated simultaneously for their drug dependence and their mental illness in psychiatric units of general hospitals or in psychiatric hospitals. They are often referred to as *multi-disabled* or *mentally ill chemical abusers—MICAs,* and psychiatric nursing is assuming an increasing responsibility for their care.

Emotional processes. The substance-dependent client who no longer has access to drugs inevitably will express a great deal of anxiety. It is helpful to him if the nurse takes his feelings seriously and encourages him to explore their source. For example, the client may share the fact that sitting in a room with a group of other people makes him "nervous." Although the nurse may find this difficult to believe because he appears to be confident and competent, she needs to understand that his use of drugs is a powerful indicator that he, in fact, does feel insecure without their blunting or stimulating effect. Therefore, it is helpful to explore with the client his worst fears about what may happen in the group and then assist him to problem solve a functional solution if his fears become reality.

Another feeling that is often displayed by individuals undergoing treatment for substance abuse or dependence is anger. Since it is often very anxiety producing for substance dependent clients to express anger, their ability to do so is often indicative of increasing ego strength. To the extent that the client's anger is reality based, it is therapeutic for the nurse to acknowledge his feelings and help him discover productive outlets for them. However, sometimes the client uses his anger about real or fantasized wrongs that he experienced in the past as a means of avoiding dealing with the present or planning for the future. In this situation, the nurse can be most therapeutic by listening in a matter-of-fact manner, but then insisting that the client get on with the task at hand. The tendency for substance-dependent clients to ruminate about problems in their past is the basis for the famous Serenity Prayer used so successfully by Alcoholics Anonymous.

Interpersonal processes. It is important for the nurse to fully appreciate that substance-dependent clients are likely to have a great deal of difficulty with conduct/impulse processes. Understanding this, however, does not mean that the nurse should condone unacceptable behavior. Early in the treatment regimen the client needs to be confronted in a nonjudgmental and nonpunitive way with the fact that he will be held responsible for his behavior. Therefore, the consequences of behavior such as lying, taking drugs, or being verbally or physically assaultive need to be made clear to him. Needless to say, it is imperative that all staff behave toward the client in a consistent manner when and if these infractions occur.

The client needs to be helped to plan realistically for a future life without drugs. The first step in this process is to help him explore what drugs meant to him and to identify and grieve about the losses he will experience without them. These losses may be very concrete, such as friends and activities, or they

NURSING CARE PLAN

A heroin-dependent individual

CASE FORMULATION

David S. is a 24-year-old, single man who was admitted to a long-term residential drug rehabilitation program, following a 2-week inpatient stay on a detoxification unit for withdrawal from heroin. David began using marijuana and then heroin when he was a junior in high school because his 14-year-old girlfriend refused to date him any longer. About the same time, David was sent by his mother, who lived in New York City, to attend high school in a distant southern city because his parents were getting a divorce.

According to David, marijuana made him feel excited, stimulated, and happy. Everything seemed more pleasant, and he enjoyed his daydreams. He was also sexually stimulated by the drug. About the same time, he tried taking barbiturates, which made him sleepy. Because he did not enjoy their effect, he did not continue them. He got drunk a few times, but alcohol failed to produce the calmness and contentment he was seeking. Since marijuana did not completely satisfy him either, he was convinced that his willpower would be great enough to allow him to stop using this drug when he wanted to be free of it.

David first took heroin in the vein. He described feeling a "flash," which was accompanied by a flush of blood from the abdomen to the head and a feeling of happiness. Although the "flash" passed away, a constant feeling of euphoria remained. For the first time in his life he experienced a feeling of deep contentment. He said, "It didn't affect my intellect, only my emotions. I was happy and content." From that time on he took heroin to assist him in facing any situation that caused him to be tense or anxious. Heroin helped him feel independent of his mother and reduced his nervousness when he was out with a girl. Although heroin gave him a feeling of contentment, it lessened his sexual desire and made it impossible for him to reach a sexual climax.

After David discovered the contentment heroin could achieve for him, he became involved in crimes to support his drug habit. As his need for larger and larger quantities of heroin grew, making his habit more costly, his crimes became more frequent and more serious. His mother repeatedly intervened to keep him out of jail by paying his fines. He entered several colleges but because of his drug habit was never able to stay in any of them for more than a semester.

Finally David tried to withdraw himself from heroin. He thought he could achieve this by himself, since he had been withdrawn twice before in treatment centers. He was not able to accomplish his goal and finally at 24 years of age signed himself into a detoxification unit in the hope of stopping the drug so that he could return to college. He had set for himself the goal of becoming an engineer.

Following the 2-week detoxification program, staff members recommended to David that he admit himself to a long-term residential treatment setting, due to the chronic nature of his difficulties and his past inability to remain abstinent when confronted by stressful life events.

The residential drug rehabilitation program was staffed by a variety of professional and nonprofessional staff, including recovered drug addicts. The staff worked with David to develop a plan of care designed to meet his individual needs and enhance his strengths. On admission to the center, David was drug free. He appeared undernourished, but was in no acute physical distress. He initially gave evidence of being highly motivated and tested in the superior range on a standardized intelligence test.

During the admission interview, David recounted the following information about his early childhood. He stated that his parents were married when his mother was 16 years old. David was their first child, and he recalled his mother often reminding him that his birth had been traumatic for her. During his formative years his father suffered from tuberculosis and spent many months in a sanitarium. David remembered that when he was 3 and 4 years old

Continued.

NURSING CARE PLAN—cont'd

his mother fondled his genitals when she bathed him. As he grew older, she allowed him to observe her dressing and bathing but scolded him if he evidenced interest in her body.

Nursing assessment

David's history reveals a number of factors that potentially contributed to his dependence on heroin for a sense of well-being. He described the feelings of happiness, contentment, relief of anxiety, and independence that he experienced when using heroin.

David's relationship with his mother was a highly ambivalent and conflicted one. From the time he was a child he had been given the message that he was unwanted and unloved. Owing to her own difficulties in adjustment, David's mother was unable to provide him with a healthy environment in which to develop and grow. Her sexually provocative behaviors contributed to David's poor psychosexual adjustment and his anxieties in relation to intimacy with women. David's attempts to separate from his mother were unsuccessful. Her continual interventions on his behalf with the police enabled him to continue his substance dependence while maintaining his unhealthy and dependent relationship with her. The absence of a healthy male role model further hindered David's ability to develop effective adaptations to stress. He seemed to rely solely on drugs for a sense of well-being and autonomy and used drugs to deal with all anxiety-provoking situations.

David failed to develop a healthy sense of self as an autonomous male individual. His dependence on drugs may have been a substitute for the dependence he experienced in relation to his rejecting and controlling mother. The adaptation was dysfunctional in that his use of drugs further impeded his ability to negotiate the adolescent tasks of separation and identity development.

David appeared undernourished, probably due to his use of funds to purchase heroin rather than food. His work history was poor, as was his school performance, and he had begun to rely on stealing to purchase heroin. David's strengths included his superior intelligence, as well as his apparent motivation to remain free of drugs and to pursue a career. His willingness to commit himself to a long-term rehabilitation center indicated his emerging recognition of the severity of his drug dependence and his desire for change.

Nursing diagnosis

Based on the nursing assessment that included prior knowledge of the family dynamics and an understanding of the dynamics underlying substance abuse and dependence, the nurse formulated the following three pairs of nursing diagnoses for David S. The first of each pair is from the Classification of Human Responses of Concern for Psychiatric–Mental Health Nursing Practice; the second is from the approved NANDA Diagnostic Categories.

7.7.2   Altered Nutrition Processes related to inadequate food and fluid intake

OR

1.1.2.2   Altered Nutrition: Less than body requirements related to inadequate food and fluid intake

5.5.3   Ineffective Individual Coping related to long-term reliance on drugs to cope with stressful life events

OR

5.1.1.1   Ineffective Individual Coping related to long-term reliance on drugs to cope with stressful life events

5.7.2   Altered Social Interaction related to fear of rejection and psychosexual conflicts

OR

3.1.1   Impaired Social Interaction related to fear of rejection and psychosexual conflicts

Planning and implementing care for *David S.*

The plan of nursing care for David S. is summarized in the box on pp. 322-323. The team working with David consisted of a variety of professional and nonprofessional members and included a primary nurse, the team psychiatrist, a psychiatric social worker, and an occu-

NURSING CARE PLAN—cont'd

pational therapist. In addition, David attended Synanon meetings daily. These meetings were held each evening at the center and were attended by several persons recovering from drug dependence, one of whom served as David's sponsor.

The staff members assigned to David were mature individuals experienced in the treatment of clients with substance dependence. They approached David in a hopeful, caring, and supportive fashion, while clearly maintaining boundaries of separateness and setting firm limits. The initial task of treatment was to assist David to recognize and accept his heroin addiction as a problem, thereby breaking through the massive defense of denial common to drug-dependent individuals. Despite David's high motivation to be drug free, the treatment team expected that David eventually would express ambivalence in relation to treatment, and they would need to help him remain abstinent at that time. Finally, treatment would focus on assisting David to develop alternative coping methods to handle stressful life events and uncomfortable feelings to prevent a return to reliance on drugs as a coping style.

The treatment approach consisted of a variety of modalities, including group therapy; peer groups; milieu therapy; peer pressure; recreational and expressive-creative therapies; and assistance with developing social and vocational skills. A contract developed by David and the team outlined mutual expectations for treatment participation. In addition, David was expected to do his share of housekeeping and meal preparation as outlined by the community in weekly meetings. David agreed to the plan as written and was given his final copy of the contract. He agreed to remain in the program for 1 year, to remain drug free as evidenced by daily urine screens, and to follow the contract as written. David was assigned a primary nurse whose plan was to establish a supportive but firm relationship, to develop a climate of acceptance that allowed for the expression of feelings, and to facilitate David's full participation in the program as

outlined. Violation of the treatment plan would constitute grounds for immediate review and potential discharge.

Evaluation

David's participation and progress were reviewed by all staff members with David present on a biweekly basis. While he made steady progress, his course of treatment was not without difficulty. After 2 months at the center, it was felt that David was ready to handle an all-day pass to visit with his mother. David had verbalized the hope that he could use some of his new knowledge and behaviors, and that the meeting would go well. On David's return, his urine drug screen revealed that he had used marijuana while on pass, despite his earlier denial of any drug use. He began to challenge staff when confronted and vehemently denied that the action had any meaning, stating, "It doesn't mean anything . . . it wasn't heroin, just pot. What's the big deal?" David was confronted by his peers in group therapy the following day and became withdrawn, sullen, and nonverbal for several weeks. He then began to discuss his fears related to a "life without drugs" with his primary nurse, who encouraged him to discuss and explore these issues in the various groups he attended. David responded to this suggestion by accusing the nurse of being rejecting, just like his mother. The nurse remained accepting of these feelings and encouraged David to discuss them. Gradually he began to use groups and peers for increased support and became particularly close to a group of men close to his age. They relied on one another for support and encouragement.

Each new anxiety-producing circumstance David confronted led to a desire to return to drug use. As he began to explore career avenues, his anxiety again increased, as did the desire to rely on drugs. David feared each new step toward an independent and drug-free existence. He often expressed the feeling that others were "forcing" him to quit drugs and was frequently reminded by peers that he had voluntarily chosen to make a commitment to treatment.

Continued.

NURSING CARE PLAN—cont'd

David slowly continued to progress toward recovery. He gradually developed an interest in pottery and became quite skilled. He began to expand his support network and develop new relationships. He became particularly helpful with individuals new to the program. In addition, he began to discuss and explore his angry but dependent feelings toward his mother. He began to attend a local university parttime to pursue his interest in engineering and was permitted increased time away from the center in an effort to encourage independent living and to confront stress while support was available.

As the time of David's discharge drew near, many separation issues arose. David's fears about living independently emerged in full force. He angrily stated that he felt as if he was being "thrown out." He expressed the wish to remain longer. David was assisted in coping with these feelings by peers and staff. He was encouraged to continue his involvement with support groups in the community, and contracted to volunteer at the center once a week. At the time of discharge, staff members were hopeful that David had made much progress and would continue to make gains with available supports, meetings with his sponsor, and weekly visits to his therapist. He had not made much progress in the area of heterosexual relationships and continued to be quite anxious and fearful when he contemplated dating and intimacy. It was hoped that David would begin to explore this issue in the future with his therapist.

NURSING CARE PLAN FOR *David S.*

Nursing diagnosis		Objective	Nursing actions	Outcome criteria
7.7.2	Altered Nutrition Processes related to inadequate food and fluid intake	To increase client's nutritional status	Monitor client's intake, encouraging three well-balanced meals each day	Within 1 week client will gain 5 pounds
OR			Supplement daily meals with high-calorie nutritional snacks between meals	Within 1 month client will show evidence of adequate nutrition in hair, skin, eyes, and mucous membranes
1.1.2.2	Altered Nutrition: Less than body requirements related to inadequate food and fluid intake			
5.5.3	Ineffective Individual Coping related to long-term reliance on drugs to cope with stressful life events	To assist client to abstain from drug use	Convey a caring but firm attitude Conduct daily urine screens for drugs Encourage daily participation in Synanon groups Encourage frequent meetings with sponsor	Within 2 weeks client will: Obtain urine for drug screens without reminder, and remain drug free Attend Synanon meetings daily without reminder

NURSING CARE PLAN—cont'd

OR 5.1.1.1 Ineffective Individual Coping related to long-term reliance on drugs to cope with stressful life events	To assist client to recognize and accept his drug addiction as a problem	Offer positive appraisals for abstinence. Convey hope and support while confronting emerging evidence of the use of denial. Encourage participation in Synanon, peer groups, and community discussions	Within 2 weeks the client will: Willingly attend Synanon, peer group, and meet with sponsor daily without reminder. Initiate discussions of behaviors related to addiction and the negative impact of these behaviors on life goals
	To assist the client to develop alternative coping methods to deal with stressful life events and uncomfortable feelings	Accept expressions of fear related to loss of heroin as a coping method. Assist with the exploration of new coping styles. Encourage and monitor attendence of biweekly group therapy. Encourage participation in expressive activities (that is, art, music, poetry)	Within 1 month the client will: Begin to discuss ways to deal with uncomfortable feelings. Plan and begin a creative project. Attend group therapy without reminder
	To assist client to develop and follow through with career and educational plans	Discuss educational and career interests, conveying hope and support. Offer positive appraisals for success. Refer to vocational counselor	Within 1 month the client will: Initiate discussion related to career plan. Meet with vocational counselor
5.7.2 Altered Social Interaction related to fear of rejection and psychosexual conflicts OR 3.1.1 Impaired Social Interaction related to fear of rejection and psychosexual conflicts	To assist client to develop a sense of trust in close relationships as well as the belief that identity can be simultaneously maintained	Establish trusting relationship, conveying support and acceptance of client as an individual with value, in daily meetings. Encourage autonomous and healthy behaviors and independent decision making	Within 2 weeks the client will initiate conversation in meetings with primary nurse
	To assist client to explore and discuss anxieties related to intimate relationships with women	Encourage discussion by use of reflective listening, conveying acceptance and support	Within 2 weeks the client will identify feelings and fears related to intimacy

may be more abstract, such as a way of life. After the grieving process has taken place, practical issues such as where he is going to live, what kind of work he wants to prepare for, and how he is going to develop a social network with people who do not use drugs are topics that need to be addressed.

The client's family is in need of as much help as is the client. Not only do they have many issues to deal with about events in the past, but they must also adjust to changes in the client. The nurse can be most helpful to the family by ensuring that they become involved in group counseling, either through the mental health facility or with the appropriate self-help organization.

Perception processes. The substance-dependent person is an individual with very low self-esteem. Thus, the nurse is most therapeutic when she focuses on the client's strengths, acknowledges them, and helps him build upon them. For example, having the client participate in decision making about his activities and providing opportunities for success can be important interventions if the nurse also acknowledges his wise judgments and achievements. The client also needs to be helped to see that one achievement can lead to another, and that each is not an isolated event.

Physiological processes. When the client is intoxicated or being withdrawn from a substance, meeting his physical needs is of paramount importance. Every body system is likely to be in a greater or lesser state of disequilibrium, and, in some instances, the client may be in danger of dying. It is important that the nurse be particularly alert to the client's level of consciousness, the maintenance of a patent airway, adequate fluid intake and output, and prevention of injury.

Once the client is drug free, the nurse will find that it is likely that he will have some residual physiological alterations resulting from his substance dependence. As previously stated, malnutrition is common among all substance abusers. In addition, there may be other problems specific to the effects of the drug he abused or its mode of transmission, such as skin infections in the opiate-dependent individual and peripheral neuropathy in the alcohol-dependent person. The nurse needs to address these problems as she would with any person who exhibited the same alterations.

> The nurse is most therapeutic when she focuses on the client's strengths and helps him see that one achievement can lead to another.

END NOTE

This chapter focuses on the nursing care needs of individuals who abuse or are dependent upon chemical substances. The effects of abuse of or dependence on six categories of substances are discussed and the causes of substance abuse and dependence are explored. The chapter concludes with a plan of nursing care for a young adult who is dependent upon heroin to cope with the stresses of daily living.

SUGGESTED SOURCES OF ADDITIONAL INFORMATION

Adams FE: Drug dependency in hospital patients, Am J Nurs 88(4):477, April 1988.
Arneson SW, Schultz M, and Triplett JL: Nurses' knowledge of the impact of parental alcoholism on children, Arch Psychiatr Nurs 1(4):251, August 1987.

Bean-Bayog M: Alcoholism as a cause of psychopathology, Hosp Commun Psychiatr 39(4):352, April 1988.

Berger F: Alcoholism rehabilitation: a supportive approach, Hosp Commun Psychiatr 34(11):1040, 1983.

Betemps E: Management of the withdrawal syndrome of barbiturates and other central nervous system depressants, J Psychosoc Nurs Ment Health Serv 19:31, September 1981.

Bingham A and Bargar J: Children of alcoholic families, J Psychosoc Nurs Ment Health Serv 23(12):13, 1985.

Bissell L and Jones R: The alcoholic nurse, Nurs Outlook 29:96, February 1981.

Boyd C and Mast D: Addicted women and their relationships with men, J Psychosoc Nurs Ment Health Serv 21:10, February 1983.

Busch D, McBride AB, and Benaventura L: Chemical dependency in women: the link to OB/GYN problems, J Psychosoc Nurs Ment Health Serv 24(4):26, 1986.

Cadoret RJ, Troughton E, O'Gorman TW, and Heywood E: An adoption study of genetic and environmental factors in drug abuse, Arch Gen Psychiatr 43:1131, December 1986.

Caroselli-Karinja M: Drug abuse and the elderly, J Psychosoc Nurs Ment Health Serv 23(6):25, 1985.

Carruth GR and Pugh JB: Grieving the loss of alcohol: a crisis in recovery, J Psychosoc Nurs Ment Health Serv 20:18, March 1982.

Cohn L: The hidden diagnosis, Am J Nurs 82:1862, 1982.

Compton P: Drug abuse: a self-care deficit, J Psychosoc Nurs Ment Health Serv 27(3):22, March 1989.

Eells MAW: Interventions with alcoholics and their families, Nurs Clin N Am 21(3):493, September 1986.

Ellison Hough ES: Alcoholism: prevention and treatment, J Psychosoc Nurs Ment Health Serv 27(1):15, January 1989.

Jefferson L and Ensor B: Help for the helper: confronting a chemically impaired colleague, Am J Nurs 82:574, 1982.

Khantzian EJ: The self-medication hypothesis of addictive disorders: focus on heroin and cocaine dependence, Am J Psychiatr 142(11):1259, November 1985.

Loweree F, Freng A, and Baines B: Admitting an intoxicated patient, Am J Nurs 84:616, 1984.

McCoy S, Rice M, and McFadden K: PCP intoxication: psychiatric issues of nursing care, J Psychosoc Nurs Ment Health Serv 19:17, July 1981.

McKelvy MJ, Kane JS, and Kellison K: Substance abuse and mental illness: double trouble, J Psychosoc Nurs Ment Health Serv 25(1):20, 1987.

Mittleman H, Mittleman R, and Elser B: Cocaine, Am J Nurs 84:1092, 1984.

Naigle M: The nurse and the alcoholic: redefining an historically ambivalent relationship, J Psychosoc Nurs Ment Health Serv 21:17, June 1983.

Nighorn S: Narcissistic deficits in drug abusers: a self-psychological approach, J Psychosoc Nurs Ment Health Serv 26(9):22, 1988.

Nubel AS and Solomon LZ: Addicted adolescent girls: familial interpersonal relationships, J Psychosoc Nurs Ment Health Serv 26(1):32, 1988.

O'Brien CP, Woody GE, and McLellan T: Psychiatric disorders in opioid-dependent patients, J Clin Psychiatr 45(12):9, December 1984.

Pugh JB: My love: the story of an addiction, J Psychosoc Nurs Ment Health Serv 20:22, March 1982.

Scherwertz P: An alcohol treatment team, Am J Nurs 82:1878, 1982.

Schickit M: Alcoholism and other psychiatric disorders, Hosp Commun Psychiatr 34:1022, 1983.

Schloemer N and Skidmore J: Opiate withdrawal with clonidine, J Psychosoc Nurs Ment Health Serv 21:8, October 1983.

Smith J: Diagnosing alcoholism, Hosp Commun Psychiatr 34(11):1017, 1983.

Spring G and Rothgery J: The link between alcoholism and affective disorders, Hosp Commun Psychiatr 35(8):820, 1984.

Sullivan EJ: A descriptive study of nurses recovering from chemical dependency, Arch Psychiatr Nurs 1(3):194, June 1987.

Trevelyan J: The forgotten addicts, Nurs Times 84(16):16, April 1988.

Twerski A: Early intervention in alcoholism: confrontational techniques, Hosp Commun Psychiatr 34(11):1027, 1983.

Vandegaer F: Cocaine: the deadliest addiction, Nurs 89 19(2):72, February 1989.

Wegscheider S: Another chance, Palo Alto, Calif, 1981, Science and Behavior Books.

Individuals with personality disorders

20

LEARNING OBJECTIVES

After studying this chapter the student will be able to:

○ Describe the characterisitics exhibited by a person with the medical diagnosis of personality disorder.

○ Discuss the causative factors associated with personality disorders.

○ Describe behaviors the nurse is most likely to observe in an adult with borderline personality disorder.

○ State examples of nursing diagnoses likely to be applicable to an adult with borderline personality disorder.

○ Discuss nursing interventions likely to be effective with an adult with borderline personality disorder.

○ Describe behaviors the nurse is most likely to observe in an adult with antisocial personality disorder.

○ State examples of nursing diagnoses likely to be applicable to an adult with antisocial personality disorder.

○ Develop a hypothetical plan of nursing care for an adult with antisocial personality disorder.

Personality has been defined as *the aggregate of the physical and mental qualities of the individual as these interact in characteristic fashion with his environment.* When an individual's personality is characterized by an identifiable trait or style that is relatively enduring regardless of the circumstances, that individual may be seen as "odd" or "different." For example, some persons are suspicious in most situations in which they find themselves, others overreact with a great deal of emotion to everyday events, and still others are fearful most of the time. For many people these personality traits do not cause personal distress or interfere with their ability to live satisfying and satisfactory lives. Some persons, however, are distressed by the way in which they characteristically relate to the world around them but are unable to alter their behavior. In other instances, the individual may see nothing unusual about his behavior, but others find it objectionable. Such persons may be suffering from a personality disorder even though they do not exhibit the flagrant symptoms lay persons usually associate with mental disorders.

Although nurses often come in contact with individuals with personality disorders in work and social settings, they are unlikely to be in the position of providing care to these persons, since they rarely seek treatment for this disorder alone. However, there are two exceptions. Individuals with borderline personality disorder and those with antisocial personality disorder may require hospitalization for varying periods of time. Therefore, this chapter focuses on the care of individuals with these personality disorders.

HISTORICAL PERSPECTIVE

Although individuals with borderline personality disorder undoubtedly have existed throughout history, this disorder was not officially considered to be a distinct syndrome until 1980 when this diagnosis first appeared in the Diagnostic and Statistical Manual of Mental Disorders III (DSM-III). This does not mean to say that borderline personality disorder had been unknown until 1980. In fact, one of the foremost authorities on treating persons with borderline personality disorder, Dr. Otto Kernberg, has been writing about this syndrome since the 1960s. However, since the official recognition of borderline personality disorder there has been an abundance of both professional and lay literature that addresses the characteristics, dynamics, and interventions associated with this disorder.

In contrast, the phenomenon of antisocial personality disorder has been well known for years, although such individuals were labeled *sociopaths* or *psychopaths* in the past. Although this terminology is no longer used, the characteristics and numbers of these persons remain the same as they have throughout history.

PERSONALITY DISORDERS

Personality traits are those characteristics of an individual which make him unique and form the basis for the way he perceives the world and how he relates to others. Individuals with a personality disorder exhibit an extreme manifestation of a personality trait. For example, if a shyness interferes with his ability to live a satisfying and satisfactory life, he would be considered to have a schizoid personality disorder.

The DSM-III-R groups personality disorders into three clusters. Cluster A includes paranoid, schizoid, and schizotypal personality disorders. People with these disorders often appear odd or eccentric. Cluster B includes antisocial, borderline, histrionic, and narcissistic personality disorders. People with these disorders often appear dramatic, emotional, or erratic. Cluster C includes avoidant, dependent, obsessive-compulsive, and passive-aggressive personality disorders. People with these disorders often appear anxious or fearful.

Because persons with borderline personality disorder and those with antisocial personality disorder are likely to require psychiatric treatment, these disorders will be discussed in depth.

Borderline personality disorder

For reasons that are not known, the vast majority of individuals with borderline personality disorder are women. Some authorities believe that this disorder is a precursor to dissociative disorders, particularly multiple personality disorder, which is seen almost exclusively in women.

Individuals with borderline personality disorder have not developed an integrated sense of self. Even though they are chronological adults, they are unable to define who they are and what values and goals undergird their lives. For example, they are likely to vacillate widely among career choices, values, and goals for their life, first making one set of decisions and then shifting to another set that is in marked contrast to the first. This inability to develop an integrated sense of self results in erratic behavior as well as feelings of "emptiness," which is often expressed as boredom.

> Individuals with borderline personality disorder have not developed an integrated sense of self, have a deep fear of being alone, and experience exreme shifts in mood over a short period of time.

Not surprisingly, individuals with borderline personality disorder have a deep fear of being alone because they look to others to fill the void in their sense of self. Consequently, they are continuously establishing intense relationships, each of which initially is seen as the answer to their problems. Unfortunately, these relationships are doomed to fail because individuals with borderline personality disorder seem to be unable to realistically view themselves and others as human beings with strengths and limitations. Rather, persons are seen as being totally good or totally bad. This phenomenon is based on the primitive defense mechanism of "splitting." It is not unusual for the very same person who is beloved to become the object of intense hatred less than a week later because he or she was found deficient in meeting the individual's inordinate needs. For example, if the newly found friend arrives 5 minutes late for a date, the individual with borderline personality disorder might very well construe this as evidence that her friend doesn't really care about her. Needless to say, this perception of interpersonal interactions leads to a great deal of overt and covert manipulation by the individual with borderline personality disorder.

The third prominent characteristic of individuals with borderline personality disorder is extreme shifts in mood over a very short period of time. When they are experiencing stress, especially that related to real or perceived abandonment, these individuals are likely to respond with massive amounts of anxiety, depression, or anger. While the nature of this reaction may be understandable, the extent of it is out of proportion to the stressor. What is even more surprising is the fact that within hours or a few days the person's mood may change to one of cheer and pleasure, often associated with having "found a new friend."

During periods of depression and anxiety, these persons often make suicidal gestures, characteristically scratching or gouging their wrists and arms. It is not clear whether this behavior is an attempt to gain attention or an effort to inflict pain to confirm the existence of self, or both. During periods of anger they tend to provoke fights and may injure themselves and others. They also engage in real and symbolic self-destructive, impulsive behaviors such as casual sex, shopping sprees, and substance abuse.

Antisocial personality disorder

Individuals with antisocial personality disorder are persons who have a long history of dysfunctional behavior in the areas of interpersonal relationships and occupational endeavors. In addition, they often have a criminal record, may be dependent upon alcohol or drugs, and frequently engage in sexually deviant behavior. What is so outstanding about these persons, however, is not their history or even their behavior, but rather the initial impression they make. Even when his past is known, such an individual easily impresses a stranger with his articulate expression, his ability to rationalize or justify his behavior, his fantasized exploits, and his general appearance. The casual acquaintance quickly succumbs to this charisma and becomes his staunch supporter.

Individuals with antisocial personality disorder are incapable of valuing other people and manipulate them to achieve their own purposes.

Behind this effective facade of charm is a personality that is incapable of valuing other people. Rather, this person views others as objects to be manipulated to achieve his purposes. These individuals are characterized by a total lack of responsibility and an inability to conform to even the minimal moral and legal standards of society if these conflict with the fulfillment of their desires. They possess poor judgment and insight, do not profit by experience or punishment, and are notoriously unreliable. They consciously fabricate stories to impress the listener and have an uncanny ability to rationalize contradictions in their stories. In addition, they seem incapable of experiencing guilt or remorse for their behavior, although they will express these feelings if they believe it will be to their advantage to do so.

For reasons that are unknown this personality disorder occurs almost exclusively in men. In addition, these persons are always of at least average intelligence, with many having superior intellectual abilities. Because of their criminal behavior many of these persons are found in the jails and prisons of the country. It is unlikely, however, that the professional criminal suffers from an antisocial personality. A successful life of crime requires long-range, careful planning. This is impossible for an individual with an antisocial personality because his behavior is characterized by impulsiveness and a low tolerance for frustration.

CAUSATIVE FACTORS OF PERSONALITY DISORDERS

The causative factors of personality disorders are essentially unknown. However, since many behaviors of these individuals would be considered normal at a much earlier stage of personality development, some authorities believe that the basis of these disorders lies in the arrested psychosexual development of the individual. Even if future research confirms this hypothesis, questions still remain about what factors contribute to fixation at an earlier stage of psychosexual development.

Many authorities believe that the fundamental problem of individuals with borderline personality disorder is their earlier inability to resolve the separation-individuation process in infancy. During early infancy, the infant and the mothering one have a symbiotic relationship whereby they are emotionally fused. This stage of development is an extension of the physical symbiosis experienced when the infant was in utero. By the age of 5 months, however, the infant has developed sufficiently to be able to begin the process of separating from the mothering one and embark on the long process of establishing his own identity as a separate, distinct human being. This is a gradual process that takes years to achieve, although success in the stages of infancy and early childhood is necessary to provide the foundation upon which the tasks of later childhood and adolescence can be built. For example, one of the earliest signs of the separation process is when the infant visually and tactilely explores the mother's face and can recognize her among a group of adults, thereby indicating that he is beginning to differentiate her from himself and others. If this does not occur, in later stages of development he is unlikely to be able to comfortably leave the mothering one even for short periods of time.

A fundamental problem of persons with borderline personality disorder stems from their inability as infants to separate themselves from their mother.

A major goal of the separation-individuation process is the development of a unified sense of self in which the total personality is integrated. Although this is not fully achieved until late adolescence or early adulthood, the beginnings of a unified self-concept are apparent in healthy children by age three. For reasons that are unknown, individuals with borderline personality disorder have been unable to develop this unified, integrated self-concept and continue to use the primitive defense mechanism of splitting whereby they view themselves and others as all good or all bad.

Studies of the histories of individuals with antisocial personality disorder reveal that they were emotionally impulsive and maladjusted children. In fact, adjustment difficulties before age 15 is one criterion of this diagnosis. Some authorities believe that careful history taking would indicate antisocial behavior before age 12 in most, if not all, individuals who develop antisocial personality disorder as adults. These adjustment difficulties include poor school perfor-

Persons with antisocial
personality disorder have
failed as children to make
a positive identification
with parents or parental
substitutes.

mance related to frequent truancy, petty crimes including thefts and arson, and a uniform lack of satisfactory relationships with family, peers, and authority figures.

These individuals have apparently failed to develop a socialized superego. The personality appears to be dominated by the primitive demands of the id. The ego has failed to establish a mature identity or to evolve socially useful adaptations and controls. In some way these individuals have failed to make a positive identification with parents or parental substitutes who could have provided the love, security, recognition, and respect that a child requires if he is to develop into an emotionally healthy adult. Failure to make a positive identification and to develop socially acceptable controls on his own behavior may have been the result of faulty parent-child relationships.

Social scientists who have conducted longitudinal studies of these individuals report that they frequently come from home environments in which there is only one parent, who is likely to be alcohol or drug dependent or who has an antisocial personality, or both. As a result, the child has little or no supervision, and the rules of conduct that are established are enforced inconsistently. The child is, in essence, left to fend for himself, often on the streets of the slums of large cities.

Although these familial factors are present often enough to be noteworthy, it is important to understand that not every child who is a product of such a background develops an antisocial personality disorder. Furthermore, some adults who have antisocial personality disorder do not have this family background. Therefore it must be concluded that there are other, as yet unknown, factors that are necessary for the development of antisocial personality disorder.

NURSING CARE OF INDIVIDUALS WITH BORDERLINE PERSONALITY DISORDER
Nursing assessment

The following discussion is organized around the human processes introduced in Chapter 9. Although behaviors in each category are presented as separate entities, it should be understood that they are highly interrelated and are adaptations to similar stressors. Further, in many instances behavior designed as an adaptation to one stressor becomes a stressor itself in another dimension. Therefore, nursing care directed at altering one behavior will inevitably have an effect on others.

Activity processes. Although motor behavior is usually not altered, the individual with borderline personality disorder who is ill enough to require psychiatric treatment will invariably display impulsivity, which may be exhibited through motor behavior. This is especially likely when the client feels angry because of some real or imagined slight, at which time she may lash out at others, the environment, or at herself. The inexperienced nurse commonly views the client's impulsive motor behavior as unpredictable, since she has not yet learned to fully appreciate the depth of reaction these clients experience in response to untoward events and people who do not do exactly the "right" thing at the right time. For example, one client was known to spontaneously assault an aide who announced that a planned unit picnic had to be cancelled because of thunderstorms.

Recreation patterns may be antisocial and involve substance abuse and sexual promiscuity. Individuals with borderline personality disorder have a great deal of difficulty being alone, so they seek activities that involve other people. However, they also have an inability to delay gratification, so they are likely to become impatient and irritable when involved in recreational activities that are characterized by rules and competition, as is true of many games.

Self-care in regard to grooming and hygiene may or may not be altered. However, many clients with borderline personality disorder have alterations in eating patterns, often binging and purging.

Cognition processes. Cognition processes are often altered in regard to decision making and judgment. As previously discussed, these clients suffer from a diffused identity and thus are unable to make decisions based on long-term goals and deeply held values. Their poor judgment is evidenced by the spontaneity of their decisions without reference to long-term consequences. Although delusions are not present, their thought processes indicate a highly personalized interpretation of the actions of others. For example, the previously mentioned client who assaulted the aide after he cancelled the picnic exclaimed, "How could he have done that to me?"

Ecological processes. Ecological processes, in and of themselves, are usually not altered.

Emotional processes. Altered feeling states and feeling processes are prime characteristics of clients with borderline personality disorder. These persons experience an extreme depth of emotion, especially anger, anxiety, elation, and sadness in response to what others see as relatively trivial events. As previously discussed, these extreme emotions are accompanied by mood swings, which are almost always preciptiated by an external factor. For example, it is not unusual for one nurse to report to another that the client is exceptionally depressed, only for the second nurse to discover the client in the day room laughing and joking with others.

Interpersonal processes. Altered conduct/impulse processes are another of the major characteristics of clients with borderline personality disorder. Their impulsivity and feelings of emptiness and boredom, combined with their rage at themselves and others, often result in physical assaults on the environment, others, and themselves. Suicidal or self-destructive acts are common in those clients who are hospitalized and are likely to be the factors that made hospitalization necessary.

The client with borderline personality disorder becomes involved in intense but superficial interpersonal relationships. As previously discussed, these relationships are always short-lived because of the client's tendency to view others as all good or all bad and consequently to idealize or devalue others. Therefore, the client's interpersonal experience is turbulent.

Of particular note is the fact that the client's behavior seriously strains family relationships. It is not unusual for the client to consciously or unconsciously relate to one family member as her savior and to another as the source of all her difficulties. It does not take much imagination to see how this situation can result in one family member's being pitted against another.

Role performance is seriously altered, and the client is likely to have a long history of failure in both school and work situations. It should be understood, however, that the client is characteristically unable to appreciate the part she played in creating these failures. Rather, she will convincingly relate long, involved stories about how she was the victim of others' inadequacies.

Perception processes. Perhaps the most fundamental problem of clients with borderline personality disorder is their undeveloped self-concept. As previously discussed, these individuals have not developed a sense of self and therefore appear to "try on" self-concepts, often based on the identity of the individual who is currently idealized. Therefore, the nurse will observe a great deal of mimicking behavior, reminiscent of the normal behavior of 3–6-year-olds.

Physiological processes. Physiological processes are not necessarily altered in clients with borderline personality disorder. However, this condition does not provide immunity to physiological alterations, so a complete physical examination must be completed and any physiological problems addressed.

Because of the client's self-destructive behavior the nurse should be particularly alert for signs of wound infection and indications of malnourishment.

Valuation processes. Closely related to the client's identity diffusion is the client's unclear value system. Because the client has not been able to develop a value system to guide her behavior, it is not unusual for her to engage in antisocial behavior such as sexual promiscuity but then feel great remorse about her actions.

Nursing diagnosis

As with all nursing diagnoses, the nursing diagnoses for the individual with borderline personality disorder are based on the themes identified during the assessment phase of the nursing process. Categories of human responses from the ANA Classification of Human Responses of Concern for Psychiatric–Mental Health Nursing Practice that may be specifically applicable to individuals with borderline personality disorder include the following:

1.1.2   Altered Motor Behavior
1.2.2   Altered Recreation Patterns
1.3.4   Altered Self-Care
2.1.2   Altered Decision Making
2.2.2   Altered Judgment

Margin note: Assessment of the individual with borderline personality disorder often reveals impulsivity; antisocial recreation patterns; fear of being alone; altered eating patterns of binging and purging; poor judgment in relation to long-term consequences; extreme depth of emotions accompanied by mood swings; physical assaults on the environment, others, and herself; intense but superficial interpersonal relationships; strained family relationships; history of failure in school and work situations; undeveloped self-concept; and an unclear value system.

4.1.2   Altered Feeling States

4.2.2   Altered Feeling Processes

5.3.2   Altered Conduct/Impulse Processes

5.4.2   Altered Family Processes

5.5.2   Altered Role Performance

5.7.2   Altered Social Interaction

6.3.3   Undeveloped Self-Concept

8.3.2   Altered Values

NANDA nursing diagnostic categories that may be specifically applicable to the individual with borderline personality disorder include:

1.2.1.1   Potential for Infection

1.6.1   Potential for Injury

3.1.1   Impaired Social Interaction

3.2.1   Altered Role Performance

3.2.2   Altered Family Processes

5.1.1.1   Ineffective Individual Coping

7.1.3   Personal Identity Disturbance

9.2.2   Potential for Violence: Self-directed or directed at others

9.3.1   Anxiety

To develop a nursing diagnosis that fulfills its function of providing direction for planning nursing care, the nurse is encouraged to postulate and state etiologic or antecedent factors for each human response and connect the two phrases by using the term "related to." For example:

6.3.3   Undeveloped Self-Concept related to unresolved
        separation-individuation process

Planning and implementing nursing care

The plan for nursing care is derived from the nursing diagnoses and includes the objectives of the care, the nursing actions, and outcome criteria. To be effective the plan needs to be highly individualized. The suggestions that follow should be seen as general guidelines to be used if they are appropriate to the client's needs.

In general, the objectives of all nursing care for the individual with borderline personality disorder should relate to helping her learn to develop an integrated sense of self and perception of others and to control impulsive behaviors.

Since the client's nursing diagnoses are often interrelated, stemming as they do from similar etiologies or antecedents, the student will see that the appropriate nursing actions are also interrelated. In other words, by intervening in one dimension, the nurse will also affect other dimensions.

Activity processes. Prevention is the key to helping the client deal with impulsive motor behavior. Rather than viewing the client's behavior as unpredictable, the nurse is encouraged to understand that the client often experiences an

The nurse is most helpful to the client with borderline personality disorder when she teaches the client socially acceptable ways of showing anger, makes a written contract with the client, helps the client learn words to describe her feelings, and helps the client develop an integrated sense of self and perception of others.

extreme amount of rage over which she has little control. The fact that the client cannot control what she feels does not mean that she cannot learn to control her behavior. Rather than focusing on the inappropriateness of the anger, the nurse can be most helpful to the client by teaching her socially acceptable ways of discharging this emotion. For example, the client can learn to punch a pillow rather than hitting another person when she feels as if she will explode with anger.

Cognition processes. Because clients with borderline personality disorder are in contact with reality and their memory is not affected, a written contract between the nurse and the client has proven to be a very useful tool. This contract is developed by the client and the nurse together, specifies the goals to be achieved, and delineates the behaviors and actions in which both the client and the nurse will engage. For example, the contract may specify that the client will keep a journal of those situations which anger her and that she will not act on this anger but rather approach her assigned nurse to discuss the situation. The nurse's responsibility would be to inform the client of when she will be available to discuss the journal and then meticulously adhere to that time frame.

Emotional processes. Learning to develop personally and socially acceptable outlets for the client's emotions is one of the biggest challenges that face the nurse and the client. Often the nurse initially must help the client to identify and label the emotion she is feeling. Unless the client can be helped to learn the words that describe her feelings, she will not be able to talk about her emotions to others and will be more likely to act them out. Once the client can identify the emotion she is experiencing, she can be helped to learn how to identify the themes and patterns that precipitate various feelings. For example, even though it may be obvious to the staff, it may come as a surprise to the client that every time she has a visit from her mother she responds with sadness and a desire to mutilate herself. Once the precipitants of emotions are identified, it becomes possible for the client to learn adaptive coping mechanisms through such techniques as role playing and problem solving.

Interpersonal processes. Because the client uses the defense mechanism of splitting, thereby seeing everything and everyone as all good or all bad, the staff needs to be keenly alert to preventing the dissension that occurs among staff when the client tells her "favorite" nurse how badly she is treated by another nurse. Only by developing an in-depth understanding of the dynamics underlying the behavior of clients with borderline personality disorder and a heightened sense of self-awareness can the nurse hope to avoid the pitfall of believing that only she understands the client, or that only she can be of help to the client. This is necessary not only to prevent the client from manipulating the staff by pitting one against the other but also to present a unified stance so that the client will have the opportunity to experience consistent limit setting and learn that it is possible for the staff to care about her while still enforcing the rules.

Ironically, the more the staff is successful in enforcing uniform limits on the client's behavior, the greater the initial likelihood that the client will attempt to mutilate herself or otherwise act out. This behavior should be seen as testing. Although the staff has the responsibility to protect the client at all times, they should resist the temptation to focus on the acting out behavior but rather should continue to focus on the feelings that precipitated the behavior. For example, one client approached the nurse carrying a light bulb, which she smashed on the counter once she got the nurse's attention. The client then stated that she was going to cut her wrist. Because the nurse knew this client well, she made no attempt to get the jagged glass from her, nor did she comment about it. Rather, she asked the client what she was feeling and was not surprised when the client placed the glass on the counter a few minutes into the discussion.

Perception processes. As previously stated, the goal of all nursing care for the client with borderline personality disorder includes assisting her to develop an integrated sense of self and perception of others. The nurse can be most helpful in assisting the client to achieve this goal by relating to her with meticulous consistency, demonstrating acceptance of her as an individual with value and worth regardless of her behavior, and helping her to view herself and others in a realistic light by discussing the reality of situations with her. Obviously this takes a great deal of time, patience, and commitment on the part of the nurse.

NURSING CARE OF INDIVIDUALS WITH ANTISOCIAL PERSONALITY DISORDER
Nursing assessment

Activity processes. Motor behavior of an individual with antisocial personality disorder is not necessarily altered. However, his recreation patterns are likely to consist of activities that are antisocial. For example, substance abuse and prostitution are common.

A combination of lack of material resources and little motivation often lead to self-care alterations in grooming, hygiene, and health-seeking behaviors. Therefore, the individual with antisocial personality disorder may be unclean and unkempt. In other instances, however, he may present quite the opposite picture.

Cognition processes. Although cognition process are not altered in and of themselves, the individual with antisocial personality disorder consistently uses judgment and makes decisions that reflect his total lack of concern for the rights of others or the rules of society. He is concerned only about short-term gratification of his needs and is willing to risk almost any consequence to meet these needs. As a result, he often has a long history of arrests, often for petty thievery, vandalism, and vagrancy.

Ecological processes. Ecological processes are markedly altered in that the person with antisocial personality disorder is not concerned about such things as home or community. He is satisfied if he has a bed to sleep in and is not necessarily appreciative or even understanding of the efforts of a wife or parent in the unlikely event that such a person might attempt to maintain a comfortable, clean environment.

Emotional processes. Individuals with antisocial personality disorder are incapable of experiencing any depth of emotion, despite the fact the feeling tone they convey is often appropriate to the situation. It is this fact that inexperienced nurses initially find so confusing. In reality, the individual has learned appropriate emotional responses as a means of influencing the reactions of others. Because he is actually incapable of feeling anxiety, guilt, fear, or remorse, threats of retribution are useless in motivating him to change his antisocial behavior.

Interpersonal processes. Individuals with antisocial personality disorder have a long history of alterations in interpersonal processes, particularly in regard to conduct/impulse processes. Because they have engaged in many antisocial acts and because they ultimately alienate everyone with whom they come in contact, they experience social isolation. In fact, when individuals whose friendships they have cultivated realize how they were used, their anger may be so great that the physical safety of the person with antisocial personality disorder may be in real jeopardy. It is for this reason that these persons are transferred from unit to unit if they are hospitalized for a long time. Certainly, those who are serving prison terms require periodic transfers to maintain their safety.

Of almost diagnostic significance is the nurse's reaction to the person. Despite all she may know about him, this individual is able to "con" the inexperienced nurse into defending and supporting his antisocial actions and believing that she alone can help him. These feelings are termed a *rescue fantasy* and nurses, who are inclined to be nuturing, are particularly vulnerable to the development of this phenomenon.

It goes without saying that the individual's role performance is seriously compromised. It is likely that he never finished high school, although he may speak as if he has a great deal of knowledge. If he ever had a job, it is unlikely that he was able to hold it for very long.

Perception processes. Despite much evidence to the contrary, the person with antisocial personality disorder views himself in the most positive light while seeing others as inadequate. A testimony to this alteration in perception processes is the individual's ability to convincingly explain his history on the basis of deficiencies in others or unfortunate circumstances over which he had no control.

Physiological processes. Physiological processes are not altered by the personality disorder itself but are almost always altered secondary to the life-style adopted by the individual. For example, there are likely to be physiological sequelae to substance abuse, sexual promiscuity, homelessness, inadequate nutrition, and physical aggression. Therefore, the individual with antisocial personality disorder should have a complete physical examination upon admission to a mental health facility.

Assessment of the individual with antisocial personality disorder often reveals antisocial recreation patterns, lack of concern for the rights of others and rules of society, lack of concern for home or community, inability to experience any depth of emotion, a feeling of social isolation, a positive perception of himself and a negative perception of others, and values in conflict with the social order.

Valuation processes. A prominent characteristic of the individual with anti-social personality disorder is the fact that his values are in conflict with the social order. As previously stated, he will go to any length to gratify his needs, regardless of the consequences or who is hurt in the process. At the same time, he seems incapable of internalizing values that are socially acceptable.

Nursing diagnosis

Categories of human responses from the ANA Classification of Human Responses of Concern for Psychiatric–Mental Health Nursing Practice that may be specifically applicable to individuals with antisocial personality disorder include the following:

1.2.2	Altered Recreation Patterns
1.3.4	Altered Self-Care
2.1.2	Altered Decision Making
2.2.2	Altered Judgment
3.3.2	Altered Home Maintenance
4.1.99	Feeling States NOS (not otherwise specified)
5.3.2	Altered Conduct/Impulse Processes
5.5.2	Altered Role Performance
5.7.2	Altered Social Interaction
6.3.2	Altered Self-Concept
8.3.2	Altered Values

NANDA nursing diagnostic categories that may be specifically applicable to the individual with antisocial personality disorder include:

1.6.1	Potential for Injury
3.1.1	Impaired Social Interaction
3.1.2	Social Isolation
3.2.1	Altered Role Performance
6.5.2	Bathing/Hygiene Self-Care Deficit
7.1.3	Personal Identity Disturbance

To develop a nursing diagnosis that fulfills its function of providing direction for planning nursing care, the nurse is encouraged to postulate and state etiologic or antecedent factors for each human response and connect the two phrases by using the term "related to." For example:

5.7.2   Altered Social Interaction related to manipulation of others

Planning and implementing nursing care

The plan for nursing care is derived from the nursing diagnoses and includes the objectives of the care, the nursing actions, and outcome criteria. To be effective the plan needs to be highly individualized. The suggestions that follow should be seen as general guidelines to be used if they are appropriate to the client's needs.

In general, the objectives of all nursing care for the individual with antisocial personality disorder should relate to assisting him to alter his behavior so that he does not infringe on the rights of others and recognizes his responsibility for his own actions.

Since the client's nursing diagnoses are often interrelated, stemming as they do from similar etiologies or antecedents, the student will see that the appropriate nursing actions are also interrelated. In other words, by intervening in one dimension, the nurse will also affect other dimensions.

Activity processes. Because individuals with antisocial personality disorder lack a well-developed social conscience, they usually function poorly in group activities. However, insofar as possible, it is suggested that they be helped to accept a role in some of the available group functions.

Interpersonal processes. Some nurses feel that an individual who behaves in an antisocial way is a criminal and therefore should not be treated within the health care system. Other nurses believe that little, if anything, is wrong with these persons and therefore they do not require treatment. Both these extreme attitudes can prove detrimental to the individual who engages in antisocial acts.

Although the current trend is to keep as many individuals as possible out of institutions, many authorities still believe that persons with antisocial personality disorder require hospitalization if they are to be treated with any hope of success. The institution should provide a friendly, accepting, humane environment, where firm, reasonable, consistent limits and controls are placed on behavior. A permissive atmosphere is usually not helpful for these individuals. They need to be helped to develop a socialized superego, and such growth may be fostered by an organized, structured, controlled environment.

The treatment goals should include helping them to accept and use more socially approved attitudes and standards in their relationships with other people. To achieve this they must be helped to trust other people. It is hoped that this can be achieved through the development of a therapeutic relationship with one of the members of the professional treatment team. Since the psychiatrist is usually the ultimate authority in the treatment team, it would probably be helpful if the therapeutic relationship could be developed with a psychiatrist who could provide the necessary discipline.

The treatment goals can be promoted through a system of rewards and prohibitions, with socially acceptable behavior being rewarded with privileges and less acceptable behavior being responded to by the withholding of privileges.

If the client's behavior has developed out of negative social and cultural influences, the individual should be helped to seek a more acceptable social situation. Certainly he should be encouraged not to return to the same environment.

Because the individual with antisocial personality disorder is often attractive, intelligent, and an interesting conversationalist, he easily gains control of the situation by manipulating others. It is helpful to remember that although

The nurse is most helpful to the client with an antisocial personality disorder when she assists him to accept a role in available group functions; provides an organized, structured, and controlled environment; assists him to develop a therapeutic relationship; helps the client achieve a more acceptable social environment; uses a helpful, friendly, yet consistent approach with regard to responsibilities; and provides him with challenging activities.

these individuals are usually clever in manipulating others, they frequently use extremely poor judgment. They are likely to be troublemakers among other clients and have been known to organize psychotic individuals for the purpose of accomplishing their antisocial plans.

Although the nurse can be most effective if she uses a helpful, friendly approach when dealing with the individual who exhibits antisocial behaviors, she also needs to be constantly alert to the possibility of his attempting to gain control of the situation. The clinical team should identify approaches they believe will be most effective in dealing with this individual and should list the responsibilities that he will be expected to fulfill. When these decisions have been made, it is of primary importance for all hospital personnel to be consistent in carrying them out and in holding the individual to fulfilling his obligations.

These individuals do not profit by being scolded or lectured. Such an approach is never helpful and will serve only to arouse angry feelings. Since it is thought that these individuals learn little from experience, punishing them accomplishes nothing. Limits must be set on their behavior, since they frequently indulge in temper tantrums or destructive activities to achieve their objectives.

When the individual engages in antisocial behavior, it is important to treat him in such a manner that he will know that the staff want to help him even though he cannot be allowed to continue the behavior he is exhibiting.

Individuals with antisocial personality disorder need a variety of challenging activities throughout the day. They are likely to plead for special privileges, but the nurse should be cautious about granting such requests. Like all other individuals they should be rewarded for acceptable behavior. If possible, these individuals should be placed in situations in which they can obtain socially acceptable satisfactions. Thus success in some type of vocational therapy is ideal. It is essential to insist these individuals fulfill the responsibilities expected of them, since they are likely to cooperate only at their own convenience.

Due to the personality characteristics of the individual that result in behavior that is superficially pleasing, staff misjudge persons with antisocial personality disorder more often than any others with whom they come in contact. Inexperienced staff are likely to feel that a perfectly normal person is being detained for treatment without justification; in this case it is important that a more experienced health professional be consulted for clarification.

END NOTE

The focus of this chapter is the nursing care of individuals with personality disorders. Individuals with borderline personality disorder and antisocial personality disorder are discussed in depth, since it is these clients for whom the nurse is most likely to provide care. A case formulation from which a hypothetical nursing care plan is derived, implemented, and evaluated is presented for an individual with antisocial personality disorder.

NURSING CARE PLAN

An individual with antisocial behavior

CASE FORMULATION

James B. is a 30-year-old, unmarried man who was admitted to the state psychiatric hospital after being arrested for vagrancy and following children as they walked to school in the morning. He is the oldest child of a woman who divorced his father after many episodes of abuse to both her and the child. Shortly after leaving her husband, James' mother took him and his two younger siblings to live in a rooming house, the only accommodations she could afford. Within a week she was befriended by another tenant, an unemployed, alcohol-dependent man 20 years her senior. This man moved in with the Bs, ostensibly to save money, and within a month convinced Mrs. B. to move with him to the rural area in which he had been reared. Even though they had no financial resources they were successful in renting a rundown shack on several acres of land. This property was owned by an absentee landlord. It was in this environment that James remained until he was 15 years old.

Upon moving to the rural community, the family was befriended by well-meaning members of the local church. However, James was unable to curb his antisocial behavior, which included truancy, dismembering a dead cat, setting small fires in the bedrooms of the home, and stealing money from Sunday school offerings. Amazingly, he was never held back in school even though he was functionally illiterate. In fact, his teachers routinely appeared at the home on Christmas Eve with many gifts for all the children. When his mother asked to have him repeat a grade, the school authorities stated their belief that such an action would hinder the progress the teachers felt he was making.

James became involved with the law for the first time at age 12 when he volunteered to solicit money for a church benevolence. He was successful in collecting 70 dollars, which he spent on candy, cigarettes, and arcade games.

The minister of the church brought legal charges against James, who was placed on 1 year's probation in the custody of his mother, although Mrs. B. was incapable of controlling him.

When James was 15 years old the landlord evicted the family from their home because they had not paid rent for the past 3 years. The landlord indicated he would have been willing to wait for the rent if they had maintained the house and land. However, since the house was in a state of extreme disrepair and the acreage was strewn with garbage and machine parts, he felt he had no choice but to evict them. The social service agency to whom the family was well known found them an apartment in a community 20 miles away. On the trip to this apartment the family stopped in a public rest area. James ran out of the back door of the rest room and hitchhiked 400 miles to a large metropolitan area. His mother never notified the police that he was missing, and they have not seen each other since.

Upon arriving in the city, James quickly became prey to a "pimp" who fed, housed, and clothed him in return for his services as a prostitute for businessmen whose sexual preference was young boys. He was so endearing that several businessmen gave him money and personal gifts, in addition to the fee they paid for his services. When his "pimp" discovered this extra source of income, he was so enraged that he almost beat James to death.

James fled this situation and since then has been drifting in the "skid row" section of another large city. He has a lengthy criminal record for petty crimes and has been committed to a psychiatric hospital four times.

Upon admission, he appeared malnourished but was in no acute physical distress. The mental status exam indicated no psychosis or organic disturbance. He stated he was following the children to protect them from predators.

NURSING CARE PLAN—cont'd

Nursing assessment

This case history demonstrates rather clearly many of the characteristics of an individual with antisocial personality disorder. As a young child James was severely abused by his father and probably a witness to this man's abuse of his mother. It is not unreasonable to assume that he adapted to his fear through repression. James' mother seemed incapable of providing the support or structure necessary for a child to develop in a mentally healthy way. The fact that she became involved with an older, unemployed, alcohol-dependent man indicates her poor judgment.

James' childhood behavior indicates a wide range of antisocial behaviors. Of significance is the fact that despite these behaviors and his lack of academic achievement, there is evidence James was well liked by his teachers. It is also significant that his first known act of stealing occurred in defiance of the church that had befriended him and his family.

Certainly this man failed to develop a socialized superego. Thus his behavior was dominated by instinctual demands, he failed to develop a constructive identity, and he had not incorporated socially useful controls. Like other individuals who are said to possess antisocial behaviors, he seemed incapable of conforming to social or legal standards. Even though he was previously treated at several psychiatric hospitals, he did not profit by this experience or by his encounters with the law.

Despite his dirty clothing and malnourished physique, the nurse found him quite charming and convincing in his explanations of his behavior.

Nursing diagnoses

The assessment data, including present behavior, past experiences, and an understanding of the underlying dynamics, led to the development of the following two pairs of nursing diagnoses for James B. The first of each pair is from the Classification of Human Responses of Concern for Psychiatric–Mental Health Nursing Practice; the second is from the approved NANDA Diagnostic Categories.

7.7.2   Altered Nutrition Processes related to inadequate food and fluid intake

OR

1.1.2.2   Altered Nutrition: Less than body requirements related to inadequate food and fluid intake

5.3.2   Altered Conduct/Impulse Processes related to lack of impulse control

OR

5.1.1.1   Ineffective Individual Coping related to lack of impulse control

Planning and implementing nursing care for *James B.*

The plan of nursing care developed for James B. is summarized in the box beginning on pp. 344-345. It should be noted that no psychotropic medications were prescribed.

The team psychiatrist assumed primary responsibility for James' treatment in the belief that this client would respond best to the member of the team who has the most authority.

The nursing staff who gave care to James B. were mature, experienced individuals. They strove to develop a friendly, accepting, humane environment while at the same time establishing firm, consistent, reasonable controls. Because they had previous experience working with clients with antisocial personality disorder, they were alert to James' manipulative behavior and were not fooled by his charm.

James was assigned a single room to prevent his influencing other clients in private. A schedule of activities, which included O.T., R.T., and reading classes, was developed. A plan of specified rewards and withholding of privileges was designed to accompany each activity and was implemented depending upon James' participation. A copy of this schedule and reward structure in the form of a contract was given to James. He and the psychiatrist both signed it. This contract specified that no excuses would be accepted as

Continued.

NURSING CARE PLAN—cont'd

reasons for James' lack of attendance at the scheduled activities.

Evaluation

The contract specifying James' behavior was reviewed by all staff and rigidly adhered to. He showed little difficulty in fulfilling the terms of the contract and therefore received a number of rewards. For example, he was allowed to stay in the day room and watch the television until midnight for each activity he attended and participated in for a week. This resulted in his staying up late for four nights a week.

An unanticipated negative outcome of James' treatment was the fact he bragged to other clients about how special he was as evidenced by his private room and television privileges. Three weeks after admission he found his room ransacked and his few personal belongings gone or destroyed. Another client quickly admitted he had done this to "teach him a lesson." James was very distraught and apparently fearful about this event, and a number of nursing staff freely sympathized with him.

At this point, a team conference was called to evaluate James' progress and current status. The absolute necessity of pointing out the part James played in this incident was stressed. His apparent distress and fear were viewed as ungenuine and as an attempt at manipulation. In addition, the contract was revised to make it more stringent. It was the team's consensus that the only real progress James had made in 3 weeks was a return to a sound nutritional status.

James remained in the hospital for another 3 weeks before he was discharged to a transitional living situation. Although his presence on the unit created identifiable tension, some staff were sad to see him leave. His behavior on the unit had become more acceptable, but the staff had little hope he would be able to maintain this level of functioning in the community.

NURSING CARE PLAN FOR *James B.*

Nursing diagnosis		Objectives	Nursing actions	Outcome criteria
7.7.2	Altered Nutrition Processes related to inadequate food and fluid intake	To increase client's nutritional status	Make sure client eats 3 well balanced meals each day as served in cafeteria Supplement meals with high calorie, nutritionally sound snacks (for example, malted milk) 3 times/day until 20 pounds have been gained	Within 1 week client will gain 5 pounds Within 1 month client's hair, skin, eyes, and mucous membranes will show evidence of adequate nutrition
OR				
1.1.2.2	Altered Nutrition: Less than body requirements related to inadequate food and fluid intake			

NURSING CARE PLAN—cont'd

5.3.2	Altered Conduct/ Impulse Processes related to lack of impulse control	To teach impulse control through behavior modification techniques	Assign to a single room Plan schedule of activities designed to increase number of skills Enforce client's participation in scheduled activities by rewards and withholding privileges as specified in contract	Within 2 weeks client will attend and participate in three of the four scheduled daily activities spontaneously and without complaint
OR 5.1.1.1	Ineffective Individual Coping related to lack of impulse control			
			Do not allow staff to be drawn into client's manipulation (for example, all requests for privileges must be made directly to Dr. F; all decisions about nursing care to be made by Ms. R.)	Within 1 month client will give evidence of attempting to gain rewards by altering behavior
		To increase sense of responsibility for accountability for own actions	As situation arises teach client socially acceptable behaviors and consequences to himself and others of ignoring these. For example, stealing other client's property hurts both persons	Within 1 month client is able to repeat consequences to himself and others of his behavior
			Enforce rewards and withholding privileges as outlined in contract with meticulous consistency	Within 1 month client gives evidence of attempting to gain rewards by altering behavior

SUGGESTED SOURCES OF ADDITIONAL INFORMATION

Barile L: A model for teaching management of disturbed behavior, J Psychosoc Nurs Ment Health Serv 20:9, November 1982.

Brobyn LL, Goren S, and Lego S: The borderline patient: systemic versus psychoanalytic approach, Arch Psychiatr Nurs 1(3):172, June 1987.

Frosch JP: The treatment of antisocial and borderline personality disorders, Hosp Commun Psychiatr 34(3):243, 1983.

Gallop R: Escaping borderline stereotypes, J Psychosoc Nurs Ment Health Serv 26(2):16, 1988.

Gallop R: The patient is splitting: everyone knows and nothing changes, J Psychosoc Nurs Ment Health Serv 23(4):6, 1985.

Hickey BA: The borderline experience: subjective impressions, J Psychosoc Nurs Ment Health Serv 23(4):24, 1985.

Kaplan CA: The challenge of working with patients diagnosed as having a borderline personality disorder, Nurs Clin North Am 21(3):429, September 1986.

Kernberg O and Haran C: Interview: milieu treatment with borderline patients: the nurse's role, J Psychosoc Nurs Ment Health Serv 22(4):29, 1984.

Lion JR, editor: Personality disorder: diagnosis and management, Baltimore, 1974, The Williams & Wilkins Co.

McEnany GW and Tescher BE: Contracting for care: one nursing approach to the hospitalized borderline patient, J Psychosoc Nurs Ment Health Serv 23(4):11, 1985.

O'Brien P, Caldwell C, and Transeau G: Destroyers: written treatment contracts can help cure self-destructive behaviors of the borderline patient, J Psychosoc Nurs Ment Health Serv 23(4):19, 1985.

Pelletier LR and Kane JJ: Strategies for handling manipulative patients, Nurs 89(5):81, May 1989.

Reid WH: The antisocial personality: a review, Hosp Commun Psychiatr 36(8):831, 1985.

Rowe J: The student nurse and the borderline patient, Issues Ment Health Nurs 6:311, 1984.

Populations at risk
The elderly

LEARNING OBJECTIVES

After studying this chapter the student will be able to:

o Discuss three social factors that affect the ability of elderly persons to successfully achieve ego integrity.

o Discuss life review, loneliness, and loss and grief as these are manifested by elderly persons.

o Describe nursing interventions designed to prevent or alter depression, suspiciousness, and dementia in elderly persons.

o Describe the symptoms exhibited by a person with the medical diagnosis of Alzheimer's disease.

o Discuss the causative factors associated with Alzheimer's disease.

o Describe behaviors the nurse is most likely to observe in an individual with Alzheimer's disease.

o State examples of nursing diagnoses likely to be applicable to an individual with Alzheimer's disease.

o Develop a hypothetical plan of nursing care for an individual with Alzheimer's disease.

Old age is an integral part of the life cycle, not one stage separated from the rest of life. Unfortunately, the United States is a youth-oriented society, and the elderly are viewed as a homogeneous group to which predominantly negative characteristics are ascribed. For example, a common but erroneous belief is that once a person has reached the arbitrarily established age of retirement he becomes at best, useless, or at worst, a burden to his family and to society. It is also believed that individuals over 65 or 70 years of age inevitably become forgetful and confused. While the elderly share much in common with each other, as do persons in any other developmental stage, the reality is they are also individuals who continue to adapt in the ways they have learned in earlier years. Elderly individuals have the potential to learn and develop. Survival with esteem—not mere physical survival—is the goal of the aged person.

HISTORICAL PERSPECTIVE

Throughout history there has always been an occasional individual who has lived to reach the age of 80, 90, or even 100. However, never before has the life expectancy of the average individual been as long as it currently is. For example, white males born in 1900 had a life expectancy of 48 years; white females born in the same year had a life expectancy of 51 years. In contrast, white males born in 1978 had a life expectancy of 70 years and white females had a life expectancy of 78 years. Therefore, until the twentieth century it was the unusual individual who lived beyond 50 years of age. Many women died in childbirth; the general population was vulnerable to epidemics of respiratory infections and other communicable diseases; and there were few effective treatments for such life-threatening illnesses as cancer and cardiovascular disease. In addition occupational hazards took their toll and the death rate from accidents was high. These factors combined with few preventive measures resulted in what is now seen as a short life expectency. Therefore illnesses associated with old age were rarely experienced and poorly understood.

Because of the increased life expectancy and effective treatment of illness and injuries, the number of persons 65 years of age or older is larger than ever before. It is projected that more than 13% of the total population will be over age 65 by the year 2005, representing a 60% increase in this age group from 1980. As the number of people who live longer increases, there is a concomitant increase in the health care needs of this population, including mental health needs. Until recently it was assumed that a person who lived long enough would eventually become "senile" and that the symptoms of confusion and regression associated with this diagnosis were inevitable outcomes of the aging process. As the number of persons in this age group increases, this assumption can no longer be made without being validated by research.

Research about mental disorders of the elderly has led to the identification of Alzheimer's disease, which is discussed in depth in this chapter. It was first discovered in 1906 by a German neurologist, Alois Alzheimer. Dr. Alzheimer treated a 51-year-old woman who exhibited all the symptoms associated with senility of the elderly. He became curious about her symptoms in light of her young age. After her death he examined her brain and discovered that parts of it contained clumps of twisted nerve-cell fibers that he called "neurofibrillary tangles." Although he did not understand what caused these abnormal nerve-cell configurations, he felt certain their existence created the patient's behavior.

Alzheimer's disease was assumed to be rare and to affect only the relatively young, leading to it being called a "presenile dementia."

With the advent of the electron microscope in the 1960s, scientists discovered the same neurofibrillary tangles in elderly persons diagnosed as having senile dementia. Thus it is now concluded that Alzheimer's disease is not rare or confined to the relatively young, but rather accounts for over 50% of the cases of dementia in the aged.

THE AGING PROCESS

There is no exact definition of old age. It is a developmental stage defined by complex physiological, psychological, and sociological factors. It has been defined by some gerontologists as the period marked by the relinquishing of midlife roles (career, parenting), combined with the view of oneself as being elderly.

The elderly population is a diverse group. Elderly persons have as many individual differences as do those in earlier developmental stages. The negative stereotyping that has been applied to elderly individuals is called *ageism,* a term representing the discriminatory practices against the elderly in our culture. The stereotype that describes all elderly persons as irritable, forgetful, rigid, regressed, and confused is a distorted and limited view. Most elderly individuals can be healthy and productive and continue to learn and develop when they are allowed to do so.

Although elderly persons are individuals with diverse needs and strengths, they share some commonalities, as do persons in other developmental stages. Physiological changes often occur as a result of normal aging, but the rate of change varies with each individual and with each organ system. These changes include increasing perceptual difficulties, diminished psychomotor abilities, and memory deficits that are reflected by difficulty in recall. However, these physiological changes appear to create little difficulty in the achievement of life goals for most elderly persons. In contrast, social and psychological changes profoundly affect the aged person.

Elderly persons have as many individual differences as do those in earlier stages. In addition, there are commonalities of experience for elderly individuals in our society.

Social factors

While the aged are beset by the same social problems as the young, their options for dealing with such problems are more limited. One example is economic inflation, during which the value of savings and pensions is eroded and there are very few opportunities for employment even if an older person were physically able to hold a job. In our society the elderly as a group are poor. In certain groups—American Indian and blacks—over 75% of the elderly live below the poverty level. Poverty not only deprives persons of the means to fulfill their basic needs adequately, it also deprives them of a powerful social tool. It takes money to look one's best and to attend many social functions.

Another example of a social phenomenon that affects the elderly is the

Social and psychological forces in our culture affect the mental health of the elderly, including the negative attitudes held toward aging.

change from small stable communities to large mobile urban centers. This change affects people of all ages and often results in a feeling of powerlessness. Older persons in particular are left without family to help cope with the bureaucracies necessary to survival in a complex society. The result often is a sense of alienation and worthlessness.

The accelerating rate of social change, as well as technological change, has subjected human beings to an unprecedented need to adapt. The ability of the elderly to make effective adaptations is dramatically impeded by a society that puts no value on age. Simple cultures value older persons because this group passes on the legends of the culture. In contrast, in an industrialized society mythology that remains important is written down, printed, and sold. Therefore in a society characterized by the nuclear family and printed and electronic communication media, there is no role for the elderly. In a society such as this it is obvious that the achievement of Erikson's psychosocial task of aging—the achievement of ego integrity versus despair—might be difficult to achieve, especially since the negative attitudes of society toward aging often have been internalized by the elderly themselves.

Psychological factors

As a result of normal aging the characteristic personality of the individual often becomes more prominent. Thus the suspicious individual may become even more so in old age. Habitual ways of behaving continue, as do social skills, verbal skills, judgment, and comprehension.

The elderly exhibit a number of characteristic behaviors while confronting the tasks of aging. The nurse caring for the elderly in any setting can offer assistance and enhance this process by recognizing the normal tasks and facilitating their resolution. The following are experiences and behaviors of the elderly frequently encountered by the nurse, with suggestions for possible interventions.

Life review is a nearly universal occurrence in older persons as they face the prospect of impending death.

Life review. Life review is the process of thinking about the meaning of one's life. Most authorities believe that life review is a nearly universal occurrence as older persons face the prospect of impending death. On the one hand, life review facilitates achieving closure to one's life. On the other hand, it leads to personal growth by bringing unresolved crises to consciousness, allowing them to be talked about at length in such a way as to facilitate their resolution.

The life review process involves almost obsessive reminiscence—remembering the significant events, people, and places in the past that helped to shape and provide meaning to the individual's life. When an individual is engaged in life review, he finds this an all-engrossing task. Small wonder that he has little interest in the events of the present, while the events of the past are recalled and recounted in minute detail.

Because it is likely that all elderly people reminisce, whether alone or with another person, it is vital that the nurse facilitate this process as a means of providing interpersonal feedback. Furthermore, planning for nursing intervention will become more individualized to the needs of the client if the life review process is used both as an aspect of assessment and as a means for intervention. At the very least, the nurse giving care to an elderly person must allow time to actively listen to his reminiscences and provide appropriate feedback.

Loneliness. More than any other group, aged persons often experience loneliness. Moustakos observes:

> Elderly citizens in our society are particularly affected by the social and cultural changes and by the separation, urbanization, alienation, and automation in modern living. There is no longer a place for old age, no feeling of organic belonging, no reverence or respect or regard for the wisdom and talent of the ancient. Our elderly citizens so often have feelings of uselessness, so often experience life as utterly futile. Old age is fertile soil for loneliness and the fear of a lonely old age far outweighs the fear of death in the thinking of many people. Loss of friends and death of contemporaries are realities. The mourning and deep sense of loss are inevitable, but the resounding and lasting depression which results and the emptiness and hopelessness are all a measure of the basic loneliness and anxiety of our time.*

To combat the loneliness of the elderly, nurses need to reach out consistently to the older person. Five minutes daily for 5 days is a louder message of concern and caring than is 20 to 30 minutes once in a while. Attempts to involve the older person in a relationship must be persistent. Nurses need to be aware of their own feelings of loneliness that may be triggered by the loneliness they sense in the older person. Younger nurses in late adolescence often experience profound loneliness as they seek their own identity and thus often want to move away from others who are experiencing loneliness. Therefore the withdrawal of the older person may evoke a mutual feeling of withdrawal in the nurse. The nurse must be conscious of her own feelings and aware of her needs when she is tempted to withdraw from the older person.

Nurses need to be aware of their own feelings of loneliness that may be triggered by the loneliness they sense in the older person.

Loss and grief. When a major interpersonal loss occurs, physical changes that the individual had not been previously aware of are often brought to awareness and perceived as losses. This phenomenon, in turn, intensifies the significance of the interpersonal loss. For example, it is not unusual to hear an elderly women remark, "If my husband had died 10 years ago, I could have managed this house by myself, but now I'm not physically able to keep the place up."

The need to grieve for losses may not be seen as necessary by the older person, and grieving may be avoided because of the pain associated with this process. Many aged persons develop physical problems rather than grieving, thereby directing their attention and the attention of others away from the loss and its attendant emotions to the somatic concerns. Consequently, the crisis associated with the loss is not resolved.

The need to grieve for losses may not be seen as necessary by the older person and may be avoided because of the pain associated with this process.

---

*Moustakos, Clark: Loneliness, Englewood Cliffs, N.J., 1961, Prentice-Hall, Inc., p. 26.

The older person's limited energy level and reluctance to experience pain and resentment allow him to deal with these feelings only for short periods. The nurse must observe for signs that the older person has had enough for now, but the willingness to return again and again to the painful area both by the nurse and by the older person is necessary for the resolution of the crisis. One 89-year-old man who had experienced a major illness was talking about the loss of his mother when he was 7 years old. He paused and said, "There are losses that everyone expects as they go through life and those you get through. However, there are losses that you feel that, in some way, you caused or that it was your fault, and those are much harder to bear. And the worst losses are those that refresh old wounds—they bring the pain of other losses to the surface. These are very hard losses to bear."

The nurse can be most effective in helping the elderly person resolve his grief about a major interpersonal loss by:

1. Assisting the person to accept the pain of the loss by validating that it is appropriate to feel pain over losses.
2. Encouraging the expression of sorrow and sense of loss by commenting on nonverbal communication, such as a shaky voice or teary eyes.
3. Facilitating the expression of hostility by viewing it as a sign of the older person's feeling of vulnerability.
4. Facilitating the expression of guilt. When the person says, "If only I had done . . .," it is helpful if the nurse restates this comment by saying, "I sense you blame yourself for . . .." Only if the person is able to acknowledge that he feels guilty can the reality of the situation be explored.
5. Assisting the older person to talk about the person who has died. Asking questions about how they met and the experiences they shared is most facilitative of helping the bereaved person to relive meaningful experiences.

The process of grieving over a major interpersonal loss may take as long as 2 years in the elderly. Signs that the individual is beginning to resolve his grief in a healthy way include indications that he is beginning to see himself as separate from the deceased person. The most common indicator of this differentiation is a movement away from talking about "we" to referring to "I." In addition, the healthy resolution of grief is indicated by behaviors indicating adaptations to an environment that acknowledges the absence of the deceased person. For example, the widow who disposes of her husband's clothing to use his closet for storing her sewing materials has made a constructive environmental adaptation that acknowledges the death of her husband. Finally, the person who is successfully resolving his grief over a major loss is able to form new relationships that are mutually satisfying and rewarding.

BEHAVIOR DISTURBANCES OF THE ELDERLY

Like younger individuals, elderly persons have widely varying needs and strengths. Most elderly persons are able to lead active and productive lives and continue to develop and learn during this developmental period. A person who has successfully completed earlier developmental tasks has a higher possibility of successfully completing the task of aging, and a helpful and supportive environment certainly contributes to its successful resolution. Nevertheless, difficulties sometimes arise.

Depression

Some elderly individuals manifest the characteristic symptoms of depression, which often go unrecognized. The physiological symptoms of depression—constipation, slow movements, insomnia—are expected signs of age, so they tend to be ignored. Apathy and lack of interest in the environment are characteristics of depression in the aged but are stereotypically viewed by most persons as characteristic of the aging process itself.

The frequency of depression in the elderly appears to be significantly greater than in other age groups. There is a decided increase in the severity and the number of depressions in the aged and a close relationship between physical illness and depression. The nurse who helps older persons maintain and sustain an interest in controlling those factors that keep them healthy, such as diet, helps to prevent depression.

Suicide prevention is an important aspect of nursing care when working with the depressed elderly (see Chapter 16). Nurses must be aware that some elderly, physically ill persons are unwilling to see any alternative except death. The fear of the process of dying, experiencing unremitting pain, being alone, and not being in control of their lives are frequently cited factors in the choice of suicide as means of coping. Common life-threatening behaviors of older people are refusal of medication, failure to follow prescribed medical regimen, and refusal to eat or drink.

Developing a therapeutic relationship with the depressed elderly person will allow him to begin to express and explore feelings and reestablish a sense of self-worth. The individual must feel safe and secure, and the environment should convey empathy and concern. In addition to intervening therapeutically on an individual basis with the elderly depressed person, group activities are often very useful in helping to alleviate depression. Although traditional group psychotherapy is rarely appropriate, remotivation groups and other quasi-social, task-oriented groups have been successfully used by nursing personnel in helping the depressed older person.

In addition to the nurse's intervening therapeutically on an individual basis with the elderly depressed person, group activities are also very useful in helping to alleviate depression.

Suspiciousness

Extreme suspiciousness or outright paranoia is frequently encountered in older persons, particularly in those individuals who were not trusting in their earlier years. When this personality structure is compounded by the hearing and sight losses that accompany aging, the person is likely to misinterpret others and the environment and conclude that the world and the people in it are hostile. To be sure, all persons experience instances in which they are the object of hostility or discrimination, but the suspicious elderly person overgeneralizes these isolated events so that his view of the environment becomes consistent with his preconceived ideas of persecution. The necessity for change that accompanies relocation sets a fertile stage for the onset of a paranoid reaction in the elderly. The following case illustrates such a situation.

> Mrs. Daniels is a 75-year-old widow who had lived by herself in the inner city apartment she shared with her husband until his death 5 years ago. Mrs. Daniels's daughters who live in the suburbs became increasingly concerned about their mother's safety in the inner city. They prevailed on her to move and finally, after 6 months, were able to convince her that she would be better off living in a newly constructed apartment complex for senior citizens in a better section of the city. Shortly after she moved Mrs. Daniels began to suspect that people were stealing her belongings. She also began hearing voices that told her they were going to "get her" in retaliation for the way she had behaved when she was a child. Mrs. Daniels told her daughters about these experiences. The community mental health nurse was called in to assess the situation.

The consistent presence and availability of the nurse is of great value in helping the aged person give up feelings of suspiciousness.

Appropriate goals when working with older persons who are exhibiting unwarranted suspiciousness include reducing the individual's anxiety level by establishing a relationship with him, helping him to restructure his environment to maximize his sense of control, and minimizing his sight and hearing deficit by the use of prosthetic devices or by adapting the environment to better accommodate the sensory loss. Throughout all these interventions the consistent presence and availability of the nurse is of inestimable value in helping the aged person give up his feelings of suspiciousness.

Dementia

Dementia is an organic mental disorder characterized by impairments in short- and long-term memory, abstract thinking, and judgment accompanied by personality change.

Dementia is an organic mental disorder characterized by impairments in short- and long-term memory, abstract thinking, and judgment, accompanied by personality change. These impairments and personality change must significantly interfere with the individual's work, usual social activities, or relationships to warrent the medical diagnosis of dementia. Dementia may be reversible or progressive, depending on the specific organic cause. For example, brain tumors and hypothyroidism are the cause of some dementias. In these instances, the mental symptoms are alleviated when the underlying cause is treated. Unfortunately, over 50% of individuals with dementia are suffering from Alzheimer's disease, which at this point cannot be prevented or cured. Therefore, the dementia associated with this illness is irreversible and progressive.

Although 1% of all behavioral problems of the elderly result from nonorganically caused (functional) mental disorders, research indicates that the diagnosis of dementia is often misapplied to those suffering from depression and from dysfunctional adaptations to the normal process of aging interacting with the inordinate stressors experienced by the elderly. Thus it is essential that the assessment of elderly individuals manifesting the symptoms of dementia be multidimensional and include psychosocial and environmental factors as well as biophysiological aspects.

Individuals suffering from dementia are in obvious need of intervention. Initially, the nurse might attempt to orient the person by introducing herself and proceeding in the least threatening manner to elicit only the information needed to help with the immediate problem. For instance, the nurse might say, "My name is Miss Jones. You seem afraid of something on the wall, Mrs. Smith. Would you tell me what is frightening you?" Hospitalization for any reason is a time of high risk for increased confusion and therefore an appropriate time for the nurse to begin preventive intervention. While all persons need to know what is going to happen to them when they are hospitalized, when a person with dementia is hospitalized, knowledge and support are critical to the prevention of confusion and to keeping him accessible to intervention when confusion does occur. Demands placed on all elderly persons who are hospitalized should be kept to a minimum. This is particularly true for those suffering from dementia. Young technicians need to learn that x-ray films, blood tests, and other tests cannot be hurried because this creates a situation where the client feels highly anxious, incompetent, and out of control.

> When a person with dementia is hospitalized, knowledge and support are critical to the prevention of confusion and to keeping the person accessible to intervention when confusion occurs.

All staff members should be aware of basic strategies of care. For example, the individual should be approached slowly to avoid startling him. He should be called by name at all times, and the nurse should use her name often. Elderly persons who close their eyes often are not asleep. The nurse needs to get as near as possible to keep eye contact at the person's level. Touch contact should be initiated carefully and gently, perhaps by taking the individual's hand at first. If he pulls away, attempts to establish touch contact should be made later.

All unnecessary stimuli should be closed out when the nurse is trying to engage the individual in conversation. If the person is frightened, someone should stay with him. This is where a member of the family could be very helpful if this person understands what is expected and receives some positive reinforcement.

Basic reality orientation is very helpful and should be part of the therapeutic relationship from the beginning. For instance, the nurse might say, "You are in the hospital for your broken hip, and in a few minutes we're going to help you sit in a chair where you can watch the *Today Show.*" It is important to keep the routine in the hospital as near to the usual life-style as possible. The more the life-style is changed, the greater the risk of confusion. Medications, especially those for control and sedation, should be used with caution, and systematic monitoring for response to treatment should be frequent.

Whatever the person is able to do alone should be encouraged and help given only to ensure success with the task. Food should be placed so that the person can see it and smell it. The elderly person with dementia often needs to be told what the food is. If he is not eating well, high-caloric drinks offered frequently help to maintain nutrition. The nurse should encourage the family to help with nutritional problems because they may know and be able to supply some favorite foods.

Family members may be very helpful if they are taught how to deal with the individual with dementia. For example, the family should be made aware that it is not helpful to withhold information from the person. Sometimes family members and staff members think they are sparing his feelings. In reality, the person almost always knows that something is amiss but does not know how to deal with mixed communication and thus becomes confused, often acting bewildered. When the dementia is advanced, individuals need to know what day it is, where and when the meals are served, where the bathroom is, and what time of day it is—morning, afternoon, or evening.

It is truly a fine thing to see a nurse model creative care of an elderly person with dementia. Often she must use her whole being to explore the meaning of his behavior and to respond in a way that is helpful and dignified to him. Modeling excellence in terms of caring for aged persons with dementia is the best way to teach staff and families.

ALZHEIMER'S DISEASE

Alzheimer's disease is an irreversible progressive and degenerative dementia that accounts for over 50% of all the dementias of old age.

Alzheimer's disease is a degenerative brain disease, causing a dementia that is progressive and irreversible. The DSM-III-R diagnosis of this dementia is termed *primary degenerative dementia of the Alzheimer type.* This illness accounts for over 50% of all persons with dementia and represents the fourth leading cause of death among the elderly. It is estimated that by the year 2030, over 2 million persons will be afflicted with this disease.

Alzheimer's disease most commonly occurs after age 65 but may occur as early as age 40. Its course from onset to death ranges from 2 to 20 years, with the usual course being 5 years. Previously, it was referred to as presenile dementia when it occurred in individuals below age 65 and as senile dementia in those 65 and older. These terms and the age distinctions they imply are no longer used.

Alzheimer's disease is devastating for victim and family alike. Its onset is insidious, and there follows a uniformly progressive deterioration. Early signs include loss of memory, difficulty with language, poor attention span, and personality changes. Later, poor judgment, confusion, agitation, incontinence, and severe personality changes are evident. Finally, the individual is no longer able to walk or to control elemental functions and gradually sinks into coma and death.

Causative factors of Alzheimer's disease

When it was known as senile dementia, the dementia associated with Alzheimer's disease was felt to be an inevitable consequence of the aging process that resulted from impaired blood circulation to the brain. Today it is known that such is not the case. Although the cause of Alzheimer's disease is not known, biopsy of brain tissue reveals characteristic neurofibrillary tangles and neuritic plaques. In addition, recent research reveals that victims of Alzheimer's disease have reduced levels of acetylcholine, possibly related to a loss of neurons in the basal ganglia.

It is felt that genetics may play a role in transmission of Alzheimer's disease, since children of victims have a 50% risk of developing this disorder. Furthermore, it is known that Down's syndrome predisposes the individual to the development of this form of dementia. Therefore, it is likely there may be several related causes. There is a current national commitment in both the public and private sectors to uncover the cause of Alzheimer's disease through research.

NURSING CARE OF INDIVIDUALS WITH ALZHEIMER'S DISEASE
Nursing assessment

The following discussion is organized around the human processes introduced in Chapter 9. Although behaviors in each category are presented as separate entities, it should be understood that they are highly interrelated and are adaptations to similar stressors.

Activity processes. The motor behavior of an individual with Alzheimer's disease is always affected. In the early stages of the illness there is likely to be activity intolerance because of reduced energy. Psychomotor agitation is common as the illness progresses, and, in later stages, gait is impaired because of increased neurological involvement. Ultimately, the person becomes bedridden.

Self-care is markedly altered. Initially, the individual may not care for himself because of his memory deficit. For example, he may forget to brush his teeth or eat his lunch, although he is still capable of engaging in both these activities. Later in the course of the illness, the individual may not only forget to carry out activities of daily living but also be unable to do so when reminded.

For reasons that are not known, sleep and arousal patterns are also affected by Alzheimer's disease. It is not unusual for the individual with this illness to awaken during the night and roam about the house, not realizing it is still nighttime. Even more potentially dangerous is the likelihood that he will go outdoors and wander away, perhaps inadequately dressed for the weather.

Cognition processes. Since Alzheimer's disease stems from a progressive brain degeneration, the cognition processes of decision making, judgment, knowledge, learning, memory, and thought processes all are markedly affected. In fact, alterations in cognition processes are the first sign of the illness, particularly alterations in memory. In the early stage of the illness the individual and those close to him are aware of his loss of memory, particularly for short-term events. Many persons try to adapt to this memory loss by writing innumerable notes to themselves, the location of which they may also forget.

The cause of Alzheimer's disease is not known.

Assessment of the individual with Alzheimer's disease usually reveals an intolerance for activity; lack of self-care and home care; altered sleep and arousal patterns; memory loss; depression, anger, and mood swings; progressive deterioration leading to social isolation and withdrawal; alteration of all physiological processes; and helplessness, hopelessness, and powerlessness.

Ecological processes. Understandably, individuals with Alzheimer's disease are unable to care for their home in a purposeful, sustained manner. Furthermore, their environment may indirectly pose many threats to their safety. For example, they may set their house on fire because they forgot to turn off the gas burner, which ignited a nearby pot holder.

Emotional processes. In the early stage of the illness the individual is aware of his deterioration and is likely to experience a severe depression. Anger also is often expressed due to frustration at not being able to remember the names of people or to identify common objects. Mood swings are common in the later stages of the disease.

Interpersonal processes. Interpersonal processes are always affected. Families of the affected individual must witness the deterioration of their loved one, who gradually does not recognize them and who eventually behaves like a total stranger. Unfortunately, the frustration experienced by family members sometimes leads to their verbally and even physically abusing the individual with Alzheimer's disease. Any abuse often goes unreported because the individual is fearful of doing so or does not remember its occurrence.

Because of his memory deficit, the person with Alzheimer's disease often confabulates. Confabulation is the unconscious "filling in" of memory gaps by imaginary and often complex experiences, which are recounted in a detailed and plausible way as though they were factual.

Since the individual and his family are aware of his progressive deterioration, social isolation and withdrawal often occur early in the illness as a means of protecting everyone from embarrassment. Unfortunately, early social isolation seems to enhance mental deterioration.

Perception processes. The individual with Alzheimer's disease has a great deal of difficulty concentrating on any one thing and therefore is easily distracted. Until his memory and awareness completely fail, he must struggle with the feelings associated with diminished self-esteem. Unfortunately, this is often a losing battle, since others, friends and strangers alike, are likely to treat him in a condescending, derisive manner.

Physiological processes. In the final stages of the illness, all physiological processes are altered. Incontinence, abnormal reflexes, and seizures are common terminal symptoms. Throughout the entire course of their illness, individuals with Alzheimer's disease are unusually subject to infection and injury, probably secondary to other factors such as poor hygiene and nutrition and memory loss.

Valuation processes. For the length of time the individual remains aware of his deterioration, he experiences profound helplessness, hopelessness, and powerlessness. These feelings form the basis for depression and low self-esteem. Individuals who have had a well-defined spiritual life in earlier years also commonly express spiritual despair and distress.

Nursing diagnoses

As with all nursing diagnoses, the nursing diagnoses for the individual with Alzheimer's disease are based on the themes identified during the assessment phase of the nursing process. Categories of human responses from the ANA Classification of Human Responses of Concern for Psychiatric–Mental Health Nursing Practice that may be specifically applicable to individuals with Alzheimer's disease include the following:

1.1.2	Altered Motor Behavior
1.3.4	Altered Self-Care
1.4.2	Altered Sleep/Arousal Patterns
2.1.2	Altered Decision Making
2.2.2	Altered Judgment
2.3.2	Altered Knowledge Processes
2.4.2	Altered Learning Processes
2.5.2	Altered Memory
2.6.2	Altered Thought Processes
3.3.2	Altered Home Maintenance
4.1.2	Altered Feeling State
4.2.2	Altered Feeling Processes
5.1.2	Altered Abuse Response
5.2.2	Altered Communication Processes
5.3.2	Altered Conduct/Impulse Processes
5.4.2	Altered Family Processes
5.5.2	Altered Role Performance
5.7.2	Altered Social Interaction
6.1.2	Altered Attention
6.3.2	Altered Self-Concept
6.4.2	Altered Sensory Perception
7.1.1	Potential for Alteration in Circulation
7.2.1	Potential for Alteration in Elimination
7.4.1	Potential for Alteration in Gastrointestinal Processes
7.5.1	Potential for Alteration in Musculoskeletal Processes
7.6.2	Altered Neuro/Sensory Processes
7.7.1	Potential for Alteration in Nutrition Processes
7.8.1	Potential of Alteration in Oxygenation
7.9.1	Potential for Alteration in Physical Integrity
7.10.1	Potential for Alteration of Physical Regulation Processes
8.1.2	Altered Meaningfulness
8.2.1	Potential for Alteration of Spirituality

NANDA nursing diagnostic categories that may be specifically applicable to the individual with Alzheimer's disease include:

1.1.2.2	Altered Nutrition: Less than body requirements
1.2.1.1	Potential for Infection

1.2.2.1	Potential Altered Body Temperature
1.3.1.3	Bowel Incontinence
1.3.2.1.5	Total Incontinence
1.6.1	Potential for Injury
1.6.1.3	Potential for Trauma
1.6.1.4	Potential for Aspiration
1.6.2.1.2.2	Potential Impaired Skin Integrity
2.1.1.1	Impaired Verbal Communication
3.1.1	Impaired Social Interaction
3.1.2	Social Isolation
3.2.1	Altered Role Performance
3.2.2	Altered Family Processes
4.1.1	Spiritual Distress
5.1.1.1	Ineffective Individual Coping
5.1.2.1.1.	Ineffective Family Coping: Disabling
6.1.1.1	Impaired Physical Mobility
6.1.1.2	Activity Intolerance
6.2.1	Sleep Pattern Disturbance
6.4.1.1	Impaired Home Maintenance Management
6.5.1	Feeding Self-Care Deficit
6.5.1.1	Impaired Swallowing
6.5.2	Bathing/Hygiene Self-Care Deficit
6.5.3	Dressing/Grooming Self-Care Deficit
6.5.4	Toileting Self-Care Deficit
7.1.2	Self-Esteem Disturbance
7.2	Sensory/Perceptual Alterations (specify) (visual, auditory, kinesthetic, gustatory, tactile, olfactory)
7.3.1	Hopelessness
7.3.2	Powerlessness
8.3	Altered Thought Processes
9.3.1	Anxiety

To develop a nursing diagnosis that fulfills its function of providing direction for planning nursing care, the nurse is encouraged to postulate and state etiologic or antecedent factors for each human response and connect the two phrases by using the term *related to*. For example:

2.5.2   Altered memory related to degenerative brain process

Planning and implementing nursing care

The plan for nursing care is derived from the nursing diagnoses and includes the objectives of the care, the nursing actions, and outcome criteria. To be effective the plan needs to be highly individualized. The suggestions that follow should be seen as general guidelines to be used if they are appropriate to the client's needs.

In general, the objectives of all nursing care for the individual with Alzheimer's disease should relate to helping him maintain physiological homeokinesis and mental acuity for as long as possible.

Since the client's nursing diagnoses are often interrelated, stemming as they do from similar etiologies or antecedents, the student will see that the appropriate nursing actions are also interrelated. The nursing interventions must reflect the stage of disease progression. The client who enters a long-term health care facility has usually progressed to a later stage of the disease, and many impairments are likely to be severe.

Activity processes. The client needs to be encouraged and helped to perform as many activities of daily living as he can. The longer he can feed, bathe, and dress himself, the more the deterioration can be slowed. Since assisting and reminding the client require a great deal of time and patience, nurses often find it easier and quicker to do these tasks for the client. This practice is deleterious to his well-being and should be avoided if at all possible.

Interventions for sleeplessness include warm baths, soft music, warm milk, light exercise, and a small amount of wine. When the individual is agitated, it is important to be aware of safety factors. At times small doses of antipsychotic agents are utilized for acute disturbed states and extreme restlessness. Care must be taken in the administration of these medications because of the prolongation of drug elimination in the elderly.

Cognition processes. The nurse can help improve the cognitive functioning of the individual through communication techniques and sensory stimulation. The therapeutic relationship can provide a forum for the discussion of feelings, opinions, and the facilitation of daily life decisions. In the early stages of the disease both individual and group techniques can be utilized. Group discussions can focus on stimulating topics and encourage active participation. The creative therapies are useful, including art, creative writing, and poetry. Later in the disease process more individual approaches are indicated.

Encouraging life review is a frequently utilized therapeutic tool. By assisting the individual to reminisce, long-term memory is stimulated and the opportunity to resolve earlier life crises is made available.

Ecological processes. Memory impairment can be impeded through the use of environmental aids and clues. One family utilized signs to remind their relative of routine tasks and safety factors. Simple lists may be of assistance, as well, in the early phase. Precautions can be taken to ensure environmental safety, such as installing gates, rearranging furniture, and removing dangerous objects.

Interpersonal processes. The client with symptoms of the later stages of Alzheimer's disease is assisted by many of the interventions discussed earlier in this chapter. Clear and consistent communication is utilized. The individual is

Appropriate nursing interventions for victims of Alzheimer's disease address the cognitive deterioration and include communication techniques and sensory and environmental intervention. The family is offered the support and education needed to care for their loved one, to develop future plans, and to work through the grieving process.

NURSING CARE PLAN

A victim of Alzheimer's disease

CASE FORMULATION

Mr. Chall is a prominent 65-year-old attorney who was admitted to a local inpatient mental health facility for a diagnostic work-up. He had recently been experiencing memory loss that had seriously affected his professional performance, until he had felt forced to take a leave of absence. He admitted that he had been attempting to disguise these difficulties for some time but lately had been finding these attempts more and more difficult. He described finding himself standing in the middle of a room at home having no idea why he was there or how he got there.

In addition, Mr. Chall was finding it more and more difficult to conduct conversations and found himself practicing and rehearsing. He described having to think carefully about every word he said. He reported feeling depressed and wishing to withdraw from social interactions.

Although Mr. Chall was known for his pleasant personality, his wife reported recent disturbing changes. He had begun losing his temper at his wife and daughters at the slightest provocation. The family felt that they had to "walk on eggs" when he was nearby.

Mr. Chall had always been most meticulous about his personal hygiene and grooming. Recently, however, he had begun to find routine tasks more difficult. His wife noted that his grooming was often poor. At times he dressed in the same suit for a number of days in a row, and his shirts and ties were spotted with food stains. Such behavior was highly unusual for such a meticulous man.

Both Mrs. Chall and his family were extremely concerned. After a thorough assessment and diagnostic work-up, he and his family were informed that he had the medical diagnosis of Alzheimer's disease. Upon learning of the diagnosis Mr. Chall became deeply disturbed and manifested further evidence of withdrawal behaviors. The family was devastated and turned to the staff for support and assistance.

Nursing assessment

Mr. Chall appeared to be experiencing many of the behaviors manifested by individuals in the early stages of Alzheimer's disease. Fading memory was evident, as were attempts to mask this symptom. Mr. Chall was experiencing difficulties with language and some trouble with the performance of the routine tasks of daily living. These symptoms were impairing his work and social life.

Personality changes were among Mr. Chall's predominant symptoms. Abrupt temper tantrums were noted by the family members, despite a previously pleasant personality. Feelings of depression and a desire to withdraw from social interactions were reported by Mr. Chall.

As a result of Mr. Chall's behaviors, the family was experiencing a very difficult time. Both Mr. Chall and his family were further devastated when the diagnosis of Alzheimer's disease was learned.

Nursing diagnoses

The assessment data—including present behavior, past life experiences, and an understanding of the underlying physiology—led to the development of the following five pairs of nursing diagnoses for Mr. Chall. The first of each pair is from the Classification of Human Responses of Concern for Psychiatric–Mental Health Nursing Practice; the second is from the approved NANDA Diagnostic Categories.

2.6.2   Altered Thought Processes related to memory impairment and cognitive deterioration

OR

8.3   Altered Thought Processes related to memory impairment and cognitive deterioration

5.2.2   Altered Communication Processes related to organic brain disease

OR

2.1.1.1   Impaired Verbal Communication related to organic brain disease

NURSING CARE PLAN—cont'd

1.3.4	Altered Self-Care related to cognitive deterioration
OR	
6.5.2	Bathing/Hygiene Self-Care Deficit related to cognitive deterioration
4.1.2	Altered Feeling State related to awareness of cognitive deterioration and diminished sense of self-worth
OR	
5.1.1.1	Ineffective Individual Coping related to awareness of cognitive deterioration and diminished sense of self-worth
5.4.2	Altered Family Processes related to impairment of family member
OR	
3.2.2	Altered Family Processes related to impairment of family member

Planning and implementing nursing care for Mr. Chall

The plan of nursing care for Mr. Chall is summarized on pp. 364-365. Interventions were based on the present behaviors. However, the progressive nature of this disorder was kept in mind and appropriate revisions made as changes in Mr. Chall's status occurred. It was decided that Mr. Chall would return home in 2 weeks, allowing time for the family to prepare to offer the needed support and assistance. Long-term plans were postponed for the present time, although the potential inevitability of placement in a long-term care facility was recognized.

A therapeutic relationship was established with Mr. Chall's primary nurse, who treated him with respect and dignity and approached him in a clear, consistent fashion on a regular basis. Mr. Chall was encouraged to communicate his feelings and his interests to the nurse, who listened in a caring, supportive, and interested manner. Mr. Chall was encouraged to review his life's achievements and memories, as well as to discuss his present-day concerns and ideas. Participation in a discussion group was encouraged, where stimulating topics were explored. In addition,

Mr. Chall was encouraged to participate in creative therapies, such as art and creative writing.

The nurse assisted Mr. Chall to develop memory aids to help him to recall daily tasks and routines. He developed lists and reminders to help him structure his daily activities. It has been found that such aids are very successful in improving self-care and autonomy.

A daily routine was planned to assist Mr. Chall with bathing and hygiene. Clothes were laid out the night before, with the assistance of the nurse when necessary.

Finally, the nurse directed some of her energy toward the needs of the family who felt devastated as a result of Mr. Chall's deterioration and poor prognosis. Education was provided, as was support and assistance with crisis resolution. The family was referred to the local chapter of the Alzheimer's Disease and Related Disorders Association, an organization that could provide much support and assistance in planning for the future.

Evaluation

Evaluation of the plan of nursing care and its implementation was based on the outcome criteria developed.

Mr. Chall showed some improvement while in the inpatient setting. He reported that he felt less depressed, although he continued to feel embarrassed and fearful of social interactions. However he was able to discuss the feelings related to the loss of his health and continued his efforts to communicate with others. Mr. Chall found the memory aids extremely helpful as reminders for the tasks of the day, and felt more control over his actions as a result. He continued to experience changes in mood, including mild temper tantrums.

The family became involved in the local chapter of ADRDA and reported that they were receiving much assistance from this organization. Although unable to make long-term plans, they received many helpful suggestions about how to best provide for Mr. Chall's needs once he re-

Continued.

NURSING CARE PLAN—cont'd

turned home. It was felt by the nursing staff that the family continued to experience denial related to Mr. Chall's prognosis but that with the support of the services they had engaged they would eventually come to terms with the inevitability of Mr. Chall's deterioration and death. At the time of Mr. Chall's discharge, the family appeared able to receive him warmly into the home for the present. They were advised to utilize the recommended support services as they took on the physical and emotional task of caring for their loved one.

NURSING CARE PLAN FOR *Mr. Chall*

Nursing diagnosis	Objective	Nursing action	Outcome criteria
2.6.2 Altered Thought Processes related to memory impairment and cognitive deterioration OR 8.3 Altered Thought Processes related to memory impairment and cognitive deterioration	To assist the client to maintain environmental contact and interaction	Establish therapeutic relationship with client Interact with client in a clear, consistent manner Assist with the development of memory aids (signs, lists) Provide reality orientation and sensory stimulation Ensure client safety	Within 2 weeks the client will: List routine daily tasks Develop appropriate memory aids
5.2.2 Altered Communication Processes related to organic brain disease OR 2.1.1.1 Impaired Verbal Communication related to organic brain disease	To facilitate and enhance the client's ability to maintain communication with others	Accept and respect client's attempts to communicate Encourage discussion of life review and present day events Encourage participation in group discussion Facilitate family discussions and interactions	Within 2 weeks the client will: Spontaneously discuss daily events with the nurse Actively participate in group discussions
1.3.4 Altered Self-Care related to cognitive deterioration	To assist the client to perform tasks of bathing and dressing	Establish and implement bathing and dressing routine Encourage client to perform own hygiene as able	Within 2 weeks the client will: Follow the established bathing and dressing routine

NURSING CARE PLAN—cont'd

OR 6.5.2	Bathing/Hygiene Self-Care Deficit related to cognitive deterioration		Assist with dressing as necessary	Accept assistance as needed
4.1.2	Altered Feeling State related to awareness of cognitive deterioration and diminished sense of self-worth	To encourage the client to discuss his feelings and problems	Meet regularly to allow client opportunity for ventilation Convey empathy and support Utilize reflective listening techniques to facilitate conversation Sit in silence and offer acceptance if the client does not wish to talk	Within 2 weeks the client will spontaneously discuss feelings and recent losses with the nurse
OR 5.1.1.1	Ineffective Individual Coping related to awareness of cognitive deterioration and diminished sense of self-worth			
5.4.2	Altered Family Processes related to impairment of family member	To assist the family to cope with the present crisis and to prepare for and accept prognosis	Meet with family members weekly Offer education and refer to local support services Offer support and encourage the expression of feelings Facilitate problem solving	Within 2 weeks family will be able to discuss present and future plans for the care of Mr. Chall
OR 3.2.2	Altered Family Processes related to impairment of family member			

approached calmly, and always addressed by name. Basic reality orientation is helpful.

In the course of the disease process the client may become quite agitated and combative. The nurse must be prepared to intervene and to accept these behaviors in a nonjudgmental fashion. The nurse must continue to afford the individual the respect and dignity that she would show to any client.

The families of the victims of Alzheimer's disease are in desperate need of assistance and support. Efforts should be made to maximize their strengths, allow for the expression of feelings, provide education, and mobilize social supports. The nurse can help the family to prepare for the time when the institutionalization of their loved one may be necessary. The Alzheimer's Disease and Related Disorders Association (ADRDA) is an organization with over 100 chapters in the United States that has much to offer the victims of Alzheimer's disease and their families. These services include hot lines, self-help groups, and respite care programs. The nurse can educate the family about this organization and other local services.

Physiological processes. The nurse caring for the client with Alzheimer's disease must be aware that the disease is progressive and irreversible. The individual will eventually become bedridden and helpless, and it will be necessary to meet his most basic needs.

END NOTE

This chapter focuses on the elderly as a population at risk for mental illness. The effects of the devaluation of the elderly in our society are discussed, and social and psychological changes that affect the mental health of the elderly are described. Nursing interventions designed to prevent or address depression, suspiciousness, and dementia in the elderly are discussed. Alzheimer's disease is discussed in detail as a prevalent form of dementia. A hypothetical case formulation of an individual suffering from this illness is presented, along with nursing diagnoses from which a plan of care is derived, implemented, and evaluated.

SUGGESTED SOURCES OF ADDITIONAL INFORMATION

Baldwin BA: Community management of Alzheimer's disease, Nurs Clin North Am 23(1):47, March 1988.

Batt LJ: Managing delirium: implications for geropsychiatric nurses, J Psychosoc Nurs Ment Health Serv 27(5):22, May 1989.

Beck C and Heacock P: Nursing interventions for patients with Alzheimer's disease, Nurs Clin North Am 23(1):95, March 1988.

Bozian MW and Clark HM: Counteracting sensory change in the elderly, Am J Nurs 80:473, March 1980.

Bracey R: Time for talk, Nurs Times 85(10):40, March 8, 1989.

Britnell J and Mitchell K: Inpatient group psychotherapy for the elderly, J Psychosoc Nurs Ment Health Serv 19:19, May 1981.

Buchanan D: Psychodrama: a humanistic approach to psychiatric treatment for the elderly, Hosp Commun Psychiatr 33(3):220, 1982.

Bumagin VE and Hirn KF: Aging is a family affair, New York, 1980, Lippincott and Crowell.

Chaisson M, Beutler L, Yost E, and Allendar J: Treating the depressed elderly, J Psychosoc Nurs Ment Health Serv 22:25, May 1984.

Cohen S and Bunke Sr E: Programmed instruction: sensory changes in the elderly, Am J Nurs 81:1851, 1981.

Duffey BD: Demented, old, and alone, Am J Nurs 89(2):212, February 1989.

Ettlinger R, Binkowski N, and Zaiser A: A senior citizens' center and a geriatric transitional house at a state psychiatric hospital, Hosp Commun Psychiatr 35:1029, October 1984.

Farran CJ and Keane-Hagerty E: Communicating effectively with dementia patients, J Psychosoc Nurs Ment Health Serv 27(5):13, May 1989.

Given CW, Collins CE, and Given BA: Sources of stress among families caring for relatives with Alzheimer's disease, Nurs Clin North Am 23(1):69, March 1988.

Hall GR: Care of the patient with Alzheimer's disease living at home, Nurs Clin North Am 23(1):31, March 1988.

Harvis KA and Rabins PV: Dementia: helping family caregivers cope, J Psychosoc Nurs Ment Health Serv 27(5):6, May 1989.

Held M, Ransohoff P, and Goehner P: A comprehensive treatment program for severely impaired geriatric patients, Hosp Commun Psychiatr 35:156, February 1984.

Janforum: The practical management of the Alzheimer's disease patient in the hospital setting, J Adv Nurs 12(4):531, July 1987.

King KS: Reminiscing psychotherapy with aging people, J Psychosoc Nurs Ment Health Serv 20:21, February 1982.

Maas M: Management of patients with Alzheimer's disease in long-term care facilities, Nurs Clin North Am 23(1):57, March 1988.

O'Donovan S: Why bother? Nurs Times 84(15):43, April 13 1988.

Roberts BL and Algase DL: Victims of Alzheimer's disease and the environment, Nurs Clin North Am 23(1):83, March 1988.

Simpson S and Wilson L: Meeting the mental health needs of the aged: the role of psychiatric emergency services, Hosp Commun Psychiatr 33:833, October 1982.

Stevens GL and Baldwin BA: Optimizing mental health in the nursing home setting, J Psychosoc Nurs Mental Health Serv 26(10):27, October 1988.

Teusing JP and Mahler S: Helping families cope with Alzheimer's disease, Hosp Commun Psychiatr 35:152, February 1984.

Thornton JE, Davies HD, and Tinklenberg JR: Alzheimer's disease syndrome, J Psychosoc Nurs Mental Health Serv 24(5):16, May 1986.

Vander Zyle S: Psychotherapy with the elderly, J Psychosoc Nurs Ment Health Serv 21:25, October 1983.

Whall AL and Conklin C: Why a psychogeriatric unit? J Psychosoc Nurs Mental Health Serv 23(5):23, May 1985.

Populations at risk
Children and adolescents

LEARNING OBJECTIVES

After studying this chapter, the student will be able to

o Define the medical diagnosis of mental retardation.

o Describe the behaviors exhibited by a child with the medical diagnosis of pervasive developmental disorder.

o Discuss the ways in which an academic skills disorder or motor skills disorder might interfere with the development of a child.

o Describe the characteristics of two types of disruptive behavior disorder in children.

o Differentiate between separation anxiety disorder and overanxious disorder in children.

o State general guidelines for meeting the needs of disturbed children.

o Describe the characteristics of an adolescent suffering from the eating disorders of anorexia nervosa or bulimia nervosa.

o State general guidelines for meeting the needs of an adolescent suffering from anorexia nervosa or bulimia nervosa.

o Describe the characteristics of a suicidal adolescent.

o State general guidelines for meeting the needs of an adolescent who is suicidal.

o Develop a hypothetical plan of nursing care for an adolescent who is suicidal.

There probably is no other group for which the title "Populations at Risk" is more appropriate than the group represented by the children and adolescents of this country. About one-third of the nation's population is under 18 years of age, and it is estimated that over 11% of this group is suffering from a mental disorder. Furthermore, many authorities forecast that the incidence and prevalence of mental disorders and dysfunctional behavior among this population will increase over the next two decades. Despite this dire situation, there is a gross shortage of health care professionals who are educationally and experientially prepared to address these problems. The seriousness of this situation can be appreciated if one remembers that the children and youth of a society are that society's future.

The identification and treatment of mental disorders of children and adolescents are recognized as an area of specialization in both medicine and nursing. Thus this topic deserves more attention than can possibly be provided in one chapter of a textbook devoted primarily to the field of adult psychiatric nursing. Nevertheless, this chapter is included to present a brief overview of the field in the hope that all students will become sensitized to the needs of disturbed children and adolescents and their families and that some will become interested in pursuing further preparation in this specialty.

HISTORICAL PERSPECTIVE

Interest in the prevention and treatment of emotional disorders of children and adolescents did not develop until recently. In fact, before 1920 many authorities believed that mental illness was limited to adults. The occasional emotionally disturbed child who came to the attention of physicians was thought to be a clinical curiosity. This view reflected limited knowledge about the nature of childhood and adolescence.

A number of factors led to an increased interest in childhood and adolescence as stages of development distinct from adulthood. In preindustrial societies the progression from childhood to adulthood was rapid and accompanied by limited choices. Children were taught to take over the tasks and chores required to meet the basic needs of the family. Formal education was limited for the vast majority of children. However, the emergence of the industrial society created numerous social changes that postponed the age at which the passage into adulthood occurred. Since industrialization and expanding technology required increased education and training to prepare for a productive adulthood, the stage of adolescence was delineated as a transitional period between childhood and adulthood during which this specialized training should occur. Therefore, the student role set adolescents apart as a distinct and separate population.

The post–World War II baby boom created a very large subgroup of adolescents in the 1960's and 1970's. A distinct adolescent culture emerged, and interest in its unique development and distinct problems led to a more careful examination of this age group.

The role of the nurse in the treatment of emotionally disturbed children and adolescents has traditionally been minimal, often limited to the provision of physical care and the administration of medications. However, as more nurses pursued graduate education in psychiatric nursing through funds made available by the National Mental Health Act of 1946, the therapeutic potential of nurses in the care of children and youth became evident. In 1954 the first graduate program in child psychiatric nursing was opened at Boston University. Although there are a number of such programs today, there are fewer graduates than necessary to provide the required leadership in the prevention and treatment of emotional disorders of children and adolescents.

DISORDERS BEGINNING IN INFANCY OR CHILDHOOD

This discussion is limited to those disorders which commonly have their onset during infancy or childhood. However, it should be noted that the major mental disorders of adulthood, such as depression and schizophrenia, do occur, although infrequently, in infants and children.

Developmental disorders

Mental retardation. Since mental retardation is not a mental illness, its relevance to psychiatric nursing is often questioned. However, the mentally retarded individual is three to four times more likely than others to develop a mental disorder, the treatment of which must take into account the individual's intellectual limitations. Therefore, it is important for the psychiatric nurse to have an understanding of what is meant by mental retardation.

> Though mental retardation is not a mental illness, the individual who is mentally retarded is much more likely than others to develop a mental disorder.

The term *mental retardation* is used to describe a condition in which there is a general delay in the individual's intellectual and social development during the early years of life. If the person's development is normal before age 18, mental retardation is not an appropriate diagnosis.

The diagnosis of mental retardation is made only after a multifaceted assessment of the individual. This includes a study of his physical, social, cultural, educational, vocational, and emotional capacities. However, the determination of mental retardation leans heavily on the results of a battery of psychometric tests from which a definitive score is derived. Although authorities continue to call attention to the limitations and weaknesses of the several psychological tests currently in use, intelligence testing continues to be one of the major tools in categorizing individuals in relation to intellectual functioning. Such categorization is useful for many practical reasons, especially in planning educational programs.

A score called the intelligence quotient (IQ) is calculated by use of a formula in which the mental age (MA) is divided by the chronological age (CA) and multiplied by 100. Therefore the formula is:

$$IQ = \frac{MA}{CA} \times 100$$

Obviously, an IQ cannot be determined in infancy, and the diagnosis of mental retardation is not made in many individuals until they reach school age. However, the existence of characteristic physical features or severe physical impairment in many profoundly and severely retarded individuals sometimes allows this diagnosis to be made at birth or shortly thereafter.

The DSM-III-R categorizes mental retardation into four degrees of severity as follows:

Degree of severity	IQ
Mild	50-55 to approx. 70
Moderate	35-40 to 50-55
Severe	20-25 to 35-40
Profound	Below 20 or 25

Most individuals with an IQ below 20 or 25 are too retarded to benefit from educational programs on even the simplest level. These individuals require care not unlike that provided for infants. They also need to be safeguarded against ordinary physical danger. Some individuals who are severely mentally retarded can learn to talk and be trained in basic hygiene skills, although it may take years of effort for them to achieve these skills. Fortunately, persons with profound or severe mental retardation account for only about 5% of all individuals who are mentally retarded.

Individuals who exhibit moderate mental retardation can learn to talk and eventually master the skills necessary to take care of themselves. Although they will always require supervision for their own safety and protection, by adulthood it is possible for them to function well in familiar settings, perhaps even becoming employed in unskilled jobs.

Individuals who are mildly mentally retarded account for the largest proportion of mentally retarded persons. These individuals may not be distinguishable from others until childhood. These persons benefit from educational programs that emphasize concrete academic skills, social adjustment, and vocational preparation. Many become gainfully employed at jobs that require simple repetitive tasks and can live independently if supportive services are available.

The cause of mental retardation is unknown; however, some hereditary and perinatal factors are known to result in impaired intellectual capacity.

Although the cause of mental retardation is unknown in approximately 75% of the individuals so diagnosed, certain hereditary and perinatal factors are known to result in impaired intellectual capacity. For example, a genetic abnormality within the twenty-first chromosome results in Down's syndrome; maternal alcohol or drug use during pregnancy may result in prenatal damage reflected by mental retardation; and postnatal head injury or ingestion of toxins such as lead often lead to mental retardation.

The care of mentally retarded individuals in this country has undergone a dramatic revolution over the last two decades. Legislation and government funding have enabled all but the most profoundly retarded to live at home and to attend local schools where an individualized program of study to meet their specific needs is designed by specialists in special education. This program may call for classes separate from those attended by nonretarded children, or it may require that the child be "mainstreamed" with all other children, or it may dictate a combination of both types of learning experiences. As adults, most mentally retarded persons are able to live in the community, either independently or in group home situations where appropriate supervision is provided.

Pervasive developmental disorders. Until recently the illnesses known as pervasive developmental disorders were thought to be psychoses of infancy and childhood and have had the diagnostic labels of atypical development, symbiotic psychosis, or childhood schizophrenia. A pervasive developmental disorder of infancy or childhood is a condition in which the individual's entire development is severely and markedly impaired, particularly in developmentally appropriate social interaction, communication and imaginative activity, and range of activities and interests. In addition, there are often abnormalities in cognitive skills, posture and motor behavior, responses to sensory input, eating, drinking, and sleeping patterns, and in mood. Self-injurious behaviors are common. The most severe form of pervasive developmental disorder is autistic disorder.

Autistic disorder is often recognized by the end of the first year of age and usually by 3 years of age. It is far more common in boys than girls and may be misdiagnosed as mental retardation. Children with this disorder seem to be living in a world of their own and show little or no ability to relate to other human beings, including their mother. In fact, they appear not to recognize their mother as different from other people. They do not communicate in any meaningful way, and although they may use words, they do so in a highly personalized manner that only family members are likely to understand. Many of these children are obsessively attached to some inanimate object such as a doll or teddy bear with which they may play for hours on end. In addition, they are likely to become very upset and have temper tantrums if their environment is altered in any way. Many engage in self-destructive motor behaviors such as head banging and biting their own limbs. Interestingly, they frequently twirl around at an amazing speed without becoming dizzy and seem to enjoy music.

The cause of autistic disorder is not known, although research indicates that brain dysfunction is likely to be a predisposing factor. The earlier belief that parental rejection was the major causative factor has not been supported by research.

Specific developmental disorders. Unlike pervasive developmental disorders that affect the entire being of the individual, a variety of developmental disorders are specific to impaired development in a particular area. Among these are academic skills disorders and motor skills disorder. Even though treatment of children with these disorders usually takes place within the school system, they are mentioned here because their existence often impacts the self-esteem of the child and affects the family system, perhaps bringing them to the attention of the mental health system. For example, a child who is not able to read at grade level is in danger of being held back in school, thereby separating him from his peers and impeding successful completion of other developmental tasks. On the

A *pervasive developmental disorder* of infancy or childhood is a condition in which the individual's entire development is severely and markedly impaired.

other hand, if the child is promoted into the next grade without being able to adequately deal with the academic demands of that grade, he or she is likely to develop feelings of inadequacy brought on by continual failure.

The *academic skills disorders* include impairment in arithmetic skills, expressive writing skills, reading skills, articulation (pronunciation) skills, expressive language skills, or language comprehension. For a child to be diagnosed with one of these disorders, it must be demonstrated that there is no physiological basis for their existence, such as mental retardation or a congenital anatomical abnormality. These disorders are not uncommon, and with the specialized help now available in all public schools, almost all children who have them can be greatly helped.

Motor skills disorder is characterized by impairment in motor coordination not explained by a physical disorder such as cerebral palsy. Although the clumsiness exhibited by a child with this disorder greatly interferes with his ability to function effectively, much help is available through the special education programs in the public schools.

Disruptive behavior disorders

Of great concern is the disruptive behavior disorders, which are characterized by behavior that is socially disruptive and usually very distressing to the individuals with whom the child associates.

Attention-deficit hyperactivity disorder is diagnosed in children who are overactive, both physically and verbally. These children are unusually distractible and therefore unable to concentrate on any one task or to sit still. These characteristics result in their being unable to complete tasks, follow directions, or to respond appropriately in social situations. For example, they frequently interrupt others, often with comments that are extraneous to the topic. Being around these children has been described as being in the middle of a whirlwind. As a result of their behavior, they often alienate others and do poorly in school. Consequently, their initial problems are likely to be compounded by low self-esteem.

Children with a *conduct disorder* display a pattern of behavior that is antisocial. This almost always involves physical aggression toward others and purposeful cruelty to animals, deliberately damaging or destroying property, truancy, lying, stealing, sexual offenses, and the abuse of drugs. As is true of adults with antisocial personality disorder, these children apparently feel no remorse or guilt over their behavior and therefore are very difficult to treat.

Anxiety disorders

Although all children display signs of anxiety on occasion, some children experience anxiety continuously or with predictability in specific situations. For example, children with *separation anxiety disorder* suffer extreme anxiety when they are actually or potentially separated from significant adults, usually their

---

Two types of *specific developmental disorders,* those specific to impaired development in a particular area, are *academic skills disorders* and *motor skills disorder*.

Children with disruptive behavior disorders display behavior that is socially disruptive and distressing to those with whom the child associates.

Children with anxiety disorders display anxiety continuously or predictably in specific situations.

mother. They often display "clinging" behavior, experience an upset stomach or headache, and understandably refuse to go to school or to stay overnight at a friend's house. Needless to say, this disorder markedly interferes with their successfully achieving the developmental tasks appropriate to their age.

Some children are not anxious about a particular event but rather experience generalized anxiety continuously. When this anxiety is maintained for over 6 months, they may warrant the diagnosis of *overanxious disorder*. Children with this disorder worry about everything that is occurring both to them and to others in their family. For example, an elementary school child may be distraught about having to participate in a school concert, or an older child may express fear that her father will be laid off from work after reading in the newspaper about layoffs in another company. Furthermore, these children are particularly adept at conjuring up tragedies that might befall them or their family. One 10-year-old who developed the symptoms of this disorder when his mother took a job outside the home expressed fear about her being killed in an automobile accident, his burning the house down when he turned the oven on as instructed to prewarm it for dinner, and the house being burglarized while it was empty during the day.

GUIDELINES FOR MEETING THE NEEDS OF DISTURBED CHILDREN

Providing therapeutic care for disturbed children is one of the greatest challenges a nurse can face. Yet it is one that she must meet, since she is most likely to have both initial and sustained contact with these children, particularly as she functions in community mental health treatment centers. The behavior of children with emotional problems is frequently more baffling and more difficult to understand than the behavior of adults who are mentally ill. If the care provided for disturbed children is to be therapeutic, it must be based on the individual needs of the child. The nurse, like all other individuals working with disturbed children, will find it necessary to study the child and the symptoms he displays to identify his immediate needs and to respond to them in a realistic and helpful way. In so doing, an attempt is made to offer the child experiences that can correct, in some measure, the negative experiences that have been a part of his life.

As the nurse understands that the behaviors the child exhibits are symptoms of more basic problems, she will learn to be sensitive in the manner in which she responds to the disturbed behavior. There is no question that the disturbed behavior requires a response; however, if this becomes the primary focus of intervention, one runs the risk of reinforcing the behavior with the result that it may not only continue but actually worsen. Rather, the goal should be an attempt to discover the nature of the underlying problem, and the intervention should be directed toward its resolution, not merely toward the obliteration of the symptom. For example, it is commonly known that attempts to stop a child from nail biting are generally unsuccessful when this behavior is the sole focus

The goal of the nurse in dealing with disturbed children should be an attempt to discover the nature of the child's underlying problem. Intervention should be directed toward resolution of the problem not just toward alleviating the symptoms.

of concern. To intervene on a level more basic than the presenting symptom, the nurse needs to work collaboratively with the therapist, the pediatrician, and the social worker.

Since many of these children are highly sensitive to their environment and the people who are a part of it, nurses need to examine their feelings, attitudes, and behaviors in an attempt to understand their own reactions to the child. In this way they can modify their behavior for the benefit of the child.

Disturbed children require attention and guidance in the same areas of personal care that mothers usually provide. Thus the adult working with disturbed children will need to be involved actively in the child's bathing, toileting, feeding, dressing, and play activities. In addition, these children require organization and supervision in a variety of play activities, protection from potentially dangerous situations, and, at times, appropriate limit setting. Like normal children, each disturbed child is unique and occasionally needs special understanding and attention. It is a demanding task to respond as a wise adult to all the situations that may arise from the activities of daily living. The cooperation of all involved in the situation is required to assist each child to express his needs and find satisfying ways of meeting them.

Sometimes disturbed children, like all children, need to be held, cuddled, rocked, or comforted. Such an activity is clearly within the role of the nurse and necessitates a good deal of knowledge, sensitivity, and mature judgment to realize when and how much of such gratification is therapeutic for each child.

When admission to a treatment center is recommended for disturbed children, it is done in the hope that the climate of the center will provide greater opportunities for ego development than can be provided elsewhere. Thus the goal for the treatment of every child is the development of a climate that will encourage the adaptive aspects of the child's ego so that he will experiment with methods for coping with the environment and for developing more effective ways of dealing with people.

Disturbed children are frequently unclear about simple aspects of reality and need to have repeated clarification about these confusions. Thus the nurse-child interactions should logically focus on the reality of the situation, with emphasis being placed on verbal communication about reality matters.

Inappropriate response to environmental stimuli is a frequent problem for the disturbed child. The nurse needs to help the child recognize more appropriate responses to stimuli. Opportunities should be provided for him to test and use these new responses.

Consistency in dealing with any child is of major importance and is especially necessary in providing care for disturbed children. When several people are involved in providing care for children, consistency is difficult to achieve but is nonetheless important. Assuring a consistent approach depends on adequate communication among all people involved. Thus frequent staff meetings involving all the adults who come in contact with the child are essential. Every

Disturbed children need attention and guidance in the same areas of personal and emotional care that mothers usually provide.

Consistency in dealing with a disturbed child is especially important when a number of people are providing care in a hospital setting.

adult involved must understand what approach is being made to each child, why it has been adopted, and what it is expected to achieve. Repeated clarification of the treatment goals for each child is essential. Each staff member must have frequent opportunities to share with the group personal experiences in caring for the child. Thus all will be equally aware of the child's progress, and inconsistencies in the treatment approach can be eliminated.

Disturbed children sometimes become hyperactive and exhibit destructive behavior. Establishing and enforcing reasonable limits for children is an important responsibility of all staff. It may be necessary to restrain these children to avoid injury to themselves or to others. Restraint can best be accomplished by holding the child firmly until the outburst has subsided. Assuring the child that the staff is not frightened by his behavior may be reassuring to him because the child may fear his own angry feelings. It may also be reassuring to the child to tell him that he will not be allowed to hurt himself or other people.

The nurse frequently has an opportunity to talk with the parents of disturbed children. Most parents of disturbed children are themselves working with a therapist and thus have opportunities to discuss their concerns and anxieties. However, the nurse is frequently the most available professional person to whom they can turn to share the concerns that may have arisen or to ask advice about some aspect of behavior the child has developed. The nurse's interest in their child and willingness to listen to their fears and doubts are therapeutic for the parents.

In addition, many nurses have had the experience of finding that when they focus on the family in assisting them to explore and resolve familial conflicts, the child's disturbed behavior improves. The theoretical basis for this phenomenon is that the family is a system and that the disturbed behavior used by the child is a symptom reflecting dysfunction within the family unit. As the family unit becomes more functional, the child is likely to have more of his needs met and to feel more secure and therefore have less need to use disturbed behavior.

Another important function of the nurse that cannot be overemphasized is her role in providing anticipatory guidance to families to prepare them for the behaviors that can be expected as the child progresses through each developmental stage. Many parents, particularly mothers, feel most comfortable in sharing their concerns with a nurse. Appropriate reassurances and instruction can be of inestimable value in helping parents to provide acceptance and guidance for an emotionally disturbed child. In addition, appropriate anticipatory guidance of parents may play an important role in the prevention of behavioral disturbances in children who are basically healthy.

Play therapy is almost universally employed in the treatment of children with emotional problems. Its use is based on the knowledge that play is the medium through which children normally express themselves. Therapists use the child's play as a means of gaining insight into his unconscious feelings and attitudes about life as he is experiencing it. Play therapy has the additional function

The nurse is therapeutic in dealing with the parents of a disturbed child by listening to their fears and doubts and by providing anticipatory guidance.

of enabling some children to work through some of the problems they are experiencing. The therapy room is furnished with a variety of toys and other equipment the child may choose to play with. The therapist remains in the playroom with the child and spends time in getting acquainted with the child and in developing a relationship of trust. The therapist observes the child carefully and listens attentively to his comments. If the therapist and the child have developed a trusting relationship, the therapist may ask the child to tell something about the meaning of the play in which he is engaging. Usually a complete dollhouse and a family of dolls are part of the equipment in a play therapy room. This equipment is purposefully included because the way the child plays with the family of dolls provides insights into the relationships the child is experiencing with the members of his own family. Since the child's emotional life revolves around the members of his family, these insights are significant.

It is important that play therapy, which enables the therapist and the child to communicate with one another, be appropriate to the developmental level at which the child is functioning.

When children are questioned about spanking or punishing one of the child dolls excessively, one learns much about the punishment the child has experienced or fantasizes that he should have experienced. Children sometimes try to destroy an offending child doll or one of the adult members of the doll family. When asked to talk about these occurrences, the child may explain some of his unconscious fears or his feelings toward a sibling or a parent. Thus play therapy helps the therapist and the child to communicate with one another. Even when the child is essentially nonverbal, much can be learned from observing the child at play.

It is important that the form of play therapy chosen be appropriate to the developmental level at which the child is functioning. For example, finger painting and other forms of artwork may be used in therapy. This type of activity may appeal more to some children than does playing with toys. This is especially true in the case of an older child. Much can be learned from the child's choice of color, the topic featured in the artwork, and the story the child may tell about the painting when it has been completed.

DISORDERS BEGINNING IN ADOLESCENCE

Adolescence is the term used to describe the period of life that falls between the ages of 12 and 18. This period spans the developmental phase between childhood and adulthood that is marked by intense biological, cognitive, intrapsychic, and interpersonal changes. One of the major tasks of adolescence is separation from the family as a means of establishing an independent identity and assuming an adult role in society. This struggle for independence is often awkward and at times stormy as the individual experiences confusion and fear regarding his ability to master the tasks of this stage. The adolescent wrestles with the desire to stay close to protective parental figures and the simultaneous desire for freedom and autonomy. This ambivalence is often manifested by continual conflicts between the adolescent and his parents.

The adolescent is engaged in an intrapsychic struggle in an attempt to establish a new psychological equilibrium. In addition, the individual is exerting much effort to control new desires and impulses that come about as a result of biological maturation. The outcome of these struggles is largely determined by the success with which earlier developmental tasks have been achieved.

Today's adolescent confronts this critical developmental period during a time of great stress generated by the highly complex postindustrial society in which he lives. The stresses of contemporary Western culture may contribute to the distress, alienation, loneliness, and despair that at times characterize the adolescent experience. The number and severity of emotional problems of adolescents continue to increase. Adolescent suicide has been described as an epidemic in the United States; the rate has tripled in the last 20 years. Self-destructive behaviors such as drug abuse, alcoholism, eating disorders, and sexual promiscuity are also on the rise.

Adolescents may develop many of the mental disorders described earlier in this chapter as beginning in childhood and infancy. Major mental illnesses such as schizophrenia may also first develop during adolescence. However, two serious emotional problems are most likely to develop during adolescence and deserve special attention, namely, eating disorders and adolescent suicide.

Eating disorders: anorexia nervosa and bulimia nervosa

The incidence and awareness of the eating disorders known as anorexia nervosa and bulimia nervosa have risen dramatically in recent years. Both disorders most commonly begin in adolescence and young adulthood and primarily affect females. Although much has been written on eating disorders in recent years in both professional and popular literature, there is disagreement among authorities about the cause and treatment of these disorders.

Anorexia nervosa is the term used to describe a disorder characterized by extreme weight loss, behavior designed to effect weight loss, an intense fear of fat, a distorted body image, and peculiar patterns of eating and handling food. The term *anorexia* is a misnomer in that it means loss of appetite. However, the anorectic rarely experiences loss of appetite until late in the illness.

The individual with anorexia nervosa usually comes to the attention of the health care system after a drastic reduction in weight. Therefore she has an emaciated appearance. She has drastically reduced her total food intake, most specifically those foods containing carbohydrates. There are ritualistic and bizarre eating habits, such as hiding and hoarding foods, collecting recipes, dawdling and methodically rearranging food on the plate, and refusing to eat with family or in public. These individuals have an intense fear of getting fat, despite their often emaciated appearance. Symptoms of depression are often evident, such as sleep disturbances, crying spells, and suicidal ideation. They usually have amenorrhea and a lack of interest in sexual activity. The individual often engages in excessive exercising and is preoccupied with food and weight loss. Physical signs include hypothermia, bradycardia, dependent edema, dehydra-

Anorexia nervosa is a disorder occurring most commonly in adolescents and is characterized by extreme weight loss, behavior directed toward weight loss, an intense fear of fat, distorted body image, and peculiar ways of handling food.

tion, hypotension, and lanuga, a fine downy hair covering the body. Laboratory tests reveal electrolyte imbalances, including hypokalemic alkalosis secondary to self-induced vomiting and laxative abuse. These individuals are often withdrawn and socially isolated. They are described by family members as having been perfect children with above-average scholastic achievement and fear of failure.

Bulimia nervosa is the term to describe a disorder marked by episodic, uncontrolled, and rapid consumption of food over a short period of time (binge eating), inconspicuous eating during a binge, and termination of the binge by abdominal pain, sleep, social interruption, or self-induced vomiting. The bulimic individual makes repeated attempts to lose weight by severe dieting, fasting, laxative abuse, or self-induced vomiting. She is aware of the fact that her eating behaviors are abnormal and is plagued by self-deprecating thoughts and depressed moods.

The individual with bulimia nervosa often appears healthier than the client with anorexia nervosa because the behavior is generally less incapacitating. This person is usually of normal body weight or slightly overweight but may report frequent fluctuations in weight. While the individual with anorexia nervosa is often shy and withdrawn, the client with bulimia nervosa is frequently an extrovert. The individual will often report low self-esteem and self-loathing, symptoms of depression, and a fear of losing control. She is able to describe the binge episodes and will report frequent attempts to lose weight through fasting or severely restricted diets, laxative abuse, or self-induced vomiting. There is usually an excessive fear of fat and a preoccupation with weight and weight loss. At times, other self-destructive behaviors such as suicide attempts, kleptomania, and sexual promiscuity are present. Individuals with bulimic behaviors are often described as perfectionists, high achievers scholastically and professionally, and highly dependent on the approval of others to maintain self-esteem. They fear rejection and loss of control. Physical signs usually relate to the behaviors of self-induced vomiting and laxative abuse and include electrolyte imbalances, cardiac irregularities, edema, dehydration, swollen salivary glands, broken blood vessels in the eyes, tooth decay from erosion of the enamel, broken nails and scars on the knuckles from self-induced vomiting, and general gastrointestinal distress. The individual with bulimic behaviors often describes a loss of control. If the binge-purge behaviors are excessive, the victim becomes socially isolated and dominated by these behaviors. Family relationships are often strained and disturbed, and the individual and her family both feel helpless, angry, and rejected.

Early psychodynamic theorists suggested anorexia nervosa symbolized a wish to be pregnant and fantasies of oral impregnation, which the individual rejects by starvation. Today a number of theories exist that propose other possible causes of this disorder. It seems that an understanding of bulimia nervosa and anorexia nervosa demands an openness to numerous views because the

Bulimia nervosa is a disorder commonly occurring in adolescence and is marked by episodic, uncontrollable, and rapid consumption of food over short periods of time (binge eating) and termination of the binge by abdominal pain, sleep, social interruption, or self-induced vomiting.

study of these disorders is relatively new and the causative factors are likely to be many.

Some theorists propose a behavioral perspective and suggest that these behaviors are learned patterns. Others utilize a psychodynamic framework and suggest that these behaviors reflect a developmental arrest in the very early years of childhood around issues of trust, autonomy, and separation-individuation. Family theorists propose that the behaviors take place within the context of disturbed family relationships, faulty communication, and lack of boundaries between family members.

Social theorists point to the dramatic rise in the incidence of these disturbances in recent years. Some relate this rise to societal pressures to be thin, to the changing role of women and the conflicting messages given to females, and to the absence of a clear set of values and norms that guided the behavior of adolescents of previous generations. Still others believe that these disorders are biological in origin or that a biological predisposition exists.

There is general consensus among experts that an appropriate model for the treatment of these disorders must integrate biological, psychological, and social perspectives. These disorders manifest themselves in disturbances in all subsystems. The symptoms are physiologic, psychologic, and social. Appropriate interventions clearly must address the whole person, and a plan of nursing care must be individualized to meet the needs of the client.

> Appropriate treatment for anorexia nervosa and bulimia nervosa must address the whole person, and a plan of nursing care must be individualized to meet the needs of the client.

Guidelines for meeting the needs of adolescents with eating disorders. Individuals with eating disorders pose specific challenges to professionals, who often feel frustrated and helpless in their efforts to nurture those who reject their attempts. Food and eating are quite symbolic in this culture, often representing love and nurturance. Individuals with eating disorders have conflicts that specifically focus on these symbols, and their behaviors may be viewed by some as rejecting and hostile. In caring for clients with such disorders, one must keep in mind the powerful sense of ineffectiveness that seems to grip them and work toward building a relationship of collaboration and trust.

Numerous treatment modalities have evolved to treat clients with anorectic and bulimic behaviors. The nursing care plan should be developed in collaboration with the client in an effort to capitalize on strengths as well as to intervene in dysfunctional behaviors. The meanings of the behaviors must be understood if a therapeutic plan is to be developed. Although diverse opinion exists as to the most appropriate method of treatment, there is general consensus that consistency and agreement among the health care workers must exist for treatment to be effective. Thus collaboration and communication within the team are imperative for the effective care of these clients.

> Immediate short-term goals for the individual with an eating disorder usually focus on a restoration of normal nutritional status, while long-term goals aim toward the establishment of more functional coping mechanisms and healthy relationships.

Immediate interventions and short-term goals generally focus on a restoration of normal nutritional status because complications of malnourishment may be serious and eventually lead to death. The various inpatient treatment programs are derived from a number of models, including those based on behavioral interventions where positive reinforcements are used to reward weight gain and/or stabilization and an appropriate intake of a balanced daily diet. During this phase of treatment it is imperative that staff offer support as well as consistency. An attitude of firm caring has been found helpful. In addition, treatment must address such potentially dangerous behaviors as suicidal gestures and other acting-out behaviors that sometimes exist.

Long-term goals and interventions are aimed at the underlying issues as previously discussed, as well as at the establishment of more functional coping mechanisms and healthy relationships. In an attempt to help the individual develop a sense of autonomy the nurse might help the client plan and test new independent behaviors. The client with an eating disorder often possesses a sense of ineffectiveness. The nurse might assist the individual to identify and express these feelings and then facilitate situations in which the client might achieve a sense of mastery and success. One treatment unit offers art and poetry therapy, which gives the client the chance to express feelings while simultaneously experiencing a sense of achievement when projects are completed.

Group therapies and support groups are often utilized to assist individuals to improve social skills and reduce the social isolation they experience. These groups also encourage autonomous and independent behavior in a population that is struggling to separate from family and achieve identity. Group cohesiveness and activities often facilitate this process.

Family therapy is often employed with clients and their families to try to alleviate family stress and achieve effective communication and healthy relationships. The nurse might individually encourage the client, as well, to identify family stressors and recognize the dysfunctional behaviors previously used to cope with stress.

Educational groups are utilized in the treatment of these individuals. Information is provided about healthy nutrition, the physical consequences of anorectic and bulimic behaviors, and the social pressures exerted on women of today to remain unhealthily thin. In addition to providing information, it is likely that such groups facilitate sharing and help these individuals to recognize that they are not alone in their struggles.

Psychotherapy with a qualified individual is aimed at helping the individual to discover the underlying causes of her problems and the source of the anorectic and bulimic symptoms. In addition, some psychopharmacological agents have been shown to be helpful in the treatment of these disorders.

Nurses who work with individuals who have anorexia nervosa or bulimia nervosa can tell many stories about the challenges and frustrations they confront. The client is ambivalent, confused, and in conflict about the task of separation and often manifests his conflict in anger directed at the nurse. In addition, the individual often rejects the nurse's efforts to nurture. Nursing is a predominantly female profession, faced with the same issues that all women in our society are confronting. Thus there may be a tendency for the nurse to identify with the female who is experiencing an eating disorder. This is especially true of

Therapies for the individual with an eating disorder include group therapy and support groups, family therapy, educational groups, and psychotherapy.

young nurses who have only recently made the passage into adulthood. On the other hand, the very nature of the profession puts the nurse in an ideal position to develop new insights about the feminine nature of eating disturbances. Therefore nursing is in the position to make many contributions to the understanding of these individuals.

Adolescent suicide

Suicide is one of the major causes of death for persons between the ages of 10 and 24. The adolescent suicide rate has increased rapidly in the last two decades. It is frightening to realize that authorities believe that the real incidence of adolescent suicide is even greater than the statistics indicate.

Authorities on adolescent development are defining this problem as catastrophic and epidemic. Understanding of and knowledge about adolescent suicide remains limited, and experts are struggling to define methods of prevention and intervention. Much of what was said in Chapter 16 about the individual contemplating suicide applies to the suicidal adolescent as well. However certain factors are unique to the adolescent population.

Although the shocking rise in the incidence of adolescent suicide is recognized, the causes of such behavior are not clearly understood. Studies of adolescent suicide behavior indicate individual, familial, and sociocultural issues as factors influencing this behavior.

Some studies indicate a familial tendency toward suicidal behavior, which possibly is learned. Major psychiatric disorders such as depression and schizophrenia seem to be linked to suicidal attempts in some adolescents. An impulsive personality trait has also been identified in some adolescents who have attempted or committed suicide. It has also been suggested that adolescents do not have a clear and realistic sense of death or of the finality of the act of suicide. Therefore suicidal behavior may be an effort to express anger or hostility toward loved ones or to make others feel sorry for real or imagined offenses.

Confusion over emerging sexual impulses and gender identity is common during adolescence, and suicide may represent an effort to resolve such conflicts. Substance abuse has also been linked to teenage suicide.

In terms of family dynamics a number of factors seem to relate to suicidal behaviors. Such factors include broken homes, family disorganization, overly strict parental discipline, lack of communication, and suicidal behavior in family members.

Much attention has been focused recently on the sociocultural factors that contribute to suicidal behavior in adolescence. The dramatic rise in incidence points to the influence of social change. A number of researchers cite the fact that violence has become acceptable in our society and that the adolescent has become numb to violence. In addition, authorities point to increased family mobility and rootlessness that lead to a sense of alienation and loneliness at a time when group affiliation is vital. Social isolation often precedes a suicidal act.

A number of authorities discuss the prevailing stress found in our Western

Suicides among adolescents in this country have rapidly increased in the last two decades; it is felt that the rising incidence may reflect sociocultural factors and stressors.

culture as a factor contributing to the incidence of adolescent suicide. In addition, adolescents in our society do not really have a place—they are neither child nor adult. They are often segregated into educational institutions where strong relationships with adults are lacking at a time when guidance and support are required.

It is also believed that the media have, at times, sensationalized or romanticized the act of suicide. Such idealization of the act may contribute toward suicide among those already contemplating the act. For example, epidemics of suicide have been reported in certain schools, reflecting the communicable nature of the behavior. If suicide is glorified or seen as a plausible method of coping with the life crises of adolescence, the number of suicides is likely to increase.

Although studies of suicidal behavior in adolescents indicate that it is determined by numerous and diverse individual, familial, and social factors, one factor is almost always present. This central issue is a sense of invisibility—a feeling that one is not recognized or appreciated, and a belief that one has very little impact on the world around him.

Characteristics of the suicidal adolescent. It is believed that many adolescents contemplating suicide give clues of their plans and intentions. Some of these clues and behaviors have been identified in Chapter 16. The nurse must be sensitive to such clues, which include preoccupation with themes of death, the expression of suicidal ideas, and the giving away of valued possessions. For example, one adolescent boy worked part-time for years to buy a sports car. The day before he attempted suicide he offered the car to his older brother.

Changes in sleeping patterns are often noted. The suicidal adolescent sleeps either too much or too little. Changes in eating patterns and resultant weight gain or loss may occur. A withdrawal from family and friends is common. The individual often has changes in school performance including lowered grades and truancy. Extreme fluctuations in mood, such as outbursts of anger alternating with crying spells, often occur. Finally, drug or alcohol abuse is often found in suicidal adolescents.

A previous suicidal attempt increases the likelihood of a later attempt. In addition, the recent suicide of a friend or family member increases the probability that the adolescent will act on his suicidal impulses.

Although clues to suicide are often given by the potentially suicidal adolescent, the nurse must be cautioned that the absence of clues does not eliminate the possibility of suicidal behavior. If any suspicion of suicidal ideas is present, it is far better to risk confronting these than to ignore this potential problem.

Guidelines for meeting the needs of an adolescent who is suicidal. The nurse caring for the suicidal adolescent should be familiar with the principles outlined in Chapter 16 on the care of the suicidal adult. An environment that facilitates a sense of worthiness and conveys a caring attitude is vital. There should be opportunities for the suicidal adolescent to participate safely in activities that en-

One central issue related to adolescent suicide is a sense of invisibility—a feeling that one is not recognized or appreciated and a belief that one has very little impact on the world around him.

Adolescents contemplating suicide often give clues to their plans and intentions: preoccupation with themes of death, the expression of suicidal ideas, and the giving away of valued possessions.

The nurse is therapeutic when she provides opportunities for the adolescent to develop a sense of worthiness, belonging, mastery, self-esteem, safety, and security.

hance a sense of mastery and self-esteem. The individual must be safe and secure while able to engage in adolescent group activities. The therapeutic relationship offers the opportunity for the suicidal adolescent to express and explore feelings in a climate of empathy and concern.

In the event of a successful adolescent suicide the nurse must deal with the anguish of many affected individuals. At times the nurse may be able to offer assistance to family members, school counselors, and others involved. It has been said that the true victims of suicide are the survivors. Surviving family members experience intense remorse and feelings of guilt. In addition, such a crisis will magnify any existing problems in marital and family relationships. The principles of crisis intervention, as outlined in Chapter 24, are useful in such situations. Siblings must be observed carefully because suicide in one family member may precipitate such behavior in others.

The nurse may also be consulted by school officials concerned about the potential epidemic nature of the problem. Education that focuses on the realistic aspects of death and the impact of the behavior on loved ones is often enormously beneficial. Peers must be helped through the grieving process and the stages of shock and denial, developing awareness, and eventual acceptance.

It is imperative that the nurse be concerned with the prevention of adolescent suicidal behavior. As nurses assume roles in varied settings, many opportunities for involvement in this aspect of care present themselves. Research indicates that early recognition of the warning signs is vital. Once again, education seems to be a valuable tool. The nurse may be asked to collaborate with school officials and other professionals in providing education about suicide, as well as assistance for adolescents in coping with stress and depression.

Experiences that offer the adolescent opportunities to develop a sense of belonging and mastery might be the best way to prevent suicidal behavior. Recreational activities and centers, clubs, and church groups may help prevent the desperate sense of loneliness and alienation that contributes to all of the disturbances of adolescents. Ongoing adult involvement in the lives of adolescents enhances the probability of successful resolution of this developmental phase, and nurses have a responsibility to provide some of this involvement.

END NOTE

Although nursing care of disturbed children and adolescents is acknowledged as a specialty area, this chapter presents an introduction to the subject in the hope that all students will become sensitized to the needs of these clients and that some will become interested in pursuing further preparation in this specialty. Disorders beginning in infancy and childhood, such as developmental disorders, disruptive behavior disorders, and anxiety disorders, are discussed. Eating disorders and adolescent suicide are discussed as problems commonly beginning during adolescence. General guidelines for meeting the needs of these clients

NURSING CARE PLAN

A suicidal adolescent

CASE FORMULATION

Jennie B., a 15-year-old girl, was referred to the community mental health center by the school counselor with the approval of her mother after having been treated for taking 15 aspirins. She came to the center willingly and described herself as unhappy, upset, and without friends. The school counselor was concerned about Jennie, who had entered the school as a new student only a few months earlier. Her concern focused on the following problems: Jennie had made no friends, was receiving failing grades, was absent from school almost half the time, and was involved in almost no school clubs or extracurricular activities. She made the referral after learning of Jennie's suicidal gesture.

Jennie talked freely to the nurse at the mental health center and stated she could not study because she did not sleep well at night. She described nightmares that frightened her and kept her awake, the content of which featured an older man who molested her sexually.

In discussing her family she spoke of the frequent fights between herself and her mother over her mother's drinking and her mother's boyfriend. About a year ago Jennie's mother and father had separated, and they were in the process of getting a divorce when she came to the clinic. After her parents separated, Jennie's father moved to another city and rarely found time to come back and visit with his three children, of whom Jennie was the oldest. She blamed her mother for the separation and the move from their old neighborhood and the school she had attended all her life.

Jennie's two brothers had become her responsibility since her mother's interest in her boyfriend had increased. Thus she was expected to supervise her younger brothers, get their meals, and do the laundry. With this amount of work expected of her, Jennie stated she was too tired to attend school more than half the time. Jennie's brothers did not follow her directions and re-

sented her attempts to supervise them. Thus there was conflict among the children in this family and no adult to act as a buffer in such conflicts. Jennie felt unloved and unwanted.

Her mother's boyfriend was a large, middle-aged taxi driver who teased Jennie a good deal. She told the nurse that she disliked him intensely and stated that she was afraid of him. In addition, she did not want anyone taking her father's place in the home because she loved her father very much.

Jennie was somewhat smaller in stature than most girls of her age. Her breasts had not yet begun to develop, and she was extremely anxious about this fact. She viewed her flat-chested appearance as a serious defect that made her different from other girls. Also, she had not yet begun to menstruate, which increased her belief that she was different and lacking in feminine appeal. Unfortunately, Jennie was not physically attractive because her hair was dull and unkempt and her complexion sallow.

Jennie's mother was invited to come to the clinic to discuss the treatment plans for her daughter. She found it difficult to arrange a convenient time because she held a part-time job. However, she finally kept the appointment and gave much of the same information about the family situation as did Jennie. However, Jennie's mother stated that the conflict among the children was caused by Jennie's attempt to boss her brothers. She felt that Jennie's resentment of her boyfriend was the cause of many of their disagreements and declared that her dates were none of her daughter's business. According to her mother, Jennie was her father's favorite child, but he did not deserve her devotion.

Jennie's developmental history, as related by her mother, was uneventful except that she had been enuretic until the age of 9. This problem reappeared after the separation of the parents and was present even now. Her mother also reported that Jennie had responded to discipline by hav-

NURSING CARE PLAN—cont'd

ing temper tantrums. These began when she was being toilet trained and continued until she was 9. Although she no longer had what could be described as temper tantrums, she did fly into rages. These rages seemed to be related to the mother's boyfriend and the approaching divorce. The mother stated that because of her job and home responsibilities she had not been able to work with the school counselor.

Nursing assessment

Jennie appeared to be experiencing difficulties in resolving the tasks of normal adolescent development, as a number of factors impinged on her life. Such factors included the loss of a close relationship with her father, a recent move, increased responsibilities at home, family conflicts, a perceived lack of attention and love, and the recent presence of her mother's boyfriend whom Jennie feared and resented. All of these factors might have contributed to the difficulties in adjustment that Jennie was experiencing, which culminated in a suicidal gesture. Adolescence is a time when the individual experiences ambivalent feelings toward the parents, which include a desire for love and affection along with a seemingly conflicting desire for autonomy and emancipation from the parents. The loss of her father at such a time might have made Jennie feel abandoned and guilty. In addition, her mother did not appear able to provide the love and support required during this period. Jennie might be blaming her mother for the loss of her father.

Jennie moved at a time when peer relationships and group involvement are important, and she found it necessary to enter a strange school and develop new relationships—something she had always found difficult. Her responsibilities at home might have prevented her from performing well at school, establishing successful relationships with peers, and engaging in extracurricular activities, which are all potential sources of self-esteem for adolescents. Jennie had not developed the physical characteristics of a woman and felt different and unloved.

Jennie's mother might have been ill-equipped to offer Jennie the love and support she needed for the successful resolution of earlier developmental tasks. The presence of enuresis and temper tantrums in childhood might have indicated the anger and frustration that Jennie felt toward her mother in early years and an effort to gain control and autonomy. The reappearance of enuresis when Jennie's father left home might represent the revival of these old childhood feelings toward her mother because Jennie now blamed her for the loss of her father.

Jennie's behavior disturbances reflected the difficulties she was experiencing with the tasks of adolescent development. Her rages might have reflected feelings of rejection and were directed toward her mother for saddling Jennie with home responsibilities, withholding love, and introducing an unwanted man into the home. The increase in Jennie's nightmares might relate to the introduction into the family of her mother's new boyfriend. Her social isolation might indicate feelings of low self-esteem and a fear of competition and failure. These feelings of inadequacy seem to have been reinforced by Jennie's slow sexual development.

Nursing diagnosis

Based on the nursing assessment that included prior knowledge of the family dynamics and an understanding of the dynamics underlying adolescence, the nurse formulated the following four pairs of nursing diagnoses specific to Jennie's emotional response. The first of each pair is from the Classification of Human Responses of Concern for Psychiatric–Mental Health Nursing Practice; the second is from the approved NANDA Diagnostic Categories.

5.3.2 Altered Conduct/Impulse Processes related to anger at mother

Continued.

NURSING CARE PLAN—cont'd

OR

9.2.2 Potential for Violence: Self-directed related to anger at mother

5.7.2 Altered Social Interaction related to low self-esteem and fear of competition and failure

OR

3.1.1 Impaired Social Interaction related to low self-esteem and fear of competition and failure

5.5.2 Altered Role Performance related to disturbed family relationships

OR

3.2.1 Altered Role Performance related to disturbed family relationships

1.3.4 Altered Self-Care related to poor body image and feelings of worthlessness

OR

6.5.3 Dressing/Grooming Self-Care Deficit related to poor body image and feelings of worthlessness

Planning and implementing nursing care for Jennie B.

The plan for nursing care for Jennie is summarized in the box on pp. 389-390.

Jennie was admitted to a residential treatment setting for adolescents with behavior disturbances where many opportunities for corrective experiences were available. After assessing her needs and formulating the nursing diagnoses, a plan of care was developed. An appointment was made for a physical examination to determine any specific cause of her slow sexual development. The examination revealed no significant findings.

A trusting therapeutic relationship was established with Jennie's primary nurse, who treated Jennie with respect and dignity and listened carefully to whatever she said. Her opinions were accepted, and the nurse avoided judging and moralizing.

The nurse attempted to convey a firm and caring attitude. She encouraged Jennie to function independently by establishing fair and reasonable limits while also praising autonomous behaviors, encouraging participation in extracurricular activities, and including Jennie in decisions regarding her care and treatment.

It was felt that Jennie's problems at school were a partial reflection of her problems at home. Continued efforts were made to involve Jennie's mother in treatment, although her resistance indicated that Jennie might have to learn to accept her mother's limitations and develop independent coping skills to deal with family stress.

Finally Jennie was encouraged to participate in age-appropriate activities in an effort to assist her to develop healthy peer relationships and a sense of belonging.

Evaluation

Evaluation of the plan of nursing care and its implementation was based on the outcome criteria developed in the planning phase.

Jennie made steady progress in the residential treatment setting, where ample opportunities were provided for healthy relationships and corrective experiences with both adults and peers. Her rages disappeared, and verbal hostility diminished. A tutor assisted Jennie to focus on school work, and improvement was noted. It seemed that her external controls improved, and her self-esteem was enhanced.

Discharge to outpatient services was recommended, where Jennie would continue in psychotherapy with a clinical nurse specialist.

NURSING CARE PLAN—cont'd

NURSING CARE PLAN FOR *Jennie B.*

Nursing diagnosis	Objective	Nursing actions	Outcome criteria
5.3.2 Altered Conduct/Impulse Processes related to anger at mother OR 9.2.2 Potential for Violence: Self-directed related to anger at mother	To assist client to direct anger and hostility into socially acceptable activities	Encourage participation in age-appropriate expressive and physical activities, for example, sports, art, music, and physical exercise Comment positively on successful participation	Within 1 month client will: report absence of suicidal ideation spontaneously and independently participate in alternative activities
	To encourage client to explore feelings	Utilize reflection to encourage expression of feelings Convey acceptance of angry feelings Convey interest Encourage problem solving	Within 1 month client will: spontaneously verbally express feelings of anger show evidence of problem-solving behaviors
5.7.2. Altered Social Interaction related to low self-esteem and fear of OR 3.1.1 Impaired Social Interaction related to low self-esteem and fear of competition and failure	To encourage the client's involvement in age-appropriate occupational and recreational activities	Encourage participation in activities, for example, clubs, church groups, recreational and occupational therapies Accept feelings of frustration Comment positively on successful participation	Within 2 weeks client will: spontaneously involve self in one group activity weekly report success in one activity
competition and failure	To encourage the client's involvement in adolescent group therapy	Refer to group therapy Encourage biweekly attendance Comment positively on attendance and involvement Accept expressions of frustration and fear	Within 2 weeks client will: attend group therapy biweekly spontaneously express her feelings

Continued.

NURSING CARE PLAN—cont'd

NURSING CARE PLAN FOR *Jennie B.*

Nursing diagnosis	Objective	Nursing actions	Outcome criteria
5.5.2 Altered Role Performance related to disturbed family relationships OR 3.2.1 Altered Role Performance related to disturbed family relationships	To facilitate interest in school subjects and assignments To encourage independent functioning To encourage the identification of family stressors and encourage problem-solving techniques	Discuss school topics with client and encourage and reinforce interests; offer positive appraisals for success Suggest and encourage involvement in extracurricular activities View the family as a system Recognize that as client's behavior alters the system will enter disequilibrium Assist with identification of stressors in family	Within 1 month client will: report interest in school topic earn improved school grades identify family stressors and demonstrate efforts to problem solve
1.3.4 Altered Self-Care related to poor body image and feelings of worthlessness OR 6.5.3 Dressing/ Grooming Self-Care Deficit related to poor body image and feelings of worthlessness	To encourage improved hygiene and grooming	Encourage client to engage in daily routines of hygiene and grooming Offer compliments for improved appearance	Within 2 weeks client will show interest in grooming, for example, combing hair, age-appropriate dress

are presented. The chapter concludes with a hypothetical plan of nursing care for a disturbed adolescent who attempted suicide.

SUGGESTED SOURCES OF ADDITIONAL INFORMATION

Barlow DJ: Therapeutic holding: effective intervention with the aggressive child, J Psychosoc Nurs Ment Health Serv 27(1):10, January 1989.

Cerrato PL: Nutritionist on call: helping food addicts kick the habit, RN 50(8):75, August 1987.

Deering CG: Developing a therapeutic alliance with the anorexia nervosa client, J Psychosoc Nurs Ment Health Serv 25(3):10, March 1987.

Dippel NM and Becknal BK: Bulimia, J Psychosoc Nurs Ment Health Serv 25(9):12, September 1987.

Dizon MA: The use of attachment theory in a clinical situation: secure attachment anxious attachment, J Psychosoc Nurs Ment Health Serv 22(3):27, March 1984.

Edmands MS: Overcoming eating disorders: a group experience, J Psychosoc Nurs Ment Health Serv 24(8):19, August 1986.

Evans D: Explaining suicide among the young: an analytic review of the literature, J Psychosoc Nurs Ment Health Serv 20:9, August 1982.

Federation S: Sexual abuse: treatment modalities for the younger child, J Psychosoc Nurs Ment Health Serv 24(7):21, July 1986.

Fox K: Adolescent ambivalence: a therapeutic issue, J Psychosoc Nurs Ment Health Serv 18:29, September 1980.

Freeberg S: Anger in adolescence, J Psychosoc Nurs Ment Health Serv 20:29, March 1982.

Geary MC: A review of treatment models for eating disorders: toward a holistic nursing model, Holistic Nurs Pract 3(1):39, November 1988.

Gilead M and Mulaik J: Adolescent suicide: a response to a developmental crisis, Perspect Psychiatr Care 22:94, July-September 1983.

Hodgman C: Current issues in adolescent psychiatry, Hosp Commun Psychiatr 34(6):514, 1983.

Jacobson J: Speculations on the role of transitional objects in eating disorders, Arch Psych Nurs 2(4):110, April 1988.

Keltner NL: Bulimia: controlling compulsive eating, J Psychosoc Nurs Ment Health Serv 22(8):24, August 1984.

Lilly GE and Sanders JB: Nursing management of anorexic adolescents, J Psychosoc Nurs Ment Health Serv 25(11):30, November 1987.

McBride AB: Coming of age: child psychiatric nursing, Arch Psych Nurs 2(2):57, April 1988.

Mellencamp A: Adolescent depression: a review of the literature, with implications for nursing care, J Psychosoc Nurs Ment Health Serv 19:15, September 1981.

Miles MW: Bulimia nervosa and gender identity: symbols of a culture, Holistic Nurs Pract 3(1):56, November 1988.

Oehler JM and Burns MJ: Anorexia, bulimia, and sexuality: case study of an adolescent inpatient group, Arch Psych Nurs 1(3):163, June 1987.

Pothier PC: Child mental health problems and policy, Arch Psych Nurs 2(3):165, June 1988.

Pothier PC: Child psychiatric nursing, J Psychosoc Nurs Ment Health Serv 22(3):11, March 1984.

Pothier PC Norbeck JS and Laliberte M: Child psychiatric nursing: the gap between need and utilization, J Psychosoc Nurs Ment Health Serv 23(7):18, July 1985.

Puskar K: Structure for the hospitalized adolescent, J Psychosoc Nurs Ment Health Serv 19:13, July 1981.

Reed G and Sech EP: Bulimia, J Psychosoc Nurs Ment Health Serv 23(5):16, May 1985.

Rosenfield S: Family influence on eating behavior and attitudes in eating disorders: a review of the literature, Holistic Nurs Pract 3(1):46, November 1988.

Rubin RL: Assisting adolescents toward mental health, Nurs Clin North Am 21(3):439, September 1986.

Sanger E: Eating disorders: avoiding the power struggle, Am J Nurs 84(1):31, January 1984.

Smith C and Murphy KE: Developing a children's inpatient psychiatric unit, J Psychosoc Nurs Ment Health Serv 22(3):31, March 1984.

White JH: Bulimia: utilizing individual and family therapy, J Psychosoc Nurs Ment Health Serv 22(4):22, April 1984.

Worthington-Roberts B: Eating disorders in women, Focus Crit Care 12(4):32, August 1985.

Populations at risk
The physically ill

23

LEARNING OBJECTIVES

After studying this chapter the student will be able to:

○ State general guidelines for meeting the emotional needs of persons who are physically ill.

○ Describe common emotional reactions precipitated by the use of mechanical devices in treating persons who are physically ill.

○ Describe common emotional reactions precipitated by organ transplants.

○ Describe common emotional reactions precipitated by the loss of a body part.

○ Describe common emotional reactions precipitated by cardiac surgery.

○ Describe common emotional reactions precipitated by an untoward obstetrical experience.

○ Describe common emotional reactions precipitated by an abortion.

○ Describe common emotional reactions of individuals with Acquired Immune Deficiency Syndrome (AIDS).

○ Discuss the emotional aspects of death and dying as described by Kübler-Ross.

○ Develop a hypothetical plan of nursing care for an individual who is dying.

Many individuals who are physically ill are in a state of crisis precipitated by the nature of their illness or its treatment, or both. Consequently, nursing has a tremendous opportunity to promote the mental health of a large number of persons if it will reclaim its heritage of meeting the emotional needs of persons who are physically ill. Unfortunately, all too often the emotional needs of these individuals are given little attention, and student nurses frequently look to their psychiatric nursing experience to provide them with direction in giving more comprehensive care to physically ill individuals. Therefore this chapter is devoted to helping the nurse develop an understanding of some common emotional needs of the individual who is physically ill, although no situation in this chapter can be discussed in depth.

HISTORICAL PERSPECTIVE

Before the current advances in the medical and nursing sciences nurses could do little to assist individuals who were physically ill other than helping them meet their most basic physical needs. However, the time-honored nursing actions of bathing and feeding patients certainly must have met many of their emotional needs as well.

As medical science developed, physicians delegated to nurses procedures they no longer had time to perform. An example of such a procedure is the assessment of vital signs. Some nurse authors believe that as an occupation nursing eagerly embraced these delegated technical procedures in an attempt to gain higher status by mimicking physicians. Whether this interpretation is true or not, it is a fact that current nursing care of persons who are physically ill is characterized by the execution of an increasing number of highly technical procedures, often to the neglect of attempts to meet the person's emotional needs. In fact, it is not unusual for a patient to report that the most understanding person he encountered while in the hospital was an aide or cleaning lady.

Growing dissatisfaction with nursing care has been the subject of numerous studies. These studies indicate that only a few complaints are related to physical care. The large majority of dissatisfactions has to do with the failure of professional nurses to establish satisfying interpersonal relationships with individuals receiving their services. The nurse is frequently said to lack warmth, to fail to give individuals a feeling of being important human beings, to fail to listen empathically to the concerns of individuals being cared for, or to fail to ask enough questions to gather the necessary data to make wise decisions about individual needs.

The utilization of the psychiatric liaison nurse, a relatively recent resource, can immeasurably enhance achieving the goal of meeting the emotional needs of patients who are physically ill. The subspecialty of psychiatric liaison nursing was developed in the 1970s and requires preparation at the master's degree level. Psychiatric liaison nurses have particular expertise in developing nursing interventions based on their assessment of the responses of physically ill individuals who have emotional responses that are seen as problematic by the nurses who care for them. Therefore, many of the activities of the liaison nurse focus on consultation with the nursing staff and working with the patient's family and significant others, as well as working with the patient himself.

GUIDELINES FOR MEETING THE EMOTIONAL NEEDS OF PERSONS WHO ARE PHYSICALLY ILL

Individuals who are physically ill experience a variety of feelings, which may include intense anxiety, hostility, depression, elation, fear, anger, and sorrow. These are the same feelings that may be expressed by persons who are mentally ill. Perhaps one of the few differentiations that can be made between the reactions of these two groups is the presumed ability of physically ill individuals to maintain conscious control of their behavior and to use better judgment than individuals who are mentally ill. However, even these expected differences are not always observed.

It is often difficult and more challenging to recognize and cope with the emotional needs of physically ill persons than it is to effectively address the emotional needs of persons who are mentally ill. Because part of a mentally ill individual's problem is his lack of emotional control, he sometimes expresses needs openly and directly. The mentally ill individual's needs may be difficult to understand, but their existence is obvious. Because he is said to be mentally ill, the nurse realizes that part of the task is to help him cope with his emotional problems. In contrast, the individual who is physically ill usually tries to control his feelings and to solve his own problems, and nurses frequently expect him to do so! They sometimes fail to recognize that in addition to his need for physical care the person who is physically ill needs the same acceptance, understanding, and concern as does the person who is mentally ill.

Good physical care is always the first place to start in meeting the emotional needs of persons who are physically ill. The nurse can demonstrate a caring attitude about the individual by an unhurried approach; attentive, perceptive listening; and anticipation of physical needs. It is also important that the nurse not respond to the client's anger with an angry response. The nurse will not be tempted to respond in an angry manner if she understands the frustration and fear that are the bases for the client's outburst. Likewise, she will not attempt to minimize the client's concerns by using hollow phrases such as, "Tomorrow will be a better day."

The very occurrence of a physical illness serious enough to warrant hospitalization interrupts the normal life-style of the individual and his family. As a result some degree of stress is produced to which the individual and his family may or may not be able to adapt successfully. In addition any physical illness for which hospitalization is necessary forces the individual to assume a dependent role that may be disturbing to him. Although society's view of masculinity and femininity is becoming less stereotyped, a dependent role is still seen as particularly problematic for men, who are often expected to portray an image of strength and independence and who may see physical illness as an expression of weakness. Inability to accept the forced dependency required in many hospitals is one reason for the uncooperative behavior of some individuals.

The modern hospital is a highly organized creation of a mechanized world.

Any physical illness that requires hospitalization forces the individual to assume a dependent role that may be disturbing and may cause him to react with uncooperative behavior.

Regardless of the nature of the illness that brings the individual to the hospital, he is expected to submit to a variety of procedures without always understanding what they are or why they are being done. He often believes they are being performed without his consent or without his having been given any explanation about them. Many procedures that seem common-place to health professionals, such as enemas, catheterizations, and intravenous injections, may be viewed by others as intrusions into their bodies. Not only may the individual have no understanding of the reasons for the procedure, he may also feel that he has lost control over his body. At the same time, he frequently is covertly given the message by personnel that he should be thankful to them for performing these procedures. This conflict may result in an increase in his anxiety level, which, paradoxically, decreases the effectiveness of the procedure itself. Therefore it is imperative for the individual's physical and emotional well-being that the nurse provide him with an opportunity to explore his feelings about the procedure as well as giving him an appropriate explanation of its nature.

Although the individual may have signed an operative permit, he is not likely to realize that this may cover a variety of tests and procedures before the actual surgery is performed. The physician may have explained the preoperative tests, but the anxiety level of many individuals is so high that they are unable to comprehend what the physician is saying. Even when individuals are able to concentrate on the physician's words, they do not always understand the full meaning of them, and the preoperative procedures may still come as a shocking surprise. It is not difficult to understand that a newly admitted surgical patient may be frightened and feel that he has lost his identity. Such a situation could be eased if nurses understood the importance of giving reassurance, if they could identify the basis for the anxiety, and if they were skillful in giving emotional support. Sometimes reassurance requires only a few minutes of time spent listening, answering questions, and recognizing that the individual is a unique human being reaching out for understanding and help.

People who are newly admitted to general hospitals may feel frightened and may develop a sense of having lost their identity.

Sometimes the results of hospital procedures, especially surgical procedures, precipitate an emotional crisis. Such a crisis is overwhelming for a person who has already developed the feeling that he is lost, forgotten, and reduced to a childlike state of dependence in the hospital. These feelings may actually impede his recovery and may cause him to view his hospitalization as an extremely traumatizing experience.

Self-help groups

The nurse should make an effort to become aware of the increasing number of community-based organizations designed to provide information and support to individuals and their families who have experienced certain medical or surgical procedures or the death of a family member. For example, there are ostomy clubs throughout the country whose members are people who have had ileostomies or colostomies and who meet regularly to discuss with each other the ways in which they have solved the problems they encounter. In some parts of the country similar groups are available for persons who have undergone mastectomies, laryngectomies, abortions, or myocardial infarcts. By being aware of the availability of these organizations in the community the nurse will be able to inform others of them. Although these clubs are not designed to substitute for medical supervision, the value of the support and understanding that can be gained from persons who have had similar experiences is inestimable in helping individuals and families to regain or attain a state of positive mental health.

Emotional reactions precipitated by the use of mechanical devices

Advances in biomedical science have provided several life-sustaining devices that make it possible to prolong the lives of many individuals who would be doomed to death otherwise. One of the most commonly used is the hemodialysis machine.

The hemodialysis machine may produce a profound emotional response from the individual. The individual who must rely on such a machine recognizes how dependent he is on the device for life itself. He also becomes aware of the fact that his activities are circumscribed by his need to be attached to the machine for 8 to 10 hours, two or three times each week. This schedule interferes with his work, his ability to make a living, his social life, and his family life.

Individuals who must rely on mechanical devices often feel that they have lost control of their bodies and of their destinies. This may lead to a loss of confidence and self-esteem. Such a loss of confidence results in behavior that requires emotional support and understanding.

Dependency on a mechanical device to sustain life creates anxiety in almost all individuals. It causes many individuals to feel dehumanized and to be concerned about the maintenance of their personal autonomy. In addition the individual may be resentful and angry, or he may be depressed and respond by being tearful, uninterested in his surroundings, and uncommunicative. On the other hand, the individual may express his anger and frustration at the situation by speaking sharply to the nurses or to his family. He may express fear by demanding constant attention and that the nurse remain with him at all times. He may express his disturbed emotional feelings by being critical of the hospital or clinic where he must go for the dialysis. He may fear that the device will fail to function properly and thus end his life abruptly.

Because the hemodialysis machine must be attached to the individual so often, a permanent arteriovenous shunt is frequently implanted in an arm or leg to provide access to an artery or vein whenever necessary. Individuals with these shunts have been known to tear them out, losing a great deal of blood. This action is usually considered a suicidal gesture: The rate of suicide among individuals who resent their dependence on hemodialysis machines is high.

Family members have been taught to operate portable dialysis machines

Individuals who must rely on mechanical devices for maintaining their physical health often feel that they have lost control of their bodies and of their destinies.

and thus free the individual from constantly returning to a hospital or clinic to have his blood cleansed. However, this practice makes it necessary to teach a family member to operate the machine and requires that the family member be available when the treatments are scheduled. This amount of dependence on another person is also cause for hostility and resentment among some individuals and has not provided the solution to the time-consuming dialysis procedure that it was originally intended to do.

In summary, the currently available life-saving biomedical devices are capable of improving the physical health of the individual but do not always improve emotional health. Specifically, those individuals who must rely on hemodialysis machines are chronic worriers. They worry about all the daily problems of living that confront everyone. They require nurses who are skilled in understanding that their behavior is sometimes an expression of anger, fear, and depression brought on by their resentment of being dependent for life on a mechanical device and being unable to control the situation. They require a great deal of reassurance and emotional support.

Emotional reactions precipitated by organ transplants

Organ transplants are viewed by medical scientists as providing a viable alternative for individuals with seriously damaged organs, especially hearts and kidneys. As increasingly effective drugs are developed to combat the problem of tissue rejection, the number of organ transplants is likely to increase.

Almost from the initiation of organ transplant surgery, it was recognized that providing an organ for an individual from the body of another could be an emotionally disturbing experience both for the person donating the organ and the recipient. Thus psychiatric evaluation of the donor as well as the recipient was begun soon after some of the earliest kidney transplants were performed. Since there were more individuals awaiting transplant surgery than there were appropriate organs available, it was possible to choose the organ recipients carefully. Those who were thought to be able to accept an organ from another individual without being emotionally disturbed were chosen. Likewise, donors should be stable individuals before agreeing to supply an organ for another. One mother who donated a kidney to a son was heard to shout at him, "What do you expect from me? Wasn't it enough that I gave you life? Do you also demand a part of my body?"

Organ transplant procedures are long and involved surgical techniques. Individuals who are the focus of such procedures are aware of their physical condition and that they are seriously ill. They realize that without a transplant their lives would end within a short time and that the only hope for the future lies in the replacement of the damaged organ. Thus they are willing to undergo the procedure even though they recognize the seriousness of the situation and the possibility that the organ may be rejected. These individuals are understandably fearful of what the future will bring. Although many of the recipients of such surgery have been able to cope successfully with their anxieties and fears, a few have responded with full-blown psychiatric reactions. There are few situations in which an individual is placed under so much stress as when he undergoes an organ transplant. Nurses working with these individuals need to be sensitive to their emotional responses, to be realistically reassuring, and to provide as much emotional support as they require. The individual should be encouraged to discuss his concerns and fears about death, dependency on others, and loss of self-esteem.

Providing an organ for an individual from the body of another can be an emotionally disturbing experience, both for the person donating the organ and for the recipient.

The fact that an individual who was close to death would grieve over the loss of a useless body part comes as a surprise to many nurses. Nevertheless, such is often the case, and if she is to be helpful the nurse must assist the individual with the grieving process. In general, the nurse needs to express concern for the individual and interest in his future welfare.

Emotional reactions precipitated by the loss of a body part

Every person has a mental image of his own body that is called the *body image*. This body image may be realistic, or it may be part of the individual's wish-fulfilling fantasy about himself. To a large extent, an individual functions within the boundaries of this unconscious image. A young man once said in a hopeless voice, "I can never marry. What woman would want a man with one short leg?" This man's body image was so misshapen and ugly that he was scornful of it. Because he could not accept his own body he was convinced that no one else could. He was especially convinced that no woman could want him as a marriage partner. Although he was reasonably attractive, his reaction to all aspects of life was in keeping with this attitude of being worthless and of having an unacceptable body.

Some people maintain an unrealistic image of themselves that was realistic at an earlier period in their lives. For example, it is not uncommon to hear a large, matronly woman ask a saleswoman for a size 12 dress. Without making a comment the understanding clerk brings out the required large size and helps the customer try on the garment.

Surgical removal of a breast or the uterus are among the most emotionally disturbing surgical procedures that women must face. It is unfortunate that many nurses have not been helped to understand the meaning these experiences have for some women and have not been assisted in helping with the feelings precipitated by such surgical procedures.

Although people respond in highly individual and unique ways to the same surgical procedures, almost all women unconsciously feel that they have been mutilated by a breast amputation or the removal of the uterus. If given an opportunity after such a surgical procedure, many women will express feelings about not being a whole woman or about being of less value to the world than they were before the operation. They may express fears about losing the acceptance of their sexual partners.

Many women pass through a period of mourning for the lost part of the body. Nurses need to understand the realistic reasons that underlie the frequent tears shed by women hospitalized in a gynecological unit of the hospital and should accept this as an expression of a normal emotional response about an extremely upsetting experience. Crying is probably one of the most helpful ways of expressing grief. Unfortunately, some women cannot cry about this kind of problem. Instead, they may repress their feelings of despair and sadness and respond in other ways that may be more difficult for the nurse to understand and cope with. After breast surgery one woman turned her face to the wall, refused to see any visitors, and requested that even her husband be excluded from the room.

Sadness and mourning may be expressed in a reaction that appears to an observer as an outburst of anger. The individual may respond as does a child when something of value is taken away. This response may be an expression of underlying depression, but the external reaction is one of anger at having lost something that was highly valued. Another frequent response to such a surgical loss is an unconscious feeling on the part of the woman that she is being punished for some real or fantasized transgression that may have occurred years before. This feeling may lead the woman to respond as if she were unworthy of attention from friends or relatives.

The possible reasons for the many emotional reactions to breast amputation and hysterectomy are as varied as the women who require these procedures. The important thing for the nurse to remember is that these experiences are difficult for women to accept, that individuals respond to them in highly individual ways, depending on their life situation and personality, and that the nurse needs to demonstrate an understanding and caring attitude about the woman and her feelings.

Women are not the only people who are unable to accept an altered body image. All individuals who submit to disfiguring surgery of any type have a variety of fears that focus on their concern about being acceptable to other people, especially to their sexual partners. Operations involving amputation of a leg or disfiguring facial surgery are especially difficult for individuals to accept. However, it has been noted that people are able to accept body mutilation more readily when the location is such that it is evident to everyone. This phenomenon may result from the fact that something that is obvious must be recognized and talked about. Some individuals refrain from mentioning a problem that is hidden under clothing. They are therefore burdened with a tremendous amount of unresolved sensitivity for years. Perhaps the much joked about American habit of discussing one's operation and exhibiting the surgical scar at social gatherings has some psychologically healing attributes. It is therapeutic to help individuals discuss the way they feel about the surgical procedure they have experienced.

Nurses should avoid censuring individuals who blame the surgeon for their

> Individuals who submit to disfiguring surgery of any type have a variety of fears that focus on their concern about being acceptable to other people, especially their sexual partners.

disfigured bodies. It is a natural human response to relieve anxiety by blaming someone else for an unhappy situation that the individual cannot control with his usual defenses.

One example of this kind of reaction was a man who was hospitalized for plastic reconstruction of a thumb that was lost in an accident involving high-voltage electricity. After several skin grafts and months of repeated hospitalizations, the man was disturbed when he saw the reconstructed thumb. It was many times larger than a normal thumb and was covered with short hair because the skin graft had been taken from his thigh. He had expected a normal-looking thumb and had looked forward to having a functioning hand as a reward for the frequent boring hospitalizations. He was bitterly disappointed and disgusted at the appearance of the thumb. He remarked to the nurse, "Look at that! It's obscene. I am going to sign myself out of this hospital and have my own doctor cut this thing off." The nurse reported this reaction to the head nurse who said, "He should be ashamed of himself for criticizing his doctor, who is the best plastic surgeon in this part of the country. The doctor has worked terribly hard on that thumb."

The individual did leave the hospital against medical advice. He was angry and disappointed. If someone had explained that the surgeon planned to shape the thumb to normal proportions after the body had established effective circulation to the new tissues, he might have been helped to wait for a few more weeks for the surgeon to complete the delicate and tedious work. Unfortunately, the nurse with whom the client had developed a positive relationship did not know enough about plastic surgery to use the opportunity to be helpful at the time when he needed reassurance. This incident highlights the importance of the nurse's possessing and using scientifically correct knowledge concerning the nature of the illness and treatment.

A colostomy is another emotionally disturbing experience for individuals. In our culture the emphasis placed on cleanliness and fastidiousness in personal hygiene creates a serious conflict for those who find it medically necessary to resort to a colostomy. Cultural attitudes toward toileting, which are taught early in a child's life, sometimes cause the adult to rebel at the thought of caring for a colostomy. Probably no surgical procedure has the potential for presenting individuals with more emotional and social problems than does a colostomy. Although hundreds of individuals have been able to adjust successfully to colostomies, the nurse should not forget that the person who is just beginning to cope with the problems presented by the loss of normal bowel function has many hurdles ahead of him. Individuals who have undergone a colostomy worry about their acceptability to their friends and their sexual partners. Persons who have received support in working through their feelings about their colostomies report that they have been able to maintain satisfying sexual relations. Unfortunately, others find that it becomes emotionally impossible for them to do so.

It is helpful if individuals with colostomies are encouraged to express their feelings, attitudes, and questions about their condition. Individuals are not helped by nurses who insist on the light, gay approach and refuse to involve themselves in serious conversation about these problems. The person with a colostomy deserves a nurse who will give his situation thoughtful, empathic, realistic consideration.

The nurse is being therapeutic when she helps individuals to talk about their feelings regarding the surgical procedure they have experienced.

Such procedures as colostomy operations are performed only when they are necessary to save the individual's life. The nurse cannot alter the problems that such an operation presents, but she can help the individual to talk about the problem, to accept the reality of this situation, and to learn all he can about his condition so that he can handle it as effectively as possible. The following clinical report illustrates the effect that a colostomy can have on some people.

> A fastidious man who understood English poorly entered the hospital with a diagnosis of far-advanced carcinoma of the rectum. He had suffered a great deal before coming to the hospital and was grateful when surgery relieved the pain. A colostomy opening was established. His physical recovery was rapid. When he was discharged, he left many gifts for the hospital staff. In every way he appeared to be happy and grateful. The surgeon had attempted to explain the seriousness of the problem to the patient before surgery. The hospital staff believed that the man understood the nature of his operation and the need for a permanent colostomy. One week after discharge he returned to the surgical clinic and requested admission to the hospital to have the colostomy opening closed. Again the surgeon explained the nature of the operation and the permanent character of the surgery. The individual left the clinic without appearing to be upset. The next day the newspapers carried a notice of his suicide.

The problems experienced by this individual undoubtedly grew out of his inability to understand the English language and his attitude toward the importance of physical cleaniness. Although his response to the colostomy was unusual, many individuals will admit that in the beginning of their experience with a colostomy, they occasionally wondered if life was worthwhile under such circumstances. Of particular significance in this situation was the individual's lack of expression of any negative feelings. If the health care personnel truly understood and appreciated the huge emotional significance of a colostomy, they would have viewed this man's behavior as an untoward response and could have intervened in a way that might have prevented the suicide.

Surgical operations on the male genitourinary tract sometimes cause severe emotional conflicts. Occasionally such an operation precipitates a psychotic reaction. The following clinical report presents an example of such a situation.

> A middle-aged gentleman who was a devoted church member was admitted to a surgical unit because of symptoms of prostatic hypertrophy. A successful operation was performed to relieve the distressing symptoms. Within 1 or 2 days he was complaining of suggestive pictures on the walls of his room, which he said the hospital authorities had placed there for the purpose of tormenting him. The

nurses were confused by these complaints because no pictures were hanging in his room. The patient told the psychiatrist who was called to talk with him that the annoying pictures were of young nude women. The gentleman stated that a man of his principles should not be surrounded by such lewd art.

The psychiatrist concluded that the individual was not able to accept the fact that a man of his social standing would indulge in such an active fantasy life dealing with sexual material. To relieve his own anxiety about his unconscious sexual longings, which were dramatically brought to light by his complaint about the nude pictures, he unconsciously used the mechanism of projection. It was more acceptable to him and safer to his self-esteem to blame the hospital for hanging pictures of nude women around the room than to accept the explanation that the pictures represented his own fantasies.

This unusual reaction was undoubtedly precipitated by the surgical procedure, but it would not be accurate to say that the procedure caused the response. During most of this individual's life he probably had exerted a great deal of emotional energy to repress unacceptable sexual thoughts. The emotional crisis presented by the surgical experience combined with the effects of the anesthesia were apparently enough to make it impossible for him to continue to repress his unacceptable thoughts.

Emotional reactions precipitated by cardiac surgery

Individuals respond to life-threatening situations uniquely, depending on the coping mechanisms they have developed and the attitude of personal security they maintain. In view of this, it is difficult, if not impossible to predict how a specific individual will respond to any surgical procedure, especially one that is potentially as dangerous as cardiac surgery.

No matter how well the individual appears to be anticipating the procedure, the nurse must realize that cardiac surgery is a major crisis and that the person is struggling to control feelings of anxiety and fear. He cannot avoid being concerned about the possibility of death and the separation from family and friends.

Individuals who have accepted the fact that they must undergo cardiac surgery have come to this decision after months or years of cardiac symptomatology. They may have been semi-invalids because of these symptoms, or the surgery may have been planned in the hope of preventing future invalidism. Thus the individual's fear of the outcome of the procedure is coupled with his anticipation of great improvement in his health in the immediate future.

The nurse assigned to the individual before cardiac surgery should be prepared to anticipate any number of reactions, depending on the individual's personality. He may deny the seriousness of the situation and avoid discussing it. This attitude probably suggests that he finds it difficult to bear the burden and thus copes by avoiding the topic. A different person may discuss his fears, may become tearful, and, by identifying many personal needs, may insist that the nurse stay with him. A third individual may appear to be angry and sarcastic and may be critical of the way the nurse performs the necessary nursing procedures. Each of these individuals deserves a calm, empathic nurse who is a good listener and who understands that the individual's emotional response is his way of coping with a crisis situation. The nurse should encourage him to express his feelings and concerns and should respond to his questions in an honest, straightforward manner without alarming him. The individual deserves to be assured that he will be cared for by a team of physicians and nurses who are knowledgeable, skillful, and deeply interested in his welfare and comfort.

After the surgical procedure the individual will be helpless and dependent for a short time. As he becomes aware of his dependence on others and on mechanical devices, he may respond in a variety of ways. He may be depressed and hopeless or angry and sarcastic. The postsurgical response is dependent to a large extent on the coping mechanisms the individual has used in the past.

Just as during the preoperative period, these patients require a quiet, calm, reassuring nurse who listens carefully to their comments and encourages them to express their anxieties and concerns. Reassurance is essential for these individuals, as is focusing on the reality of the improvement they are making.

Emotional reactions precipitated by an untoward obstetrical experience

Many nurses choose to work in obstetrics because the obstetrical unit is said to be a happy place. In talking about their work, obstetrical nurses frequently emphasize the great happiness of mothers and fathers when a new baby is born. It is true that there is much happiness among new parents, but nurses should not overlook the fact a few new mothers are emotionally distressed and in great need of understanding and reassurance because they have delivered imperfect babies or their babies have failed to survive. Women who deliver imperfect babies may be as troubled as mothers whose babies are stillborn.

Mothers of imperfectly formed or premature babies may be distressed by doubts concerning their own adequacy as women or by guilt concerning their own responsibility for the problem.

Production of perfect babies has traditionally been thought to be one of the most important tasks performed by women. When a woman fails in this effort, she sometimes wonders about her effectiveness and her intrinsic value. Therefore mothers of imperfectly formed babies or premature infants are frequently distressed by doubts concerning their own adequacy as women and by guilt about their responsibility for the existence of the problem. It may surprise some nurses to learn that almost all mothers whose babies are born prematurely or congenitally imperfect respond with questions that reflect concern about themselves. They ask questions such as, "What did I do to cause this?" or "Why has this happened to me?" Since the cause of prematurity and many congenital imperfections is not fully understood, scientific explanations of these events often cannot be given. Even when scientific explanations are available, they do little to remove the personal sense of failure these mothers often feel.

Guilt causes people to feel uncomfortable. When a mother feels guilty about her baby's imperfections, she may reject it outright or may spend the rest of her life punishing herself for failing to give her child a perfect body. This punishment might take the form of slavishly serving the child in an attempt to make up in every possible way for the child's poor start in life. This reaction is one of the disguised forms that rejection may take.

As in many other situations, the nurse cannot alter the reality of the difficult situation but can encourage the mother to talk about her feelings. If the mother can be helped to discuss some of these feelings, she may come to feel less guilty and may be able to clear away some of the emotion about the problem so that constructive steps can be taken and solutions can be planned.

Some women who have set high achievement goals for themselves find it particularly difficult to accept an imperfect baby. The following clinical report demonstrates this point.

> An English professor from a large midwestern university found that she was pregnant for the first time at the age of 40. She and her husband were moderately happy about this new development in their lives. However, they were sorry to have to give up their plans for a sabbatical leave and a trip abroad. When the baby boy was born, he had a bilateral harelip and a cleft palate. When the nurse brought the baby to the mother, she looked at him and said, "That can't possibly be my child," The nurse assured the mother that it was her little boy. She said to the nurse, "Don't bring that baby in here again. I won't have a baby that looks like that!" In 5 days the mother left the hospital without asking to see her baby again. The father arranged for a nurse to help him take his son to a distant city where he had an appointment with a famous surgeon who specialized in repairing harelips. Within a few weeks the mother began to experience overwhelming feelings of anxiety and guilt for which she saw no cause. These feelings became so intense that she sought professional help. Through psychotherapy this mother eventually was able to understand the highly personalized meaning that the birth of her imperfect baby had for her.

Emotional reactions precipitated by an abortion

Few situations in a woman's life have such a potential for producing a variety of emotional responses as does abortion. The response on the part of the woman involved is a highly individual one dependent on many factors. Some of these factors include her religious beliefs and cultural background. Some religious groups are explicit in their teaching against abortion, whereas others are more inclined to leave such a decision to the woman and her physician. Some cultures emphasize the relationship between a woman's intrinsic value to society and her ability to produce children; others place more importance on the quality of life that can be provided for the mother and child. Another factor is the woman's relationship with the father. If the relationship is a stable one and the man agrees that abortion is a wise decision, the reaction of the woman may be less emotionally distressing than if he wishes her to maintain the pregnancy. If the pregnancy is unwanted because of the circumstances surrounding conception (such as rape) or if the fetus has been identified as being seriously defective, the opportunity for abortion may be greeted with relief.

Some individuals may be convinced that they have discarded the early religious instructions that they received and the attitudes taught within the family about such controversial questions as abortion. However, these attitudes are difficult to discard and may greatly influence the woman's emotional response even though they are not recognized consciously.

Many women are able to accept an abortion without experiencing any untoward emotional reaction. However, it is not uncommon for certain individuals to express feelings of serious personal loss, deep regret, shame, guilt, a loss of self-esteem, and sadness. Such individuals may have difficulty sleeping, experience a loss of appetite, exhibit a lack of interest in their home and work, express resentment toward the man involved, and cry frequently.

Unless the nurse visits in the home or works with women in a clinic situation there is little opportunity to be helpful to these individuals since abortion is usually a procedure that is completed within an 8- or 10-hour period and usually does not require overnight hospitalization.

If opportunities are available, it is helpful to encourage the woman to discuss her feelings and how she perceives the situation. In certain individuals an abortion may precipitate a crisis. In this case the person should be treated as any other individual who is overwhelmed by a problem of daily living.

Women anticipating an abortion should have an opportunity to think the situation through with the help of a nurse therapist. Because abortion is irreversible, alternatives should be thoroughly explored before a choice is made.

Common feelings in some women following an abortion include serious personal loss, deep regret, shame, guilt, a loss of self-esteem, and sadness.

Emotional reactions of individuals with acquired immune deficiency syndrome (AIDS)

No other illness in recent memory has evoked the type and amount of widespread reaction seen in response to the disease of AIDS. At this point, there is no cure for AIDS, it is associated with a life-style that is stigmatized by society, and it is increasing in incidence. Therefore, the patient, his social group, his family, and the society all are profoundly affected by this illness.

The professional literature abounds with current information about the comprehensive care of the patient with AIDS; the reader is referred to these articles for specifics. In general, however, it is necessary for all nurses to understand that the diagnosis of AIDS, in itself, precipitates a situational crisis of catastrophic proportion. Because many of these persons acquired this illness secondary to a life-style that is stigmatized by society, namely, homosexual or bisexual behavior or intravenous drug use, they are confronted not only with the loss of health and likely death but also with the potential losses of a job and financial security, housing, sexual activity, and social acceptance. If the nurse is to be truly helpful to the person with AIDS, she must examine her own beliefs, value system, and fears so that she does not inadvertently contribute to the all too frequent discrimination experienced by these persons. Furthermore, she needs to develop the ability to differentiate between the individual's emotional responses to the illness and his responses to the reactions of others if she is to provide individualized care.

The first stage of the crisis is characterized by denial alternating with overwhelming anxiety, anger, and acute emotional turmoil. To fully appreciate this normal response, the nurse needs to understand that many of these individuals are at a point in their life when they are just beginning to actualize their future. The diagnosis of AIDS represents a death sentence that creates a massive assault on their total stability. Therefore, denial is accurately interpreted as a healthy defense mechanism that should be supported unless doing so increases danger to the patient. Concomitant with denial is the person's inability to understand or remember what he is being told, including instructions. Therefore, the nurse is most helpful when she writes out information the individual must have, such as names and telephone numbers of referrals.

In marked contrast to denial, some persons newly diagnosed with AIDS express a temporary sense of relief when told of their diagnosis, since they had experienced symptoms prior to seeking medical help and had privately feared this diagnosis. Therefore, the confirmation of this dreaded diagnosis makes public what was a private terror and enables discussion about it.

As the illness progresses and the individual experiences physiological symptoms that markedly interfere with his ability to function, he is likely to become very depressed, perhaps even suicidal. Once again, this response is understandable in that he is experiencing some very real losses about which he must grieve. In addition to the losses resulting from the illness itself, it is unfortunately not unusual for the individual with AIDS to find himself rejected by family and friends, to be at risk for eviction and loss of employment, and to be the object of many other forms of social ostracism. This societal response often precipitates feelings of isolation, guilt, anger, and low self-esteem.

When providing care for the patient with AIDS the nurse can be of inestimable help by treating him with the same skill, sensitivity, and respect as she would extend to any other patient who is critically ill. This means making frequent contact, encouraging him to talk about his feelings and listening nonjudgmentally, reaching out to touch him, and limiting her use of isolation precautions only to those which are necessary. The specter of a patient with AIDs lying in a private room having contact only when necessary with a fully gowned, gloved, and masked nurse is truly frightening.

> The nurse is most therapeutic in her care of the patient with AIDS when she treats him with the same skill, sensitivity, and respect that she would extend to any other critically ill patient.

If possible, another helpful intervention is to assist the person to become involved in a support group where the reality basis for his responses can be validated and where he can receive assistance in planning to meet his needs.

In the final phase of the illness, the individual is likely to accept the diagnosis and simultaneously attempt to live each day constructively within the limits imposed by his physical debility while also preparing for his death. The nurse needs to be aware, however, that each instance of opportunistic infection as well as each news bulletin about a new medication thrusts the person into another crisis. Many patients with AIDS report that one of the most difficult aspects of living with their illness is the "roller coaster" of emotions that they experience as hope vacillates with despair.

As persons with AIDS receive more effective symptomatic care and live longer, many develop dementia related to the invasion of the virus into the central nervous system. Thus, the patient may display symptoms of cognitive impairment and psychomotor retardation or agitation. Some become blatantly psychotic. Therefore, it is likely that an increasing number of patients with AIDS will be seen in psychiatric units or in hospitals for the mentally ill.

Emotional aspects of death and dying

No discussion of the emotional needs of persons who are physically ill would be complete without addressing the needs of the individual who is dying. With the development of complex medical technology the ability to prolong life has increased. This ability has raised questions about the quality of life and in the opinion of some has contributed to the unconsciously held belief that death occurs only as a result of the failure of the individual or the health care team to "try hard enough."

It is important for all health care personnel to understand that death is an inevitability and that dying persons have a right to be treated humanely. It is not humane to surround a dying person by machines and technicians so that the family cannot even reach him. The opposite often occurs as well, namely, that the terminally ill person is figuratively abandoned. Individuals in this situation are often relegated to rooms farthest away from the nurse's station, receive only cursory attention from medical and nursing staff, and may have few visitors.

The nurse must be concerned about remedying both of these extreme situations. Nursing, more than any other health care profession, has the opportunity and the obligation to assist the dying person and his family to achieve a satisfactory resolution of this last phase of life. To fulfill this responsibility the nurse needs to develop an understanding of the emotional needs of the terminally ill person.

Dr. Elisabeth Kübler-Ross, a pioneer in thanatology, has studied the responses of hundreds of terminally ill persons. Her subjects included persons of all ages, socioeconomic levels, and cultural backgrounds. These persons also represented a wide variety of illnesses and injuries, both acute and chronic. Regardless of their differences, Dr. Kübler-Ross found that all dying persons progress through a similar process of emotional response. Her formulation, which is probably familiar to most nurses, delineates five stages of dying.

Denial is the initial response caused by the person not being able to deal emotionally with the reality of his impending death. To deal with the intense

Dr. Elisabeth Kubler-Ross has delineated five stages in the dying process: denial, anger, bargaining, depression, and acceptance.

anxiety that this news engenders, the person uses the ego defense of denial. As a result, persons in this stage often express the belief that a mistake has been made in laboratory reports or that the physician is incompetent. As with any person who is using the defense of denial, the nurse will be most helpful if she understands that this defense is operative because the individual has sustained a massive emotional assault that he cannot handle directly without endangering the integrity of his personality. Consequently, the wise nurse intervenes in a manner that allows the individual to maintain this defense while simultaneously not avoiding the reality of the situation. For example, the nurse would not encourage a person who is in this stage of the dying process to make plans for his funeral, but she would encourage him to take his medications as they were prescribed. Because the reality of the situation is such that the individual soon becomes sicker, the length of this stage is relatively short in individuals who are mentally healthy. It should be noted that illnesses that initially do not have symptoms that cause incapacitation, such as chronic lymphocytic leukemia, may enable even mentally healthy persons to cling to the denial of the fact that they are dying.

Anger characterizes the second stage of the dying process. During this stage individuals often feel as if they are victims of fate, circumstances, medical incompetence, or a vengeful God. Their thoughts and verbalizations center around the question of, "Why me?" They fear the dependency their illness creates and often resent their family and the health care workers who try to be of help. Since feeling and expressing anger are not acceptable to many people, some dying persons may express their anger in covert, rather than overt, ways. Most nurses recognize the anger and underlying anxiety in terminally ill individuals who complain about everything and everyone. Only the sensitive, insightful nurse recognizes the same dynamics in the individual who expresses his anger in passive ways, such as "forgetting" to take his medication and then asking the nurse what he should do.

Bargaining is the third stage of the dying process characterized by the individual attempting to gain more time by trading off "good" behavior. Most commonly, the dying individual bargains with supernatural powers—God, fate, or whatever higher Being he believes can effect a change in his condition. Bargaining takes the form of, "If you (let me live until Christmas) then I (will bequeath half of my money to the church)." The behavior that the person "trades off" is highly individualized and is probably related to earlier unresolved conflicts. The bargaining stage is helpful to the dying person in that it temporarily eases his anxiety and enables him to deal with the pain and dependence that may accompany his illness.

The *depression* stage follows bargaining. Depression begins when the reality of the situation can no longer be ignored and the uselessness of denial, anger, and bargaining is apparent. The depression that the individual feels is a response to an overwhelming sense of anticipated loss—the loss of his entire world. At this stage the dying person looks and acts depressed and often has no need to talk with others about how he feels. He must use his energy to confront the fact that what is done is done, and what is undone will remain so. Because he is depressed, the person in this stage of dying makes few demands. Consequently his behavior is often misinterpreted as "cooperative."

Acceptance is the final stage of the dying process when the individual has come to peace with himself about the fact that his death is imminent. Acceptance is characterized by an affective void; the person is not happy, nor is he depressed. His interests, even in his own care, narrow. During this time only those persons who are most significant to him are able to elicit a positive response. The presence of others is merely tolerated. This does not mean, however, that the dying person cannot receive comfort from the nursing interventions of a warm, caring nurse. It does mean that the most effective interventions are likely to be nonverbal in the form of physical comfort measures delivered in a competent, compassionate way.

The nurse is most therapeutic in her care of the dying person if she first develops self-awareness about dying and death.

Understanding the emotional needs of the dying person is of value to the nurse only if she is able to combine this knowledge with self-awareness. Since death and dying are not viewed by our culture as natural phenomena, nurses, like most people, have been taught since early childhood to avoid the subject. This cultural attitude may be compounded by the nurse's own developmental stage. The developmental stages of adulthood and middle age are the stages most nurses are in and may prove to be particularly problematic in regard to the issues of death and dying. The stage of adulthood, especially early adulthood, is a time when people view all things as being possible. As a result, the nurse in this stage may be prone to view the terminally ill person as representative of the failure of the health care team. The nurse who is dealing with the developmental tasks of middle age may be actively dealing with the awareness of her own mortality reinforced by the declining health of her parents. The terminally ill person may represent the nurse's vulnerability to the prospect of her own death.

In either instance, the nurse may feel anxious and guilt ridden and avoid dealing with her feelings by avoiding the patient. During those times when the nurse cannot avoid the person, she avoids the reality of the situation by assuming a false air of cheerfulness, by changing the subject when the person or his family start to talk about death, or by not answering the client's questions. Other nurses may respond angrily to the dying person, as if his dying were his fault. This counterproductive response seems especially justifiable to the nurse when the dying person's poor health habits, such as smoking, have obviously contributed to his terminal illness. Only if the nurse can be helped to explore and confront her own feelings about the dying process will she be able to give the skilled, compassionate care the dying person deserves.

NURSING CARE PLAN

An individual who is dying

CASE FORMULATION

Mrs. Harper is a 78-year-old widow who has chronic lymphocytic leukemia, the treatment of which now requires her to go to the hospital for blood transfusions on a monthly basis.

Mrs. Harper lived in her mother's home until she married at age 25. She and her new husband had wanted to marry earlier, but Mrs. Harper was needed at home to help care for her father who was ill and ultimately died of cancer. Mrs. Harper was an executive secretary. Despite her marriage and no economic need to do so, she worked continuously until her retirement at age 62. She and Mr. Harper had two daughters, the first when Mrs. Harper was 30 and the second 10 years later. Mrs. Harper responded to the birth of her second daughter by becoming seriously depressed for 2 years. Although she was still able to work during this time, she was completely unable to care for the children or the house. As a result, her widowed mother moved in with the Harpers to care for the family and the home. Ten years later she had a stroke and required a great deal of care until she died. Both daughters studied professions and are now working and living with their families in other states.

When the Harpers retired, they sold the family home and bought a much smaller home in another area of the country that had been Mr. Harper's boyhood home. Although Mrs. Harper knew no one in the community, she agreed to the move to placate Mr. Harper, a domineering and demanding person. Five years after the move, Mr. Harper died after a lengthy illness related to complications of diabetes. Throughout his illness, Mrs. Harper devoted herself exclusively to meeting his needs, even to the extent of staying in the hospital around the clock for weeks on end.

After Mr. Harper's death the daughters were worried about how Mrs. Harper would manage by herself. As a result, they telephoned her every other day and were often worried, since she was seldom home. Finally, the older daughter asked her mother where she went so frequently. Mrs. Harper responded by saying that she wasn't about to answer for her whereabouts, since this was the first time in her life that she was free of responsibility and could do as she wished. For the next 8 years Mrs. Harper lived comfortably and happily, associating frequently with the many friends she made and visiting her daughters on holidays.

Mrs. Harper discovered that she had chronic lymphocytic leukemia 2 years ago as a result of bloodwork that she had done at a community health clinic that offered free screening exams and laboratory tests to senior citizens. The results of her bloodwork were mailed to her by certified mail accompanied by a letter strongly urging her to consult her physician. Even though her physician's tests confirmed the diagnosis and she was referred to an oncologist for treatment, Mrs. Harper confided in her daughters that she never felt better and that she was sure there was some sort of mixup—probably in the laboratory. Despite her denial of her illness, she kept her appointments with the doctor and conscientiously took the prescribed medication.

Within 18 months Mrs. Harper became increasingly tired and resistant to the effects of the chemotherapy. As a result, she now requires blood transfusions along with medication.

One month ago Mrs. Harper spent a week with her older daughter to attend the high school graduation of one of her granddaughters. Several other family members also were house guests for the occasion, including Mrs. Harper's younger daughter and her 8-year-old daughter. This child was very active and talkative, probably due to fatigue and boredom, since there were no other children present. Mrs. Harper alarmed and surprised everyone by responding to the child and her mother with thinly concealed rage, frequently yelling at the child to behave herself and telling her daughter

Continued.

NURSING CARE PLAN—cont'd

that she wasn't any better a mother than she had been a child.

When Mrs. Harper arrived for her transfusion this morning, the nurse asked how she was feeling. Although the nurse was undoubtedly inquiring about her physical health, this question precipitated an outpouring of anger about how "bad" her young granddaughter was and how her own daughter didn't know how to control the situation.

Nursing assessment

Mrs. Harper's background and her current illness give many clues as to why she may be reacting the way she is. Although her early family history of living with her parents and not marrying until she fulfilled her responsibilities to care for her dying father is not unusual for a woman of her age, the fact that she worked continuously outside of the home as an executive secretary is uncommon for a woman of her generation. Therefore, Mrs. Harper likely was meeting a need for independence while simultaneously attempting to behave dutifully in the manner appropriate for a women at that time. When she gave birth to a second child at age forty, she may have perceived this event as a potential loss of independence to which she responded with depression. The ego strength of this woman and the importance of her job as a coping mechanism are attested to by the fact that she was able to continue work despite her depression. It also appears that she suppressed many of her needs for independence after she retired as evidenced by her willingness to move to a strange area and to devotedly care for her husband during his long illness. However, once these responsibilities were met, she asserted her strong need for independence as evidenced by her response to her children's questions about her activities.

Mrs. Harper's response of denial to the news that she had a life-threatening illness is congruent with what is known about the first stage of dying. This response is particularly common in situations when the illness does not cause major symptoms or dysfunction. Since she complied with the doctor's treatment regimen, it was possible to support her denial and thereby allow her to gradually adjust to the inevitability of failing health. However, once the medication became ineffective and transfusions were necessary, it was no longer possible for Mrs. Harper to deny the gravity of her situation and, most important, her impending loss of independence. Therefore, the nurse assessed Mrs. Harper's anger at her 8-year-old granddaughter as being displaced rage about her own feelings of loss of control, characteristic of the second stage of the dying process. It is also interesting to note that Mrs. Harper's anger extended to the child's mother, whose birth 40 years earlier had precipitated Mrs. Harper's depression. It is likely that she was now outwardly expressing the anger that she had turned inward for so many years.

Nursing diagnosis

Based on the nursing assessment that included prior knowledge of the family dynamics and an understanding of the dynamics underlying the dying process, the nurse formulated the following pair of nursing diagnoses specific to Mrs. Harper's emotional response. The first is from the Classification of Human Responses of Concern for Psychiatric–Mental Health Nursing Practice; the second is from the approved NANDA Diagnostic Categories.

4.1.2   Altered Feeling State related to anger at impending loss of independence due to illness

OR

9.3.1   Anxiety related to impending loss of independence due to illness

Planning and implementing care for *Mrs. Harper*

A sample nursing care plan for Mrs. Harper is found in the boxed material that follows.

The nurse's immediate objective was to allow

NURSING CARE PLAN—cont'd

and encourage Mrs. Harper to talk about her feelings, which might enable her to see that the anger she felt toward her granddaughter's and daughter's behavior was a displacement of her own rage about having a terminal illness. The nurse also knew it was important to take this time if Mrs. Harper were to have an emotionally corrective experience by being able to express her anger about the birth of her second daughter. The nurse was careful to respond to Mrs. Harper in an accepting, empathic way even though many people might not understand how one could be currently angry about an event that happened 40 years ago and a situation that was yet to occur. Since the nurse was not surprised or frightened by Mrs. Harper, as was her family, she was able to effectively implement this approach.

Evaluation

Mrs. Harper talked so long about her feelings that the transfusion had to be rescheduled for later in the week. Although she gave no evidence that she understood the relationship between her current anger and the impending loss of independence due to her illness, she did express the insight that she had always been "furious" with her younger daughter because she felt she was too old to deal with a baby when she became pregnant.

The nurse made sure that she would be on duty when Mrs. Harper came for her next appointment so they could continue their discussion during the transfusion. She also noted on the care plan the necessity to contact the daughters about Mrs. Harper's future care with the goal of helping them explore ways in which they could assist their mother to remain as independent as possible for as long as possible.

NURSING CARE PLAN FOR *Mrs. Harper*

Nursing diagnosis	Objective	Nursing actions	Outcome criteria
4.1.2 Altered Feeling State related to anger at impending loss of independence due to illness OR 9.3.1 Anxiety related to impending loss of independence due to illness	Help patient see her anger stems from her impending loss of independence and repressed rage at younger daughter	Listen in an accepting, empathic way Reflect back patient's content and tone Encourage patient to make all decisions that are possible Contact daughters to plan for continuing independence of patient for as long as possible	Within 1 month patient will verbalize relationship of her anger to impending loss of independence and repressed rage at younger daughter Within 6 months patient will begin to grieve loss of independence Patient will continue to schedule appointments and comply with medical instructions indefinitely Daughters will confer with nurse

END NOTE

This chapter focuses on the nursing care necessary to meet the emotional needs of individuals who are physically ill. In addition to presenting general guidelines, also discussed are emotional reactions commonly precipitated by the use of mechanical devices and organ transplants, the loss of a body part, cardiac surgery, untoward obstetrical experiences, and abortion. The emotional reactions of individuals with AIDS and those who are dying are examined. The chapter concludes with a hypothetical plan of nursing care for a widow who is dying.

SUGGESTED SOURCES OF ADDITIONAL INFORMATION

Baer JW, Hall JM, Holm K, and Lewitter-Koehler S: Challenges in developing an inpatient psychiatric program for patients with AIDS and ARC, Hosp Commun Psychiatr 38(12):1299, December 1987.

Bennett K: AIDS: a generation of children at risk, J Psychosoc Nurs Ment Health Serv 25(12):32, December 1987.

Bernstein SB: Breaking the vicious circle of noncompliance, Nurs 89 19(1):74, January 1989.

Billings C: Emotional first aid, Am J Nurs 80:2006, 1980.

Flaskerud JH: AIDS: neuropsychiatric complications, J Psychosoc Nurs Ment Health Serv 25(12):17, December 1987.

Flaskerud JH: AIDS: psychosocial aspects, J Psychosoc Nurs Ment Health Serv 25(12):8, December 1987.

Grabbe LL and Brown LB: Identifying neurologic complications of AIDS, Nurs 89 19(5):66, May 1989.

Grant SM: The hospitalized AIDS patient and the psychiatric liaison nurse, Arch Psych Nurs 2(1):35, February 1988.

Hall JM and Stevens PE: AIDS: a guide to suicide assessment, Arch Psych Nurs 1(2):115, April 1988.

Henderson KJ: Dying, God, & anger: comforting through spiritual care, J Psychosoc Nurs Ment Health Serv 27(5):17, 1989.

Icenhour ML and Calvert H: EBV: managing the physiological and psychosocial implications of the Epstein-Barr virus, J Psychosoc Nurs 27(4):20, 1989.

Kübler-Ross E: Questions and answers on death and dying, New York, 1974, Macmillan Publishing Co., Inc.

Nichols SE: Psychosocial reactions of persons with the acquired immunodeficiency syndrome, Ann Int Med 103(5);765, November 1985.

MacNeil-Zimberg M: Helping cancer patients cope, J Psychosoc Nurs Health Serv 23(6):31, June 1985.

Pheifer WG and Houseman C: Bereavement and AIDS: a framework for intervention, J Psychosoc Nurs Ment Health Serv 26(10):21, October 1988.

Rubinow DR: The psychosocial impact of AIDS, Topics Clin Nurs 6(2):26, July 1984.

Ryan LJ: AIDS: a threat to physical and psychological integrity, Topics Clin Nurs 6(2):19, July 1984.

Salisbury DM: AIDS: psychosocial implications, J Psychosoc Nurs Ment Health Serv 24(12):13, December 1986.

Stewart RS: Psychiatric issues in renal dialysis and transplantation, Hosp Commun Psychiatr 34(7):623, 1983.

Streltzer J: Psychiatric aspects of oncology: a review of recent research, Hosp Commun
    Psychiatr 34(8):716, 1983.
Trusley M: The use of family therapy in terminal illness and death, J Psychosoc Nurs
    Ment Health Serv 20:17, January 1982.
Valente SM and Saunders JM: Dealing with serious depression in cancer patients, Nurs
    89 19(2):44, February 1989.
Worth C: Handle with care, Am J Nurs 89(2):196, February 1989.
Wright LK: Life threatening illness, J Psychosoc Nurs Ment Health Serv 23(9):6, 1985.

Crisis theory and intervention

24

LEARNING OBJECTIVES

After studying this chapter, the student will be able to:

○ Define the term *crisis*.
○ Differentiate between developmental and situational crises.
○ Discuss the characteristics of a crisis state.
○ Discuss the sequential phases of a crisis state.
○ State the goal of crisis intervention.
○ Discuss in sequence the steps of crisis intervention.

Crisis intervention is a subject of interest to all health professionals. It is a technique that is used successfully by persons with a variety of backgrounds to aid individuals and families in understanding and effectively coping with the intense emotions that characterize a crisis state. Once the client is able to deal with his emotions, he often is able to make appropriate decisions regarding behavior that may be required for resolution of the problems that surround the crisis. Although the responsibility for crisis intervention does not fall into the province of any one health care discipline, a discussion of it is included in this text because nurses are often in the position to engage in this technique or to counsel other health care professionals in its use. Furthermore, psychiatric nurses are expected to have particular expertise in understanding and managing emotional problems and are often looked to by their colleagues as consultants in crisis states.

HISTORICAL PERSPECTIVE

As is true of many other contemporary innovations in American psychiatry, crisis theory and intervention had their foundation in the experiences of the military during World War II. During that war there were more psychiatric casualties than physical, even after an attempt had been made to screen out those persons with a history of mental illness. Many of the casualties were precipitated by the soldier's experiences in combat. Psychiatrists in the medical corps, led by Dr. William Menninger, treated some of these soldiers close to the front, primarily because of a shortage of personnel and the inaccessibility of other treatment settings. Much to the surprise of all, those who received immediate, reality-oriented, supportive intervention and were returned to combat as soon as possible fared better emotionally than did their counterparts who were evacuated to treatment centers and treated with psychoanalytically oriented interventions.

After the war the techniques used so successfully were applied with equal success to civilians who were victims of diasters. Perhaps the most famous of these was the fire in 1942 at the Cocoanut Grove, a nightclub in Boston. The emotional reactions of the survivors of this disaster were studied in depth over a period of years by Eric Lindemann. His findings about the symptoms and management of acute grief remain the classical work in the field.

Despite its use earlier, crisis intervention did not become a recognized treatment modality until the 1960s. During that time Gerald Caplan made numerous contributions to the literature on the subject and was instrumental in developing a theory to explain the manifestations of a crisis in essentially healthy people as well as postulating intervention techniques. Since that time numerous others from all health care disciplines have contributed to the growing body of knowledge about the subject.

DEFINITION OF CRISIS

The term *crisis* is often used by laypersons to describe a situation or a feeling state. It is not unusual to hear an individual say about an event, "It was a crisis." If in fact the event referred to was a turning point in a situation, the use of the term is correct according to the dictionary definition of the word. When referring to a feeling state, persons often report that they are in a crisis when they are very upset. Almost always this is an incorrect use of the word according to its technical definition.

Mental health authorities define a crisis as *a state of disequilibrium resulting from the interaction of an event with the individual's or family's coping mechanisms, which are inadequate to meet the demands of the situation, combined with the individual's or family's perception of the meaning of the event.* Therefore a crisis refers to an interactional process among these three variables that is reflected in the feeling state of the individual or family. Although anxiety usually underlies the feeling state, the individual may feel depression, anger, fear, or any

An event, its *meaning* to the individual or family and their inability to cope interact to produce a crisis.

other of a wide range of emotions. However, it is not the emotion that is unique to a crisis, nor is it the event. Rather, it is the meaning of the event to the individual or family and their inability to cope with it that produces the crisis. Therefore not every person who is anxious, depressed, angry, or fearful is in a crisis, nor does a traumatic event necessarily produce a crisis in those whom it affects.

Health professionals are greatly interested in crisis intervention for a number of reasons. First, more people are voluntarily seeking mental health care for problems that are not necessarily indicative of long-standing dysfunction. In the past, because of the social stigma associated with mental illness, mental health counsel was sought only if the person was severely disturbed and exhibiting bizarre symptoms such as hallucinations or delusions. Although there is still more stigma associated with mental illness than with physical illness, society is gradually becoming more accepting of the value of mental health treatment so a larger number of people voluntarily seek help for less severe problems. These problems are often individual or familial crises.

Second, as professionals have gained more experience in dealing with persons in a crisis, they have realized that former unresolved crises often emerge to consciousness in conjunction with the present crisis. Therefore intervention can be directed toward both the present and past situations, providing a unique opportunity to help the client resolve long-standing problems in a relatively short period of time.

Finally, crisis intervention is of great interest to mental health professionals because it provides a specific opportunity to prevent mental illness and to promote mental health. Prevention of mental illness is achieved by helping the client to use already established coping mechanisms that he has successfully used in the past or by assisting him to develop new, healthy defenses. If this can be achieved, the necessity for the client to resort to pathological defense mechanisms, even mental illness, can be avoided.

Promotion of mental health through crisis intervention has been documented by researchers who have engaged in follow-up studies of individuals and families who have experienced crises. It has been demonstrated that there are three possible outcomes of a crisis state: (1) the client may reintegrate at a lower or less healthy level of functioning than the one prior to the crisis, (2) the client may reintegrate at the same level of functioning as previously, probably as a result of completely repressing the crisis situation and its attendant emotions, or (3) the client may reintegrate at a higher, healthier level of functioning than the level prior to the crisis experience. This last possible outcome was a startling realization at the time it was first described because the goal had always been prevention of mental illness. The idea that people could actually grow and benefit from an emotionally traumatic experience opened vast potential for increasing the level of mental health in a large population. In fact some authorities see a crisis as a catalyst that disturbs old habits, evokes new responses, and

Because society is more accepting of mental health treatment, more people voluntarily seek help for problems that are not indicative of long-standing dysfunction.

Following a crisis, an individual may reintegrate at a lower level of functioning, at the same level, or at a higher, healthier level than before the crisis.

becomes a major factor in charting new developments. Therefore the challenge that a crisis provokes may bring forth new coping mechanisms that serve to strengthen the individual's adaptive capacity and thereby, in general, to raise his level of mental health.*

Research studies have further documented that, although any one of the three outcomes can occur with or without skilled intervention, resolution of the crisis resulting in a lower level of functioning or the same level of functioning is more likely to occur without intervention, and resolution of the crisis resulting in a higher level of functioning is more likely to occur with intervention. Consequently, to promote mental health as well as to prevent mental illness, an increasing number of communities have established crisis intervention centers. These centers may take the form of mental health emergency rooms, suicide prevention clinics, family guidance clinics, or telephone crisis services. Whatever the name, these centers are always staffed by personnel skilled in crisis intervention.

TYPES OF CRISES

Two types of events may precipitate a crisis state: developmental and situational events. Developmental events are those situations which naturally occur during the lifetime of an individual and his family—for example, the birth of a child. Therefore, developmental events are predictable. Situational events, on the other hand, do not inevitably occur to all individuals or families and therefore are unexpected. An example of a situational event is an automobile accident. It should be understood, however, that very few events inevitably produce a crisis state in all persons. If the reader reviews the definition of crisis, it will be clear that the nature of the event is only one factor in the production of a crisis. In addition to the event, the other two necessary factors are the personalized meaning of the event to the individual and family and the nature and extent of their coping mechanisms. These must interact in such a way as to produce a state of disequilibrium. For example, a hysterectomy may be well received by a 50-year-old unmarried career woman who sublimates her maternal needs through the children of friends and relatives and whose emotional energy is directed toward her profession. Another 50-year-old woman experiencing the same surgical procedure may be plunged into a state of crisis because her identity unconsciously has been formed around her role as mother and homemaker, and the hysterectomy marks the end of her child-bearing years, thus threatening her sense of self. To take this example one step further, the same career woman may enter a state of disequilibrium or crisis if she loses her job or retires, whereas the homemaker might respond to a loss of her outside job with an inner sense of relief.

Events that may precipitate crises are developmental (predictable) or situational (unexpected).

---

*Rapaport L: The state of crisis: some theoretical considerations. In Pared HJ, editor: Crisis intervention: selected readings, New York; 1965, Family Service Association of America.

Developmental crises

Developmental crises are well documented. The reader will remember that each stage of development has its own developmental task, the achievement of which requires the individual to emphasize certain behaviors and to minimize others. Consequently, the family as a unit is called on to adjust and adapt to the changes experienced by each of its members. Although these changes in individuals are most pronounced during infancy and early childhood, they occur throughout the entire life cycle. Therefore any family unit is likely to have members who represent at least two different developmental stages. Many families have members who may be experiencing one of five or six different developmental stages, each stage having its own needs and manifestations. When this is the case, it is common to find family disequilibrium occurring because behaviors that meet the needs of one or more of its members may be in direct opposition to the needs of other members. An increasingly common example of such a situation is the phenomenon of adult children who return to the home of their parents to live after having been away for a few years. This phenomenon is occurring more often today, related in part to problems in the society at large. A scarcity of jobs and economic inflation make it difficult if not impossible for some young adults to become economically independent. Nevertheless, the young adult is developmentally ready to work on establishing his independence but is in a position of dependence on his parents. On the other hand, his parents are developmentally ready to address their generativity needs by engaging in community activities, not by nurturing a family. It does not take much imagination to appreciate the nature and extent of the family disequilibrium that may result from this situation.

Developmental crises are characterized by their predictability. For example, behavioral scientists know that a young married couple will have new demands placed on them when their first child is born. No matter how eagerly they may anticipate this event, many young parents react with depression and frustration when the dependency needs of the infant cause them to alter their previous spontaneous life-style. During midlife this couple may go through an anxiety-laden period when they question the value of the direction they have taken in their marriage, family, and work. Finally, the same couple might become depressed and frustrated once again when they find that their long-anticipated freedom from responsibility for childrearing is limited by the financial and physical limitations of old age. Although the transition from one developmental phase to another is always fraught with a certain degree of increased individual and familial tension, these transitional periods can be prevented from becoming crises through the use of anticipatory guidance.

Anticipatory guidance is primarily an educative process that helps prepare the individual and family for behavioral changes likely to occur in the near future. This process has been greatly aided by the proliferation of information about behavior during each developmental phase now available in newspapers,

Developmental crises can be prevented through *anticipatory guidance,* which helps prepare the individual and family for behavioral changes likely to occur in the near future.

magazines, and paperback books. Therefore many families successfully engage in their own anticipatory guidance without requiring the assistance of health care professionals.

Public health nurses are in a unique position to provide anticipatory guidance. As they visit families in their homes, they have the opportunity to assess the entire family situation, even though they might be present to give care to only one member. For example, the nurse might counsel the mother of a 2-year-old in regard to the meaning of his negativistic behavior while visiting the home to administer a parenteral diuretic to the grandmother. The opportunities for anticipatory guidance by nurses are not limited to home visits. The nurse is in a position to assess the family dynamics when a member is hospitalized for a physical illness and visitors seek out the nurse to covertly ask advice about their problems rather than those of the patient. The astute nurse will recognize these clues and respond in a helpful way.

Situational crises

Situational crises cannot be as accurately predicted as can developmental crises. Situational events that can precipitate a state of crisis include such major catastrophes as the unexpected death of a family member due to accident, the loss of a home through fire or flood, and sudden widespread economic depression as occurred in the 1930s. The event does not have to be as catastrophic as these to precipitate a state of crisis. Any event, no matter how minor or even how desirable it may superficially appear, may combine with the individual's or family's perception of it to produce a situation that is felt to be *hazardous* to the equilibrium of the system. If the event is perceived as hazardous, and the individual or family does not have adequate coping mechanisms available to ward off such a threat, a state of crisis will ensue. Although most people would understand why a family might enter into a state of crisis after their home was burned in a fire that killed their infant daughter, few laypeople would understand why a family might enter a state of crisis after the father receives a major promotion to the position for which he has been striving for many years. In this example, the promotion might represent a threat to a satisfying life-style, a change in social class and social group, and increased responsibility for all family members. Therefore although the family would undoubtedly gain many things they desire and have worked for, to do so they must give up the familiarity of the life they have known, and they may not have immediately available the coping mechanisms necessary to make a smooth adjustment.

Whether the type of event that precipitated the crisis is developmental or situational, the characteristics of the crisis state remain essentially the same.

CHARACTERISTICS OF A CRISIS STATE

A crisis state is not an illness but rather an upset in the steady state of the system. Although the behaviors displayed by those experiencing the crisis may vary, a massive amount of free-floating anxiety is at the basis of these behaviors.

A crisis state is not seen as an illness but rather as an upset in the steady state of the system in which there are massive amounts of free-floating anxiety.

The anxiety may be perceived as such, or it may take the form of depression or anger at various points in the crisis state. Since great amounts of anxiety cannot be sustained by the human being without serious damage to the personality organization, the individual consciously and unconsciously actively seeks to reorganize his personality in such a way that he rids himself of this unbearable emotion. Therefore *a state of crisis is self-limiting,* usually from 4 to 6 weeks in length. It is almost always resolved in this time frame, although not always in the healthiest way. If new, more adequate coping mechanisms are not developed within this period, the individual is likely to repress the events and emotions surrounding the crisis to avoid the further personality disorganization that would result from a prolonged high level of anxiety. Thus a pseudoresolution to the state of crisis is achieved.

A state of crisis is self-limiting, usually from 4 to 6 weeks' duration.

As previously discussed, a crisis state seems to be a response to an event, whether developmental or situational, that is perceived as hazardous. Consequently, a crisis state is highly individualized, and an event that may precipitate a crisis in one individual or family may not necessarily have the same effect on another individual or family. Hazardous events are further categorized into three groups: (1) those which represent a *threat* to fundamental instinctual needs or to the person's sense of integrity, (2) those which represent a real or perceived *loss,* and (3) those which represent a *challenge.*

A crisis state seems to be a response to an event perceived as hazardous—a threat, a loss, or a challenge.

Another characteristic of the crisis state is that *it rarely affects an individual without also affecting those significant others who comprise the individual's social support system.* In most instances, this system is the family group. Therefore it is usually inappropriate to view an individual as being in a state of crisis without also taking into consideration the fact that it is highly likely that the family is also in a state of crisis. This point has numerous implications for intervention. Obviously any resolution to the crisis achieved by an individual in isolation from his previously established social system may be short-lived if it is not workable within the system as a whole.

Because of the mobility of the population in this country and the subsequent demise of the large, extended family, many persons have developed support systems that are not limited to and in fact may not include, family members. Therefore it is important to recognize that friends and neighbors may serve as significant others to an individual even though these persons may not be relatives in the traditional sense. This social pattern is increasingly seen in older persons whose spouses have died and whose married children live at a great distance. In all instances, the individual being counseled should be the one who defines his significant social system, not the crisis counselor who may be misled into making assumptions based on traditional societal patterns.

A crisis state affecting an individual usually also affects the significant others who constitute his social support system.

PHASES OF A CRISIS STATE

Whether it be an individual or a family in a state of crisis, the crisis seems to run through a series of definable, although overlapping, phases.

The initial phase is *denial,* which usually lasts for a period of hours. Denial

The first four phases of a crisis state are experienced by all persons: denial, increased tension, disorganization, and attempts to reorganize.

is a defense mechanism that the mind unconsciously employs to protect itself from the sudden assault of intense anxiety. Denial is evident in the situation where a 55-year-old executive calmly returns to his usual business activities after being informed by the corporate president that he has been fired. In most mentally healthy persons, the reality of the situation quickly becomes apparent and leads into the next phase of crisis, which is characterized by increased tension.

During the phase of *increased tension,* the persons involved make valiant efforts to continue their activities of daily living but do so while attempting to cope with ever-increasing amounts of anxiety. During this phase, therefore, the individual or family remains functional, although those who know them can easily see indications of increased tension in the form of hyperactivity or psychomotor retardation. A common example of this phase is seen in persons who are successfully making funeral arrangements for a loved one who has just died unexpectedly. The phase of increased tension is followed by disorganization.

During the phase of *disorganization,* those in a crisis seem to "fall apart." They can no longer continue with activities of daily living, become obsessively preoccupied with the event, and may remember earlier events they thought they had forgotten and that, unbeknownst to them, have a symbolic link to the current situation. During this phase the person is consciously flooded by a great deal of anxiety and fears that he may be "losing his mind." The fact that he is in a state of crisis may or may not be apparent to him. If it is not, as is often the case, it is usual for the person to become highly anxious about his anxiety, thereby compounding the problem. Therefore it is during this phase that most persons seek professional help, if this has not been done earlier.

The next phase of a crisis is characterized by *attempts to reorganize.* With or without assistance, the individual or family attempts to bring previously used coping mechanisms to bear on the current situation. At this point the mechanisms used are likely to be short-range and directed specifically at the immediate problem. For example, the homemaker who has not been able to mobilize sufficient energy to wash the dishes for the last 3 days may wheel the portable television into the kitchen in an attempt to divert her mind sufficiently to get through the increasingly large stack of dirty dishes. The mental mechanism the woman in this example is using is suppression. If attempts at reorganization are successful at this point, they tend to build on one another and lead to general reorganization, the ultimate goal of crisis resolution. The affected persons gradually resume their normal activities of daily living, becoming anxious and depressed only when specific stimuli are present to remind them of the crisis situation. The attempt at reorganization lasts for weeks, if successful.

An attempt to escape the problem occurs if initial attempts to reorganize are unsuccessful. Failure to escape is followed by local reorganization and finally general reorganization.

A phase characterized by an *attempt to escape the problem* occurs within a matter of days if initial attempts to reorganize are unsuccessful. Without appropriate intervention, during this phase blaming commonly occurs. The persons involved tend to "escape the problem" by projecting responsibility for its existence onto other people, societal institutions, or a supernatural phenomenon such as God or fate. Blaming behaviors, at the very least, create increased tension in a system already overwhelmed by stress and at worst lead to actions that ultimately compound rather than relieve the problem. For example, the husband who blames his wife's lack of supervision for their son's juvenile delinquency may initiate divorce proceedings only to find himself totally alone and still highly anxious a year later when the divorce becomes final. A couple who blames the rigid narrow-mindedness of the community in which they live for their failure to be accepted into the local country club may decide to move to a distant state only to find that they have left behind their primary support system in the form of co-workers. A highly religious person in this phase of crisis may officially leave his church as a means of publicly rejecting the God whom he blames for his problems. In so doing, he may also cut himself off from the human social system whose support he has used in the past and could benefit from now.

Regardless of whether the persons involved in the crisis resort to blaming behaviors or whether they attempt to escape the problem by consciously pretending it does not exist (as opposed to denial, which is an unconscious defense mechanism), this phase rarely results in a successful resolution to the crisis.

After failing at attempts to escape the problem, the individual or family moves into the phase of *local reorganization*. This phase has characteristics similar to the phase "attempts to reorganize" previously described.

After the local reorganization phase, the final phase of *general reorganization* occurs. It may take up to a year before new patterns of behavior are sufficiently well integrated into the individual's personality organization or the family's interactional structure and communication system to withstand additional stress on the system. However, the acute phase of the crisis is usually over within the 6-week period previously mentioned.

Unsuccessful resolution of a crisis state occurs when during any phase, the individual or family adopts pathological means of adaptation, which serve to obscure and compound the crisis. This is most likely to occur when the ego strength of the individual is already weakened or when the family has been using dysfunctional adaptations prior to the crisis. The outlook is particularly dim when skilled intervention is not sought or available and the persons involved resume functioning on a level lower than the one at which they had previously been functioning.

Pseudoresolution occurs when the crisis is repressed and the individual or family have learned nothing from the experience, returning to their former level of functioning. Although all may appear well, these people have missed a valuable opportunity to increase their repertoire of adaptive responses. Furthermore, future crises are likely to be compounded by the reemergence of the conflicts surrounding the previously unresolved repressed one. See

Unsuccessful resolution of a crisis state occurs when pathological adaptations are used at any phase of the crisis state. Pseudoresolution occurs when the crisis experience is repressed and leads to no change in the level of functioning.

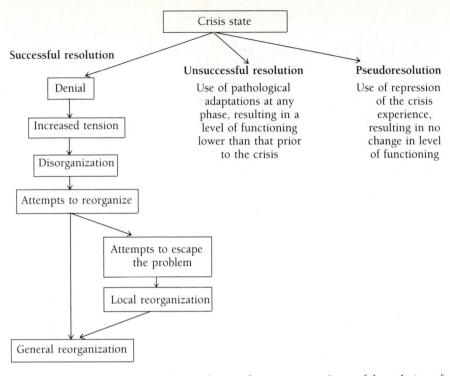

FIGURE 24-1 Processes leading to resolution of a crisis state. Successful resolution of such a state follows a series of phases before culminating in the ultimate goal of general reorganization. The initial four phases are experienced by all persons. Some persons may then move directly from attempts to reorganize to general reorganization. Others may need to take a temporary detour and attempt to escape the problem. When this attempt fails, they proceed to local reorganization, eventually reaching the goal of general reorganization. Successful resolution results in functioning at a level higher than that before the crisis.

Fig. 24-1 for a schematic representation of the processes leading to successful, unsuccessful, or pseudoresolution of a crisis state.

TECHNIQUES OF CRISIS INTERVENTION

The goal of crisis intervention is to assist the individual to seek new and useful adaptive mechanisms within the context of his social support system. By so doing, the crisis counselor aids involved persons to reorganize their individual personalities and their social system on a higher level of functioning than that which they had previously experienced. If this goal is achieved, these persons are better able to deal successfully with future developmental and situational events that inevitably will occur within their lifetimes.

It is important to note that many people who are in a state of crisis are not aware of this fact. They may come to, or telephone, a crisis intervention center with vague, diffuse complaints such as, "I can't sleep," "I'm afraid I'm losing my

The goal of crisis intervention is to assist the individual to seek new and useful adaptive mechanisms within the context of his social support system.

mind," or "I'm afraid that something dreadful is going to happen." On the other hand, friends or relatives may bring a person for treatment, stating that he is "not behaving like himself."

The initial step in intervention is to take the time to thoroughly assess the situation. Direct questions are appropriate, since the individual or family is likely to be in the phase of disorganization during which it is very difficult for them to focus their thoughts and feelings. In addition to collecting identifying data, it is important to ask specifically who else is involved in the problem.

The next step is to define the event. It is not unusual for the persons involved to initially state that nothing unusual has occurred. If they respond in this way, it is not because they are lying but rather because they are truly unaware of the significance of the event in their lives. To elicit this information, it is helpful to ask the person to review in detail what has occurred in his life over the past 2 weeks. If this account indicates nothing unusual, even with specific questioning, the interviewer asks the clients to go back 1 week further. Rarely is it necessary to go back further than 4 weeks. In the course of the narrative, the precipitating event will probably become clear to the interviewer and sometimes to the client as well. If the client is still unaware of the hazardous event, the interviewer can repeat back the situation she has identified from the narrative and suggest that many people would find this situation troublesome. This intervention almost always elicits a surprised emotional response on the part of the client. The following is an example:

> Mrs. Curry received a regularly scheduled monthly visit from the public health nurse. Instead of finding her in the kitchen cleaning up after breakfast as was usually the case, the nurse found Mrs. Curry sitting on the living room couch, still in her nightgown and robe, crying and wringing her hands. The nurse sat down next to her and asked what was wrong. Mrs. Curry replied, "I don't know. I don't know. I just feel awful—as if something horrible is happening to me. Please help me." The nurse then asked if something unusual had happened since her last visit. Mrs. Curry replied, "No, nothing except I am going crazy." The nurse asked Mrs. Curry to tell her what the days had been like for her starting with 2 weeks ago. Although Mrs. Curry protested mildly at having to go through the last 2 weeks in such detail, she complied with gentle questioning from the nurse. The nurse was not surprised to hear that Mrs. Curry's mother-in-law had moved into the home 6 days ago. After 1 or 2 days of settling-in activities, the mother-in-law requested to cook the meals "for my son" so that she would feel useful. Mrs. Curry stated that she felt resentful about turning over the meal preparation to her husband's mother but in turn felt guilty about her reaction, since she would now have more free time. As a result, she dismissed her feelings as "unreasonable," agreed to her mother-in-law's request, and made arrangements to go clothes shopping with a friend late the following afternoon. When the following afternoon arrived, Mrs. Curry could not meet her friend because she was immobilized by anxiety, the source of which was unknown to her. Since that time she had been relatively sleepless and decreasingly involved in the household activities. The above narra-

tive was related by Mrs. Curry in a matter-of-fact way and with no particular emotion until the nurse said, "Many people find that when a new member of the family moves in, there is a major adjustment to make. I wonder if that's what could be troubling you?" At that point, Mrs. Curry began to sob but stopped wringing her hands.

Once the event and those involved have been identified, they are helped to develop a plan for coping with the crisis situation. To be effective in this step, the crisis counselor needs to explore with the clients the resources that are available and known to them as well as to suggest resources available in the community about which they might not know. Most mentally healthy people have numerous interpersonal, social, and community resources available to them but may need help to identify the appropriate ones to use and to accept aid from. For clients to benefit from this step they need to be encouraged to make as many arrangements for help as possible by themselves. However, since high levels of anxiety often interfere with cognitive comprehension and retention of information, it is important to write out information. For example, if it is decided that the clients could benefit from a talk with a representative of a social service agency, the name and telephone number of the agency and a suggested day and time for the clients to call for an appointment should be clearly written out.

> An effective plan for coping with the crisis situation must include awareness of available resources.

These steps in crisis intervention are designed to help the clients achieve a correct cognitive perception of the situation, which is enhanced by the counselor's seeking the facts surrounding the situation and by her helping the clients to keep the problem in their consciousness.

Another vital aspect of crisis intervention is assisting the clients in managing their feelings. To achieve this goal, the clients need to develop an awareness of their feelings. Appropriate verbalization of them, assisted by the reflection of the crisis counselor, leads to desensitization and mastery of the feelings that seem overwhelming. In helping clients deal with their feelings, it is important not to give them false reassurance, although it is helpful to tell them that they are likely to feel better in 1 or 2 months despite the fact that it may seem impossible at this point. As previously stated, it is also important not to encourage them to blame others. If the counselor falls into this trap, the result is to support the clients' natural avoidance of looking at their own behavior, thereby decreasing their opportunities to develop more mature patterns of coping.

> To successfully manage their feelings, clients need to develop an awareness of them.

All these steps are usually gone through in the initial contact with persons in a crisis. Obviously such an interview may take longer than the traditional 50-minute therapy hour. Since the best results in crisis situations seem to be achieved through intensive but short-term intervention, it is advisable to spend as much time as necessary, as often as necessary, with the clients without engendering unwarranted dependency. At the end of the first visit the crisis counselor will make a specific appointment to see the clients again, preferably in a few days but no longer than a week later. In the meantime the clients should know how they can contact her and should be encouraged to do so if they feel it is necessary. Often the knowledge that help is readily available is sufficient to enable the clients to manage without a telephone call until the next appointment.

During subsequent contacts the clients are assisted to go through the same steps all over again. In addition, the plan that was made in the previous session needs to be evaluated in terms of its effectiveness. If it seems to be working, it should be reinforced by supporting the clients' efforts at implementation. If the plan is not working or if new factors have altered the situation, the plan needs to be revised accordingly, but always with the mutual agreement of those involved.

In summary, crisis intervention is designed to help essentially healthy persons who are in a state of disequilibrium to help themselves. This goal is facilitated by assisting them to achieve correct cognitive perception of the situation and to gain effective management of their emotions. Successful resolution of crisis situations results in the clients' developing a larger repertoire of adaptive mechanisms, which in turn enables them to function on a level higher than the level on which they were functioning prior to the crisis state. In this way, effective crisis intervention prevents mental illness and promotes mental health.

END NOTE

This chapter discusses crisis theory and intervention as a potent means for promoting mental health and preventing mental illness in essentially mentally healthy individuals and their families. Although crisis intervention is a technique employed by members of all mental health disciplines, the nurse is often in a position to engage in its use and to consult with other health care professionals about those in a crisis state.

SUGGESTED SOURCES OF ADDITIONAL INFORMATION

Aguilera DC and Messick JM: Crisis intervention: theory and methodology, ed 5, St Louis, 1986, CV Mosby Co.

Britton JG and Mattson-Melcher DM: The crisis home: sheltering patients in emotional crisis, J Psychosoc Nurs 23:18, December 1985.

Ching J, Gordon R, and O'Mahoney M: Crisis intervention following severe psychological trauma in late pregnancy, Hosp Commun Psychiatr 32:53, January 1981.

Crisis intervention, Adv Nurs Sci 6: 1984.

Gaston S: Death and midlife crisis, J Psychosoc Nurs Ment Health Serv 18:31, January 1980.

Grier AM and Aldrich CK: The growth of a crisis intervention unit under the direction of a clinical specialist in psychiatric nursing, Perspect Psychiatr Care 10:73, April-June 1972.

Harrison DF: Nurses and disasters, J Psychosoc Nurs Ment Health Serv 19:34, December 1981.

Hatch C and Schut L: Description of a crisis-oriented psychiatric home visiting service, J Psychosoc Nurs Ment Health Serv 18:31, April 1980.

King JM: The initial interview: basis for assessment in crisis intervention, Perspect Psychiatr Care 9:247, November-December 1971.

Mitchell CE: Identifying the hazard: the key to crisis intervention, Am J Nurs 77:1194, 1977.

Murphy S: After Mount St. Helens: disaster stress research, J Psychosoc Nurs Ment Health Serv 22:8, July 1984.

Norman E: PTSD: the victims who survived, Am J Nurs 82:1696, 1982.

Parad HJ, editor: Crisis intervention: selected readings, New York, 1965, Family Service Association of America.

Sheehy G: Passages: predictable crises of adult life, New York, 1976, EP Dutton & Co.

Group theory and intervention

25

LEARNING OBJECTIVES

After studying this chapter the student will be able to:

○ Discuss the characteristics of groups.

○ State the goal of a therapeutic group.

○ Discuss the developmental phases of a therapeutic group.

○ State examples of the role of the leader in each phase of group development.

○ Discuss the characteristics of socialization groups.

○ Describe psychodrama, transactional analysis, and gestalt therapy as group interventions.

Human beings spend most of their time in group situations. They live, work, play, learn, and worship in groups. Group association is a prominent part of everyone's life because human beings are inherently social and because in complex, technological societies individuals are interdependent and must rely on each other for services. Therefore the nature of our humanness and the nature of the society in which we live dictate the necessity for a social structure organized around groups.

The individual's first experience with groups occurs in infancy when he is incorporated into his family—a specialized type of natural group. The second major group situation most people experience is school. In fact, significant group associations continue throughout the entire life span. Despite the pervasiveness of groups in our society, however, few persons give any thought to the nature and function of groups.

HISTORICAL PERSPECTIVE

Interestingly, the intervention known as group therapy did not originate within the mental health delivery system. Rather, it began in 1905 as a technique to assist patients with tuberculosis to learn about their illness and to receive emotional support from each other. The success of these groups soon led to their use with patients suffering from "nervous disorders." It was not until World War II that group therapy became a standard intervention for the treatment of persons diagnosed as mentally ill.

During World War II many members of the civilian population as well as large numbers of Armed Forces personnel required psychiatric help. It became obvious that the traditional treatment methods utilized at that time could not provide the help required by the large population of individuals who were mentally ill. To make maximum use of psychiatrically trained personnel a plan was initiated through which patients were encouraged to talk out their problems in groups. As psychiatrists worked with this method and developed an effective technique that could be taught to others, it became obvious not only that group therapy was a more efficient means by which relatively few personnel could treat a large number of patients but also, more important, that this mode of therapy had effects that could not be achieved through individual, one-to-one therapy. Some theorists believe that one reason for this positive effect is that groups tend to simulate the familial situation, wherein the leaders are seen in the role of parent figures and group members are seen as siblings. Therefore it becomes possible for persons who have had difficulty in their early family relationships to experientially work through many problems as a result of their interaction with other group members. Group members also find support and reassurance in the realization that others have problems that are similar to theirs. Consequently, group intervention is seen as the treatment of choice for some individuals.

CHARACTERISTICS OF GROUPS

Group
An identifiable system composed of three or more individuals who engage in certain tasks to achieve a common goal.

A group is not a mere collection of individuals. Rather, a group is an identifiable system composed of three or more individuals who engage in certain tasks to achieve a common goal. Furthermore, to be a group the members must relate to each other, usually around the tasks and goals of the group. The individuals who ride the elevator in a skyscraper office building to get to their offices may share the common goal of getting to work, but they rarely relate to each other about this goal. Therefore they would not be considered a group. If, on the other hand, the elevator stalled between floors and its occupants expressed their fears to each other, offered each other emotional support, made plans to get themselves out of their predicament, or otherwise began relating to each other, they would quickly become a group in the technical sense of the word.

To be a group, members must relate to each other, usually around the tasks and goals of the group.

As identifiable systems, groups share certain characteristics regardless of their differences in size, task, or goal. Since nursing care is often rendered in group situations, it is important for the nurse to develop an understanding of these characteristics.

Groups can be composed of as few as 3 or as many as 20 members. The upper limit of membership size is determined by the number of individuals who can easily relate to each other at the same time. In most group situations it is not possible for more than 20 people to meet this criterion, and even then difficulty is encountered. When a group is larger than the number of individuals who can comfortably relate to one another simultaneously, *subgroups* are formed. For example, the 100-member senior class at the local high school cannot possibly function as a total group but is likely to be an aggregate of subgroups. Groups that are very small (3 or 4 members) also are not likely to be the most effective, since there may be insufficient membership to fulfill all the roles necessary for the achievement of the group's goal.

All groups have goals. These may be multiple or single. Multiple goals may have equivalent importance, or they may be prioritized according to their value. Group members may or may not be equally aware of and supportive of the goals of the group. However, the group's effectiveness is strongly related to the degree to which the members are aware of and supportive of the goals. When the goals have been achieved, the group either disbands or determines new goals. Natural groups, such as families, tend to remain as groups by redefining their goals. Groups that have been formed around a single goal tend to disband after achievement of that goal. An example of such a group is the aforementioned senior high school class. The graduating seniors commonly feel a strong group association and promise to maintain contact with each other after graduation, but because the group has achieved its goal and disbands, the group members rarely follow through on their promise.

A group is a system and as such functions in a manner designed to maintain its equilibrium. Therefore the behavior of any one member affects and is affected by all other group members and must be seen as reflective of group behavior. Learning to view group behavior from a holistic perspective, rather than as a summation of individual interactions, is a difficult task for most students. A commonly used example that may be helpful in this regard is that of a symphony orchestra. If the listener attends to only the notes played by each individual, he will have a distorted impression of what the finished piece sounds like, because each musician contributes only a part of what is necessary to the completed piece. However, when the listener attends to the contributions of all the musicians put together, a synchronized, harmonious piece is heard. This example not only illustrates the concept that the whole is different from and greater than the sum of its parts but also implies that each part is necessary and of great value. In a group individuals have great value, but the result of their interactions is a product that can be best appreciated only when viewed from a group perspective.

The interactional behavior of the group's members has a great deal to do

An effective group is large enough to fulfill all the roles necessary to achieve the group's goals and small enough so that its members can comfortably relate to one another at the same time.

All groups have goals; in effective groups the members are aware of and support the group's goals.

Individuals have great value in a group, but the result of their interactions is best appreciated when viewed from a group perspective.

with the group's ability to achieve its goal. The term used to designate the behavior of group members is *role*. A role is the characteristic behavioral pattern employed by a group member and is determined by the personality of the individual and the needs of the group. At any point in time the group has a need to address the tasks necessary to achieve its goal, while simultaneously maintaining its life. Addressing the task is achieved through roles that have a content orientation, and group maintenance is achieved through roles that have a process orientation.

The content of a group is the overt verbal exchange, while the process is the underlying meaning the content has to the group, not to the individual. For example, Mr. Jones might say, "I'm not sure how to proceed." If Mr. Jones is viewed as an individual rather than as a group member, the content of his statement could lead one to believe that he feels insecure, a somewhat negative assessment. If this same content is viewed within the context of a group, it would be more appropriate to interpret the process as a need of the group for orientation and Mr. Jones as fulfilling the role of orienter. This interpretation not only conveys a positive tone, but is more accurate than the individually based one.

The roles assumed by group members relate to either the content or to the process of the group. Task- or content-oriented roles as suggested by Robert Bales* include coordinator, orienter, recorder, observer and commentator, opinion seeker or giver, elaborater, information seeker or giver, and initiator. Roles related to group maintenance or a process orientation include energizer, encourager, dominator, aggressor, compromiser, blocker, harmonizer, and rejecter.

These lists of roles are not intended to be reflective of all the possible roles a group member could assume. However, they do represent the most commonly seen behaviors of group members, and they also illustrate the reciprocal nature of content and process interactions (for example, information seeker or giver, encourager or blocker).

Since human beings have numerous experiences in many groups, by the time they reach adulthood most have developed a large repertoire of group behaviors. Therefore any one individual may assume different roles in different groups and different roles at different times in the same group, dependent in part on the needs of the group. Consequently, it is impossible to predict with complete assurance the role any individual will assume in a group. Furthermore, since the behavior of any group member affects and is affected by all other group members, it is not unusual for an individual to behave in a group in a way that is quite different from the way he behaves when relating to only one other individual.

To function effectively, groups develop rules or *norms* that govern their op-

The group needs to address the tasks necessary to achieve its goal while also maintaining its life.

An individual may assume different roles in different groups and different roles at different times in the same group.

---

*Bales R: Interaction process analysis: a method for the study of small groups, Reading, Mass, 1950, Addison-Wesley Publishing Co.

eration. Some norms may be externally imposed, but the norms that have the most meaning are those which have emerged from within the group. For example, group members are much more likely not to smoke if that norm was established by themselves rather than by the superintendent of the building in which they meet. Norms are sometimes fully known to all members and therefore can be explicitly stated. Other norms are not consciously formulated by the group but rather have evolved as a result of the group's experience. Whether the group norms are explicit or implicit, their purpose is to influence the behavior of the group. Since implicit norms cannot be overtly conveyed, individuals who join an established group may be in a precarious position because they may unknowingly violate an implicit norm and receive a negative, nonverbal reaction from the others. The violation of implicit group norms is the basis of many social faux pas. The power of implicit norms is attested to by the excruciating embarrassment experienced by the person who has committed a social error, even when the reality of his error does not warrant such a reaction.

> To function effectively, groups develop norms that govern their operation. Norms that have the most meaning are those which have emerged from within the group.

Another characteristic of groups is that each group has a unique identity, while at the same time sharing much in common with all other groups. The student will recognize this characteristic as also being true of individuals. The uniqueness of each group is based on the specific interactional combination of its size, its goals and the tasks designed to achieve its goals, the roles its members characteristically assume, and the norms the members establish to govern its operation. On the other hand, all groups share enough in common that an individual is able to apply that which he has learned in previous group associations to new group experiences. When a group is first formed, its members tend to behave in the ways they found to be successful in previous groups. As the group develops its own unique characteristics, its members modify their behavior to a greater or lesser degree to adapt to the group's uniqueness, thereby further enlarging their repertoire of group behaviors.

> Each group has a unique identity while also sharing much with all other groups. Members modify their behavior to adapt to the group's uniqueness.

The unique identity of a group is often recognized by both members and nonmembers. The reader is familiar with the "in-group, out-group" phenomenon where two superficially identical groups are valued very differently by their members. The group term for the value placed on a group by both its members and nonmembers is *attractiveness*. An in-group is seen as being attractive, an out-group unattractive. The degree of attractiveness a group has is determined to a large extent by its unique identity; the mere altering of a few members, goals, or norms does not succeed in altering the group's identity or resultant attractiveness.

Finally, all groups, just like individuals, go through predictable developmental phases. However, the time at which the group moves from one phase to another is not as uniform as it is with individual development. Rather, the speed of group development is determined by a number of factors unique to the group, such as the anticipated duration of the group's life, the developmental strengths and weaknesses of its members, the importance the group places on its goal, the relevance of its norms to its goals, and the group's attractiveness. In addition, groups may skip developmental phases for a variety of reasons. However all groups must go through a beginning and ending phase. These and the intermediate phases of group development are described in conjunction with the discussion of group therapy in this chapter.

GROUP THERAPY
Considerations in establishing a therapy group

Group psychotherapists differ in their approach when establishing a therapeutic group. Questions involving the size of the membership, the frequency of meetings, and the characteristics of the participants must be decided. As might be expected, authorities answer these questions according to their personal treatment philosophies.

Some group psychotherapists insist on a balanced group, which means that only individuals of the same age, sex, and diagnostic category should be included. Others do not believe that a balanced group is necessary or even conductive to the best possible group interaction. Another consideration is whether to include persons with different levels of intelligence or verbal skills. Since group therapy depends on effective communication skills, this may be an important consideration.

Certainly a decision must be made as to how large the group will be. Most authorities agree that a group should not be larger than 10, but many group leaders prefer a group no larger than 6. They also agree that the membership of a group should be stable.

A definite place in which to hold the group meeting must be identified. It should be quiet, comfortable, and private. The frequency and time of meeting must be decided as well as the date when group meetings will begin and end. When these decisions have been made and the group has come together for the first time, these norms should be shared with the members so that they will understand the nature of the contract they have with each other and with the group leader.

Some group leaders prefer to talk with potential group members before the actual group meetings begin. In this way each individual is acquainted with the nature of the sessions prior to the first meeting.

Characteristics of group therapy

The therapeutic group, like other groups, has a specific goal. It differs from a social group because its goal is to assist individuals to alter their behavioral patterns and to develop new and more effective ways of dealing with the stresses of daily living. To achieve this goal, individuals meet together regularly for a stated period to express their ideas, feelings, and concerns; to examine their current ways of behaving; and to develop new patterns of behavior.

The group leader works to develop among the group members a sense of

Margin note (left, upper): Before group meetings are initiated, decisions are made about the size of membership, frequency of meetings, time and place of meetings, and characteristics of members.

Margin note (left, lower): The goal of the therapeutic group is the alteration of the behavioral patterns of group members through the development of new and more effective ways of coping with stress.

trust in her as an individual and as a group leader. She avoids being critical or judgmental of the behavior of individual members of the group and relies on group action to control unacceptable behavior. The group leader strives to convey to the group members her acceptance of them as individuals and her respect for them as people. She avoids exerting undue control over the group or being the authority in the situation.

For a group to have maximum therapeutic effect it is essential that members learn to know and trust not only the leader but also each other. Therefore this becomes an important goal, the achievement of which is facilitated by the leader when she refers questions to the group, encourages participation from all members, and shows acceptance and respect for each individual. By engaging in these behaviors, the leader acts as a role model for the members. The inexperienced group leader will be surprised at how quickly the group members learn to act toward each other in the manner suggested by her behavior.

Group development

Every group, like every individual, progresses through several developmental phases. The first developmental phase of a group is the *preaffiliation* or *getting acquainted phase*. During this time group members behave toward each other as strangers and are obviously distrustful of each other and of the leader. Their expectations of the group activity are, of necessity, determined by experiences they have had in other groups. Although members are likely to be overtly polite to each other, their behavior also indicates an approach-avoidance dilemma. That is, most members are eager to become involved with each other but simultaneously fear the risks that such involvement may entail. During this stage the leader is most effective when she provides structure, protects members from embarrassment by not allowing them to prematurely reveal highly personal information, and gently invites trust.

The second developmental period is the *phase of experiencing intragroup conflict* and is characterized by power and control issues. Unavoidably, conflict will emerge during this time, since the members are in the process of establishing their positions in the group relative to the positions of other members and the leader. Often group members look to the leader for sanction or condemnation of another member. If the leader falls into this trap, she is likely to find the group critical of her because of her decision. In this instance it is always wise to deflect the question about a member's behavior back to the group by a comment such as, "I wonder what the rest of you think about Mr. Jones's question?" During this second phase of group development the group attempts to formalize relationships through the establishment of explicit norms. These attempts should be supported as long as they do not infringe on the rights or safety of one or more members. Throughout the group process the leader has the responsibility of protecting the safety of individuals and property, but the necessity for doing so becomes greatest during this second phase of group development. During the second phase group sessions may seem nonproductive in that the members alternate competitive, aggressive behavior with apathetic withdrawal. Interrelated with this phenomenon is the great danger of membership dropout.

If the leader can help the group safely navigate through this phase, characteristics of the third phase will emerge. This is called the *working phase* or the *phase of intimacy and differentiation*. During this phase the work of the group is achieved. It is a period of relatively high communication in which members appropriately share personal feelings and concerns about emotional problems.

During the working phase of the group the members' sense of belonging, or group *cohesiveness,* is at its highest. When a group is cohesive, its members tend to feel emotionally close to one another, and individuals respond well to advice offered by other members. Consequently, during this period there is an opportunity for emotional reeducation and relearning. The members discover through the reactions of the other group members that there are many different reactions to their feelings and behavior. They come to realize how universal their problems are and that they are not as unique in their difficulties as they may have believed.

The last developmental phase is precipitated by the approaching time for the group to conclude its meetings. Thus it is the *termination phase* and may require a number of meetings to work through the feelings of the individuals involved. The goal of the termination phase is to help group members integrate what they have learned about themselves and the behavioral changes they have made so that they can use these in the future. If the termination phase is not handled skillfully, not only will this goal not be achieved but the group members may also leave the group feeling that the only thing to be gained by group association is more emotional pain. During this period the members relive previous periods when they experienced personal loss of someone very close to them. They may express feelings of being abandoned, rejected, or forsaken. The expression of these feelings provides an excellent opportunity to help individual members of the group deal with these feelings and work through them.

Four phases of group development have been described. It should be noted, however, that these phases overlap one another and that only the first and the last are seen in all groups. Groups that meet for only a few sessions or groups whose members have a great deal of difficulty in trusting others are not likely to be able to move through the phase of experiencing intragroup conflict and the working phase. Consequently, the termination phase will not be as meaningful and therefore not as difficult as when the group has traveled successfully through all developmental phases.

Role of the leader

The group leader is the key to a successful group therapy experience. The leader needs to be aware of her own behavior and its effect on others. The effectiveness of the getting acquainted phase for the group is largely dependent on

Each group progresses through several developmental phases including getting acquainted, experiencing intragroup conflict, working, and termination.

An effective group leader is essential to successful group therapy.

the way in which the leader orients the members to the group process, to each other, and to herself. The phase of experiencing intragroup conflict can be successfully resolved if the group leader is able to be supportive to the members and successfully establishes a feeling of acceptance and respect for all. As the group moves into the working phase, the leader is able to involve the less verbal members by redirecting questions to them or by asking them for their perceptions of a situation. The leader sometimes provides essential factual information that is important to the resolution of an issue. On occasion the leader may help a member learn what others think about his behavior or his responses. The leader assist members in exploring situations they bring to the group from the outside and helps them to think through and test out more appropriate ways of responding.

As the group develops the leader will be confronted with a variety of specific problems in group interaction that will necessitate her intervention. Problems such as silence, monopolizing behavior, tardiness, and acting out on the

OF SPECIAL INTEREST

Why is group therapy helpful? Dr. Irvin D. Yalom believed that it was necessary to answer this question if the practice of group psychotherapy were to have a scientific basis rather than being determined by the fads of the day. Furthermore, he believed that the effective training of group psychotherapists depended on an answer to this question. In 1970, the first edition of his text, *The Theory and Practice of Group Psychotherapy,* was published. The following "curative factors"* of group therapy are identified and discussed in this text.

1. Imparting of information
2. Instillation of hope
3. Universality
4. Altruism
5. The corrective recapitulation of the primary family group
6. Development of socializing techniques
7. Imitative behavior
8. Interpersonal learning
9. Group cohesiveness
10. Catharsis

You may wonder how Dr. Yalom determined that these factors were curative. Dr. Yalom describes his methodology in Chapter 1 of his book. He reports that he engaged in a systematic research approach, correlating a series of in-therapy variables with ultimate patient outcome in therapy. In addition, he asked the opinions of practicing group therapists. Finally—and most astoundingly—he asked patients what they found helpful!

Perhaps we could learn a great deal more about what is helpful in psychiatric nursing if, in addition to engaging in research and relying on the experiences of expert psychiatric nurses, we were to ask clients to share their perceptions of what they found helpful about our interventions.

*Yalom ID: The theory and practice of group psychotherapy, New York, 1970, Basic Books, Inc.

part of members are common and require the skill of the leader if the group session is to be effective. It is beyond the scope of this text to discuss these problems and possible appropriate interventions, but the student should be aware that a number of excellent references are available that will provide specific direction. It should be noted, however, that the most effective group leader is one who is able to vary her style of intervention based on her assessment of the needs of the group.

Skillful termination of a group requires first and foremost that the leader recognize her own feelings of loss. If she recognizes her own feelings she is less likely to act them out by doing such things as "forgetting" the final meeting, acting punitively to members who express a sense of loss, or promising members that she will continue to contact them when this is not possible or desirable. The skillful group leader will understand that the anger at her and other members commonly expressed during this phase is a reflection of the severity of the loss the members are experiencing. She will not respond to anger with anger but will help the group members to acknowledge their sadness about the disbanding of the group.

Finally, the skillful group leader will help the group members to identify what they have gained through their association. If they identify these gains, the members will be able to take away something concrete that helps to offset the emotional loss.

Many group therapists believe that it is most beneficial to the group if two staff members act as co-therapists. In this situation one therapist is able to concentrate on the content being expressed while the other therapist focuses primarily on the group process. Although the co-therapists may change their function from one group session to another, it is believed that co-leaders who are experienced and comfortable with each other can view the group more comprehensively and therefore provide the group with helpful direction in regard to both content and process.

SOCIALIZATION GROUPS: A REMOTIVATION TECHNIQUE

Group interaction is one of the most successful ways of stimulating persons who have lost interest in their surroundings.

Psychiatric hospitals are frequently heavily populated with mentally ill persons who appear to have lost interest in reality, to have lost a sense of personal value, and who seem to be unaware of other persons with whom they come in daily contact. Group interaction is one of the most successful ways of stimulating these people to rekindle their interest in their surroundings.

The nurse may be the only person who is available or interested in developing some form of group experience that will encourage these individuals to begin to communicate with each other and with the staff. The primary goal of these group activities is to facilitate socialization and is most easily achieved by focusing on a task. If several persons come together as a group and carry on an activity for a few sessions, the initial attempt has been successful.

The focus of the group activity depends almost entirely on the individuals who are to be included as members. Their age, educational backgrounds, and physical health will greatly influence the choice of activities that can be suggested.

Some individuals might be interested in a current events discussion group. Others who evidence no interest in reading the newspaper or listening to the television news reports would not be interested in such a group activity. Some might be interested in forming a poetry reading group, whereas others would abhor such an activity. Some might enjoy sewing or knitting while they visit together; others would not.

In view of this wide variation in personal abilities and taste the first rule to follow in initiating any recreational or motivational activity is to be well acquainted with the individuals who will form the group membership. The leader will find that it is wise to encourage the members to participate in selecting the focus for the group meetings. Although she will formulate some tentative plans for the first meeting, these need to be flexible and easily changed in case there are suggestions from the members.

The leader will find that at first many persons will be reluctant to participate. Some individuals may require more than one friendly invitation to attend. Some who have lost interest in reality carry on an active fantasy life. Any group activity must compete with these fantasies for the individual's attention and enjoyment. Thus it is wise to offer the group members refreshments during the initial group meetings. As the group becomes cohesive, the members' interest in the group activity may become great enough to overshadow the food as the major enjoyment of the meeting.

It is wise to vary the focus of the group activity from time to time to maintain the interest of the group members. As the members become acquainted with one another, they themselves will suggest changes in the focus or the format of the meeting.

The following are some concrete suggestions for planning an effective socialization group experience:*

1. Develop a flexible plan that provides for change and spontaneity.
2. Encourage all group members to participate in planning.
3. Keep the plan practical and within achievable limits.
4. Initiate activities that group members are able to handle.
5. Provide something specific such as refreshments that will give each group member some tangible satisfaction.
6. Avoid monotony by varying the focus of group activity.
7. Maintain consistency in the feeling tone of each meeting so that group member's expectations will be fulfilled.

---

*Brown M and Fowler GR: Psychodynamic nursing—a biosocial orientation, ed 4, Philadelphia, 1972, WB Saunders Co.

PSYCHODRAMA

Another type of therapeutic experience sometimes provided for a group of clients is called psychodrama. This technique was developed by J. L. Moreno, a psychiatrist who began working with emotionally disturbed individuals in a theater in Vienna as early as 1941. Psychodrama is usually conducted by a leader who has been especially prepared to direct this type of activity. Although a variety of methods may be used, one of the more frequent techniques places the leader on a stage in front of an audience of clients and staff members. The leader identifies a situation in which interpersonal conflict is involved. He invites members of the audience to come to the stage to act out this human relations problem.

When members of the audience agree to accept parts in the drama, they are told the essential facts about the roles they are to play. The chosen situation frequently focuses on a conversation with the significant members of a family. In the role of an actor, the individual is given a specially selected part that affords him an opportunity to express his inner conflicts freely as a situation is acted out with other performers who symbolize or represent persons who are the real objects of his love or hate. For example, a son who normally represses his hostility toward his father may freely express it as an actor and may even reveal its basis. On the other hand, if he is induced to take the father role he may then be more objective and understanding about his own father's point of view. It is surprising how effectively individuals fill the roles to which they are assigned and how realistically feelings are expressed. The leader stops the action when he believes the enactment has progressed far enough to provide the audience with a basis for a fruitful discussion.

Another method that has been used productively in psychodrama is for the leader to request a volunteer from the audience to come forward and set up a situation that he wishes to portray. This person is also asked to select individuals from the audience to play the parts required and to provide the players with the necessary data about the roles they will enact. This technique focuses specially on some personal concern of the individual who volunteered to develop the psychodramatic situation. With either of these methods individuals from the audience may be asked to come forward to play the role of alter ego for the major characters in the psychodrama.

After the role playing is completed the people in the audience are given an opportunity to discuss the situation they have witnessed and experienced vicariously. The participants from the audience may focus attention on various aspects of the situation and frequently present similar life experiences.

Psychodrama provides individuals with an opportunity to express feelings and concerns that relate to a personal human relations situation that is like, but not identical to, a personal problem of their own. Thus psychodrama has somewhat the same therapeutic effect as *abreaction,* the lessening of emotional trauma by reenacting the situation. It also furnishes individuals with an oppor-

Psychodrama is a form of group therapy that allows individuals to role play problem situations by alternating various roles and to receive feedback from observers in the audience.

tunity for *catharsis,* an opportunity to freely express feelings. As in other group therapy situations, the individual is helped by the group to express feelings and consider them objectively.

The nurse is frequently involved in psychodrama as a role player or as a discussant. Skill and understanding of psychodrama are developed through continued participation in this treatment modality. Eventually the nurse may accept the role of the leader of the psychodrama sessions.

TRANSACTIONAL ANALYSIS

Transactional analysis is both a theoretical framework and a treatment method developed by Eric Berne. Its popularity and utility are attested to by the amount of literature available to laypersons on the subject. As a theory, transactional analysis postulates that each person has three elements of his personality in greater or lesser operation at any given point in time. These elements are (1) the immature, need-gratifying aspect, referred to as the Child, (2) the moralistic, rigid, standard-setting aspect, referred to as the Parent, (3) and the mature, reality-based aspect, referred to as the Adult. The student will notice the similarity between this theoretical formulation and Freud's conception of the id, superego, and ego, respectively. Unlike Freudian theory, however, Berne's construct does not imply a judgment about the existence of these personality elements. Rather, he states that problems arise only when there is an incongruency among the elements that are operating when people relate with each other. This belief is the foundation for his use of the term *transactional.* The emphasis on dysfunctional interpersonal relationships as the crux of emotional problems is reminiscent of Sullivan's theories. Consequently, Berne's theory of transactional analysis is seen by many as effectively combining the salient intrapsychic features of Freudian theory and the aspects of Sullivanian theory that provide direction for therapeutic intervention.

When persons communicate and the adult elements of their personalities are operative, it is likely that they will be effective in hearing and responding to each other. In addition, the nonverbal aspects of the process will be congruent with the verbal content and no hidden messages will be perceived by either person. Each will reality test on the basis of feedback received and each is likely to feel that the interaction has been satisfying. This is not to imply that no differences of opinion will arise during such an interaction, but the individuals will probably feel that any differences are based on content issues rather than on covert attempts to dominate, control, or otherwise minimize the value of the other person. Adult-Adult interactions are effective and therefore desirable interactional processes when the participants are engaged in problem-solving or task-oriented activities.

Another effective and desirable interactional process occurs when two or more chonological adults simultaneously have the child element of their personalities in preeminence. It is at these times they have fun "playing." Many

Transactional analysis uses the child-parent-adult framework to analyze and improve interactional patterns.

adults have had the experience of spontaneously engaging in what appear to be foolish or childlike activities with another adult, such as frolicking through a park on a beautiful autumn day instead of attending a scheduled meeting. As long as this behavior does not have major irreversible consequences and does not become a persistent pattern, it can enhance the individual's feelings of well-being and strengthen the relationship.

Problems arise when two persons characteristically relate to each other through divergent elements of their personalities. For example, a husband who relates to his wife through the parent element of his personality will feel continuously dissatisfied with their interactions unless she responds with the child element of her personality. If she does respond in this way, there may be little initial conflict because both their needs are superficially being met. However, it should be noted that neither is engaged in reality-testing behaviors and neither can change interactional elements without open conflict emerging. Therefore this pattern is growth-stifling for both partners.

The previous situation is merely one example of a common interactional problem. The reader can speculate as to the large variety of interactional problems that can occur when two or more people interact from the basis of incongruent personality elements. For more detailed explanations of transactional analysis the student is referred to the many excellent books on the subject.

Transactional analysis as a method of treatment is most effective as a form of family therapy. When this is not possible, it can be effectively implemented as a method of group therapy, in which the group members consciously and unconsciously assume characteristic familial roles. In either the family or group setting the participants can analyze their reactions and subsequent behavior in light of the Child-Parent-Adult framework and experience how they affect others and are affected by them. They also can experiment with using other elements of their personality and can receive immediate feedback.

Transactional analysis is also used for individual treatment. The effectiveness of this treatment modality is limited, however, since the client has only one other person with whom to interact, and feedback about behavioral changes in life situations is delayed. Nevertheless many therapists successfully adopt some of the concepts of transactional analysis in their treatment of individuals because these concepts are seen by many clients as easy to understand and relevant to their life situations.

Regardless of setting, the primary role of the transactional therapist is to observe and tactfully comment on the discrepancies between the personality elements of those engaged in the interactional process. The therapist often suggests and supports role playing with another personality element so that the person can experience its effects. The dynamics that underlie the person's use of one personality element as opposed to the other two are not always explored. If they are discussed, it is usually done in the context of the present rather than in terms of childhood experiences.

GESTALT THERAPY

Gestalt therapy is as much a philosophy as it is an intervention technique. Its developer is Frederic S. Perls, who has trained many others in its use. The emphasis in gestalt therapy is on treatment of the person as a holistic being, placing as much importance on somatic responses as on emotional responses. Proponents of gestalt therapy believe that many persons' problems emanate from the fact that individuals have lost touch with their feelings, both physical and emotional. If one is unaware of what one is feeling, the likelihood of being able to express these feelings is greatly diminished, and therefore one is unlikely to have one's needs met. Therefore treatment consists primarily of helping the individual increase sensory awareness of his present state. Once the individual begins the process of getting in touch with himself, his current relationships with others and with his environment are explored. The configuration of the holistic being in interaction with others and with the environment is referred to as the *gestalt* and is heavily based on systems theory. Although it is acknowledged that multiple factors produced the individual's current responses, the understanding of these factors is not believed to alleviate the present problems and they are therefore not explored.

> Gestalt therapy focuses on helping persons fulfill their potential through increased sensory awareness of themselves and their relationships with others and with the environment within the context of the present.

As with transactional analysis, the principles of gestalt therapy can be used in a one-to-one psychotherapeutic relationship but are most commonly practiced as a form of group therapy. Eight to 10 participants are seen as an ideal number for a gestalt group. The environment in which the group meets is viewed as instrumental in facilitating self-awareness. Therefore factors such as comfortable chairs, a pleasing decor, and adequate space are seen as essential. Techniques such as role playing and ventilation are used frequently. The ultimate goal of gestalt therapy is to assist the client to fulfill his potential, and therefore it is appropriately used with individuals interested in self-growth as well as with persons who are emotionally disturbed.

SELECTION OF A THERAPEUTIC GROUP

It is important to note that the type of group activity that is most appropriate for the mentally ill person depends on a number of variables including his degree of ego strength and his current insight into his problems. It is likely that a person whose contact with reality is tenuous would benefit most from a socialization group rather than from a more formal group psychotherapy session. As the client gains more ego strength, he may be introduced into a group whose primary goal is that of supportive therapy. As members progress in this type of group, the focus of the group may very well change to that of insight therapy. This is not to say that socialization groups do not have therapeutic effects, but rather that the degree of stress the person is able to tolerate should be a major determining factor in the decision as to the type of group in which he will participate. Furthermore, this determination should be made jointly by the multidisciplinary health care team, which is able to view the client from a variety of perspectives.

> The type of group activity most appropriate for persons who are mentally ill should be determined after consideration of a number of variables. As each individual progresses in treatment, the type of group activity appropriate to meet his needs will change.

GROWTH AND SELF-ACTUALIZATION GROUPS

Other types of groups such as sensitivity, encounter, and self-help groups are well known in our society. The nature of these groups will not be discussed here because expert leaders or facilitators of these groups believe that their primary goal is not and should not be therapeutic but rather educative, in the sense of self-growth, self-actualization, and increased self-awareness. Therefore these types of groups are rarely, if ever, used with mentally ill persons, and the nurse is not likely to be involved with them in a professional capacity. Nevertheless, there is much available literature about these groups that the reader may be interested in exploring.

END NOTE

It is ironic that all human beings spend most of their time in group situations, and yet few are aware of or understand the dynamics of group behavior. The psychiatric nurse cannot afford to be uninformed about the nature of groups and their behavior, since groups are used increasingly as a treatment modality for a wide variety of clients. Consequently, this chapter discusses the characteristics of a group, its developmental phases, and the role of the leader. Various types of group therapies are presented, and the student is encouraged to seek further information and experience in their use as therapeutic interventions.

SUGGESTED SOURCES OF ADDITIONAL INFORMATION

Adrian S: A systematic approach to selecting group participants, J Psychosoc Nurs Ment Health Serv 18:37, February 1980.

Bales R: Interaction process analysis: a method for the study of small groups, Reading, Mass, 1950, Addison-Wesley Publishing Co.

Beeber LS and Schmitt MH: Cohesiveness in groups: a concept in search of a definition, Adv Nurs Sci 9:1, 1986.

Birckhead L: The nurse as leader: group psychotherapy with psychiatric patients, J Psychosoc Nurs Ment Health Serv 22:24, June 1984.

Britnell J and Mitchell K: Inpatient group psychotherapy for the elderly, J Psychosoc Nurs Ment Health Serv 19:19, May 1981.

Collison C: Grappling with group resistance, J Psychosoc Nurs Ment Health Serv 22:6, August 1984.

Echternacht MR: Day treatment groups: helping patients stay out, J Psychosoc Nurs Ment Health Serv 22:11, October 1984.

Ernst C, Vanderzyl S, and Salinger R: Preparation of psychiatric inpatients for group therapy, J Psychosoc Nurs Ment Health Serv 19:28, July 1981.

Hoover R and Parnell P: An inpatient educational group on stress and coping, J Psychosoc Nurs Ment Health Serv 22:16, June 1984.

Moreno JL: Psychodrama, 1946, Beacon Press.

Neizo B and Murphy M: Medication groups on an acute psychiatric unit, Perspect Psychiatr Care 21:70, April-June 1983.

Newton G: Self-help groups: can they help? J Psychosoc Nurs Ment Health Serv 22:27, July 1984.

Pelletier L: Interpersonal communications task group, J Psychosoc Nurs Ment Health Serv 21:32, September 1983.

Rogers C: On encounter groups, New York, 1970, Harper & Row.

Small LL: Finding your leadership style in groups, Am J Nurs 80:1301, 1980.

Spetz H: Contemporary trends in group psychotherapy: a literature survey, Hosp Commun Psychiatr 35(2):132, 1984.

Von Mering O and King SH: Remotivating the mental patient, New York, 1957, Russell Sage Foundation.

Whitaker D and Lieberman M: Psychotherapy through the group process, Chicago, 1964, Aldine Publishing Co.

White E and Kahn EM: Use and modifications in group psychotherapy with chronic schizophrenic outpatients, J Psychosoc Nurs Ment Health Serv 20:14, February 1982.

Yalom ID: Inpatient group psychotherapy, New York, 1983, Basic Books, Inc.

Yalom ID: The theory and practice of group psychotherapy, ed 3, New York, 1985, Basic Books, Inc.

Family theory and intervention

26

LEARNING OBJECTIVES

After studying this chapter the student will be able to:

○ Define the term *family.*

○ Discuss the functions of the family.

○ Discuss the developmental stages of the family according to Duvall.

○ Discuss the patterns of behavior characteristic of the effective family.

○ Describe the characteristics of the child-abusing family as an example of the ineffective family.

○ Explain the rationale underlying the use of family therapy as a treatment modality.

It is commonly asserted that the family is the most basic of all societal institutions. This assertion stems from two factors. The first is the universal tendency of human beings to organize themselves around the structure of the family. Second, it is believed that the experiences a child has as a family member have the most powerful influence on the kind of adult he will become. Therefore the society as a whole is very much affected by the family, both directly and indirectly, in both the present and future. Other societal institutions, such as the school and the church, are certainly fundamental to the society but are believed to be organizational structures that fulfill functions that historically have been delegated by the family. These societal institutions have developed in the belief that the collective society can fulfill certain functions more efficiently than can the singular family. However, the question of whether the society can fulfill these functions more effectively than the family is the subject of continuous de-

The experiences a child has as a family member have the most influence on the kind of adult he will become.

bate, and dynamic fluctuations of functions between the family and other societal institutions can be observed over the course of generations.

A nurse's interactions with an individual are indirect interactions with that individual's family because the family is a system.

The nurse often deals not just with an individual but also with a family. This contact may be direct and formalized as when engaged in family therapy or direct but informal as when seeking information from or supplying information to family members. Some family theorists believe that even when the nurse is dealing only with an individual it is impossible for the interaction not to affect and be affected by that individual's family. Therefore interactions with an individual are seen as indirect interactions with that individual's family. This view stems from the belief that the family is a system. The behavior of an individual is greatly influenced by his family, and in turn, any alterations in his behavior invariably affect his family. Whether one agrees with this view or not, it is hard to deny the fact that to be effective the nurse needs to understand the family.

HISTORICAL PERSPECTIVE

Awareness of the family as a significant social institution has been present throughout history. However, it was not until the twentieth century that the family was recognized as a system and studied as such. Prior to that time the family unit was understood to be a summation of the characteristics of its members. This view resulted in ascribing praise or blame to one or more family members for the effectiveness of the family's functioning. When a member was diagnosed as being mentally ill, it was often thought to be the fault of the parents, particularly the mother.

The family unit was not studied as a system until the escalating divorce rate after World War II created national concern about the future of the family in this country. In retrospect it seems clear that the large number of divorces that occurred after World War II resulted from the fact that while husbands were serving in the Armed Forces wives were working in factories, both evolving adaptations in the absence of the other. When the husband returned, the lifestyles that each had evolved were not necessarily compatible, and no help was available to assist the marriage partners to regain system homeokinesis.

Three of the earliest proponents of family therapy were Nathan W. Ackerman at Columbia University, Gerald Caplan at Harvard, and Don Jackson at the University of California. Their earliest work was done in the 1950s. Since that time many theorists have studied the family as a system, and currently there is general agreement that effective promotion of mental health and prevention and treatment of mental illness must take place within a family context. What remains as an unresolved dilemma is how to deliver this type of care within a health delivery system designed to focus on the individual.

FAMILY STRUCTURE

The extended family is a type of family structure seen in nonindustrial societies and consists of several generations living together.

In nonindustrial societies the family pattern most commonly observed is the *extended family,* where several generations live together and leave only for the purpose of joining another extended family through marriage. Before the Industrial

Revolution families in the United States often consisted of children, parents, and grandparents and perhaps one or more unmarried aunts or uncles. This pattern of family life provided the work force necessary for the productive management of the family business, usually the farm. When daughters married, they often left their family to join the family of their husband, while the sons' wives were incorporated into their family. This traditional family structure was also the mechanism whereby family resources, primarily land, were passed from generation to generation. The advantages of the extended family structure were many—physical and emotional resources were shared among a large group, and a broad division of labor was possible.

However, there were also many disadvantages. Families whose offspring were all female had to face the possibility of all the children leaving, thereby placing the elderly parents in a very vulnerable economic and social position. Furthermore, although the prescribed roles of each family member provided stability and continuity, this prescription also thwarted individuality. The eldest boy was expected to continue the family business, leaving the younger brother, who might have been more interested and capable of so doing, the choice of either striking out on his own or working at the behest of his older sibling. The image we now have of the "good old days" as characterized by close-knit, warm, loving families is believed by most authorities to be a distortion of the reality of intense sibling rivalry and parental frustration.

The settlement of the Western frontier, which placed great value on rugged individualism, and the Industrial Revolution both contributed greatly to a dramatic change in the typical family structure. Individuals moved from settled rural areas to the unsettled West or to industrialized urban areas with the goal of making their own fortune. A pervasive belief in both instances was that more money could be earned with less labor. Initially that belief proved to be false as evidenced by the hardships of Western settlement and the horrors of the urban sweatshop. The mobility of American citizens along with waves of European immigrants combined to create cities where people lived in dense concentration. Population density and mobility mitigated against the perpetuation of the extended family, and the nuclear family structure became the norm.

The *nuclear family* is defined as a two-generational family where it is understood that the children will leave once they have achieved maturity. Therefore the nuclear family, as a family, is only a temporary arrangement. Although the nuclear family has the disadvantages of potential alienation from the family of origin and fewer emotional supports from within the family, it has the major advantage of facilitating upward social mobility because it tends not to predetermine the children's roles as inheritors of the family business.

The nuclear family is a type of family structure seen in industrialized societies and consists of two generations.

DEFINITION OF FAMILY

A family is traditionally defined as two or more people who are related by blood or by legal ties such as marriage or adoption. However, a family also has the characteristic of identifying itself and being identified by others as such. Sharing

A family is traditionally defined as two or more people who are related by blood or legal ties, although an increasing number of nonrelated groups are identifying themselves as families.

a common surname is a manifestation of this characteristic, although it is not requisite to being a family as evidenced by the increasing number of young women in our society who retain the surname of their family of origin after marriage. Another characteristic of a family is that it is a relatively permanent human affiliation. A family, therefore, has a history and a future.

In the complex, highly mobile, technological society in which we live, there are an increasing number of human groups that identify themselves as a family and that exist over a period of time, but whose members do not meet the traditional criteria of being related by blood or by legal ties. Therefore a more accurate and relevant definition of family may be one that reflects the functions of a family.

FUNCTIONS OF THE FAMILY

A family is a specialized group that bands together in pursuit of the common goal of growth and development of its members. This goal is achieved through certain functions. Although none of these functions is unique to the family, the combination of them is unique to this institution. The following is a list of functions considered by most authorities to belong to the family.

Regulation of sexual activity and reproduction. The family structure provides for socially sanctioned sexual activity between spouses, while at the same time enforcing the societal taboo against incest by defining parental and sibling relationships. Survival of the culture is ensured by systematizing reproduction within a context that is capable of providing for children who in turn become the vehicle for the transmission of cultural values and practices. Therefore a family conveys to its children its cultural heritage as a means of ensuring the culture's future.

Physical maintenance. The family structure provides a vehicle through which the physical needs of its members can be met. It provides an efficient means of organizing responsibility for meeting the needs of individuals for food, clothing, shelter, and health care. In this regard the family can be seen as an economic unit.

Protection. The family structure is designed to provide both literal and figurative protection of its members by providing a model for interacting with the society in a way that protects the family members from undesirable outside influences.

Education and socialization. Some authorities believe that the family's function of providing education and socialization is the most fundamental one in that it is through the family that children learn how to function in and relate to the world in which they live.

Recreation. Traditionally the family has been the structure in which the individual has engaged in leisure time activities that are a source of personal and group refreshment and renewal, leading to increased family cohesion. The function of recreation is feared to be rapidly waning since the advent of television and other passive or nonparticipant forms of recreation.

Status conferring. Another traditional function of the family that seems to be undergoing fundamental alteration is that of status conferring. Before the advent of industrialization in a democratic society, which places emphasis on individualism, the individual was conferred social status by virtue of the family into which he was born. Although this is no longer strictly the case today, social status is still somewhat determined by the socioeconomic level of one's family of origin.

Affection giving. Only within the family can an individual be guaranteed unconditional acceptance by the mere fact of his relationship to that family. In all other societal interactions, acceptance of an individual is determined by such things as the quality or speed of his performance, his appearance, his social class, or his occupation. In functional families acceptance is conveyed by a deep, enduring affection among the members.

• • •

A perusal of these family functions reveals that the family unit provides services that are essential to the survival and stability of the society. For example, by regulating sexual activity within the family, society is protected from the consequences of wanton mating. Simultaneously, the family unit provides essential services to its members, such as physical maintenance and affection giving.

All functions of a family are not equally prominent at any given time. Each function is more specific to certain stages of family development than others and as such becomes a developmental task of the family.

Family sociologist Evelyn Duvall* has outlined a series of developmental stages of the family. This concept is not without problems but nevertheless provides a useful frame of reference from which many traditional families can be viewed.

DEVELOPMENTAL STAGES OF THE FAMILY

The first stage of family development is divided into two phases and is represented by the childless newly married couple. The initial phase begins at the time of marriage and consists of two persons (a dyad) who have made a major commitment to each other and therefore have the task of adjusting to living together as a married pair. This period of family life is filled with great stress as the two persons negotiate to effect a union while at the same time attempting to maintain their individuality. In other words these two individuals are learning to assume the roles of husband and wife. The divorce rate during this stage is very high, probably due to the shattering of the romantic illusion fostered during the preceding courtship period. The second phase of this stage commences

Traditional families progress through a series of developmental stages that are primarily related to role changes of their members.

*Duvall EM: Family development, Philadelphia, 1962, JB Lippincott Co.

with the wife's pregnancy. The family goal during this phase is to adjust to the pregnancy, which often means a change in affective focus. Prior to pregnancy both the husband and wife are focused on each other, but during pregnancy the wife becomes increasingly self-absorbed as she emotionally prepares for the birth of the child. In addition the husband may feel an increase in responsibility, especially if the couple decides that the wife should leave an income-producing job.

The second stage of family development begins when the first child is born and generally is believed to last until this eldest child enters school. The major change experienced by the husband and wife is the expansion of their roles to include those of father and mother. The family unit is reorganized around the needs of infants and preschool children, which often require dramatic shifts in priorities and activities.

The third stage of family development begins when the eldest child enters school and ends when this child becomes an adolescent. If there are younger siblings, the family unit needs to reorganize to fit into the expanding world of school-aged children, while still meeting the needs of the preschoolers. Through the school-aged child the family is often confronted for the first time with societal values that may conflict with family values. The goal of this stage is for the family to protect school-aged children from undesirable influences while still enabling them to fit into the larger social world.

The fourth stage of a family's development begins when the oldest child becomes an adolescent. The family goal during this very tumultuous time is to loosen family ties to permit greater freedom and heavier responsibility of the members. This task is not easy because the children have a history of dependence on their parents and often overreact to their newfound independence, resulting in an increase rather than the desired decrease in the control behaviors of the parents.

The fifth stage is referred to as the *launching* stage because it is during this time that the children are preparing to or are actually leaving home. This developmental task requires the reorganization of the family into an egaletarian unit as opposed to the earlier superior and subordinate structure. At this time the family needs to be able to release its members. It superficially appears that parents would have the most difficulty with this task, but often it is equally difficult for children to assume adult responsibility and leave the family to start their own family.

The next stage is termed the *postparental family* and is characterized by the parents' having to subsume their parental roles to their marital roles. In other words, the father and mother are left with no children to parent and find themselves with only each other to relate to. This stage is commonly referred to as the *empty nest syndrome* and is successfully navigated only if the parents were able to satisfactorily maintain their marital relationship during the childbearing and childrearing years. During this stage parents often become grandparents, an event that once again requires learning a new role. Although the grandparent role has similarities to the parent role, it is fundamentally different because the ultimate responsibility for children rests with the parents, not the grandparents.

The last stage of family development is the retirement and postretirement years. During this time the couple prepares for the dissolution of the family by the death of one of the spouses. Couples who have satisfactorily achieved the earlier tasks and are able to view their families as satisfactory are able to thoughtfully prepare for this eventuality without undue anxiety.

THE CHANGING FAMILY

The structure, size, functions, and developmental stages of the family are undergoing many changes in today's society. For example, it is not uncommon for a family to consist of only one parent who is raising one or more children and fulfilling both roles of mother and father. Increasingly common are *blended* or *reconstituted families* that consist of a parent who had been previously married and has children. This parent is married to another parent who also has children from a previous marriage. Such a couple may also have children of their own so that the family's task in this instance is to "blend" together three different sets of children into a functional family structure.

> A common change in family structure is the *blended* or *reconstituted family*. The nurse must expand her view of family when dealing with individuals who live in "nontraditional" structures.

Finally we are seeing an increase in the number of people who are joining together to form a family group based on mutual respect and common interests rather than for the purpose of procreation. These persons may or may not be related by blood or by law but tend to reside in the same household. The household concept, or living under the same roof, has been the criterion used by the U.S. Census Bureau to define a family. With the multiplicity of family structures apparent in the society this criterion may prove to be the most applicable. In any event, it is important for the nurse to extend her view of family beyond the traditional nuclear or extended family structure when dealing with individuals who do not live in these structures, if she is to accurately assess the individual's familial associations and dynamics. An example is the instance in which an adult woman was admitted to the hospital for surgery and was asked to supply the name of her next of kin. She responded by stating that her only blood relative lived at a great distance and was not involved in her day-to-day affairs and that she preferred to have her housemate of 5 years listed as the person to be notified in an emergency. The admitting clerk replied that the person listed on the chart had to be related by blood or law. This situation reflects the legal and societal lag so often apparent in our society that put this woman in jeopardy by forcing her to either lie to get her needs met or to tell the truth but forego gratification of her needs—all at a time when she was already under the stress of ill health and impending surgery.

THE EFFECTIVE FAMILY

The effective family* is one that is able to facilitate the growth and development of its members while still maintaining cohesion as an identifiable system. This definition implies that the following patterns of behavior are characteristic of an effective family:

1. The family places the emotional, physical, and social needs of its members over other concerns, such as acquisition of possessions or status.
2. The family recognizes, values, and accommodates to differences among its members.
3. The family is sufficiently flexible so that changes stemming from within and outside the system can be accommodated without loss of family stability.
4. The family seeks and uses information from relevant outside sources, simultaneously maintaining its autonomy.
5. The family makes and carries out decisions, taking into account its goals and the age and experience of its members.

An effective family is not necessarily a family without problems. Rather, an effective family is one that has developed a structure and pattern of functioning that enables it to deal with its problems productively as they arise. Just as is true of individuals, families must learn these processes, and many authorities believe that helping young families to develop effective patterns of functioning is the crux of promoting mental health.

Most young people receive no preparation for establishing an effective family. Therefore they unconsciously perpetuate the only patterns of familial functioning they know—the patterns they experienced in their families of origin. If fortuitously such learned patterns of behavior are conductive to effective family functioning, effective families will perpetuate. If ineffective patterns are learned, the probability of perpetuating ineffective family patterns is greatly enhanced.

> An effective family is able to deal with problems productively when they arise.

THE INEFFECTIVE FAMILY

Families that are unable to establish and maintain a structure and patterns of behavior conducive to effective functioning often show signs of continuous and irresolvable stress. Such stress may be manifested by the entire system, as in instances where there is overt tension and hostility among members, or the stress may be focused on only one member who is covertly designated to assume and act out the family problems. In this instance the family member is often, although not always, a child. This phenomenon occurs because children are likely to be the most vulnerable, since they are so highly dependent on the family and their behavioral patterns are less firmly entrenched. Bed-wetting, learning difficulties, antisocial behaviors, and profound fears in a child are all seen to be symptoms of an ineffective family.

> Ineffective families show signs of continuous and irresolvable stress manifested by either the entire system or by one of its members.

---

*Adapted from Sedwick R: Family mental health, St Louis, 1981, The CV Mosby Co., pp. 20-24.

It is beyond the scope of this text to discuss the many types of family dysfunction. The following discussion of child abuse is presented as an example of one increasingly common and very serious form of ineffective family functioning.

THE CHILD-ABUSING FAMILY

The incidence of reported child abuse appears to be dramatically increasing. However, accurate statistics are difficult to obtain because the phenomenon is poorly defined. Child abusers often go to extraordinary lengths to conceal their actions, and friends, relatives, and health care providers are hesitant to get involved. Nevertheless, it is known that the neglect or abuse of children occurs often enough to be of major concern to the legal and health care professions.

Child abuse can range from violent, physical attacks that result in severe injury to passive neglect that results in insidious malnutrition. Child abuse is not limited to physical maltreatment; it also includes emotional maltreatment such as continual yelling at and berating the child.

Children are the usual victims of family violence because they are relatively powerless and, until they reach adolescence are certainly physically weaker than adults. The pattern of the powerless becoming victims of violence is seen not only in child abuse but also in wife battering and the tyrannization of the elderly in their homes and on the street.

The concept of powerlessness includes not only physical weakness but also social subordination. Children, women and the elderly are all persons who traditionally have had less power in our society than has the young adult male. This situation is gradually changing. The values, needs, and rights of children, women, and the elderly are being recognized and becoming protected by law. These persons therefore are achieving a modicum of social power. Ironically some authorities believe that the very amelioration of this problem is contributing to its intensification, a phenomenon that is not socially unusual. In other words, individuals who have no power and do not assert themselves are often not overtly abused. An example is the benevolent plantation owner who had a patronizingly paternal attitude toward his compliant slaves. Once the slaves began to assert themselves, however, much more systematic and spontaneous abuse occurred. Likewise, as children, women, and the elderly achieve more power, they are more likely to constitute a threat and therefore be abused more often.

Table 26-1 lists physical and behavioral indicators of child abuse and neglect. It should be noted that the laws of most states require that health care personnel report to legal authorities situations in which child abuse or maltreatment is suspected; most state laws do not require proof before reporting child abuse or maltreatment. After a report is made the child protective agency is responsible for the actual determination of the situation.

Many health care professionals, including nurses, are very hesitant to report

Child abuse ranges from violent, physical attacks to passive neglect. Maltreatment may be physical or emotional.

Children are the usual victims of family violence because they are relatively powerless, being both physically weaker and socially subordinate.

TABLE 26-1 *Physical and behavioral indicators of child abuse and neglect**

Type of abuse/neglect	Physical indicators	Behavioral indicators
Physical abuse	Unexplained bruises and welts: on face, lips, mouth on torso, back, buttocks, thighs in various stages of healing clustered, forming regular patterns reflecting shape of article used to inflict (electric cord, belt buckle) on several different surface areas regularly appear after absence, weekend, or vacation Unexplained burns: cigar, cigarette burns, especially on soles, palms, back, or buttocks immersion burns (socklike, glovelike, doughnut shaped on buttocks or geni- talia) patterned like electric burner, iron, etc. rope burns on arms, legs, neck, or torso infected burns, indicating delay in seek- ing treatment Unexplained fractures/dislocations to skull, nose, facial structure in various stages of healing multiple or spiral fractures Unexplained lacerations or abrasions: to mouth, lips, gums, eyes to external genitalia in various stages of healing Bald patches on the scalp	Feels deserving of punishment Wary of adult contacts Apprehensive when other children cry Behavioral extremes: aggressiveness withdrawal Frightened of parents Afraid to go home Reports injury by parents Vacant or frozen stare Lies very still while surveying surroundings Will not cry when approached by examiner Responds to questions in monosyllables Inappropriate or precocious maturity Manipulative behavior to get attention Capable of only superficial relationships Indiscriminately seeks affection Poor self-concept
Physical neglect	Underweight, poor growth pattern, failure to thrive Consistent hunger, poor hygiene, inappro- priate dress Consistent lack of supervision, especially in dangerous activities or for long periods Wasting of subcutaneous tissue Unattended physical problems or medical needs Abandonment Abdominal distention Bald patches on the scalp	Begging, stealing food Extended stays at school (early arrival and late departure) Rare attendance at school Constant fatigue, listlessness, or falling asleep in class Inappropriate seeking of affection Assuming adult responsibilities and con- cerns Alcohol or drug abuse Delinquency (e.g., thefts) States there is no caretaker
Sexual abuse	Difficulty in walking or sitting Torn, stained, or bloody underclothing Pain, swelling, or itching in genital area Pain on urination Bruises, bleeding, or lacerations in external genitalia, vaginal, or anal areas Vaginal/penile discharge Venereal disease, especially in preteens Poor sphincter tone Pregnancy	Unwilling to change for gym or participate in physical education class Withdrawal, fantasy, or infantile behavior Bizarre, sophisticated, or unusual sexual behavior or knowledge Poor peer relationships Delinquent or runaway Reports sexual assault by caretaker Change in performance in school

*Heindl C et al: The nurse's role in the prevention and treatment of child abuse and neglect. DHEW Publication No. (OHDS) 79-30202, Washington, DC, 1979, US Government Printing Office, p. 10.

TABLE 26-1   *Physical and behavioral indicators of child abuse and neglect—cont'd*

Type of abuse/neglect	Physical indicators	Behavioral indicators

Emotional maltreatment	Speech disorders
	Lags in physical development
	Failure-to-thrive
	Hyperactive/disruptive behavior
		Habit disorders (sucking, biting, rocking, etc.)
		Conduct/learning disorders (antisocial, destructive, etc.)
		Anxiety disorders (hysteria, obsession, compulsion, phobias, hypochondriasis, sleep disturbances, inhibition of play, unusual fearfulness)
		Behavior extremes:
		  compliant, passive
		  aggressive, demanding
		Overly adaptive behavior:
		  inappropriately adult
		  inappropriately infantile
		Developmental lags (mental, emotional)
		Attempted suicide

incidents of suspected child abuse. Commonly expressed reservations include a fear of becoming involved in legal processes and a desire to protect the familial integrity. By not reporting suspected instances of child abuse the health care worker is not only *not* protecting the family but is also indirectly contributing to the perpetuation of physical and emotionally dangerous family patterns.

Dynamics underlying child abuse

An understanding of the dynamics underlying child abuse includes societal, familial, and individual factors.

Societal factors. Dr. Harold Feldman, an expert on domestic violence at Cornell University, believes that family violence is a reflection of a society that endorses violence as a means of dealing with frustration and achieving goals. There has been a great deal of publicity regarding the amount of violence on television and in the movies. It is interesting to note that in our society a movie is more likely to be rated "X" if it portrays explicit sexual acts than if it depicts graphic details of a murder. More subtle forms of violence are socially sanctioned by the national preoccupation with such sports as football and boxing. In this way children learn that violent acts are socially acceptable outlets for anger and frustration.

Familial factors. It is a well-known fact that child abusers are people who have themselves been abused as children. Therefore there is a multigenerational pattern of child abuse. In addition many authorities believe that the nuclear family structure contributes to the incidence of child abuse. In this family structure a small group of persons, the nuclear family, is often isolated from other

> Social, family, and individual factors must be considered to understand the dynamics of child abuse.

sources of concerned support. Therefore an intensity of demands develops, and there are few outlets to meet these needs. This leads to increased tension that may explode in the form of violence or neglect directed at the most powerless member of the family—the child.

Individual factors. Whether or not ineffective family functioning will manifest itself by child abuse is largely determined by the dynamics of the family members and how these interact with each other. The box below lists behavioral indicators of abusive parents. These indicators, however, fail to reflect the very real human pain that many child-abusing parents experience. As previously stated, these individuals are most likely to have been abused children themselves. Therefore they have many unmet needs, are emotionally immature, and have limited control of their impulses. Many abusing parents, especially mothers, unconsciously look to their child as a vehicle through which their own

---

Behavioral indicators of abusive parents*

PARENTS OF ABUSED CHILDREN MAY

Lack family supports such as friends, relatives, neighbors, and community groups; consistently fail to keep appointments, discourage social contact, and never participate in school activities or events

Seem to trust no one

Have a childhood history of abuse or neglect

Be reluctant to give information about the child's injuries or condition. When questioned, are unable to explain or offer farfetched or contradictory explanations

Respond inappropriately to the seriousness of the child's condition either by overreacting, seeming hostile or antagonistic when questioned even casually, or by underreacting, showing little concern or awareness and seeming more preoccupied with their own problems than those of the child

Refuse to consent to diagnostic studies

Fail or delay to take the child for medical care, for routine checkups, for optometric or dental care, or for treatment of injury or illness. In taking an injured child for medical care they may choose a different hospital or doctor each time

Be overcritical of the child; seldom if ever discuss the child in positive terms

Have unrealistic expectations of the child, expecting or demanding behavior that is beyond the child's years or ability

Believe in the necessity of harsh punishment for children

Seldom touch or look at the child; ignore the child's crying or react with impatience

Keep the child confined, perhaps in a crib or playpen, for overlong periods of time

Seem to lack understanding of children's physical, emotional, and psychological needs

Appear to be abusing alcohol or drugs

Be difficult or impossible to locate

Appear to lack control or fear losing control

Be of borderline intelligence, psychotic, or antisocial. While such diagnoses are the responsibility of mental health professionals, even the lay observer can note whether the parent seems intellectually capable of childrearing, exhibits generally irrational behavior, or seems excessively cruel and sadistic.

---

*Child abuse and neglect: vol 1, An overview of the problem; vol 2, The problem and its management, DHEW Publication, Washington, DC, 1975, US Government Printing Office.

needs can be met. When it becomes obvious that an infant or young child takes more than it can give, these parents may react with almost uncontrollable rage at once again being disappointed and deprived. In other words, these parents have many fundamental, unmet needs themselves that they look to their children to meet. When this need fulfillment is not forthcoming, they tend to react with violence, reflecting a primitive expression of frustration.

Why is it that one child in a family is consistently abused, while others develop unscathed? This question has no definitive answer, but some hypotheses can be stated. The abused child often has characteristics that set him apart from others in the family. These include birth order (youngest or oldest), physical characteristics (resembles paternal or maternal side of the family), particular skills or deficits, and identifiable personality characteristics (more or less intelligent, more or less assertive, likes solitary activities or activities involving others). In any event, the abused child seems to have particular significance not only to the parents but also to his siblings. The question arises as to why the abused child characteristically colludes with his family in concealing the events surrounding his injuries. Many social scientists believe the answer to this question lies in the fact that children so desperately need attention from significant adults that they are willing to submit to abuse if this appears to be the only way they can gain this attention. Family therapists postulate that the child knowingly assumes a role that is necessary for the survival of the family system. Regardless of why it occurs, it is well known that abused children block attempts to divulge the reality of the situation.

Role of the nurse

Because of the multifaceted dynamics operating in the ineffective family that abuses its children, treatment is very complex. Needless to say, the physical needs of the injured or neglected child must be met before attempts are made to alter the family's pattern of functioning. During the time the child is receiving treatment the parents need a great deal of support and understanding. Health care personnel, including nurses, often have great difficulty avoiding the tendency to blame one or both parents. This attitude, which may be conveyed overtly or covertly, is counterproductive, since it reinforces the guilt and sense of worthlessness the parents already feel. It also reflects a lack of understanding that family units function as a system where each member contributes to the function or dysfunction of the unit.

The treatment of choice for the abusive family, as for all ineffective families, is family therapy. As nurses become more educationally prepared, they increasingly become responsible for using this treatment modality.

Family therapy is the treatment of choice for child-abusing families and all other ineffective families.

FAMILY THERAPY

Family therapy as such is a relatively new treatment modality, although it has been unknowingly practiced in the past by the family physician and the public health nurse. These professionals realized that the effectiveness of treatment of an individual was either enhanced or impeded by the attitudes of his family. In addition, these professionals often became quasifamily members and were consulted and included during family crises. With the explosion of medical knowledge and the increase in medical specialization, the intimate knowledge of the family history and dynamics became unknown to the physician. Simultaneously, public health nurses assumed a greater number of technical functions that consumed a larger part of their role, giving them less time to act as family confidants. Until recently it has seemed most expeditious of time and resources for the individual to be treated by professionals who were specialists. This approach has not only relegated the family to a position of second-class citizens but has also deprived the individual of a valuable resource. Nowhere is this more dramatically illustrated than in the instance of mental illnesses.

Family therapy is based on the belief that the behavior of any one family member affects and is affected by the entire family system.

    The concept of family therapy is based on the belief that the family is a social system with its own characteristic structure and pattern of communication. Although this structure and communication pattern are certainly related to the personalities of the family members, they cannot be explained by a mere summation of the traits of the individuals who comprise the family. In other words, the family as a unit is seen as a system and the family members as components of that system who influence it and are in turn influenced by it. If one accepts this concept, it becomes inappropriate to refer to one member as being mentally ill without looking at the family constellation, which, it is believed, has sanctioned the deviant behavior of one member and in turn is affected by it. In other words, the behavior of the "sick" member serves a function within the family. This belief is supported by two observations. First it is not unusual for a person to be successfully treated for mental illness on an individual basis and for another member of the family to become ill, sometimes with very similar symptoms. This phenomenon suggests that the family structure and communication pattern, if they are to be maintained, require one member to be deviant. A second observation that supports the systems approach is the frequency with which family members bring one member for treatment with the statement that all is well within the family except for the stress-producing behavior of the one member. When that member is removed from the family, either through prolonged hospitalization or by geographical relocation, it is not uncommon for the family to enter into a state of acute disequilibrium that may manifest itself by such actions as divorce of the parents. This phenomenon is equally well documented in families in which a chronically physically ill person has died.

Family therapy is based on the belief that the treatment and prevention of mental illness will occur only when the needs of the individual are considered within the context of the family system.

    Lately a growing number of mental health professionals believe that any attempt to treat individuals in isolation from their families is either futile or, if helpful to the individual, is at the expense of the equilibrium of his family system. Proponents of family therapy maintain that major strides in the promotion of mental health and the prevention and treatment of mental illness will occur only when the needs of the individual are considered within the context of the family system, which still remains as the fundamental social unit of our society. Although this may seem an extreme view, there is no doubt that family therapy is the treatment of choice when the identified client is a child or adolescent, and this treatment modality should be used in other situations when possible.

The goals of family therapy are to assist in resolving pathological conflicts and anxiety, to strengthen the individual member against destructive forces both within himself and within the family environment, to strengthen the family against critical upsets, and to influence the orientation of the family identity and values toward health. When therapy commences, the therapist assembles all family members, regardless of age, and pays as much attention to their behavior with each other as to the content of what they say. For example, the husband and wife may vehemently state how emotionally close they are while at the same time sit as far as possible from each other. It is important for the therapist to avoid blaming one or the other member, and this pitfall will be avoided if the role of each member is seen in relation to the total family functioning. In one family therapy situation the identified client was a 20-year-old daughter who had made numerous suicidal attempts. This girl was hospitalized, and the entire family came to the hospital once a week for family therapy. The parents maintained that they had an unusually good relationship and could not understand why their daughter tormented them so with her life-threatening gestures. Several times during the course of therapy, their adolescent son took the risk of contradicting his parents by observing that the parents' relationship was highly tension-laden, at which point the daughter would begin crying. This behavior on her part diverted the participants' attention to her and successfully prevented the parents from having to face, much less talk about, their differences. The therapist interpreted this behavior not as being sick, but rather as the daughter's role in maintaining the family equilibrium.

It is the prerogative of the family to determine their own destiny, and often the major role of the therapist is to comment on the interactional process as it is observed. Bringing this process to a level of consciousness allows the family to evaluate its purpose and outcome. If the family desires a change, the therapist can be instrumental in modeling behaviors that can initiate such change.

Some family therapy sessions have been held in the home. As this trend develops, it appears likely that the role of family therapist will become increasingly identified with the prepared psychiatric nurse because she is comfortable in the role of family visitor, is knowledgeable about family dynamics, and is becoming skillful in family therapy.

CONJOINT THERAPY

Conjoint therapy usually refers to therapy in which marriage partners engage in a therapeutic endeavor with a therapist. The importance of this technique is supported not only by the well-being that can be attained by the marriage partners but also because these persons are seen by family theorists as the architects

Conjoint therapy usually involves marital partners who are helped to awareness of their expectations of each other and of their marital relationship.

of the future family system. That is, treatment of the marital couple can have a profound effect on the promotion of mental health and prevention of mental illness of the growing family. Often it is found that couples who have marital conflict have incongruent expectations of each other, the most common being the expectation that each will have their dependency needs met by the other. When these expectations are simultaneously operationalized, both are disappointed. Frequently the mutual realization of these expectations moves the couple ahead to understand that both can have their needs met if they are able to compromise. Several experts have written excellent texts about conjoint therapy, which the student is encouraged to read for additional information. Particularly recommended is *Conjoint Family Therapy* by Virginia Satir.

END NOTE

The structure, functions, and development of the family as a social unit are presented in this chapter in the belief that the family directly or indirectly affects and is affected by all psychiatric nursing interventions. The characteristics of an effective family are contrasted with those of the ineffective family. The child-abusing family is discussed at length as one increasingly common example of an ineffective family. Finally, the principles of family and conjoint therapy are introduced to enable the nurse to better understand the indications for and the objectives of these treatment modalities.

SUGGESTED SOURCES OF ADDITIONAL INFORMATION

Battered women: issues of public policy, Washington, DC, 1978, US Commission on Civil Rights.

Bowen M: Family therapy in clinical practice, New York, 1978, Jason Aronson.

Bumagin VE and Hirn KF: Aging is a family affair, New York, 1980, Lippincott & Crowell.

Cain AO: Family therapy: one role of the clinical specialist in psychiatric nursing, Nurs Clinics North Am 21(3):483, 1986.

Child abuse and neglect: vol 1, An overview of the problem, DHEW Publication, Washington, DC, 1975, US Government Printing Office.

Child abuse and neglect: vol 2, The problem and its management, DHEW Publication, Washington, DC, 1975, US Government Printing Office.

Collison C and Futrell JA: Family therapy for the single-parent family system, J Psychosoc Nurs Ment Health Serv 20:16, July 1982.

Curran D: Traits of a healthy family, New York, 1983, Ballantine Books.

Danziger S: Major treatment issues and techniques in family therapy with the borderline adolescent, J Psychosoc Nurs Ment Health Serv 20:27, January 1982.

deChesnay M: Father-daughter incest, J Psychosoc Nurs Ment Health Serv 22:24, September 1984.

Gemmill F: A family approach to the battered woman, J Psychosoc Nurs Ment Health Serv 20:22, September 1982.

Gerace L: Phenomenon of early engagement in family therapy, J Psychosoc Nurs Ment Health Serv 19:25, April 1981.

Grossman J, Pozanski E, and Bonegas M: Lunch: time to study family interactions, J Psychosoc Nurs Ment Health Serv 21:19, July 1983.

Gunderson SS: Advocacy in family therapy, J Psychosoc Nurs Ment Health Serv 18:24, September 1980.

Harter L: Multi-family meetings on the psychiatric unit, J Psychosoc Nurs Ment Health Serv 26(8):19, 1988.

Heindl C et al: The nurse's role in the prevention and treatment of child abuse and neglect, DHEW Publication No. (OHDS) 79-30202, Washington, DC, 1979, US Government Printing Office.

Holfing CK and Lewis JM, editors: The family: evaluation and treatment, New York, 1980, Bruner/Mazel, Inc.

Jones S: Family therapy: a comparison of approaches, Bowie, 1980, Robert J. Brady, Co.

Jones S and Dimond M: Family theory and family therapy models: comparative review with implications for nursing practice, J Psychosoc Nurs Ment Health Serv 20:12, October 1982.

Lantz J and Treece N: Identity operations and family treatment, J Psychosoc Nurs Ment Health Serv 20:20, October 1982.

Miller S and Winstead-Fry P: Family systems theory in nursing practice, Reston, Va, 1982, Reston Publishing Co.

Miller V and Mansfield E: Family therapy for the multiple incest family, J Psychosoc Nurs Ment Health Serv 19:29, April 1984.

Minuchin S: Families and family therapy, Cambridge, Mass, 1974, Harvard University Press.

Napier AY and Whitaker C: The family crucible, New York, 1980, Harper & Row.

Palermo E: Remarriage: parental perceptions of step-relations with children and adolescents, J Psychosoc Nurs Ment Health Serv 18:9, April 1980.

Rose L, Finestone K, and Bass J: Group support for the families of psychiatric patients, J Psychosoc Nurs Ment Health Serv 23(12):24, December 1985.

Sedgwick R: Family mental health: theory and practice, St Louis, 1981, The CV Mosby Co.

So you use a systems approach in therapy: what does that mean? (editorial), Arch Psychiatr Nurs 2(2):55, April 1988.

Starkey P: Genograms: a guide to understanding one's own family system, Perspect Psychiatr Care 19:164, September-December 1982.

Steiner P: The well child and the hospitalized disabled sibling, J Psychosoc Nurs Ment Health Serv 22:23, March 1984.

Stern PN: Conflicting family culture: an impediment to integration in stepfather families, J Psychosoc Nurs Ment Health Serv 20:27, October 1982.

Swanson A and Hurley P: Family systems: values and value conflicts, J Psychosoc Nurs Ment Health Serv 21:24, July 1983.

Tamex E: Familism, machismo and child rearing practices among Mexican Americans, J Psychosoc Nurs Ment Health Serv 19:21, September 1981.

Tousley M: The use of family therapy in terminal illness and death, J Psychosoc Nurs Ment Health Serv 20:17, January 1982.

Walker L: The battered woman, New York, 1980, Harper & Row.

Weil S: The unspoken needs of families during high-risk pregnancies, Am J Nurs 81:2047, 1981.

Whall A: Nursing theory and the assessment of families, J Psychosoc Nurs Ment Health Serv 19:30, January 1981.

White J: Bulimia: utilizing individual and family therapy, J Psychosoc Nurs Ment Health Serv 22:22, April 1984.

Wilk J: Family environments and the young chronically mentally ill, J Psychosoc Nurs Ment Health Serv 26(10):15, October 1988.

Glossary

The following words are frequently used by the psychiatric nurse. Many of the definitions were taken from *A Psychiatric Glossary*.* A larger and equally useful book is the *Psychiatric Dictionary*.†

abstinence Voluntarily denying oneself some kind of gratification; in the area of alcohol or drug dependence, being without the substance on which the subject is dependent. The abstinence syndrome is equivalent to withdrawal symptoms, and its appearance suggests the presence of physiologic dependence or addiction.

abused child Child or infant who has suffered repeated injuries, which may include bone fractures, neurologic and psychologic damage, and sexual abuse at the hands of a parent, parents, or parent surrogates. The abuse takes place repeatedly and is often precipitated by the child's minor and normal irritating behavior.

acrophobia Fear of heights.

acting out Expressions of unconscious emotional conflicts or feelings in actions rather than words. The person is not consciously aware of the meaning of such acts. Acting out may be harmful or, in controlled situations, therapeutic (e.g., children's play therapy).

addiction Strong emotional and physiologic dependence on a chemical substance that has progressed beyond voluntary control.

affect Emotional feeling tone; affect and emotional response are commonly used interchangeably.

ageism Systematic stereotyping of and discrimination against elderly people to create distance from the social plight of older people and to avoid primitive fears of aging and death. It is distinguished from gerontophobia, a specific pathologic fear of old people and aging.

aggression Forceful physical, verbal, or symbolic action.

agitation Excessive motor activity, usually nonpurposeful and associated with internal tension. For example, inability to sit still, fidgeting, pacing, wringing of hands, or pulling of clothes.

agoraphobia Fear of open spaces.

Al-Anon Organization of relatives of alcoholics operating in many communities under

---

*American Psychiatric Association: A psychiatric glossary, ed 5, Washington, DC, APA, 1980.

†Campbell RJ: Psychiatric dictionary, ed 5, New York, 1981, Oxford University Press, Inc.

the philosophic and organizational structure of Alcoholics Anonymous to facilitate discussion and resolution of common problems.

Alateen   Organization of teenaged children of alcoholic parents operating in some communities under the philosophic and organizational structure of Alcoholics Anonymous. It provides a setting in which the children may receive group support in achieving a better understanding of their parents' problems and better methods for coping with them.

alcohol dependence (alcoholism)   Physical dependence on alcohol characterized by either tolerance to the agent or development of withdrawal phenomena on cessation of, or reduction in, intake. Other aspects of the syndrome are psychologic dependence and impairment in social or vocational functioning.

Alcoholics Anonymous (AA)   Group of abstinent alcoholics who collectively assist other alcoholics through personal and group support.

Alzheimer's disease   Degenerative brain disease of unknown cause marked by insidious onset and uniformly progressive deterioration. The disorder occurs most commonly in those over 65 but may occur as early as age 40.

ambivalence   Coexistence of two opposing drives, desires, feelings, or emotions toward the same person, object, or goal; may be conscious or partially conscious.

anal stage   Second stage of psychosexual development, immediately following the oral stage, marked by a shift of libidinal energy to the anus and urethra; includes both anal-expulsive and anal-retentive phases. Many adult traits, such as stinginess, hoarding, and collecting, find their prototypes here.

anorexia nervosa   Psychiatric disorder marked by severe and prolonged refusal to eat with severe weight loss, amenorrhea or impotence, disturbance of body image, an intense fear of becoming obese, and peculiar patterns of eating and handling food. Most frequently encountered in girls and young women.

antisocial personality   Personality disorder marked by a history of chronic antisocial behavior in which the rights of others are violated, with persistence into adult life of a pattern of antisocial behavior that began in adolescence, and a failure to sustain good job performance over several years. Lying, stealing, fighting, and truancy are typical early signs.

anxiety   Apprehension, tension, or uneasiness that stems from the anticipation of danger, the source of which is largely unknown or unrecognized; primarily of intrapsychic origin, in distinction to fear, which is the emotional response to a consciously recognized and usually external threat or danger.

apathy   Used by Sullivan to describe the security operation whereby the individual defends against anxiety by not experiencing the emotion associated with an anxiety-producing event; there is a manifestation of extreme indifference.

autonomy   Quality or state of being self-governing. The living organism does not represent merely an inactive element but is, to a large extent, a self-governing entity.

autism   Developmental disability caused by a physical disorder of the brain appearing during the first three years of life. Symptoms include disturbances in physical, social, and language skills; abnormal responses to sensations; and abnormal ways of relating to people, objects, and events.

autistic thinking   Form of thinking that attempts to gratify unfulfilled desires without due regard for reality; objective facts are distorted, obscured, or excluded in varying degrees.

bi-polar disorder   Major affective disorder in which there are episodes of both mania and depression; formerly called manic depressive psychosis, circular or mixed type.

blocking   Difficulty in recollection or the sudden interruption of a train of thought or speech due to emotional factors that are usually unconscious.

body image   One's sense of self as presented to others.

body language   Message(s) transmitted by one's body motion and facial expressions that are learned forms of communication and that have meaning within the context in which they appear.

bonding   Attachment and unity of two people whose identities are significantly affected by their mutual interactions. Bonding often refers to the result of the process of attachment between the mother and her child.

bulimia nervosa   Psychiatric disorder, occurring primarily in females, marked by episodic uncontrolled and rapid consumption of food over a short period of time (binges), inconspicuous eating during a binge, and termination of the binge by abdominal pain, social interruption, sleep, or self-induced vomiting.

catchment area   Geographic area for which a mental health program or facility has responsibility.

catharsis   Healthful (therapeutic) release of ideas through a "talking out" of conscious material accompanied by an appropriate emotional reaction. Also, the release into awareness of repressed material from the unconscious.

cathexis   Attachment, conscious or unconscious, of emotional feeling and significance to an idea, an object, or, most commonly, a person.

cerea flexibilitas   "Waxy flexibility" often present in catatonic schizophrenia in which the individual's arm or leg remains in the position in which it is placed.

clanging   Type of thinking in which the sound of a word, rather than its meaning, gives the direction to subsequent associations; punning and rhyming may substitute for logic, and language may become increasingly a senseless compulsion to associate and decreasingly a vehicle for communication.

claustrophobia   Fear of closed spaces.

cognitive   Refers to the mental process of comprehension, judgment, memory, and reasoning, as contrasted with emotional and volitional processes.

cognitive development   Beginning in infancy, the acquisition of intelligence, conscious thought, and problem-solving abilities. An orderly sequence in the increase in knowledge derived from sensorimotor activity has been empirically demonstrated by Piaget.

commitment   Legal process for admitting a person who is mentally ill to a psychiatric treatment program. The legal definition and procedure vary from state to state, although it usually requires a court or judicial procedure.

compensation   Mental mechanism, operating unconsciously, by which the individual attempts to make up for real or fancied deficiencies; conscious process by which the individual strives to make up for real or imagined defects in such areas as physique, performance, skills, or psychologic attributes—the two types frequently merge.

complex   Group of associated ideas that have a common strong emotional tone; these may be in part unconscious and may significantly influence attitudes and associations.

compulsion   Insistent, repetitive, intrusive, and unwanted urge to perform an act that is contrary to the person's ordinary conscious wishes or standards; a defensive substitute for hidden and still more unacceptable ideas and wishes. Anxiety results from failure to perform the compulsive act.

computerized axial tomography (CAT scan)   Technique for noninvasive radiologic examination of soft tissues. Scan of the intracranial contents allows visualization of the structure of the brain, including cerebrospinal fluid–filled spaces.

concept   Mental image.

condensation   Psychologic process often present in dreams in which two or more concepts are fused so that a single symbol represents the multiple components.

confabulation   Unconscious, defensive "filling in" of actual memory gaps by imaginary or fantastic experiences, often complex, that are recounted in a detailed and plausible way as though they were factual.

conflict   Mental struggle that arises from the simultaneous operation of opposing impulses, drives, and external (environmental) or internal demands; termed intrapsychic when the conflict is between forces within the personality; extrapsychic, when it is between the self and the environment.

confusion   Disturbed orientation in respect to time, place, or person; sometimes accompanied by disturbances of consciousness.

conscience   Morally self-critical part of one's standards of behavior, performance, and value judgments. Commonly equated with the superego.

conscious   Content of mind or mental functioning of which one is aware.

conversion   Defense mechanism, operating unconsciously, by which intrapsychic conflicts that would otherwise give rise to anxiety are instead given symbolic external expression. The repressed ideas or impulses and the psychologic defenses against them are converted into a variety of somatic symptoms involving the nervous system. These may include such symptoms as paralysis, pain, or loss of sensory function.

coping mechanism   Adaptation to anxiety based on conscious acknowledgement of a problem; the individual engages in reality-oriented problem-solving activities designed to reduce tension.

countertransference   Therapist's conscious or unconscious emotional reaction to the client.

crisis   State of disequilibrium resulting from the interaction of an event with the individual's or family's coping mechanisms, which are inadequate to meet the demands of the situation, combined with the individual's or family's perception of the meaning of the event.

decompensation   Deterioration of existing defenses, leading to an exacerbation of pathologic behavior.

defense mechanism   Unconscious intrapsychic processes serving to provide relief from emotional conflict and anxiety.

deinstitutionalization   Change in locus of mental health care from traditional, institutional settings to community-based services.

delirium   Acute organic mental disorder characterized by confusion and altered, possibly fluctuating, consciousness due to an alteration of cerebral metabolism; illusions, delusions, or hallucinations may be present. Often emotional lability, typically appearing as anxiety and agitation, is present.

delirium tremens   Acute and sometimes fatal brain disorder caused by total or partial withdrawal from excessive alcohol intake. Usually develops in 24 to 96 hours after cessation of drinking.

delusion　False belief out of keeping with the individual's level of knowledge and cultural group; the belief is maintained against logical argument and despite objective contradictory evidence.

delusions of grandeur　Exaggerated, unrealistic ideas of one's importance or identity.

delusions of persecution　Unrealistic ideas that one has been singled out for persecution.

delusions of reference　Incorrect assumption that certain casual or unrelated remarks or the behavior of others applies to oneself.

dementia　Organic mental disorder in which there is a deterioration of previously acquired intellectual abilities of sufficient severity to interfere with social or occupational functioning. Memory disturbance is the most prominent symptom.

dementia praecox　Obsolete descriptive term for schizophrenia.

denial　Defense mechanism, operating unconsciously, used to resolve emotional conflict and allay anxiety by disavowing thoughts, feelings, wishes, needs, or external reality factors that are consciously intolerable.

dependency needs　Vital needs for mothering, love, affection, shelter, protection, security, food, and warmth. May be a manifestation of regression when they reappear openly in adults.

depersonalization　Feelings of unreality or strangeness concerning the environment, the self, or both.

depression　In the psychiatric sense, a morbid sadness, dejection, or melancholy; may vary in depth; to be differentiated from grief, which is realistic and proportionate to what has been lost.

derailment　Pattern of speech seen most commonly in schizophrenic disorders, in which incomprehensible, disconnected, and unrelated ideas replace logical and orderly thought.

dereistic　Describes mental activity that is not in accordance with reality, logic, or experience; similar to autistic.

detoxification　Treatment by the use of medication, diet, rest, fluids, and nursing care to restore physiologic functioning after it has been seriously disturbed by the overuse of alcohol, barbiturates, or other addictive drugs.

developmental disability　Handicap or impairment originating before the age of 18 that may be expected to continue indefinitely and that constitutes a substantial impairment.

deviant　Any person differing markedly from what is accepted as the norm, the average, or the usual.

disorientation　Loss of awareness of the position of self in relation to space, time, or persons.

displacement　Mental mechanism, operating unconsciously, by which an emotion is transferred or "displaced" from its original object to a more acceptable substitute object.

dissociation　Psychological separation or splitting off; an intrapsychic defensive process, which operates automatically and unconsciously, through which emotional significance and affect are separated and detached from an idea, situation, or object.

dissociative disorder　Category of psychiatric disorder in which there is a sudden, temporary alteration in normally integrated functions of consciousness, identity, or motor behavior so that some part of one or more of these functions is lost.

distractibility Inability to maintain attention; shifting from one area or topic to another with minimal provocation.

dopamine hypothesis Theory that attempts to explain the pathogenesis of schizophrenia and other psychotic states as due to excesses in dopamine activity in various areas of the brain.

double bind Interaction in which one person demands a response to a message containing mutually contradictory signals while the other person is unable either to comment on the incongruity or to escape from the situation.

Down syndrome Common form of mental retardation caused by a chromosomal abnormality; formerly called mongolism.

drive Basic urge, instinct, motivation.

drug dependence Habituation to, abuse of, and/or addiction to a chemical substance.

dyad Two-person relationship, such as the therapeutic relationship between nurse and client in the nurse-client relationship.

dysarthria Impaired, difficult speech, usually due to organic disorders of the nervous system; sometimes applied to emotional speech difficulties such as stammering and stuttering.

dyslexia Inability or difficulty in reading, including word-blindness and a tendency to reverse letters and words in reading and writing.

dysphagia Difficult or painful swallowing.

dysphoria Unpleasant mood.

dystonia Acute tonic muscular spasms, often of the tongue, jaw, eyes, and neck, but sometimes of the whole body. Sometimes occurs during the first few days of antipsychotic drug administration.

ego In psychoanalytic theory, one of the three major divisions in the model of the psychic apparatus. The ego represents the sum of certain mental mechanisms, such as perception and memory, and specific defense mechanisms. It serves to mediate between the demands of primitive instinctual drives (the id), of internalized parental and social prohibitions (the superego), and of reality. The compromises between these forces achieved by the ego tend to resolve intrapsychic conflict and serve an adaptive and executive function. Psychiatric usage of the term should not be confused with common usage, which connotes self-love or selfishness.

ego ideal That part of the personality which comprises the aims and goals of the self; usually refers to the conscious or unconscious emulation of significant persons with whom one has identified.

elation Affect consisting of feelings of euphoria, triumph, intense self-satisfaction, optimism; an elated though unstable mood is characteristic of mania.

electroconvulsive treatment (ECT) Use of electric current to induce convulsive seizures. Most effective in the treatment of depression. Used with anesthetics and muscle relaxants.

emotion State of arousal determined by a set of subjective feelings (e.g., fear, anger, grief, joy, love), often accompanied by physiologic changes, that impels one toward action.

empathic linkage Sullivan's term for the relationship unique to infant and mothering one, whereby each is highly sensitive to the other's feeling states.

empathy Objective and insightful awareness of the feelings, emotions, and behavior of another person and their meaning and significance; to be distinguished from sympathy, which is nonobjective and usually noncritical.

enuresis   Incontinence of urine.

erogenous zone   Area of the body particularly susceptible to erotic arousal when stimulated, especially the oral, anal, and genital areas.

etiology   Causation, particularly with reference to disease.

euphoria   Exaggerated feeling of physical and emotional well-being, usually of psychologic origin.

extrapyramidal syndrome   Variety of signs and symptoms, including muscular rigidity, tremors, drooling, shuffling gait (parkinsonism); restlessness (akathisia); peculiar involuntary postures (dystonia); motor inertia (akinesia); and many other neurologic disturbances. Results from dysfunction of the extrapyramidal system. May occur as a side effect of certain psychotropic drugs, particularly phenothiazines.

family therapy   Treatment of more than one member of a family simultaneously in the same session.

fantasy   Imagined sequence of events or mental images that serves to express unconscious conflicts, to gratify unconscious wishes, or to prepare for anticipated future events.

fear   Emotional and physiologic response to recognized sources of danger, to be distinguished from anxiety.

fixation   Arrest of psychosexual maturation at an immature level; depending on degree, may be either normal or pathological.

flight of ideas   Verbal skipping from one idea to another before the preceding one has been concluded; the ideas appear to be continuous but are fragmentary and determined by chance associations.

forensic psychiatry   Branch of psychiatry dealing with legal issues related to mental disorders.

free association   In psychoanalytic therapy, spontaneous, uncensored verbalization by the client of whatever comes to mind.

free-floating anxiety   Severe, generalized, persistent anxiety not specifically ascribed to a particular object or event and often a precursor of panic.

functional mental illness   Illness of emotional origin in which organic or structural changes are either absent or are developed secondarily to prolonged emotional stress.

gender identity   Inner sense of maleness or femaleness that identifies the person as being male, female, or ambivalent. To be distinguished from sexual identity, which is biologically determined.

gender role   Image a person presents to others and to the self that declares him or her to be boy or girl, man or woman. Gender role is the public declaration of gender identity, but the two do not necessarily coincide.

genetic(s)   In biology, pertaining to genes or to inherited characteristics. Also, in psychiatry, pertaining to the historical development of one's psychologic attributes or disorders.

genital stage   Period of psychosexual development from the age of about 12 to 18 years, marked by a reactivation of libidinal energy and the focusing of this energy on the genital area.

geriatrics   Branch of medicine dealing with the aging process and diseases of the aging human being.

gerontology   Study of aging.

grandiose   Exaggerated belief or claims of one's importance or identity, often manifested by delusions of great wealth, power, or fame.

grief   Normal, appropriate emotional response to an external and consciously recognized loss; usually time-limited and gradually subsides.

halfway house   Specialized residence for individuals who do not require full hospitalization but who need an intermediate degree of care before returning to independent community living.

hallucination   False sensory perception in the absence of an actual external stimulus; may be of emotional or chemical (drugs, alcohol, etc.) origin and may occur in any of the five senses.

hallucinogen   Chemical agent that produces hallucinations.

holistic   Approach to the study of the individual in totality, rather than as an aggregate of separate physiologic, psychologic, and social characteristics.

homosexual panic   Acute and severe attack of anxiety based on unconscious conflicts involving homosexuality.

homosexuality   Sexual attraction or relationship between members of the same sex; active homosexuality is marked by overt activity, whereas latent homosexuality is marked by unconscious homosexual desires or conscious desires consistently denied expression.

hyperactivity   Excessive motor activity, generally purposeful. It is frequently, but not necessarily, associated with internal tension or a neurologic disorder. Usually the movements are more rapid than customary for the person.

hypomania   Psychopathologic state and abnormality of mood falling somewhere between normal euphoria and mania.

id   In Freudian theory, that part of the personality structure that harbors the unconscious instinctive desires and strivings of the individual.

ideas of reference   Incorrect interpretation of casual incidents and external events as having direct reference to oneself; may reach sufficient intensity to constitute delusions.

identification   Mental mechanism, operating unconsciously, by which an individual endeavors to pattern himself after another; plays a major role in the development of one's personality and specifically of one's superego (conscience).

identity crisis   Loss of the sense of the sameness and historical continuity of one's self and inability to accept or adopt the role one perceives as being expected by society.

idiopathic   Term applied to diseases of unknown cause, for example, idiopathic epilepsy.

illusion   Misinterpretation of a real external sensory experience.

impulse   Psychic striving; usually refers to an instinctual urge.

incorporation   Primitive mental mechanism, operating unconsciously, by which another person or parts of another person are symbolically ingested and assimilated; for example, infantile fantasy that the mother's breast has been ingested and is a part of oneself.

inhibition   Unconscious interference with or restriction of instinctual drives.

insight   Self-understanding; a major goal of psychotherapy; the extent of the individual's understanding of the origin, nature, and mechanisms of his attitudes and behavior.

insomnia Inability to fall asleep, difficulty staying asleep, and/or early morning awakening.

instinct Inborn drive. The primary human instincts include self-preservation, sexuality, and—according to some authorities—aggression, the ego instincts, and herd or social instincts.

integration Useful organization of both new and old data, experience, and emotional capacities incorporated into the personality; also refers to the organization and amalgamation of functions at various levels of psychosexual development.

intelligence Capacity to learn and to utilize appropriately what one has learned. May be affected by emotions.

intelligence quotient (IQ) Numerical rating determined through psychologic testing that indicates the approximate relationship of a person's mental age (MA) to chronologic age (CA). Expressed mathematically as $IQ = MA/CA \times 100$.

interpersonal psychiatry Theory of psychiatry developed by Sullivan, stressing the nature and quality of relationships with significant others as the most critical factor in personality development.

intrapsychic Situated, originating, or taking place in the psyche.

introjection Mental mechanism, operating unconsciously, whereby loved or hated external objects are taken within oneself symbolically; the converse of projection; may serve as a defense against conscious recognition of intolerable hostile impulses; for example, in severe depression the individual may unconsciously direct unacceptable hatred or aggression toward himself, that is, toward the introjected object within himself; related to the more primitive mechanisms of incorporation.

isolation Mental mechanism whereby the feeling is detached from the event in an individual's memory, thus enabling the event to be recalled without its attendant anxiety.

kleptomania Compulsive stealing, largely without any apparent material need for the stolen objects.

la belle indifference Literally, "beautiful indifference." Seen in certain persons with conversion disorders who show an inappropriate lack of concern about their disabilities.

labile Rapidly shifting emotions.

latency period In psychoanalysis, a phase between the phallic (or oedipal) and adolescent periods of psychosexual development; characterized by a marked decrease of sexual behavior and interest in sex.

learning disability Syndrome affecting school-age children of normal or above-normal intelligence characterized by specific difficulties in learning to read (dyslexia), write (dysgraphia), and calculate (dyscalculia). The disorder is believed to be related to slow developmental progression of perceptual motor skills.

libido Psychic drive or energy usually associated with the sexual instinct (sexual is used here in the broad sense to include pleasure and love-object seeking); also used broadly to connote the psychic energy associated with instincts in general.

life review Process of thinking about the meaning of one's life, believed to be a universal occurrence in older person as they face the prospect of impending death.

lithium carbonate Alkali metal, the salt of which is used in the treatment of acute mania and as a maintenance medication to help reduce the duration, intensity, and frequency of recurrent affective episodes, especially in bipolar disorders.

logorrhea　Uncontrollable, excessive talking.

loosening of associations　Disturbance of thinking in which ideas shift from one subject to another in an oblique or unrelated manner. The speaker is unaware of the disturbance. When loosening of associations is severe, speech may be incoherent.

LSD (lysergic acid diethylamide)　Potent hallucinogen that produces psychotic symptoms and behavior.

lust　Sullivan's term for the sexual urges first erupting in early adolescence.

magical thinking　Conviction that thinking equates with doing. Occurs in dreams, in children, in primitive peoples, and in persons with some forms of mental illness. Characterized by lack of realistic relationship between cause and effect.

mania　Mood disorder characterized by excessive elation, hyperactivity, agitation, and accelerated thinking and speaking.

megalomania　Syndrome marked by delusions of great self-importance, wealth, or power.

melancholia　Pathologic dejection, usually of psychotic depth.

mental disorder　Illness with psychologic or behavioral manifestations and/or impairment in functioning due to a social, psychologic, genetic, physical/chemical, or biologic disturbance. The disorder is not limited to relations between the person and society. The illness is characterized by symptoms and/or impairment in functioning.

mental health　State of being, relative rather than absolute. The best indices of mental health are simultaneous success at working, loving, and creating with the capacity for mature and flexible resolution of conflicts between instincts, conscience, important other people, and reality.

mental mechanisms　Also called defense mechanisms and mental dynamisms; specific intrapsychic defensive processes, operating unconsciously, that are employed to seek resolution of emotional conflict and freedom from anxiety; conscious efforts are frequently made for the same reasons, but true mental mechanisms are out of awareness (unconscious).

mental retardation　Significantly subaverage general intellectual functioning existing concurrently with deficits in adaptive behavior.

mental status　Level and style of functioning of the psyche, including a person's intellectual functioning and emotional, attitudinal, psychologic, and personality aspects. The term is commonly used to refer to the results of the examination of an individual's mental status.

methadone　Synthetic narcotic often used as a substitute for heroin producing a less socially disabling addiction and aiding in heroin withdrawal.

middle age　Conventionally considered to occur between 40 and 60 years of age and primarily defined by psychosocial rather than by physiologic events.

milieu therapy　Socioenvironmental therapy in which the attitudes and behavior of the staff of a treatment service and the activities prescribed for the client are determined by the client's emotional and interpersonal needs. This therapy is an essential part of all inpatient treatment.

mood　Pervasive and sustained emotion that in the extreme markedly colors the person's perception of the world. Mood is to affect as climate is to weather. Common examples of mood include depression, elation, anger, and anxiety.

moral treatment　Philosophy and technique of treating mental patients that prevailed in the first half of the nineteenth century and emphasized removal of restraints, humane and kindly care, attention to religion, and performance of useful tasks in the hospital.

multiple personality   Term used by Morton Prince for a rare type of dissociative reaction in which the person adopts two or more personalities.

mysophobia   Morbid fear of dirt, germs, or contamination.

narcissism   Self-love as opposed to object-love (love of another person). In psychoanalytic theory, cathexis of the psychic representation of the self with libido. An excess interferes with relations with others. To be distinguished from egotism, which carries the connotation of self-centeredness, selfishness, and conceit. Egotism is but one expression of narcissism.

narcotic   Any opiate derivative drug, natural or synthetic, that relieves pain or alters mood.

neologism   In psychiatry, new word or condensed combination of several words coined by a client to express a highly complex meaning related to his conflicts; not readily understood by others; common in schizophrenia.

object   That through which an instinct can achieve its aim; object relations theory is the psychoanalytic description of the internalization of interpersonal relations and the organizing effects of internalized human object relationships on the structure of the psyche.

obsession   Persistent, unwanted idea or impulse that cannot be eliminated by usual logic or reasoning.

obsessive-compulsive disorder   Psychiatric disorder characterized by disturbing, unwanted, intruding thoughts and ideas and repetitive impulses to perform acts that the person may consider abnormal, undesirable, or distasteful.

Oedipus complex   Situation occurring during the phallic stage of psychosexual development (approximate ages 3 to 6) in which the child shifts energies into sexual interest in parents. The child normally becomes attached to the parent of the opposite sex and develops competitive feelings toward the same-sex parent. Eventually, through identification with the same-sex parent, the child relinquishes oedipal strivings.

omnipotence   Infantile perception that the outside world is part of the organism and within it, which leads to a primitive feeling of all-powerfulness. This feeling gradually becomes limited as the ego and a sense of reality develop. Similar phenomena are found in disturbed individuals who lose contact with reality.

opiate   Any chemical derived from opium; relieves pain and produces a sense of well-being.

oral stage   Includes both the oral-erotic and oral-sadistic phases of infantile psychosexual development, lasting from birth to 12 months or longer; oral-erotic phase is the initial pleasurable experience of nursing; oral-sadistic phase is the subsequent aggressive (biting) phase; both eroticism and sadism normally continue to later life in disguised or sublimated forms.

organic mental disorder   Transient or permanent dysfunction of the brain, caused by a disturbance of physiologic functioning of brain tissue at any level of organization—structural, hormonal, biochemical, electrical, etc.

orientation   Awareness of oneself in relation to time, place, and person.

panic   In psychiatry, refers to an attack of acute, intense, and overwhelming anxiety, accompanied by a considerable degree of personality disorganization.

paranoia   Psychotic disorder that develops slowly and becomes chronic; characterized by an intricate and internally logical system of persecutory or grandiose delusions, or both; stands by itself and does not interfere with the remainder of the personality, which continues essentially normal and apparently intact; to be distinguished from paranoid schizophrenic reactions and paranoid states.

paranoid   Lay term commonly used to describe an overly suspicious person. The technical use of the term refers to people with paranoid ideation or to a type of schizophrenia or a class of disorders.

paranoid ideation   Suspiciousness or nondelusional belief that one is being harrassed, persecuted, or unfairly treated.

pedophilia   Term used to describe adults who demonstrate a pathological sexual interest in children.

penis envy   Literally, envy by the female of the penis of the male; more generally, the female's wish for male attributes, position, or advantages; believed by many to be a significant factor in female character development.

personality   Aggregate of the physical and mental qualities of the individual as these interact in characteristic fashion with the environment.

personality disorders   Deeply ingrained, inflexible, dysfunctional patterns of relating, perceiving, and thinking of sufficient severity to cause either impairment in functioning or distress. Personality disorders are generally recognizable by adolescence or earlier, continue throughout adulthood, and become less obvious in middle or old age.

phallic stage   Period of psychosexual development from the age of about 3 to 6 years during which sexual interest, curiosity, and pleasurable experience center about the penis and, in girls, to a lesser extent, the clitoris.

phobia   Obsessive, persistent, unrealistic fear of an external object or situation such as heights, open spaces, dirt, and animals; fear believed to arise through a process of displacing an internal (unconscious) conflict to an external object symbolically related to the conflict.

play therapy   Treatment technique utilizing the child's play as a medium for expression and communication between the child and therapist.

pleasure principle   Basic psychoanalytic concept that humans instinctually seek to avoid pain and discomfort and strive for gratification and pleasure; in personality development theories, the pleasure principle antedates and subsequently comes into conflict with the reality principle.

posttraumatic stress disorder   Develops after experiencing a psychologically distressing event. It is characterized by reexperiencing the event and by overresponsiveness to, or involvement with, stimuli that recall the event.

preconscious   Thoughts not in immediate awareness but that can be recalled by conscious effort.

preoccupation   State of being self-absorbed or engrossed in one's own thoughts, typically to a degree that hinders effective contact with or relationship to external reality.

pressured speech   Rapid, accelerated, frenzied speech. Sometimes it exceeds the ability of the vocal musculature to articulate, leading to jumbled and cluttered speech; at other times it exceeds the ability of the listener to comprehend as the speech expresses a flight of ideas or an unintelligible jargon.

primary gain   Relief from emotional conflict and the freedom from anxiety achieved by a defense mechanism.

projection   Mental mechanism whereby that which is emotionally unacceptable in the self is unconsciously rejected and attributed (projected) to others.

projective tests   Psychologic diagnostic tests in which the test material is unstructured so that any response will reflect a projection of some aspect of the subject's underlying personality and psychopathology.

psyche   Mind, in distinction to the soma, or body.

psychodrama   Technique of group psychotherapy in which individuals express their own or assigned emotional problems in dramatization.

psychodynamics   Systematized knowledge and theory of human behavior and its motivation, the study of which depends largely on the functional significance of emotion; psychodynamics recognizes the role of unconscious motivation in human behavior; a predictive science, based on the assumption that a person's total makeup and probable reactions at any given moment are the product of past interactions between his specific genetic endowment and the environment in which he has lived from conception onward.

psychomotor excitement   Generalized physical and emotional overactivity in response to internal and/or external stimuli, as in hypomania.

psychomotor retardation   Generalized slowing of physical and emotional reactions. Specifically, the slowing of movements such as eye-blinking; frequently seen in depression.

psychopathology   Study of the significant causes and processes in the development of mental disorders. Also the manifestations of mental disorders.

psychosexual development   Series of stages from infancy to adulthood, relatively fixed in time, determined by the interaction between a person's biologic drives and the environment. With resolution of this interaction, a balanced, reality-oriented development takes place; with disturbance, fixation and conflict ensue. This disturbance may remain latent or give rise to characterologic or behavioral disorders.

psychosis   Major mental disorder of organic or emotional origin in which a person's ability to think, respond emotionally, remember, communicate, interpret reality, and behave appropriately is sufficiently impaired so as to interfere grossly with the capacity to meet the ordinary demands of life.

psychosocial development   Progressive interaction between a person and the environment through stages beginning in infancy, as primarily described by Erikson. Specific developmental tasks involving social relations and the role of social reality are faced by a person at phase-specific developmental points. The early tasks parallel stages of psychosexual development; the later tasks extend through adulthood.

psychotherapy   Any form of treatment for mental illness, behavioral dysfunctions, and other problems that are assumed to be of an emotional nature, in which a trained person deliberately establishes a professional relationship with a client for the purpose of removing, modifying, or retarding existing symptoms, of attenuating or reversing disturbed patterns of behavior, and of promoting positive personality development and growth.

rapport   Confidential relationships between the client and the professional person who is in a helping relationship with him.

rationalization   Mental mechanism, operating unconsciously, by which the individual attempts to justify or make consciously tolerable by plausible means those feelings, behaviors, and motives that would otherwise be intolerable (not to be confused with conscious evasion or dissimulation).

reaction formation Mental mechanism, operating unconsciously, wherein attitudes and behavior are adopted that are the opposite of impulses the individual disowns either consciously or unconsciously—for example, excessive moral zeal may be the product of strong but repressed antisocial impulses.

reality principle In Freudian theory, the concept that the pleasure principle in personality development in infancy is normally modified by the inescapable demands and requirements of external reality; the process by which this compromise is effected is technically known as reality testing, both in normal development and in psychiatric treatment.

reality testing Ability to evaluate the external world objectively and to differentiate adequately between it and the internal world.

regression Partial or symbolic return to more infantile ways of gratification; most clearly seen in severe psychoses.

repression Mental mechanism, operating unconsciously; the common denominator and unconscious precursor of all mental mechanisms in which there is involuntary relegation of unbearable ideas and impulses into the unconscious whence they are not ordinarily subject to voluntary recall but may emerge in disguised form through use of the various mental mechanisms; particularly operative in early years.

resistance In psychiatry, an individual's massive psychological defense against bringing repressed (unconscious) thoughts or impulses into awareness, thus avoiding anxiety.

ritual Repetitive activity, usually a distorted or stereotyped elaboration of some routine of daily life, employed to relieve anxiety.

Rorschach test Psychological test developed by the Swiss psychiatrist Hermann Rorschach (1884-1922), that seeks to disclose conscious and unconscious personality traits and emotional conflicts through eliciting the person's associations to a standard set of inkblots.

schizophrenia, catatonic Type of schizophrenia characterized by immobility with muscular rigidity or inflexibility; alternating periods of physical hyperactivity and excitability may occur; generally there is marked inaccessibility to ordinary methods of communication.

schizophrenia, disorganized Type of schizophrenia characterized by incoherence and flat, incongruous, or silly affect, with no systematized delusions.

schizophrenia, paranoid Type of schizophrenia marked by a feeling that external reality has altered; suspiciousness; ideas of reference; hallucinations; delusions of persecution or grandiosity.

schizophrenia, residual Condition of being without gross psychotic symptoms following a psychotic schizophrenic episode.

schizophrenia, undifferentiated Type of schizophrenia characterized by prominent delusions, hallucinations, incoherence, or grossly disorganized behavior that cannot be classified in one of the other categories.

secondary gain External gain derived from any illness, such as personal attention and service, monetary gains, disability benefits, and release from unpleasant responsibility.

security operations   Sullivan's term for mechanisms such as apathy and selective inattention that, no matter how rational at first glance, are defenses against recognizing or experiencing anxiety.

selective inattention   Term for a security operation identified by Sullivan, whereby anxiety-producing aspects of a situation are not allowed into awareness.

sensorium   Synonymous with consciousness. Includes the special sensory perceptive powers and their central correlation and integration in the brain. A clear sensorium conveys the presence of a reasonably accurate memory together with orientation for time, place, and person.

separation-individuation   Psychologic awareness of one's separateness, described by Margaret Mahler as a phase in the mother-child relationship that follows the symbiotic stage. In the separation-individuation stage, the child begins to perceive himself as distinct from the mother and develops a sense of individual identity and an image of the self as object.

shame   Emotion resulting from the failure to live up to self-expectations.

sibling rivalry   Competition between siblings for the love of a parent or for other recognition or gain.

soma   Body; the physical aspect of a human as distinguished from the psyche.

somatic therapy   In psychiatry, the biologic treatment of mental disorders (e.g., electroconvulsive therapy, psychopharmacologic treatment).

somnolent detachment   Sullivan's term for the security operation with its origin in infancy, whereby the individual falls asleep when confronted by a highly-threatening, anxiety-producing experience.

speech disturbance   Any disorder of verbal communication that is not due to faulty innervation of speech muscles or organs of articulation.

stereotypy   Persistent, mechanical repetition of an activity; common in schizophrenia.

stressor   In terms of stress and adaptation theory, the stressor is any system input, which may have either positive or negative effects, depending on the way it is processed; may be classified as situational (untoward events) or developmental (anticipated events related to growth and maturation).

stupor   State in which a person does not react to or is unaware of the surroundings. Due to neurologic as well as psychiatric disorders. In catatonic stupor, the unawareness is more apparent than real.

sublimation   Mental mechanism, operating unconsciously, through which consciously unacceptable instinctual drives are diverted into personally and socially acceptable channels.

substance abuse   Pathological use of agents modifying mood, behavior, and cognition, creating an impairment in social or occupational functioning.

substitution   Mental mechanism, operating unconsciously, by which an unattainable or unacceptable goal, emotion, or object is replaced by one that is more attainable or acceptable.

suggestion   Process of influencing a client to accept an idea, belief, or attitude suggested by the therapist.

superego   In Freudian theory, that part of the mind that unconsciously identifies itself with important and esteemed persons from early life, particularly parents; the supposed or actual wishes of these significant persons are taken over as part of one's own personal standards to help form the "conscience."

supportive psychotherapy   Type of psychotherapy that aims to reinforce a client's defenses and help suppress disturbing psychologic material. Supportive psychotherapy utilizes such measures as inspiration, reassurance, suggestion, persuasion, counseling, and reeducation. It avoids probing the client's emotional conflicts in depth.

suppression   Conscious effort to overcome unacceptable thoughts or desires by forcing them out of the conscious mind.

symbiosis   Mutually reinforcing relationship between two persons who are dependent on each other. A normal characteristic of the relationship between the mothering one and infant child.

symbolization   Mental mechanism, operating unconsciously, in which a person forms an abstract representation of a particular object, idea, or constellation. The symbol carries, in more or less disguised form, the emotional feelings vested in the initial object or ideas.

tangentiality   Replying to a question in an oblique or irrelevant way.

tardive dyskinesia   Serious side effect of antipsychotic medication characterized by grimacing, choreiform, or athetoid movements of the arms, fingers, ankles, and toes, and tonic contractions of the neck and back muscles. At present it is irreversible.

therapeutic community   Term of British origin, now widely used, for a specially structured mental hospital environment that encourages clients to function within the range of social norms.

therapeutic window   Range of blood levels associated with clinical response to certain drugs.

thought disorder   Disturbance of speech, communication, or content of thought, such as delusions, ideas of reference, poverty of thought, flight of ideas, perseveration, loosening of association, etc. A thought disorder can be caused by a functional mental disorder or an organic condition.

toxic psychosis   Psychosis resulting from the toxic effect of chemicals and drugs, including those produced in the body.

tranquilizer   Medication that decreases anxiety and agitation. Preferred terms are antianxiety or anxiolytic and antipsychotic medications.

transference   Unconscious attachment to others of feelings and attitudes that were originally associated with important figures (parents, siblings, etc.) in one's early life. The transference relationship follows roughly the pattern of its prototype; the therapist uses the phenomenon as a therapeutic tool to help the client understand his emotional problems and their origin; in the client-therapist relationship the transference may be negative (hostile) or positive (affectionate).

unconscious   In Freudian theory, that part of the mind or mental functioning the content of which is only rarely subject to awareness; a repository for data that have never been conscious (primary repression) or that may have become conscious briefly and were then repressed (secondary repression).

undoing   Primitive defense mechanism, operating unconsciously, by which something unacceptable and already done is symbolically acted out in reverse, usually repetitiously, in the hope of "undoing" it and thus relieving anxiety.

volition   Will.

withdrawal   Pathologic retreat from people or the world of reality, often seen in schizophrenia.

withdrawal symptoms   Physical and mental effects of withdrawing addictive substances from clients who have become habituated or addicted to them.

word salad   Mixture of words and phrases that lacks comprehensive meaning or logical coherence, commonly seen in schizophrenic states.

working through   Exploration of a problem by client and therapist until a satisfactory solution has been found or until a symptom has been traced to its unconscious sources.

Appendix A

A patient's bill of rights

1. The patient has the right to considerate and respectful care.
2. The patient has the right to obtain from his physician complete current information concerning his diagnosis, treatment, and prognosis in terms the patient can be reasonably expected to understand. When it is not medically advisable to give such information to the patient, the information should be made available to an appropriate person in his behalf. He has the right to know, by name, the physician responsible for coordinating his care.
3. The patient has the right to receive from his physician information necessary to give informed consent prior to the start of any procedure and/or treatment. Except in emergencies, such information for informed consent should include but not necessarily be limited to the specific procedure and/or treatment, the medically significant risks involved, and the probable duration of incapacitation. Where medically significant alternatives for care or treatment exist, or when the patient requests information concerning medical alternatives, the patient has the right to such information. The patient also has the right to know the name of the person responsible for the procedures and/or treatment.
4. The patient has the right to refuse treatment to the extent permitted by law and to be informed of the medical consequences of his action.
5. The patient has the right to every consideration of his privacy concerning his own medical care program. Case discussion, consultation, examination, and treatment are confidential and should be conducted discreetly. Those not directly involved in his care must have the permission of the patient to be present.
6. The patient has the right to expect that all communications and records pertaining to his care should be treated as confidential.
7. The patient has the right to expect that within its capacity a hospital must make reasonable response to the request of a patient for services. The hospital must provide evaluation, service, and/or referral as indicated by the urgency of the case. When medically permissible, a patient may be transferred to another facility only after he has received complete information

---

and explanation concerning the needs for and alternatives to such a transfer. The institution to which the patient is to be transferred must first have accepted the patient for transfer.

8. The patient has the right to obtain information as to any relationship of his hospital to other health care and educational institutions insofar as his care is concerned. The patient has the right to obtain information as to the existence of any professional relationships among individuals, by name, who are treating him.

9. The patient has the right to be advised if the hospital proposes to engage in or perform human experimentation affecting his care or treatment. The patient has the right to refuse to participate in such research projects.

10. The patient has the right to expect reasonable continuity of care. He has the right to know in advance what appointment times and physicians are available and where. The patient has the right to expect that the hospital will provide a mechanism whereby he is informed by his physician or a delegate of the physician of the patient's continuing health care requirements following discharge.

11. The patient has the right to examine and receive an explanation of his bill regardless of source of payment.

12. The patient has the right to know what hospital rules and regulations apply to his conduct as a patient.

Appendix B

The code for nurses

1. The nurse provides services with respect for human dignity and the uniqueness of the client, unrestricted by considerations of social or economic status, personal attributes, or the nature of health problems.
2. The nurse safeguards the client's right to privacy by judiciously protecting information of a confidential nature.
3. The nurse acts to safeguard the client and the public when health care and safety are affected by the incompetent, unethical, or illegal practice of any person.
4. The nurse assumes responsibility and accountability for individual nursing judgments and actions.
5. The nurse maintains competence in nursing.
6. The nurse exercises informed judgment and uses individual competence and qualifications as criteria in seeking consultation, accepting responsibilities, and delegating nursing activities to others.
7. The nurse participates in activities that contribute to the ongoing development of the profession's body of knowledge.
8. The nurse participates in the profession's efforts to implement and improve standards of nursing.
9. The nurse participates in the profession's efforts to establish and maintain conditions of employment conducive to high quality nursing care.
10. The nurse participates in the profession's effort to protect the public from misinformation and misrepresentation and to maintain the integrity of nursing.
11. The nurse collaborates with members of the health professions and other citizens in promoting community and national efforts to meet the health needs of the public.

From American Nurses' Association: Code for nurses (with interpretive statements), Kansas City, Mo., 1985. Reprinted with permission from the American Nurses' Association.

DSM-III-R classification
Axes I and II categories and codes

All official DSM-III-R codes are included in ICD-9-CM. Codes followed by a *
are used for more than one DSM-III-R diagnosis or subtype in order to maintain
compatibility with ICD-9-CM.

A long dash following a diagnostic term indicates the need for a fifth digit
subtype or other qualifying term.

The term *specify* following the name of some diagnostic categories indicates
qualifying terms that clinicians may wish to add in parentheses after the name
of the disorder.

NOS = Not Otherwise Specified

The current severity of a disorder may be specified after the diagnosis as:

mild ┐
moderate ├ currently meets diagnostic criteria
severe ┘

in partial remission
(or residual state)
in complete remission

DISORDERS USUALLY FIRST EVIDENT IN INFANCY, CHILDHOOD, OR ADOLESCENCE

DEVELOPMENTAL DISORDERS

Note: These are coded on Axis II.

Mental Retardation

317.00	Mild mental retardation
318.00	Moderate mental retardation

Continued.

318.10   Severe mental retardation
318.20   Profound mental retardation
319.00   Unspecified mental retardation

Pervasive Developmental Disorders

299.00   Autistic disorder
          Specify if childhood onset
299.80   Pervasive developmental disorder NOS

Specific Developmental Disorders

Academic skills disorders

315.10   Developmental arithmetic disorder
315.80   Developmental expressive writing disorder
315.00   Developmental reading disorder

Language and speech disorders

315.39   Developmental articulation disorder
315.31*   Developmental expressive language disorder
315.31*   Developmental receptive language disorder

Motor skills disorder

315.40   Developmental coordination disorder
315.90*   Specific developmental disorder NOS

Other Developmental Disorders

315.90*   Developmental disorder NOS

Disruptive Behavior Disorders

314.01   Attention-deficit hyperactivity disorder

          Conduct disorder,
312.20   group type
312.00   solitary aggressive type
312.90   undifferentiated type
313.81   Oppositional defiant disorder

Anxiety Disorders of Childhood or Adolescence

309.21   Separation anxiety disorder
313.21   Avoidant disorder of childhood or ado-
          lescence
313.00   Overanxious disorder

Eating Disorders

307.10   Anorexia nervosa
307.51   Bulimia nervosa
307.52   Pica
307.53   Rumination disorder of infancy
307.50   Eating disorder NOS

Gender Identity Disorders

302.60   Gender identity disorder of childhood
302.50   Transsexualism
               Specify sexual history: asexual, homo-
               sexual, heterosexual, unspecified
302.85*   Gender identity disorder of adolescence
          or adulthood, nontranssexual type
               Specify sexual history: asexual, homo-
               sexual, heterosexual, unspecified
302.85*   Gender identity disorder NOS

Tic Disorders

307.23   Tourette's disorder
307.22   Chronic motor or vocal tic disorder
307.21   Transient tic disorder
               Specify: single episode or recurrent
307.20   Tic disorder NOS

Elimination Disorders

307.70   Functional encopresis
               Specify: primary or secondary type
307.60   Functional enuresis
               Specify: primary or secondary types
               Specify: nocturnal only, diurnal only,
               nocturnal and diurnal

Speech Disorders not Elsewhere Classified

307.00*   Cluttering
307.00*   Stuttering

Other Disorders of Infancy, Childhood, or Adolescence

313.23	Elective mutism
313.82	Identity disorder
313.89	Reactive attachment disorder of infancy or early childhood
307.30	Stereotypy/habit disorder
314.00	Undifferentiated attention-deficit disorder

ORGANIC MENTAL DISORDERS
Dementias Arising in the Senium and Presenium

Primary degenerative dementia of the Alzheimer type, senile onset,

290.30	with delirium
290.20	with delusions
290.21	with depression
290.00*	uncomplicated

(Note: code 331.00 Alzheimer's disease on Axis III)

Code in fifth digit:

1 = with delirium, 2 = with delusions, 3 = with depression, 0* = uncomplicated

290.1x	Primary degenerative dementia of the Alzheimer type presenile onset,_____

(Note: code 331.00 Alzherimer's disease on Axis III)

290.4x	Multi-infarct dementia,_____
290.00*	Senile dementia NOS

Specify etiology on Axis III if known

290.10*	Presenile dementia NOS

Specify etiology on Axis III if known (e.g., Pick's disease, Jakob-Creutzfeldt disease)

Psychoactive Substance-Induced Organic Mental Disorders

Alcohol

303.00	intoxication
291.40	idiosyncratic intoxication
291.80	Uncomplicated alcohol withdrawal
291.00	withdrawal delirium
291.30	hallucinosis

291.10	amnestic disorder
291.20	Dementia associated with alcoholism
	Amphetamine or similarly acting sympathomimetic
305.70*	intoxication
292.00*	withdrawal
292.81*	delirium
292.11*	delusional disorder
	Caffeine
305.90*	intoxication
	Cannabis
305.20*	intoxication
292.11*	delusional disorder
	Cocaine
305.60*	intoxication
292.00*	withdrawal
292.81*	delirium
292.11*	delusional disorder
	Hallucinogen
305.30*	hallucinosis
292.11*	delusional disorder
292.84*	mood disorder
292.89*	Posthallucinogen perception disorder
	Inhalant
305.90*	intoxication
	Nicotine
292.00*	withdrawal
	Opioid
305.50*	intoxication
292.00*	withdrawal
	Phencyclidine (PCP) or similarly acting arylcyclohexylamine
305.90*	intoxication
292.81*	delirium
292.11*	delusional disorder
292.84*	mood disorder
292.90*	organic mental disorder NOS
	Sedative, hypnotic, or anxiolytic
305.40*	intoxication
292.00*	Uncomplicated sedative, hypnotic, or anxiolytic withdrawal
292.00*	withdrawal delirium
292.83*	amnestic disorder

Other or unspecified psychoactive substance

305.90*	intoxication
292.00*	withdrawal
292.81*	delirium
292.82*	dementia
292.83*	amnestic disorder
292.11*	delusional disorder
292.12	hallucinosis
292.84*	mood disorder
292.89*	anxiety disorder
292.89*	personality disorder
292.90*	organic mental disorder NOS

Organic Mental Disorders associated with Axis III physical disorders or conditions, or whose etiology is unknown.

293.00	Delirium
294.10	Dementia
294.00	Amnestic disorder
293.81	Organic delusional disorder
293.82	Organic hallucinosis
293.83	Organic mood disorder
	Specify: manic, depressed, mixed
294.80*	Organic anxiety disorder
310.10	Organic personality disorder
	Specify if explosive type
294.80*	Organic mental disorder NOS

PSYCHOACTIVE SUBSTANCE USE DISORDERS

Alcohol

303.90	dependence
305.00	abuse

Amphetamine or similarly acting sympathomimetic

304.40	dependence
305.70*	abuse

Cannabis

304.30	dependence
305.20*	abuse

Cocaine

304.20	dependence
305.60*	abuse

	Hallucinogen
304.50*	dependence
305.30*	abuse
	Inhalant
304.60	dependence
305.90*	abuse
	Nicotine
305.10	dependence
	Opioid
304.00	dependence
305.50*	abuse
	Phencyclidine (PCP) or similarly acting arylcyclohexylamine
304.50*	dependence
305.90*	abuse
	Sedative, hypnotic, or anxiolytic
304.10	dependence
305.40*	abuse
304.90*	Polysubstance dependence
304.90*	Psychoactive substance dependence NOS
305.90*	Psychoactive substance abuse NOS

SCHIZOPHRENIA

Code in fifth digit: 1 = subchronic, 2 = chronic, 3 = subchronic with acute exacerbation, 4 = chronic with acute exacerbation, 5 = in remission, 0 = unspecified.

	Schizophrenia,
295.2x	catatonic,_____
295.1x	disorganized,_____
295.3x	paranoid,_____
	Specify if stable type_____
295.9x	undifferentiated,_____
295.6x	residual,_____
	Specify if late onset

DELUSIONAL (PARANOID) DISORDER

297.10	Delusional (Paranoid) disorder
	Specify type: erotomanic
	grandiose
	jealous
	persecutory
	somatic
	unspecified

PSYCHOTIC DISORDERS NOT ELSEWHERE CLASSIFIED

298.80   Brief reactive psychosis
295.40   Schizophreniform disorder
            Specify: without good prognostic features or with good prognostic features
295.70   Schizoaffective disorder
            Specify: bipolar type or depressive type
297.30   Induced psychotic disorder
298.90   Psychotic disorder NOS (Atypical psychosis)

MOOD DISORDERS

Code current state of Major Depression and Bipolar Disorder in Fifth digit:

1 = mild
2 = moderate
3 = severe, without psychotic features
4 = with psychotic features (*specify* mood-congruent or mood-incongruent)
5 = in partial remission
6 = in full remission
0 = unspecified

For major depressive episodes, *specify* if chronic and *specify* if melancholic type.

For Bipolar Disorder, Bipolar Disorder NOS, Recurrent Major Depression, and Depressive Disorder NOS, *specify* if seasonal pattern.

Bipolar Disorders

          Bipolar disorder,
296.6x   mixed,_____
296.4x   manic,_____
296.5x   depressed,_____
301.13   Cyclothymia
296.70   Bipolar disorder NOS

Depressive Disorders

          Major Depression,
296.2x   single episode,_____
296.3x   recurrent,_____

300.40   Dysthymia (or Depressive neurosis)
          Specify: primary or secondary type
          Specify: early or late onset
311.00   Depressive disorder NOS

ANXIETY DISORDERS (or Anxiety and Phobic Neuroses)

          Panic disorder
300.21   with agoraphobia
                Specify current severity of agoraphobic avoidance
                Specify current severity of panic attacks
300.01   without agoraphobia
                Specify current severity of panic attacks
300.22   Agoraphobia without history of panic disorder
                Specify with or without limited symptom attacks
300.23   Social phobia
                Specify if generalized type
300.29   Simple phobia
300.30   Obsessive compulsive disorder (or Obsessive compulsive neurosis)
309.89   Post-traumatic stress disorder
                Specify if delayed onset
300.02   Generalized anxiety disorder
300.00   Anxiety disorder NOS

SOMATOFORM DISORDERS

300.70* Body dysmorphic disorder
300.11   Conversion disorder (or Hysterical neurosis, conversion type)
                Specify: single episode or recurrent
300.70* Hypochondriasis (or Hypochondriacal neurosis)
300.81   Somatization disorder
307.80   Somatoform pain disorder
300.70* Undifferentiated somatoform disorder
300.70* Somatoform disorder NOS

DISSOCIATIVE DISORDERS (or Hysterical Neuroses, Dissociative Type)

300.14   Multiple personality disorder
300.13   Psychogenic fugue
300.12   Psychogenic amnesia
300.60   Depersonalization disorder (or Depersonalization neurosis)
300.15   Dissociative disorder NOS

SEXUAL DISORDERS
Paraphilias

302.40   Exhibitionism
302.81   Fetishism
302.89   Frotteurism
302.20   Pedophilia

> *Specify*: same sex, opposite sex, same and opposite sex
> *Specify* if limited to incest
> *Specify*: exclusive type or nonexclusive type

302.83   Sexual masochism
302.84   Sexual sadism
302.30   Transvestic fetishism
302.82   Voyeurism
302.90*   Paraphilia NOS

Sexual Dysfunctions

Specify: psychogenic only, or psychogenic and biogenic (Note: If biogenic only, code on Axis III)
Specify: lifelong or acquired
Specify: generalized or situational

Sexual desire disorders
302.71   Hypoactive sexual desire disorder
302.79   Sexual aversion disorder

Sexual arousal disorder
302.72*   Female sexual arousal disorder
302.72*   Male erectile disorder

Orgasm disorders
302.73   Inhibited female orgasm
302.74   Inhibited male orgasm
302.75   Premature ejaculation

Sexual pain disorders
302.76   Dyspareunia
306.51   Vaginismus
302.70   Sexual dysfunction NOS

Other Sexual Disorders
302.90*   Sexual disorder NOS

SLEEP DISORDERS
Dyssomnias

Insomnia disorder
307.42*   related to another mental disorder (nonorganic)
780.50*   related to known organic factor
307.42*   Primary insomnia
Hypersomnia disorder
307.44   related to another mental disorder (nonorganic)
780.50*   related to a known organic factor
780.54   Primary hypersomnia
307.45   Sleep-wake schedule disorder
Specify: advanced or delayed phase type, disorganized type, frequently changing type
Other dyssomnias
307.40*   Dyssomnia NOS

Parasomnias

307.47   Dream anxiety disorder (Nightmare disorder)
307.46*   Sleep terror disorder
307.46*   Sleepwalking disorder
307.40*   Parasomnia NOS

FACTITIOUS DISORDERS

Factitious disorder
301.51   with physical symptoms
300.16   with psychological symptoms
300.19   Factitious disorder NOS

IMPULSE CONTROL DISORDERS NOT ELSEWHERE CLASSIFIED

312.34   Intermittent explosive disorder
312.32   Kleptomania

312.31	Pathological gambling
312.33	Pyromania
312.39*	Trichotillomania
312.39*	Impulse control disorder NOS

ADJUSTMENT DISORDER

Adjustment disorder

309.24	with anxious mood
309.00	with depressed mood
309.30	with disturbance of conduct
309.40	with mixed disturbance of emotions and conduct
309.28	with mixed emotional features
309.82	with physical complaints
309.83	with withdrawal
309.23	with work (or academic) inhibition
309.90	Adjustment disorder NOS

PSYCHOLOGICAL FACTORS AFFECTING PHYSICAL CONDITION

316.00	Psychological factors affecting physical condition
	Specify physical condition on Axis III

PERSONALITY DISORDERS

Note: These are coded on Axis II.

Cluster A

301.00	Paranoid
301.20	Schizoid
301.22	Schizotypal

Cluster B

301.70	Antisocial
301.83	Borderline
301.50	Histrionic
301.81	Narcissistic

Cluster C

301.82	Avoidant
301.60	Dependent
301.40	Obsessive compulsive
301.84	Passive aggressive
301.90	Personality disorder NOS

V CODES FOR CONDITIONS NOT ATTRIBUTABLE TO A MENTAL DISORDER THAT ARE A FOCUS OF ATTENTION OR TREATMENT

V62.30   Academic problem

V71.01   Adult antisocial behavior

V40.00 Borderline intellectual functioning
(Note: This is coded on Axis II.)

V71.02   Childhood or adolescent antisocial behavior

V65.20   Malingering

V61.10   Marital problem

V15.81   Noncompliance with medical treatment

V62.20   Occupational problem

V61.20   Parent-child problem

V62.81   Other interpersonal problem

V61.80   Other specified family circumstances

V62.89   Phase of life problem or other life circumstance problem

V62.82   Uncomplicated bereavement

ADDITIONAL CODES

300.90   Unspecified mental disorder (nonpsychotic)

V71.09*   No diagnosis or condition on Axis I

799.90*   Diagnosis or condition deferred on Axis I

V71.09*   No diagnosis or condition on Axis II

799.90*   Diagnosis or condition deferred on Axis II

MULTIAXIAL SYSTEM

Axis I   Clinical Syndromes
          V Codes

Axis II   Developmental Disorders
          Personality Disorders

Axis III Physical Disorders and Conditions

Axis IV   Severity of Psychosocial Stressors

Axis V   Global Assessment of Functioning

Severity of psychosocial stressors scale: adults

| Code | Term | Examples of stressors | |
		Acute events	Enduring circumstances
1	None	No acute events that may be relevant to the disorder	No enduring circumstances that may be relevant to the disorder
2	Mild	Broke up with boyfriend or girlfriend; started or graduated from school; child left home	Family arguments; job dissatisfaction; residence in high-crime neighborhood
3	Moderate	Marriage; marital separation; loss of job; retirement; miscarriage	Marital discord; serious financial problems; trouble with boss; being a single parent
4	Severe	Divorce; birth of first child	Unemployment; poverty
5	Extreme	Death of spouse; serious physical illness diagnosed; victim of rape	Serious chronic illness in self or child; ongoing physical or sexual abuse
6	Catastrophic	Death of a child; suicide of spouse; devastating natural disaster	Captivity as hostage; concentration camp experience
0	Inadequate information, or no change in condition		

Severity of psychosocial stressors scale: children and adolescents

| Code | Term | Examples of stressors | |
		Acute events	Enduring circumstances
1	None	No acute events that may be relevant to the disorder	No enduring circumstances that may be relevant to the disorder
2	Mild	Broke up with boyfriend or girlfriend; change of school	Overcrowded living quarters; family arguments
3	Moderate	Expelled from school; birth of sibling	Chronic disabling illness in parent; chronic parental discord
4	Severe	Divorce of parents; unwanted pregnancy; arrest	Harsh or rejecting parents; chronic life-threatening illness in parent; multiple foster home placements

Severity of psychosocial stressors scale: children and adolescents—cont'd

Code	Term	Examples of stressors	
		Acute events	*Enduring circumstances*
5	Extreme	Sexual or physical abuse; death of a parent	Recurrent sexual or physical abuse
6	Catastrophic	Death of both parents	Chronic life-threatening illness
0	Inadequate information, or no change in condition		

Global assessment of functioning scale (GAF scale)

Consider psychological, social, and occupational functioning on a hypothetical continuum of mental health-illness. Do not include impairment in functioning due to physical (or environmental) limitations.

Note: Use intermediate codes when appropriate, e.g., 45, 68, 72.

CODE

90 ⎪ 81	**Absent or minimal symptoms** (e.g., mild anxiety before an exam), **good functioning in all areas, interested and involved in a wide range of activities, socially effective, generally satisfied with life, no more than everyday problems or concerns** (e.g., an occasional argument with family members).
80 ⎪ 71	**If symptoms are present, they are transient and expectable reactions to psychosocial stressors** (e.g., difficulty concentrating after family argument); **no more than slight impairment in social, occupational, or school functioning** (e.g., temporarily falling behind in school work).
70 ⎪ 61	**Some mild symptoms** (e.g., depressed mood and mild insomnia) **OR some difficulty in social, occupational, or school functioning** (e.g., occasional truancy, or theft within the household), **but generally functioning pretty well, has some meaningful interpersonal relationships.**
60 ⎪ 51	**Moderate symptoms** (e.g., flat affect and circumstantial speech, occasional panic attacks) **OR moderate difficulty in social, occupational, or school functioning** (e.g., few friends, conflicts with co-workers).
50 ⎪ 41	**Serious symptoms** (e.g., suicidal ideation, severe obsessional rituals, frequent shoplifting) **OR any serious impairment in social, occupational, or school functioning** (e.g., few friends, unable to keep a job).
40 ⎪ 31	**Some impairment in reality testing or communication** (e.g., speech is at times illogical, obscure, or irrelevant) **OR major impairment in several areas, such as work or school, family relations, judgment, thinking, or mood** (e.g., depressed man avoids friends, neglects family, and is unable to work; child frequently beats up younger children, is defiant at home, and is failing at school).
30 ⎪ 21	**Behavior is considerably influenced by delusions or hallucinations OR serious impairment in communication or judgment** (e.g., sometimes incoherent, acts grossly inappropriately, suicidal preoccupation) **OR inability to function in almost all areas** (e.g., stays in bed all day; no job, home, or friends).

Continued.

Global assessment of functioning scale (GAF scale)—cont'd

CODE

20 | **Some danger of hurting self or others** (e.g., suicide attempts without clear expectation of death, frequent violent, manic excitement) **OR occasionally fails to maintain minimal personal hygiene** (e.g., smears feces) **OR gross impairment in communication** (e.g., largely incoherent or mute).
11 |

10 | **Persistent danger of severely hurting self or others** (e.g., recurrent violence) **OR persistent inability to maintain minimal personal hygiene OR serious suicidal act with clear expectation of death.**
1 |

Appendix D

NANDA *approved nursing diagnostic categories*

Pattern 1: EXCHANGING

1.1.2.1	Altered Nutrition: More than body requirements
1.1.2.2	Altered Nutrition: Less than body requirements
1.1.2.3	Altered Nutrition: Potential for more than body requirements
1.2.1.1	Potential for Infection
1.2.2.1	Potential Altered Body Temperature
1.2.2.2	Hypothermia
1.2.2.3	Hyperthermia
1.2.2.4	Ineffective Thermoregulation
1.2.3.1	Dysreflexia
1.3.1.1	Constipation
1.3.1.1.1	Perceived Constipation
1.3.1.1.2	Colonic Constipation
1.3.1.2	Diarrhea
1.3.1.3	Bowel Incontinence
1.3.2	Altered Patterns of Urinary Elimination
1.3.2.1.1	Stress Incontinence
1.3.2.1.2	Reflex Incontinence
1.3.2.1.3	Urge Incontinence
1.3.2.1.4	Functional Incontinence
1.3.2.1.5	Total Incontinence
1.3.2.2	Urinary Retention
1.4.1.1	Altered (Specify Type) Tissue Perfusion (Renal, cerebral, cardiopulmonary, gastrointestinal, peripheral)
1.4.1.2.1	Fluid Volume Excess
1.4.1.2.2.1	Fluid Volume Deficit (1)
1.4.1.2.2.1	Fluid Volume Deficit (2)
1.4.1.2.2.2	Potential Fluid Volume Deficit

North American Nursing Diagnosis Association: NANDA Approved Nursing Diagnosis Categories, Nursing Diagnosis Newsletter 15(1):1-3, Summer 1988, The Association.

1.4.2.1	Decreased Cardiac Output
1.5.1.1	Impaired Gas Exchange
1.5.1.2	Ineffective Airway Clearance
1.5.1.3	Ineffective Breathing Pattern
1.6.1	Potential for Injury
1.6.1.1	Potential for Suffocation
1.6.1.2	Potential for Poisoning
1.6.1.3	Potential for Trauma
1.6.1.4	Potential for Aspiration
1.6.1.5	Potential for Disuse Syndrome
1.6.2.1	Impaired Tissue Integrity
1.6.2.1.1	Altered Oral Mucous Membrane
1.6.2.1.2.1	Impaired Skin Integrity
1.6.2.1.2.2	Potential Impaired Skin Integrity

Pattern 2: COMMUNICATING

2.1.1.1	Impaired Verbal Communication

Pattern 3: RELATING

3.1.1	Impaired Social Interaction
3.1.2	Social Isolation
3.2.1	Altered Role Performance
3.2.1.1.1	Altered Parenting
3.2.1.1.2	Potential Altered Parenting
3.2.1.2.1	Sexual Dysfunction
3.2.2	Altered Family Processes
3.2.3.1	Parental Role Conflict
3.3	Altered Sexuality Patterns

Pattern 4: VALUING

4.1.1	Spiritual Distress (distress of the human spirit)

Pattern 5: CHOOSING

5.1.1.1	Ineffective Individual Coping
5.1.1.1.1	Impaired Adjustment
5.1.1.1.2	Defensive Coping
5.1.1.1.3	Ineffective Denial
5.1.2.1.1	Ineffective Family Coping: Disabling
5.1.2.1.2	Ineffective Family Coping: Compromised
5.1.2.2	Family Coping: Potential for Growth
5.2.1.1	Noncompliance (Specify)
5.3.1.1	Decisional Conflict (Specify)
5.4	Health Seeking Behaviors (Specify)

Pattern 6: MOVING

6.1.1.1	Impaired Physical Mobility
6.1.1.2	Activity Intolerance
6.1.1.2.1	Fatigue
6.1.1.3	Potential Activity Intolerance
6.2.1	Sleep Pattern Disturbance
6.3.1.1	Diversional Activity Deficit
6.4.1.1	Impaired Home Maintenance Management
6.4.2	Altered Health Maintenance
6.5.1	Feeding Self Care Deficit
6.5.1.1	Impaired Swallowing
6.5.1.2	Ineffective Breastfeeding
6.5.2	Bathing/Hygiene Self Care Deficit
6.5.3	Dressing/Grooming Self Care Deficit
6.5.4	Toileting Self Care Deficit
6.6	Altered Growth and Development

Pattern 7: PERCEIVING

7.1.1	Body Image Disturbance
7.1.2	Self Esteem Disturbance
7.1.2.1	Chronic Low Self Esteem
7.1.2.2	Situational Low Self Esteem
7.1.3	Personal Identity Disturbance
7.2	Sensory/Perceptual Alterations (Specify) (Visual, auditory, kinesthetic, gustatory, tactile, olfactory)
7.2.1.1	Unilateral Neglect
7.3.1	Hopelessness
7.3.2	Powerlessness

Pattern 8: KNOWING

8.1.1	Knowledge Deficit (Specify)
8.3	Altered Thought Processes

Pattern 9: FEELING

9.1.1	Pain
9.1.1.1	Chronic Pain
9.2.1.1	Dysfunctional Grieving
9.2.1.2	Anticipatory Grieving
9.2.2	Potential for Violence: Self-directed or directed at others
9.2.3	Post-Trauma Response

9.2.3.1	Rape-Trauma Syndrome
9.2.3.1.1	Rape-Trauma Syndrome: Compound Reaction
9.2.3.1.2	Rape-Trauma Syndrome: Silent Reaction
9.3.1	Anxiety
9.3.2	Fear

Appendix E

Classification of human responses of concern for psychiatric mental health nursing practice
Draft IV-R, September 20, 1988

1. HUMAN RESPONSE PATTERNS IN ACTIVITY PROCESSES
   1.1 Motor Behavior
      1.1.1   Potential for Alteration
          *1.1.1.1   Activity Intolerance
          1.1.1.2
      1.1.2   Altered Motor Behavior
          *1.1.2.1   Activity Intolerance
          1.1.2.2   Bizarre Motor Behavior
          1.1.2.3   Catatonia
          1.1.2.4   Disorganized Motor Behavior
          *1.1.2.5   Fatigue
          1.1.2.6   Hyperactivity
          1.1.2.7   Hypoactivity
          1.1.2.8   Impulsive Motor Behavior
          1.1.2.9   Psychomotor Agitation
          1.1.2.10   Psychomotor Retardation
          1.1.2.11   Restlessness
      1.1.99   Motor Behavior Not Otherwise Specified (NOS)
   1.2 Recreation Patterns
      1.2.1   Potential for Alteration
          1.2.1.1
          1.2.1.2

O'Toole A.W. and Loomis M.E. 1989. Classifying human responses in psychiatric-mental health nursing. *Classification systems for describing nursing practice: working papers*, pp. 27-29. Kansas City, MO: American Nurses' Association. Reprinted with permission from the association.
*Approved NANDA Diagnoses.

1.2.2   Altered Recreation Patterns
       1.2.2.1   Age Inappropriate Recreation
       1.2.2.2   Anti-Social Recreation
       1.2.2.3   Bizarre Recreation
       *1.2.2.4   Diversional Activity Deficit
1.2.99   Recreation Patterns NOS

1.3   Self Care
    1.3.1   Potential for Alteration in Self Care
    *1.3.2   Potential for Altered Health Maintenance
    *1.3.3   Altered Growth and Development
    1.3.4   Altered Self Care
       *1.3.4.1   Altered Eating
          1.3.4.1.1   Binge-Purge Syndrome
          1.3.4.1.2   Non-nutritive Ingestion
          1.3.4.1.3   Pica
          1.3.4.1.4   Unusual Food Ingestion
          1.3.4.1.5   Refusal to Eat
          1.3.4.1.6   Rumination
       *1.3.4.2   Altered Feeding
          *1.3.4.2.1   Ineffective Breastfeeding
       *1.3.4.3   Altered Grooming
       *1.3.4.4   Altered Health Maintenance
       *1.3.4.5   Altered Health Seeking Behaviors
       *1.3.4.6   Altered Hygiene
       1.3.4.7   Altered Participation in Health Care
       *1.3.4.8   Altered Toileting
    *1.3.5   Impaired Adjustment
    *1.3.6   Knowledge Deficit
    *1.3.7   Noncompliance
    1.3.99   Self Care Patterns NOS

1.4   Sleep/Arousal Patterns
    1.4.1   Potential for Alteration
    *1.4.2   Altered Sleep/Arousal Patterns
       1.4.2.1   Decreased Need for Sleep
       1.4.2.2   Difficult Transition to and from Sleep
       1.4.2.3   Hypersomnia
       1.4.2.4   Insomnia
       1.4.2.5   Nightmares/Terrors
       1.4.2.6   Somnolence
       1.4.2.7   Somnambulism
    1.4.99   Sleep/Arousal Patterns NOS

2. HUMAN RESPONSE PATTERNS IN COGNITION PROCESSES
   2.1 Decision Making
       2.1.1   Potential for Alteration
       2.1.2   Altered Decision Making
       2.1.99   Decision Making Patterns NOS
   2.2 Judgment
       2.2.1   Potential for Alteration
       2.2.2   Altered Judgment
       2.2.99   Judgment Patterns NOS
   2.3 Knowledge
       2.3.1   Potential for Alteration
    *2.3.2   Altered Knowledge Processes
              2.3.2.1   Agnosia
              2.3.2.2   Altered Intellectual Functioning
           *2.3.2.3   Knowledge Deficit
       2.3.99   Knowledge Patterns NOS
   2.4 Learning
       2.4.1   Potential for Alteration
       2.4.2   Altered Learning Processes
       2.4.99   Learning Patterns NOS
   2.5 Memory
       2.5.1   Potential for Alteration
       2.5.2   Altered Memory
               2.5.2.1   Amnesia
              2.5.2.2   Distorted Memory
              2.5.2.3   Long-Term Memory Loss
              2.5.2.4   Memory Deficit
              2.5.2.5   Short-Term Memory Loss
       2.5.99   Memory Patterns NOS
   2.6 Thought Processes
       2.6.1   Potential for Alteration
    *2.6.2   Altered Thought Processes
               2.6.2.1   Altered Abstract Thinking
              2.6.2.2   Altered Concentration
              2.6.2.3   Altered Problem Solving
              2.6.2.4   Confusion/Disorientation
              2.6.2.5   Delirium
              2.6.2.6   Delusions
              2.6.2.7   Ideas of Reference
              2.6.2.8   Magical Thinking
              2.6.2.9   Obsessions
              2.6.2.10   Thought Insertion
       2.6.99   Thought Processes NOS

3. HUMAN RESPONSE PATTERNS IN ECOLOGICAL PROCESSES
   3.1 Community Maintenance
      3.1.1   Potential for Alteration
      3.1.2   Altered Community Maintenance
           3.1.2.1   Community Safety Hazards
           3.1.2.2   Community Sanitation Hazards
      3.1.99   Community Maintenance Patterns NOS
   3.2 Environmental Integrity
      3.2.1   Potential for Alteration
      3.2.2   Altered Environmental Integrity
      3.2.99   Environmental Integrity Patterns NOS
   3.3 Home Maintenance
      3.3.1   Potential for Alteration
    *3.3.2   Altered Home Maintenance
           3.3.2.1   Home Safety Hazards
           3.3.2.2   Home Sanitation Hazards
      3.3.99   Home Maintenance Patterns NOS
4. HUMAN RESPONSE PATTERNS IN EMOTIONAL PROCESSES
   4.1 Feeling States
      4.1.1   Potential for Alteration
          *4.1.1.1   Anticipatory Grieving
      4.1.2   Altered Feeling State
           4.1.2.1   Anger
         *4.1.2.2   Anxiety
           4.1.2.3   Elation
           4.1.2.4   Envy
         *4.1.2.5   Fear
         *4.1.2.6   Grief
           4.1.2.7   Guilt
           4.1.2.8   Sadness
           4.1.2.9   Shame
      4.1.3   Affect Incongruous in Situation
      4.1.4   Flat Affect
      4.1.99   Feeling States NOS
   4.2 Feeling Processes
      4.2.1   Potential for Alteration
      4.2.2   Altered Feeling Processes
           4.2.2.1   Liability
           4.2.2.2   Mood Swings
      4.2.99   Feeling Processes NOS
5. HUMAN RESPONSE PATTERNS IN INTERPERSONAL PROCESSES
   5.1 Abuse Response Patterns
      5.1.1   Potential for Alteration

    *5.4.2   Altered Family Processes
        5.4.2.1   Ineffective Family Coping
            *5.4.2.1.1   Compromised
            *5.4.2.1.2   Disabled
    5.4.99   Family Processes NOS
5.5 Role Performance
    5.5.1   Potential for Alteration
    *5.5.2   Altered Role Performance
        5.5.2.1   Altered Family Role
            5.5.2.1.1   Parental Role Conflict
        5.5.2.2   Altered Leisure Role
        5.5.2.3   Altered Play Role
        5.5.2.4   Altered Student Role
        5.5.2.5   Altered Work Role
    *5.5.3   Ineffective Individual Coping
        *5.5.3.1   Decisional Coping
        *5.5.3.2   Defensive Coping
        *5.5.3.3   Ineffective Denial
    5.5.99   Role Performance Patterns NOS
5.6 Sexuality
    5.6.1   Potential for Alteration
    5.6.2   Altered Sexual Behavior Leading to Intercourse
    5.6.3   Altered Sexual Conception Actions
    5.6.4   Altered Sexual Development
    5.6.5   Altered Sexual Intercourse
    5.6.6   Altered Sexual Relationships
    *5.6.7   Altered Sexuality Patterns
    5.6.8   Altered Variation of Sexual Expression
    *5.6.9   Sexual Dysfunction
    5.6.99   Sexuality Processes NOS
5.7 Social Interaction
    5.7.1   Potential for Alteration
    *5.7.2   Altered Social Interaction
        5.7.2.1   Bizarre Behaviors
        5.7.2.2   Compulsive Behaviors
        5.7.2.3   Disorganized Behaviors
        5.7.2.4   Social Intrusiveness
        *5.7.2.5   Social Isolation/Withdrawal
        5.7.2.6   Unpredictable Behaviors
    5.7.99   Social Interaction Patterns NOS
6. HUMAN RESPONSE PATTERNS IN PERCEPTION PROCESSES
6.1 Attention
    6.1.1   Potential for Alteration

6.1.2   Altered Attention
    6.1.2.1   Attention
    6.1.2.2   Hyperalertness
    6.1.2.3   Inattention
    6.1.2.4   Selective Attention
6.1.99   Attention Pattern NOS
6.2 Comfort
  6.2.1   Potential for Alteration
  *6.2.2   Altered Comfort Patterns
    6.2.2.1   Discomfort
    6.2.2.2   Distress
    *6.2.2.3   Pain
      6.2.2.3.1   Acute Pain
      *6.2.2.3.2   Chronic Pain
  6.2.99   Comfort Patterns NOS
6.3 Self Concept
  6.3.1   Potential for Alteration
  6.3.2   Altered Self Concept
    *6.3.2.1   Altered Body Image
    *6.3.2.2   Altered Personal Identity
    *6.3.2.3   Altered Self Esteem
      *6.3.2.3.1   Chronic Low Self Esteem
      *6.3.2.3.2   Situational Low Self Esteem
    6.3.2.4   Altered Sexual Identity
      6.3.2.4.1   Altered Gender Identity
  6.3.3   Undeveloped Self Concept
  6.3.99   Self Concept Patterns NOS
6.4 Sensory Perception
  6.4.1   Potential for Alteration
  6.4.2   Altered Sensory Perception
    *6.4.2.1   Altered Sensory Perception
      *6.4.2.1.1   Auditory
      *6.4.2.1.2   Gustatory
      *6.4.2.1.3   Kinesthetic
      *6.4.2.1.4   Olfactory
      *6.4.2.1.5   Tactile
      *6.4.2.1.6   Visual
    6.4.2.2   Illusions
  6.4.99   Sensory Perception Processes NOS
7. HUMAN RESPONSE PATTERNS IN PHYSIOLOGICAL PROCESSES
7.1 Circulation
  7.1.1   Potential for Alteration
    7.1.1.1   Fluid Volume Deficit

7.1.2   Altered Circulation
     7.1.2.1   Altered Cardiac Circulation
          *7.1.2.1.1   Decreased Cardiac Output
     7.1.2.2   Altered Vascular Circulation
          *7.1.2.2.1   Altered Fluid Volume
          *7.1.2.2.2   Fluid Volume Excess
          *7.1.2.2.3   Tissue Perfusion
               *7.1.2.2.3.1 Peripheral
               *7.1.2.2.3.2 Renal
7.1.99   Altered Circulation Processes NOS
7.2 Elimination
     7.2.1   Potential for Alteration
     7.2.2   Altered Elimination Processes
          *7.2.2.1   Altered Bowel Elimination
               *7.2.2.1.1   Constipation
                    *1.2.2.1.1.1 Colonic
                    *1.2.2.1.1.2 Perceived
               *7.2.2.1.2   Diarrhea
               7.2.2.1.3   Encopresis
               *7.2.2.1.4   Incontinence
         *7.2.2.2 Altered Urinary Elimination
               7.2.2.2.1   Enuresis
               *7.2.2.2.2   Incontinence
                    *7.2.2.2.2.1 Functional
                    *7.2.2.2.2.2 Reflex
                    *7.2.2.2.2.3 Stress
                    *7.2.2.2.2.4 Total
                    *7.2.2.2.2.5 Urge
               *7.2.2.2.3   Retention
          7.2.2.3   Altered Skin Elimination
7.2.99   Elimination Processes NOS
7.3 Endocrine/Metabolic Processes
     7.3.1   Potential for Alteration
     7.3.2   Altered Endocrine/Metabolic Processes
          7.3.2.1   Altered Growth
          7.3.2.2   Altered Hormone Regulation
               7.3.2.2.1   Premenstrual Stress Syndrome
7.3.99   Endocrine/Metabolic Processes NOS
7.4 Gastrointestinal Processes
     7.4.1   Potential for Alteration
     7.4.2   Altered Gastrointestinal Processes
          7.4.2.1   Altered Absorption

7.7 Nutrition
    7.7.1   Potential for Alteration
          *7.7.1.1   Potential for More Than Body Requirements
          *7.7.1.2   Potential for Poisoning
    7.7.2   Altered Nutrition Processes
          7.7.2.1   Altered Cellular Processes
          7.4.2.2   Altered Eating Processes
                7.7.2.2.1   Anorexia
                *7.7.2.2.2   Altered Oral Mucous Membrane
          7.7.2.3   Altered Systemic Processes
                *7.7.2.3.1   Less Than Body Requirements
                *7.7.2.3.2   More Than Body Requirements
          7.7.2.4   Impaired Swallowing
    7.7.99   Nutrition Processes NOS

7.8 Oxygenation
    7.8.1   Potential for Alteration
          *7.8.1.1   Potential for Aspiration
          *7.8.1.2   Potential for Suffocating
    7.8.2   Altered Oxygenation Processes
          7.8.2.1   Altered Respiration
                *7.8.2.1.1   Altered Gas Exchange
                *7.8.2.1.2   Ineffective Airway Clearance
                *7.8.2.1.3   Ineffective Breathing Pattern
          *7.8.2.2   Tissue Perfusion
    7.8.99   Oxygenation Processes NOS

7.9 Physical Integrity
    7.9.1   Potential for Alteration
          *7.9.1.1   Potential for Altered Skin Integrity
          *7.9.1.2   Potential for Trauma
    7.9.2   Altered Physical Integrity
          *7.9.2.1   Altered Oral Mucous Membrane
          *7.9.2.2   Altered Skin Integrity
          *7.9.2.3   Altered Tissue Integrity
    7.9.99   Physical Integrity Processes NOS

7.10 Physical Regulation Processes
    7.10.1   Potential for Alteration
          *7.10.1.1   Potential for Altered Body Temperature
          *7.10.1.2   Potential for Infection
    7.10.2   Altered Physical Regulation Processes
          7.10.2.1   Altered Immune Response
                7.10.2.1.1 Infection
          7.10.2.2   Altered Body Temperature
                *7.10.2.2.1 Hyperthermia

        *7.10.2.2.2   Hypothermia

        *7.10.2.2.3   Ineffective Thermoregulation

    7.10.99   Physical Regulation Processes NOS

8. HUMAN RESPONSE PATTERNS IN VALUATION PROCESSES

   8.1 Meaningfulness

      8.1.1   Potential for Alteration

    *8.1.2   Altered Meaningfulness

         8.1.2.1   Helplessness

       *8.1.2.2   Hopelessness

         8.1.2.3   Loneliness

       *8.1.2.4   Powerlessness

      8.1.99   Meaningfulness Patterns NOS

   8.2 Spirituality

      8.2.1   Potential for Alteration

      8.2.2   Altered Spirituality

         8.2.2.1   Spiritual Despair

       *8.2.2.2   Spiritual Distress

      8.2.99   Spirituality Patterns NOS

   8.3 Values

      8.3.1   Potential for Alteration

      8.3.2   Altered Values

         8.3.2.1   Conflict With Social Order

         8.3.2.2   Inability to Internalize Values

         8.3.2.3   Unclear Values

      8.3.99   Value Patterns NOS

ANA standards of psychiatric and mental health nursing practice

Standard I. Theory

The nurse applies appropriate theory that is scientifically sound as a basis for decisions regarding nursing practice.

Standard II. Data collection

The nurse continuously collects data that are comprehensive, accurate, and systematic.

Standard III. Diagnosis

The nurse utilizes nursing diagnoses and standard classification of mental disorders to express conclusions supported by recorded assessment data and current scientific premises.

Standard IV. Planning

The nurse develops a nursing care plan with specific goals and interventions delineating nursing actions unique to each client's needs.

Standard V. Intervention

The nurse intervenes as guided by the nursing care plan to implement nursing actions that promote, maintain, or restore physical and mental health, prevent illness, and effect rehabilitation.

Standard V-A. Intervention: Psychotherapeutic interventions

The nurse uses psychotherapeutic interventions to assist clients in regaining or improving their previous coping abilities and to prevent further disability.

Standard V-B. Intervention: Health teaching

The nurse assists clients, families, and groups to achieve satisfying and productive patterns of living through health teaching.

Reprinted with permission of the American Nurses' Association, Kansas City, 1982.

Standard V-C. Intervention: Activities of daily living

The nurse uses the activities of daily living in a goal-directed way to foster adequate self-care and physical and mental well-being of clients.

Standard V-D. Intervention: Somatic therapies

The nurse uses knowledge of somatic therapies and applies related clinical skills in working with clients.

Standard V-E. Intervention: Therapeutic environment

The nurse provides, structures, and maintains a therapeutic environment in collaboration with the client and other health care providers.

Standard V-F. Intervention: Psychotherapy

The nurse utilizes advanced clinical expertise in individual, group, and family psychotherapy, child psychotherapy, and other treatment modalities to function as a psychotherapist, and recognizes professional accountability for nursing practice.

Standard VI. Evaluation

The nurse evaluates client responses to nursing actions in order to revise the data base, nursing diagnoses, and nursing care plan.

Standard VII. Peer review

The nurse participates in peer review and other means of evaluation to assure quality of nursing care provided for clients.

Standard VIII. Continuing education

The nurse assumes responsibility for continuing education and professional development and contributes to the professional growth of others.

Standard IX. Interdisciplinary collaboration

The nurse collaborates with other health care providers in assessing, planning, implementing, and evaluating programs and other mental health activities.

Standard X. Utilization of community health systems

The nurse participates with other members of the community in assessing, planning, implementing, and evaluating mental health services and community systems that include the promotion of the broad continuum of primary, secondary, and tertiary prevention of mental illness.

Standard XI. Research

The nurse contributes to nursing and the mental health field through innovations in theory and practice and participation in research.

Index